Functional Foods and Dietary Supplements

Functional Foods and Dietary Supplements

Processing Effects and Health Benefits

Edited by

Athapol Noomhorm, Imran Ahmad and Anil Kumar Anal

Food Engineering and Bioprocess Technology,
Asian Institute of Technology, Pathum Thani, Thailand

WILEY Blackwell

Registered office
John Wiley & Sons Ltd, The Atrium, Southern Gate, Chichester, West Sussex, PO19 8SQ, UK

Editorial offices
9600 Garsington Road, Oxford, OX4 2DQ, UK
The Atrium, Southern Gate, Chichester, West Sussex, PO19 8SQ, UK
111 River Street, Hoboken, NJ 07030-5774, USA

For details of our global editorial offices, for customer services and for information about how to apply for permission to reuse the copyright material in this book please see our website at www.wiley.com/wiley-blackwell.

Library of Congress Cataloging-in-Publication Data

Noomhorm, Athapol, 1952–
Functional foods and dietary supplements : processing effects and health benefits / Athapol Noomhorm, Imran Ahmad, and Anil Anal.
pages cm
Includes index.
ISBN 978-1-118-22787-9 (cloth)
1. Functional foods. 2. Dietary supplements–Therapeutic use. 3. Natural foods–Health aspects. I. Ahmad, Imran, 1974– II. Anal, Anil. III. Title.
QP144.F85N66 2013
613.2–dc23

2013024204

A catalogue record for this book is available from the British Library.

Wiley also publishes its books in a variety of electronic formats. Some content that appears in print may not be available in electronic books.

Cover images: ©iStockphoto/dianne555 and iStockphoto/filo
Cover design by Meaden Creative

Set in 9.5/11.5pt Times Ten by Aptara Inc., New Delhi, India
Printed and bound in Singapore by Markono Print Media Pte Ltd

1 2014

Contents

List of Contributors

Imran Ahmad, Food Engineering and Bioprocess Technology, Asian Institute of Technology, Pathum Thani, Thailand

Eman M. Alissa, Faculty of Medicine, King AbdulAziz University, Jeddah, Kingdom of Saudi Arabia

Nina Karla M. Alparce, Asian Institute of Technology, Pathum Thani, Thailand

Anil Kumar Anal, Food Engineering and Bioprocess Technology, Asian Institute of Technology, Pathum Thani, Thailand

Khoomtong Atcharaporn, Asian Institute of Technology, Pathum Thani, Thailand

Gordon A. Ferns, Division of Medical Education, Brighton and Sussex Medical School, Sussex, UK

Kelvin K. T. Goh, Institute of Food, Nutrition and Human Health, Massey University, Palmerston North, New Zealand

Jiraporn Sripinyowanich Jongyingcharoen, Faculty of Engineering, King Mongkut's Institute of Technology Ladkrabang, Bangkok, Thailand

J. Jerish Joyner, Indian Institute of Crop Processing Technology, Thanjavur, Tamilnadu, India

Mandeep Kaur, Amity Institute of Food Technology, Amity University, Noida, India

Se-Kwon Kim, Marine Biochemistry Laboratory, Department of Chemistry, Pukyong National University, Busan, Republic of Korea

Maushmi S. Kumar, Department of Pharmaceutical Biotechnology, Shobhaben Pratapbhai Patel School of Pharmacy and Technology Management, SVKM'S NMIMS (Deemed-to-be University), Mumbai, India

Ramesh Kumar, Massey University (Singapore), Singapore

Kishore K. Kumaree, Food Engineering and Bioprocess Technology, Asian Institute of Technology, Pathum Thani, Thailand

Buddhi Lamsal, Food Science and Human Nutrition Department, Iowa State University, USA

Sung Je Lee, Institute of Food, Nutrition and Human Health, Massey University, Auckland, New Zealand

Shruti Mishra, Asian Institute of Technology, Pathum Thani, Thailand

Nantarat Na Nakornpanom, Faculty of Agricultural Product Innovation and Technology, Srinakharinwirot University, Bangkok, Thailand

Taslima Ayesha Aktar Nasrin, Postharvest Technology Section, Horticulture Research Centre, Bangladesh Agricultural Research Institute, Gazipur, Bangladesh

Athapol Noomhorm, Food Engineering and Bioprocess Technology, Asian Institute of Technology, Pathum Thani, Thailand

Ratih Pangestuti, Marine Bioprocess Research Center, Pukyong National University, Busan, Republic of Korea and
Research and Development Center for Marine and Fisheries Product Processing Technology, Ministry of Marine and Fisheries, Petamburan VI, Jakarta, Indonesia

Vilai Rungsardthong, King Mongkut's University of Technology North Bangkok, Bangkok, Thailand

H. K. Sharma, Food Engineering and Technology Department, Sant Longowal Institute of Engineering and Technology (Deemed-to-be-University), Punjab, India

Porntip Sirisoontaralak, Faculty of Agricultural Product Innovation and Technology, Srinakharinwirot University, Bangkok, Thailand

Anges Teo, Institute of Food, Nutrition and Human Health, Massey University, Palmerston North, New Zealand

Mridula Thapa, Food Engineering and Bioprocess Technology, Asian Institute of Technology, Pathum Thani, Thailand

Pananun Thawunporn, Charoen Pokphand Foods (CPF), Thailand

Alisha Tuladhar, Food Engineering and Bioprocess Technology, Asian Institute of Technology, Pathum Thani, Thailand

Punchira Vongsawasdi, Department of Microbiology, King Mongkut's University of Technology Thonburi, Bangkok, Thailand

Shen-Siung Wong, Massey University (Singapore), Singapore

Binod K. Yadav, Indian Institute of Crop Processing Technology, Thanjavur, Tamilnadu, India

Preface

Growing evidence supports the observation that functional foods containing physiologically active components, either from plant or animal sources, may enhance health. Health-conscious consumers are increasingly seeking out functional foods in an effort to improve their own health and well-being. Publishing in functional foods is mostly limited to the health benefits of functional foods, such as their antioxidant and anticancer activities. In fact, identification of the suitable extraction or processing techniques for these functional components is imperative in maximizing their beneficial activities. For instance, most functional plants or herbs should be dried and ground to facilitate the extraction process. In order to extract curcuminoids, which are the major antioxidant compounds in turmeric, different drying methods have been found to affect the extracted content of curcuminoids. Among hot air, vacuum, infrared, infrared-convection, infrared-vacuum and fluidized bed drying methods, significantly the highest curcuminoid content was obtained from infrared-vacuum drying. This is an example of how processing affects the physiologically active components of functional foods.

This book, therefore, is written with the aim of highlighting the processing effects on active ingredients in various functional food materials, such as turmeric, pomegranate, drumstick leaves, jackfruit seeds, brown rice, etc. The book will be of interest to food scientists and the food industry, particularly those who are working on products for which health claims are being made.

The first section of the book introduces some of the fundamentals of functional ingredients; definitions and classification; prebiotics and probiotics, biochemical pathways; critical steps in processing the functional food; product developments and industrial trends. The second part focuses on the major sources of functional foods. Here the emphasis is again on the impact of processing, for example the effect of drying temperature on the activity of isoflavones from soybeans and the changes in γ-aminobutyric acid (GABA) from germinated brown rice, etc. In the third part, the challenges faced during the extraction, processing and application of functional ingredients are addressed. Dedicated chapters cover various techniques such as extrusion, drying, thermal and non-thermal processing as well improvements to processes like, encapsulation, among others.

One of the objectives of writing this book was to compile the available evidence on the health benefits and disease prevention claims for functional foods. This is a major challenge faced by the industry today. The chapters included in the fourth section address the pharmacology of bioactive compounds and their cardioprotective effects.

Finally, we have tried to make the book interesting to people from varied scientific and clinical backgrounds with the assumption that the readers will have a basic knowledge of nutrition and food processing. We, therefore, hope that the book will be of use to those interested in dietary supplements and the development of products that have a beneficial health claim.

Athapol Noomhorm
Imran Ahmad
Anil Kumar Anal
Editors

I

Fundamentals of Functional Food Processing

1

Functional Foods, Nutraceuticals and Probiotics as Functional Food Components

Athapol Noomhorm, Anil Kumar Anal and Imran Ahmad
Food Engineering and Bioprocess Technology, Asian Institute of Technology, Pathum Thani, Thailand

1.1 Functional food

Eating food is no longer limited to just satisfying the appetite or providing basic nutrition. Consumers are driven by many issues related to health concerns, the negative effects of unhealthy food and a desire to have a healthier lifestyle, which have significantly changed modern attitudes towards food habits. Functional food can thus be summarized as the complete package of fundamental needs plus additional food ingredients that can play an important role in decreasing health risks and also improving health. The modern thirst for a healthy life through food was visualised 2500 years ago by Hippocrates in his famous doctrine 'Let food be thy medicine and medicine be thy food'.

The term 'functional food' was first used by the Japanese in the mid 1980s. But in the past decade the market has expanded to the United States, northern Europe and central European countries (Menrad, 2003). Functional foods fall into two broad categories: plant origin and animal origin.

1.1.1 Functional components from plant origin

A plant-based diet can help to cure chronic diseases, especially cancer. A review conducted in 1992 showed that the risk of cancer among people consuming fruits and

Functional Foods and Dietary Supplements: Processing Effects and Health Benefits, First Edition.
Edited by Athapol Noomhorm, Imran Ahmad and Anil Kumar Anal.

vegetables is only half that of those consuming lesser amounts of these foods (Block *et al.*, 1992). This proves that plant-based foods have some components that act against such lethal diseases. Such chemicals were classified by Steinmetz and Potter (1991) as phytochemicals. They identified a few such active plant components.

Oats Oats is the most studied dietary supplement that is capable of lowering cholesterol as it contains β-glucan. The food with the highest amount of β-glucan was reported in oats (Wood and Beer, 1998; Manthey *et al.*, 1999). Decreasing the level of low density cholesterol (LDL) can reduce the chances of coronary heart disease (CHD). Researchers have also shown that the hypocholesterolaemic effect of β-glucan can result in a 20–30% reduction of LDL-cholesterol, hence the chance of getting heart problems also decreases.

Flax seed The use of flaxseed (*Linum usitatissimum*) as a suitable additive in functional food has become more widespread because of its potential health benefits, such as reducing the risk of heart disease (cardiovascular disease, CVD) (Bloedon and Szapary, 2004), diabetes (Haliga *et al.*, 2009) and also in cancer. Phipps *et al.* (1993) have shown that the daily intake of 10 g of flaxseed can elicit several hormones which can reduce the risk of breast cancer. The health qualities of flaxseeds are mainly due to the presence of high omega-3 fatty acids; almost 57% of its oil is α-linoleic acid (ω-3). As well as this it contains a high amount of dietary fibre (both soluble and insoluble), proteins and antioxidants such as lignan. The presence of phenolic compounds in flaxseed such as lignan, secoisolariciresinol diglucoside (SDG) and ferulic acid gives flax seed its antioxidant properties (Kasote *et al.*, 2011).

Garlic This has been widely quoted as a plant with medicinal properties. The medicinal components of garlic have been shown to inhibit tumour genesis. It has also the potential to reduce the risk of cancer (Dorant *et al.*, 1993) by protecting against carcinogenic agents. The main factor contributing to this are its sulfur constituents, which can suppress tumour formation in breast, colon, skin or lung cancer (Amagase and Milner, 1993). It has been reported that garlic has ten different types of natural sugars. Garlic can help reduce blood sugar levels (Sheela *et al.*, 1995; Augusti and Sheela, 1996). It has been suggested that it is the best source of the nucleic acid adenosine, a building block of DNA and RNA (Blackwood and Fulder, 1987). Nearly 33 different sulfur compounds, enzymes, 17 amino acids and minerals have been reported in garlic (Newall *et al.*, 1996).

Fibre is also added to food products to help maintain a healthy digestive tract, for example Yugao Bijin from Tokyo Tanabe Co. is a fibre enriched pasta, and Caluche is a snack product from Nissin Foods that is rich in fibre.

1.1.2 Functional components from animal resources

A vast number of components naturally present in animal sources are potentially beneficial to health.

Fish oil Omega-3 fatty acids are a major component of polyunsaturated fatty acids (PUFA) from fish oil. Omega-3 has many health benefits. It has been found that a daily intake of docosahexaenoic acid (DHA) up to 0.5–0.7 g decreases the chances of CHD (Kris-Etherton, Harris and Appel, 2002). Omega-3 supplements can be taken if our everyday food is deficient in omega-3. Omega-3 FA also has beneficial effects in rheumatoid arthritis, inflammatory diseases such as asthma (Reisman *et al.* (2006), cystic fibrosis and bowel diseases. A high DHA content in the body can help decrease the risk of Alzheimer's disease.

Dairy products Dairy products are undoubtedly a good source of functional components, one major ingredient being calcium, a nutrient required to prevent osteoporosis and possibly also colon cancer. Milk has potential probiotic components which are a good source of food for the beneficial microbial flora inside the gut. The term probiotics was defined by Gibson and Roberfroid (1995) as 'non-digestible food that beneficially affect the host by selectively stimulating the growth of gut microbial flora'. These may include different dietary fibres, starches, sugars that do not get absorbed directly, sugar alcohols and oligosaccharides (Gibson *et al.*, 1996).

1.1.3 Examples of functional foods widely popular in the market

The development of drinks as functional foods has grown widely in and is an easy way to satisfy consumer demand for these foods. Most of these drinks contain dissolved fibres, minerals and vitamins. For example, Pocari Sweet Stevia from Ootsuka, is a sport drink that contains a glucose substitute sweetener (a glycoside from the *Stevia* plant); and Fibi, a soft drink from Coca-Cola, contains a high amount of fibre, is mainly focused on improving the digestive system.

The first probiotic product launched in market was Yakult from Yakult Honsha, a probiotic yoghurt drink, which contains *Lactobacillus* and *Bifidobacterium*. The health benefits related to these probiotic products are increased digestive control, inhibition of pathogenic flora, immune power stimulation, reduced risk of tumour genesis, production of vitamins (especially B vitamins) and generation of bacteriocins (Potter, 1990; Sanders *et al.*, 1991). For example, Yoplait's low-fat yoghurt Yo-Plus, with probiotic bacteria (*Bifidobacterium lactis*) mixed with probiotic (inulin) provides a perfect symbiotic combination, and a live active natural cheese product launched by Kraft contains probiotic strains *Lactobacillus lactis* for better digestive health.

1.2 Nutraceuticals

Nutraceuticals are a type of dietary supplement that delivers a concentrated form of a biologically active component from a food, presented in a non-food matrix, to enhance health in dosages that exceed those that could be obtained from regular food (Zeisel, 1999). A nutraceutical is a product isolated or purified from foods that is generally sold in medicinal forms not usually associated with food. A nutraceutical is demonstrated to have a physiological benefit or provide protection against chronic diseases (DeFelice, 1992).

The term 'nutraceuticals' was first coined by the Foundation for the Innovation in Medicine.

The actual boundary between functional food and nutraceuticals is not clear. It can be explained with the help of a simple example: if a phytochemical extract with medicinal value is included in a food product, i.e. 200 mg of the extract needs to be incorporated into 1 litre of orange juice, we get a new functional food. The same 200 mg extract can be marketed in the form of a capsule as a new nutraceutical.

A major source of nutraceuticals is omega-3 fatty acids (PUFA) from fish oils. These contain high amounts of eicosapentanoic acid (EPA) and docosahexaenoic acid (DHA), categories of fatty acids that have a protective effect against cardiovascular disease and inflammatory disease and also affect other chronic diseases. Fish oil mainly prohibits the end-organ effects of tumour-derived lipolytic and proteolytic factors, influencing the action of many receptors as well as enzymes which function during cellular signalling.

The non-essential amino acid arginine has received much attention as it has efficient immune stimulation properties. Arginine was also effective in some clinical conditions in improving the cellular immune system, increasing phagocytosis and the proper maintenance of T cells. Arginine enhances the suppressed immune response of individuals that have injury diseases, surgical trauma or malnutrition (Kirk and Barbul, 1990; Evoy *et al.*, 1998).

Table 1.1 lists functional components extracts and the effects of applying them in medicinal form, so that their consumption becomes easier.

Table 1.1 Functional component extracts and the effect of applying them in medicinal form

Supplement	Composition	Dose (perday) and assay period	Subjects	Effect	Reference
Grape seed extract	Oligomeric procyanidins	200–300 mg/ day; 1 year	3 patients with chronic pancreatitis	Reduction of chronic pancreatitis, vomiting and pain	Banerjee and Bagchi, 2011
Mixture of grape, bilberry and cranberry extract (capsule)	Oligomeric procyanidin	320 mg/day	13 menopausal women	Reduction of fluid retention	Christie *et al.*, 2004
Soya supplement	Isoflavones	60 mg (3 months)	33 postmenopausal women	Significant cognitive improvement	Duffy *et al.*, 2003
Red clover supplement	Isoflavones	80 mg (90 days)	60 postmenopausal women	Decrease of menopausal symptoms. Positive effect on avaginal cytology and trigylcerides	Hidalgo *et al.*, 2005
Red clover extract capsule	Isoflavones	100 mg (6 months)	30 postmenopausal women	Hypoglycaemic	Cheng *et al.*, 2004

Source: Goñi & Hervert-Hernández, 2011.

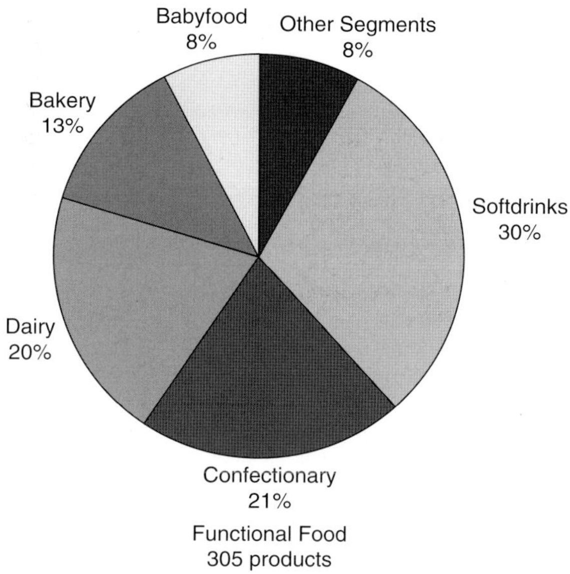

Figure 1.1 Innovations in the food and drinks market in Germany. *Source:* Anonymous, 2001

1.3 Functional food market

Research indicates that there is an estimated global market for functional foods of US$33 billion (Hilliam, 2000c). Functional foods account for 2% of the US food market. Another competing market is Japan, which focuses mainly on health claims. The concept of 'functional foods' was first introduced by Japan in 1984 (Hosoya, 1998), and between 1988 and 1998 (Heasman and Mellentin, 2001) the number of functional food products reached nearly 1700, with an estimated turnover of US$14 billion in 1999 (Hilliam, 2000). Within the European market, functional foods have a monetary value of US$4–8 billion (Hilliam, 2000). Figure 1.1 illustrates the main categories of functional foods in Germany.

Functional benefits may provide added value to consumers but cannot outweigh the sensory properties of foods. By purchasing functional foods in general consumers may achieve a modern and positive impression of themselves. These products provide consumers with an alternative way to achieve a healthy lifestyle that differs from conventional healthy diets defined by nutrition experts. In general, the attitude both to functional foods and to their consumers is positive, so such a concept represents a sustainable trend in a multi-niche market (see Table 1.2).

1.4 Probiotics

The market of functional food is growing through the continuous development of technology. Functional food with added probiotic has gained the attention of many researchers. The use of probiotics in combination with prebiotic has been very effective against several chronic diseases. Probiotics have been defined as the ingested live

Table 1.2 Some commercial examples of probiotic products

Brand/trade name	Description	Producer
Actimel	Probiotic drinking yogurt with *L. casei Imunitass*® cultures	Danone, France
Activia	Creamy yogurt containing *Bifidus ActiRegularis*®,	Danone, France
Gefilus	A wide range of LGG products	Valio, Finnland
Hellus	Dairy products containing *Lactobacillus fermentum ME-3*	Tallinna Piimatööstuse AS, Estonia
Jovita Probiotisch	Blend of cereals, fruit and probiotic yogurt	H&J Bruggen, Germany
Pohadka	Yogurt milk with probiotic cultures	Valašské Meziříčí Dairy, Czech Republic
ProViva	Refreshing natural fruit drink and yogurt in many different flavours containing *Lactobacillus plantarum*	Skåne mejerier, Sweden
Rela	Yogurts, cultured milks and juices with *L. reuteri*	Ingman Foods, Finland
Revital Active	Yogurt and drink yogurt with probiotics	Olma, Czech Republic
Snack Fibra	Snacks and bars with natural fibers and extra minerals and vitamins	Celigüeta, Spain
SOYosa	Range of products based on soy and oats and includes a refreshing drink and a probiotic yogurt-like soy–oat product	Bioferme, Finland
Soytreat	Kefir type product with six probiotics	Lifeway, USA
Yakult	Milk drink containing *Lactobacillus casei* Shirota	Yakult, Japan
Yosa	Yogurt-like oat product flavoured with natural fruits and berries containing probiotic bacteria (*Lactobacillus acidophilus, Bifidobacterium lactis*)	Bioferme, Finland
Vitality	Yogurt with pre- and probiotics and omega-3	Müller, Germany
Vifit	Drink yogurts with LGG, vitamins and minerals	Campina, the Netherlands

Source: Siró *et al.*, 2008. Reproduced with permission from Elsevier B. V.

bacteria which are responsible for providing a healthy life. The gut microflora plays an important role in maintaining stable health and disease protection (Steer *et al.*, 2000). The metabolic activity of the gut flora provides up to 50% of the energy required by the host body's gut wall through the fermentation of carbohydrates into organic acids (Figure 1.2).

1.4.1 Role of probiotics

Probiotics and prebiotics provide an alternate source for the management of different intestinal disorders. It was demonstrated that the bacterial count in the faecal matter of children is more than in adults, with high amounts of *Lactobacillus* and *Bifidobacterium.* Disorders such as gastroenteritis unbalance the biochemical environment of the gut, but the intake of probiotic functional food can stabilize the colonic microflora and also help in their maintenance against the adverse effect of antibiotics. Figure 1.3 shows a recent study of the probiotic mechanism on health enhancement.

The major contributions associated with the work of probiotics on human health are proper colonic function and increased metabolism. They are also responsible for the enhancing the expression of short chain fatty acids, the increase in faecal weight, decreased colon pH, reduced release of nitrogenous material from the body

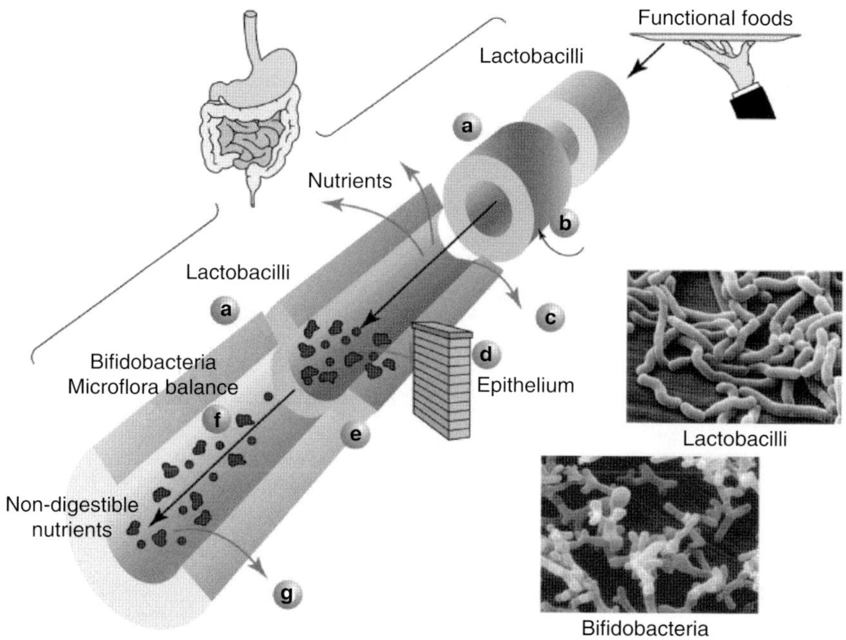

Figure 1.2 Targets throughout the gastrointestinal tract for functional food ingredients. (a) Pre- and probiotics inhibit pathogenic bacteria at various sites, from *Helicobacteria pylori* in the gastric mucosa to *Salmonella* sp. and *Clostridia* sp. in the intestine. (b) Multiple ingredients alter the rate and extent of digestion of nutrients. (c) The absorption of nutrients and anti-nutritional factors throughout the stomach and intestine is affected by the presence, form and activity of functional-food components. (d) Pre- and probiotics modify the barrier functions of the intestinal epithelium. (e) Nutrients, from vitamins and minerals to probiotics, interact with and enhance the functions of gastrointestinal immune cells and, via systemic communication, the entire body's immune system. (f) Pre- and probiotics modulate the overall ecology of the gut microflora. (g) Fermentation products of fibers or non-digestible oligosaccharides and other components from the microflora not only nourish the intestine but also improve the differentiation, maturation and overall health of colonic cells. *Source:* German *et al.*, 1999. Reproduced with permission from Elsevier. For colour details, see the colour plates section

and reductive enzymes (Bournet, Brouns, Tashiro and Duvillier, 2002; Forchielli and Walker, 2005; Qiang, YongLie and QianBing, 2009). Table 1.3 shows some contributions of probiotics.

1.5 Prebiotics

Prebiotics are foods that are beneficial but cannot be digested by the host's metabolism and can help in the growth and other activities of beneficial bacteria residing in the human gut. This indirectly improves the host's health (Gibson and Roberfroid, 1995).

Widely used prebiotics are inulin, fructo-oligosaccharide (FOS), lactulose and galacto-oligosaccharides (GOS). They improve the composition of the gut microbiota to give enhanced numbers of beneficial bacteria. Though there is no fixed recommendation for the daily intake of prebiotics, one study has shown that 4–20 g/day gives good results (K.M. Tuohy *et al.*, unpublished data). Research data on inulin

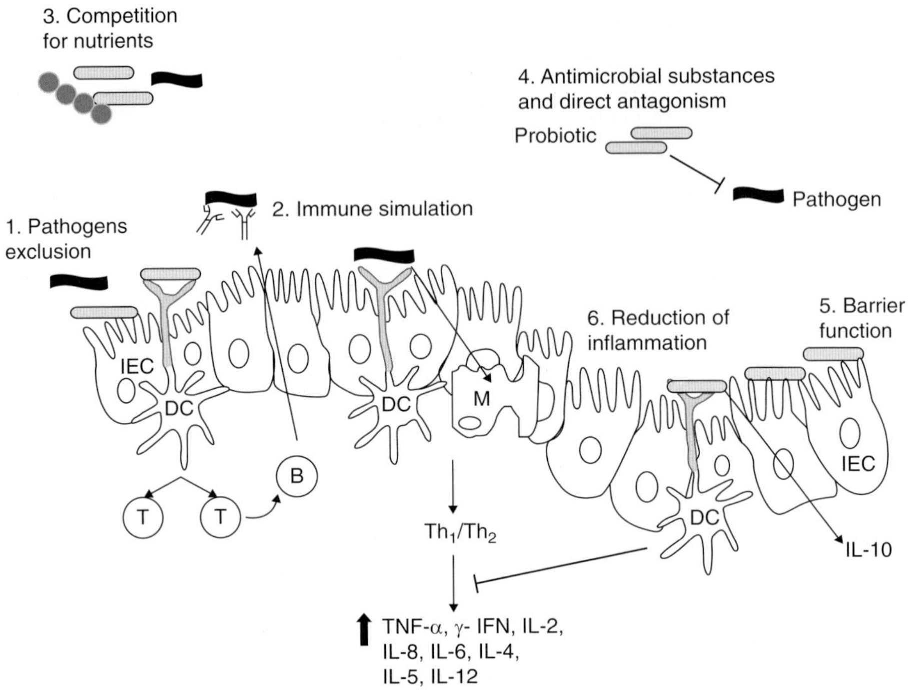

Figure 1.3 Some probiotic mechanisms that induce several beneficial host responses. Most effects consist of (1) Exclusion and competing with pathogen to epithelial cells adhesion, (2) innate immune stimulation, (3) competition for nutrients and prebiotic products, (4) production of antimicrobial substances and thereby pathogen antagonism, (5) protection of intestinal barrier integrity and (6) regulation of anti-inflammatory cytokine and inhibition of pro-inflammatory cytokine production. IEC, intestinal epithelium cells; DC, dendritic cell; IL, interleukin; M, intestinal M cell. *Source:* Saad *et al.*, 2013. Reproduced with permission from Elsevier. For colour details, see the colour plates section

or FOS intake suggest that 4 g/day is needed to increase *Bifidobacteria* (Roberfroid *et al.*, 1995).

1.5.1 Sources of prebiotic

Prebiotics are mainly obtained from plant sources and algae polysaccharides. The extraction is carried out either by a chemical process which hydrolyses the polysaccharides or by an enzymatic process of synthesis from disaccharides (Nugent, 2000; Mussamatto and Mancilha, 2007). The main prebiotics in use are FOS, GOS, isomalto-oligosaccharides (IMO) and xylo-oligosaccharides (XOS). Primarily oligosaccharides, such as soy oligosaccharides (SOS), GOS and XOS are also marketed in Japan (Ouwehand, 2007).

Currently, inulin is the major prebiotic made. It is produced by chemical synthesis using transglycosylation, which produces polysaccharides from monosaccharides and disaccharides. Figure 1.4 shows a brief description of the process of transglycosylation (Delattre *et al.*, 2005; Barreteau *et al.*, 2006).

Table 1.3 The contributions of probiotics

Disease type	Contribution by the probiotics	Reference
Intestinal flora	Inhibits the growth of pathogenic species like *S. dysenteriae, S. typhosa and E. coli* and this results in reduced diarrhoea and vomiting	Asahara *et al.*, 2001
Lactose intolerance	Lactose supplement could help in the digestion of lactose by helping in its fermentation.	Jiang and Savaiano, 1997
Immuno-modulatory effects of probiotics	Administrating probiotics has proven the activity on Payers's patches, NK cell activity, enhance of IgA production in intestine, development of GALT (gut-associated lymphoid tissue)	Palma *et al.*, 2006; Hosono *et al.*, 2003; Hoentjen *et al.*, 2005; Nakamura *et al.*, 2004; Pierre *et al.*, 1997
Preventing cancer	Recent research showed that butyric acid production by the fermentation of probiotics plays a lead role in cancer prevention. This acid helps in the chemo-prevention of carcinogenesis, and also against colon cancer by the promotion of differentiation of cell Another breakthrough is that propionate has an anti-inflammatory effect on colon cancer cells In another study, probiotics showed the inhibition of colon tumor forming azoxymethane by the probiotics in association with prebiotics (inulin)	Femia *et al.*, 2002; Pool-Zobel, 2005; Munjal *et al.*, 2009; Verghese *et al.*, 2002; Kim *et al.*, 1982
Lipid metabolism	Probiotics have been proven to show a positive effect on the hepatic lipd metabolism. Experiment of RTS has shown a decrease in cholesterol and triglycerides levels by 15% and 50% respectively due to the suppression of lipogenic enzyme activity	Delzenne *et al.*, 2002; Fiordaliso *et al.*, 1995; Delzenne and Kok, 2001; Williams and Jackson, 2002

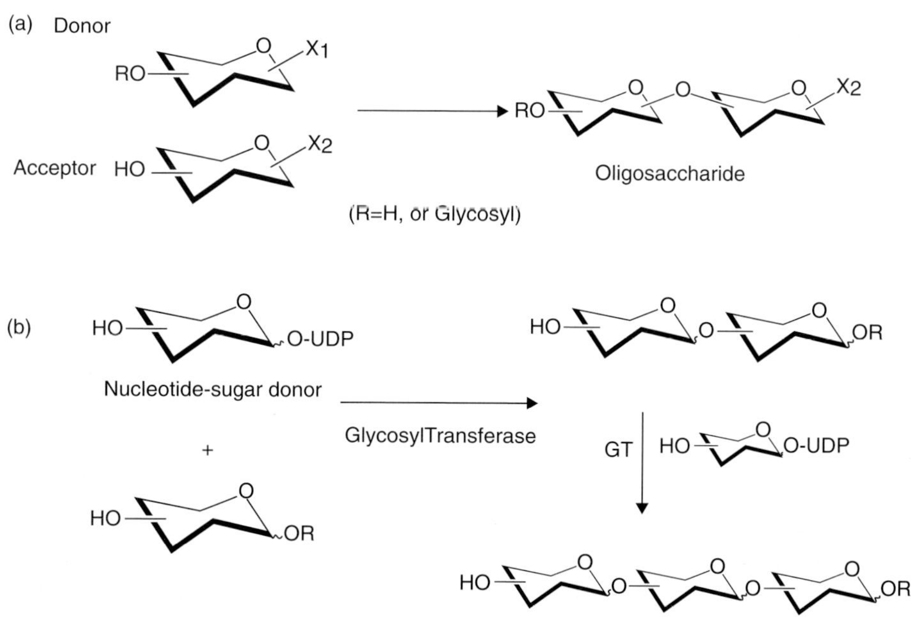

Figure 1.4 Synthesis of oligosaccharides by glycosylation using (a) a chemical process and (b) an enzymatic process with glycosyltransferases. *Source:* Saad *et al.*, 2013. Reproduced with permission from Elsevier

Table 1.4 Potential probiotic traditional fermented foods

Product	Probiotic microorganisms	Substrates	Published references
Adai	LAB	Cereal, legume	Farnworth, 2005
Agbelima	*Lb. plantarum, Lb. brevis, Lb. fermentum, Leuc. mesenteroides*	Cassava	Amoa-Awua *et al.*, 2005
Atole	LAB	Maise	Escamilla-Hurtado *et al.*, 1993
Ben-saalga	LAB	Pearl millet	Tou *et al.*, 2006
Boza	*Lb. plantarum, Lb. brevis, Lb. rhamnosus, Lb. fermentum, Leuc. mesenteroides* subsp. *dextranium*	Cereals	Hancioglu and Karapinar, 1997; Moncheva *et al.*, 2003; Botes *et al.*, 2007; Todorov *et al.*, 2008
Dosa	*Leuc. mesenteroides, Lb. fermentum, Sacch. cerevisiae*	Rice and Bengal gram	Soni *et al.*, 1986
Idli	*Leuc. mesenteroides,* LAB, yeast	Cereal, legume	Agrawal *et al.*, 2000; Aidoo *et al.*, 2006; Balasubramanian and Viswanathan, 2007
Ilambazi lokubilisa	LAB	Maize	Farnworth, 2005
Kecap	LAB	Wheat, soybeans	Roling *et al.*, 1999
Kenkey	*Lb. casei, Lb. lactis, Lb. plantarum, Lb. brevis, Lb. acidophilus, Lb. fermentum, Lb. casei,* yeast	Maize	Olsen *et al.*, 1995; Olasupo *et al.*, 1997
Kimchi	*Lb. plantarum, Lb. curvatus, Lb. brevis, Lb. sake, Leuc. mesenteroides*	Vegetables	Chin *et al.*, 2006; Lee *et al.*, 2006; Lee and Lee 2006
Kishk	LAB	Cereal and milk	Tamime and McNulty, 1999
Kisra	*Lactobacillus* sp., *Lb. brevis*	Sorghum	Mohammed *et al.*, 1991
Koko	*Lb. fermentum, Lb. salivarius*	Millet	Lei and Jacobsen, 2004
Mahewu	*Lb. bulgaricus, Lb. brevis*	Maize	McMaster *et al.*, 2005
Mawe	*Lb. fermentum, Lb. brevis, Lb. salivarius, Sacch. cerevisiae*	Maize	Hounhouigan *et al.*, 1999
Ngari	*Lactococcus lactis* subsp. *cremoris, Lactococcus plantarum, Enterococcus faecium, Lb. fructosus, Lb. amylophilus, Lb. coryniformis* subsp. *torquens*, and *Lb. plantarum*	Fish	Thapa *et al.*, 2004
Ogi	*Lb. plantarum, Lb. fermentum, Leuc. mesenteroides,* and *Sacch. cerevisiae*	Maize	Odunfa and Adeyele, 1985; Adeyemi, 1993; Ijabadeniyi, 2007; Omemu *et al.*, 2007
Sauerkraut	*Leuc. mesenteroides, Lactococcus lactis,* LAB	Cabbage	Harris *et al.*, 1992; Lu *et al.*, 2003; Johanningsmeier *et al.*, 2005
Som-fug	LAB	Fish	Riebroy *et al.*, 2007
Tarhana	*Streptococcus thermophilus, Lb. bulgaricus, Lb. plantarum*	Parboiled wheat meal and yogurt	Blandino *et al.*, 2003; Patel *et al.*, 2004; Erbas *et al.*, 2006; Ozdemir *et al.*, 2007
Tempeh	LAB, *Lb. plantarum*	Soybean	Ashenafi and Busse, 1991; Feng *et al.*, 2005
Uji	LAB	Maize, sorghum cassava, finger millet	Onyango *et al.*, 2003, 2004

Source: Rivera-Espinoza & Gallardo-Navarro, 2010. Reproduced with permission from Elsevier.

1.5.2 Functional probiotic products

Traditional probiotic products The reason for opting for probiotic food can best be explained as an easy way to maintain daily health. Eating junk foods, drinking chlorinated water, work stress and irregular diet can have a serious impact on the gastrointestinal tract by destroying the beneficial microbial flora. So the ready availability of probiotics in the market helps resolve the problem to a great extent.

Kefir is a traditional milk product containing lactic acid bacteria and yeasts, which have a symbiotic relationship. Fermented milk products (kefir, yoghurt or sour milk) have higher nutritional values and a high nitrogen content compared with milk.

Kombucha is a fermented tea product and a symbiotic culture of yeast and bacteria. It is a traditional product that has been used for centuries and has recently gained attention globally, especially in the United States.

Another traditional Japanese food with probiotics is made from soybeans – a fermented product of fungi called koji. Table 1.4 shows examples of potential probiotic traditional fermented foods.

Present day commercial products Products available in market with combined probiotics and prebiotics are now widely accepted. In 2008, Beyaz Peynir cheese from Turkey, a traditional cheese with nutritional value, was available with the addition of *Lactobacillus plantarum*.

The very first product marketed as a probiotic rather than a traditional product was Yakult by Yakult Honsha, Japan. Other commercial probiotic products available in market are shown in Table 1.5.

1.6 Probiotic market

The probiotic market is a growing industry, with lactic acid bacterial drinks accounting for 10% of the market. As health awareness increases, health-vigilant consumers are increasingly choosing probiotic functional products and as a result the market is growing at a rate of 5–30% (percentage varies with the country and product types).

The distribution of the probiotics application is shown in Figure 1.5.

The probiotic market was estimated to be around US$24.33 billion in 2011. A survey by marketsandmarkets.com (2013) says that more than 500 probiotic food and

Table 1.5 Probiotic foods in present market

Brand name	Food type
Yakult Honsha Co., Ltd.	Dairy beverage
Attune Food	Chocolate bar
Kevita	Probiotic non-diary drinks
Amul	Prolife (yoghurt and ice-cream)
GoodBelly	Probiotic fruit juice
Life way	Kefir drink
Ombar	Probiotic chocolates
Dannon	An Active dairy drink

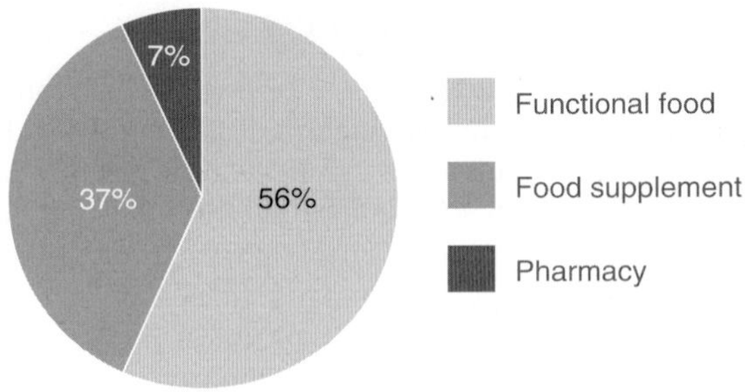

Figure 1.5 The distribution of the probiotics application. *Source:* Ubic Consulting, 2009. Reproduced with permission. For colour details, see the colour plates section

drink products have been marketed in past 10 years. Different categories of products have gained varying levels of success. The most accepted product was probiotic chocolate. The highest sales were from the food and beverage section, which makes up 85% of the total probiotic products. Among all the probiotic products, 80% of probiotic sales in 2011 came from dairy products.

According to the report published by 'Markets and Markets' (http://www.marketsandmarkets.com), 'probiotic market was valued at $24.23 billion in 2011 and is expected to grow at a CAGR [compound annual growth rate] of 6.8% from 2012 to 2017'.

The growing heath consciousness and awareness of food safety are promoting further success in an already lucrative probiotic market.

References

Adeyemi, I.A. (1993). Making the most of ogi. *Food Chain*, 8, 5–6.

Agrawal, R., Rati, E.R., Vijayendra, S.V.N. *et al.* (2000). Flavour profile of idli batter prepared from defined microbial starter cultures. *World Journal of Microbiology and Biotechnology*, 16, 687–690.

Aidoo, K.E., Nout, M.J.R. and Sarkar, P.K. (2006). Occurrence and function of yeast in Asian indigenous fermented foods. *FEMS Yeast Research*, 6, 30–39.

Amagase, H. and Milner, J.A. (1993). Impact of various sources of garlic and their constituents on 7,12-dimethylbenz[a]anthracene binding to mammary cell DNA. *Carcinogenesis*, 14, 1627–1631.

Amoa-Awua, W.K., Owusu, W.K. and Feglo, P. (2005). Utilization of unfermented cassava flour for the production of an indigenous African fermented food, agbelima. *World Journal of Microbiology and Biotechnology*, 21, 1201–1207.

Anonymous (2001). Datamonitor, Worldwide Innovations Network. www.datamonitor.com

Asahara, T., Nomoto, K., Shimizu, K., Watanuki, M. and Tanaka, R. (2001). Increased resistance of mice to *Salmonella enterica* serovar Typhimurium infection by synbiotic administration of *Bifidobacteria* and transgalactosylated oligosaccharides. *Journal of Applied Microbiology*, 91, 985–996.

Ashenafi, M. and Busse, M. (1991). Growth of Bacillus cereus in fermenting tempeh made from various beans and its inhibition by Lactobacillus plantarum. *Journal of Applied Bacteriology*, 70, 329–333.

Augusti, K.T. and Sheela, C.G. (1996). Antiperoxide effect of S-allyl cysteine sulfoxide, an insulin secretagogue, in diabetic rats.Experientia 52, 115–120.

Balasubramanian, S. and Viswanathan, R. (2007). Properties of idli batter during its fermentation time. *Journal of Food Processing and Preservation*, 31, 32–40.

Banerjee, B. and Bagchi, D. (2001). Beneficial effects of a novel IH636 grape seed proanthocyanidin extract in the treatment of chronic pancreatitis. *Digestion*, 63 (3), 203–206.

Barreteau, H., Delattre, C. and Michaud, P. (2006). Production of oligosaccharides as promising new food additive generation. *Food Technology and Biotechnology*, 44, 323–333.

Blackwood, J. and Fulder, S. (1987). *Garlic: Nature's Original Remedy*. Inner Traditions Paperback. Javelin, Poole.

Blandino, A., Al-Aseeri, M.E., Pandiella, S.S., Cantero, D. and Webb, C. (2003). Review. Cereal-based fermented foods and beverages. *Food Research International*, 36, 527–543.

Block, E. (1985). The chemistry of garlic and onions. *Scientific American*, 252, 114–119.

Block, G., Patterson, B. and Subar, A. (1992). Fruit, vegetables and cancer prevention: A review of the epidemiologic evidence. *Nutr.ition and Cancer*, 18, 1–29.

Bloedon, L.T. and Szapary, P.O. (2004). Flaxseed and cardiovascular risk. *Nutrition Reviews*, 62 (1), 18–27.

Botes, A., Todorov, S.D., von Mollendorff, J.W., Botha, A. and Dicks, L.M.T. (2007). Identification of lactic acid bacteria and yeast from boza. *Process Biochemistry*, 42, 267–270.

Bournet, F.R., Brouns, F., Tashiro, Y. and Duvillier, V. (2002). Nutritional aspects of short-chain fructooligosaccharides: natural occurrence, chemistry, physiology, and health implications. *Digestive and Liver Disease*, 34, S111–S120.

Cheng, S.Y., Shaw, N.S., Tsai, K.S. and Chen, C.Y. (2004). The hypoglycaemic effects of soy isoflavones on postmenopausal women. *Journal of Women's Health*, 13, 1080–1086.

Chin, H.S., Breid, F., Fleming, H.P., Shin, W.C. and Yoon, S.S. (2006). Identifications of predominant bacterial isolates from the fermenting kimchi using ITS-PCR and partial 16S rDNA sequence analyses. *Journal of Microbiology and Biotechnology*, 16, 68–76.

Christie, S., Walker, A.F., Hicks, S.M. and Abeyasekera, S. (2004). Flavonoid supplement improves leg health and reduces fluid retention in premenopausal women in a double-blind, placebo-controlled study. *Phytomedicine*, 11, 11–17.

DeFelice, S.L. (1992). The neutraceuticals initiative: a recommendation for U.S. Economic and regulatory reforms. *Genetic Engineering News*, 12, 13–15.

Delattre, C., Michaud, P., Courtois, B. and Courtois, J. (2005). Oligosaccharides engineering from plants and algae applications in biotechnology and therapeutics. *Minerva Biotechnology*, 17, 107–117.

Delzenne, N.M. and Kok, N. (2001). Effects of fructan-type prebiotics on lipid metabolism. *American Journal of Clinical Nutrition*, 73, 456–458.

Delzenne, N.M., Daubioul, C., Neyrinck, A., Lasa, M. and Taper, H.S. (2002). Inulin and oligofructose modulate lipid metabolis in animals, review of biological events and future prospects. *British Journal of Nutrition*, 87 (suppl. 1), 255–259.

Dorant, E., van-den-Brandt, P.A., Goldbohm, R.A., Hermus, R.J. and Sturmans, F. (1993). Garlic and its significance for prevention of cancer in humans: A critical view. *British Journal of Cancer*, 67, 424–429.

Duffy, R., Wiseman, H. and File, S.E. (2003). Improved cognitive function in postmenopausal women after 12 weeks of consumption of a soya extract containing isoflavones. *Pharmacology, Biochemistry and Behavior*, 75, 721–729.

Erbas, M., Uslu, M.K., Erbas, M.O. and Certel, M. (2006). Effects of fermentation and storage on the organic and fatty acid contents of tarhana, a Turkish fermented cereal food. *Journal of Food Composition and Analysis*, 19, 294–301.

Escamilla-Hurtado, M.L., Olguín-Lora, P. and Prado-Barragán, L.A. (1993). Lactic acid fermentation of sour corn porridge of the Tzotzil ethnic group. *Revista Española de Ciencia y Tecnologia de Alimentos*, 33, 555–565.

Evoy, D., Lieberman, M.D., Fahey, T.J. and Daly, J.M. (1998). Immunonutrition: The role of arginine. *Nutrition*, 14, 611–617.

Farnworth, E.R. (2005). The beneficial effects of fermented foods-potential probiotics around the world. *Journal of Nutraceuticals, Functional & Medical Foods*, 4, 3–4.

Feng, X.M., Eriksson, A.R.B. and Schnürer, J. (2005). Growth of lactic acid bacteria and *Rhizopus oligosporus* during barley tempeh. *International Journal of Food Microbiology*, 104, 249–256.

Femia, A.P., Luceri, C., Dolara, P. *et al.* (2002). Antitumorigenic activity of the prebiotic inulin enriched with oligofructose in combination with the probiotics *Lactobacillus rhamnosus* and *Bifidobacterium lactis* on azoxymethane-induced colon carcinogenesis in rats. *Carcinogenesis*, 23, 1953–1960.

Fiordaliso, M., Kok, N., Desager, J.P. *et al.* (1995). Dietary oligofructose lowers triglycerides, phospholipids and cholesterol in serum and very low density lipoproteins of rats. *Lipids*, 30, 163–167.

Forchielli, M.L. and Walker, W.A. (2005). The role of gut-associated lymphoid tissues and mucosal defence. *British Journal of Nutrition*, 93 (Suppl. 1), 41–48.

Gibson, G.R. and Roberfroid, M.B. (1995). Dietary modulation of the human colonic microbiotia: Introducing the concept of prebiotics. *Journal of Nutrition*, 125, 1401–1412.

Gibson, G.R., Saavedra, J.M., Macfarlane, S. and Macfarlane, G.T. (1996). Probiotics and intestinal infection. In *Probiotics: Therapeutic and Other Beneficial Effects* (ed. R. Fuller). Chapman and Hall, London.

Haliga, R., Mocanu, V., Oboroceanu, T., Stitt, P.A. and Luca, V.C. (2007). The effects of dietary flaxseed supplementation on lipid metabolism in streptozotocin-induced diabetic hamsters. *Revista Medico-chirurgicala a Societatii de Medici si Naturalisti din Iasi*, 111 (2): 472–476.

Hancioglu, O. and Karapinar, M. (1997). Microflora of boza. A traditional fermented Turkish beverage. *International Journal of Food Microbiology*, 35, 271–274.

Harris, L.J., Fleming, H.P. and Klaenhammer, T.R. (1992). Characterization of two nisin-producing *Lactococcus lactis* subsp. *lactis* strains isolated from a commercial sauerkraut fermentation. *Applied Environmental Microbiology*, 58, 1477–1483.

Heasman, M. and Mellentin, J. (2001). *The Functional Foods Revolution. Healthy People, Healthy Profits?* Earthscan Publications Ltd, London and Sterling.

Hidalgo, L.A., Chedraui, P.A., Morocho, N., Ross, S. and San Miguel, G. (2005). The effect of red clover isoflavones on menopausal symptoms, lipids and vaginal cytology in menopausal women: A randomized, double-blind, placebo-controlled study. *Gynecological Endocrinology*, 21, 257–264.

Hilliam, M. (2000). Functional food – How big is the market? *The World of Food Ingredients*, 12, 50–52.

Hoentjen, F., Welling, G. W., Harmsen, H.J. *et al.* (2005). Reduction of colitis by prebiotics in HLA-B27 transgenic rats is associated with microflora changes and immunomodulation. *Inflammatory Bowel Disease*, 11, 977–985.

Hosono, A., Ozawa, A., Kato, R. *et al.* (2003). Dietary fructooligosaccharides induce immunoregulation of intestinal IgA secretion by murine Peyer's patch cells. *Bioscience, Biotechnology and Biochemistry*, 67, 758–764.

Hosoya, N. (1998). Health claims in Japan. *Japanese Journal of Nutritional Food*, 1 (3–4), 1–11.

Hounhouigan, D.J., Nout, M.J.R., Nago, C.M., Houben, J.H. and Rombouts, F.M. (1999). Use of starter cultures of lactobacilli and yeast in the fermentation of mawe, an African maize product. *Tropical Science*, 39, 220–226.

Ijabadeniyi, A.O. (2007). Microorganisms associated with ogi traditionally produced from three varieties of maize. *Research Journal of Microbiology*, 2, 247–253.

Jiang, T. and Savaiano, D.A. (1997). *In vitro* lactose fermentation by human colonic bacteria is modified by *Lactobacillus acidophilus* supplementation. *Journal of Nutrition*, 127 (8), 1489–1495.

Johanningsmeier, S.D., Fleming, H.P., Thompson, R.L. and McFeeters, R.F. (2005). Chemical and sensory properties of sauerkraut produced with *Leuconostoc mesenteroides* starter cultures of differing malolactic phenotypes. *Journal of Food Science*, 70, 343–349.

Kirk, S.J. and Barbul, A. (1990). Role of arginine in trauma, sepsis, and immunity. *Journal of Parenteral and Enteral Nutrition*, 14, 226S–229S.

Kim, Y.S., Tsa, O.D., Morita, A. and Bella, A. (1982). Effect of sodium butyrate and three human colorectal adenocarcinoma cell lines in culture. *Falk Symposium*, 31, 317–323.

Kasote, D. M., Hegde, M. V. and Deshmukh, K. K. (2011). Antioxidant activity of phenolic components from n-butanol fraction (PC-BF) of defatted flaxseed meal. *American Journal of Food Technology*, 6, 604–612.

Kris-Etherton, P.M., Harris, W.S. and Appel, L.J. (2002). AHA Scientific Statement: Fish consumption, fish oil, omega-3 fatty acids and cardiovascular disease. *Circulation*, 106, 2747–2757.

Lee, H.M. and Lee, Y. (2006). Isolation of *Lactobacillus plantarum* from kimchi and its inhibitory activity on the adherence and growth of *Helicobacter pylori*. *Journal of Microbiology and Biotechnology*, 16, 1513–1517.

Lee, J.Y., Kim, C.J. and Kunz, B. (2006). Identification of lactic acid bacteria isolated from kimchi and studies on their suitability for application as starter culture in the production of fermented sausages. *Meat Science*, 72, 437–445.

Lei, V. and Jacobsen, M. (2004). Microbiological characterization and probiotic potential of koko and koko sour water, African spontaneously fermented millet porridge and drink. *Journal of Applied Microbiology*, 96, 384–397.

Lu, Z., Breidt, F., Plengvidhya, V. and Fleming, H.P. (2003). Bacteriophage ecology in commercial sauerkraut fermentations. *Applied Environmental Microbiology*, 69, 3192–3202.

Manthey, F.A., Hareland, G.A. and Huseby, D.J. (1999). Soluble and insoluble dietary fiber content and composition in oat. *Cereal Chemistry*, 76, 417–420.

marketsandmarkets.com (2013). Probiotics Market By Products (Functional Foods, Dietary Supplements, Specialty Nutrients, Animal Feed), Applications (Regular, Therapeutic, Preventive Health Care) And Ingredients (Lactobacilli, Bifidobacteria, Yeast) – Global Trends & Forecasts To 2017. Report Code: FB 1046. http://www.marketsandmarkets.com/Market-Reports/probiotic-market-advanced-technologies-and-global-market-69.html [accessed 26 July 2013].

McMaster, L.D., Kokott, S.A., Reid, S.J. and Abratt, V.R. (2005). Use of traditional African fermented beverages as delivery vehicles for *Bifidobacterium lactis* DSM 10140. *International Journal of Food Microbiology*, 102, 231–237.

Menrad, K. (2003). Market and marketing functional food in Europe. *Journal of Food Engineering*, 56 (2–3), 181–188.

Mohammed, S.I., Steenson, L.R. and Kirleis, A.W. (1991). Isolation and characterization of microoganisms associated with the traditional sorghum fermentation for production of Sudanese kisra. *Appled Environmental Microbiology*, 57, 2529–2533.

Moncheva, P., Chipeva, V., Kujumdzieva, A. *et al.* (2003). The composition of the microflora of boza, an original Bulgarian beverage. *Biotechnology and Biotechnological Equipment*, 17, 164–168.

Munjal, U., Glei, M., Pool-Zobel, B.L. and Scharlau, D. (2009). Fermentation products of inulin-type fructans reduce proliferation and induce apoptosis in human colon tumour cells of different stages of carcinogenesis. *British Journal of Nutrition*, 27, 1–9.

Mussamatto, S.I. and Mancilha, I.M. (2007). Non-digestible oligosaccharides: a review. *Carbohydrate Polymers*, 68, 587–597.

Nakamura, Y., Nosaka, S., Suzuki, M. *et al.* (2004). Dietary fructooligosaccharides up-regulate immunoglobulin A response and polymeric immunoglobulin receptor expression in intestines of infant mice. *Clinical Experimental Immunology*, 137, 52–58.

Newall, C.A., Anderson, L.A. and Phillipson, J.D. (1996). *Herbal Medicines: A Guide For Health-Care Professionals*, Vol. ix. Pharmaceutical Press, London, p. 296.

Nugent, M.A. (2000). Heparin sequencing brings structure to the function of complex oligosaccharides. The Proceedings of the National Academy of Sciences USA, 97, 10301–10303.

Odunfa, S.A. and Adeyele, S. (1985). Microbiological changes during the traditional production of ogi-baba, a West African fermented sorghum gruel. *Journal of Cereal Science*, 3, 173–180.

Olasupo, N.A., Olukoya, D.K. *et al.* (1997). Identification of *Lactobacillus* species associated with selected African fermented foods. *Zeitschrift für Naturforschung Section C A Journal of Biosciences*, 51, 105–108.

Olsen, A., Halm, M. and Jakobsen, M. (1995). The antimicrobial activity of lactic acid bacteria from fermented maize (kenkey) and their interactions during fermentation. *Journal of Applied Bacteriology*, 79, 506–512.

Omemu, A.M., Oyewole, O.B. and Bankole, M.O. (2007). Significance of yeasts in the fermentation of maize for ogi production. *Food Microbiology*, 24, 571–576.

Onyango, C., Okoth, M.W. and Mbugua, S.K. (2003). The pasting of lactic-fermented and dried uji (an East African sour porridge). *Journal of the Science of Food and Agriculture*, 83, 1412–1418.

Onyango, C., Bley, T., Raddatz, H. and Henle, T. (2004). Flavour compounds in backslop fermented uji (an East African sour porridge). *European Food Research and Technology*, 218, 579–583.

Ouwehand, A. (2007). Success in applying pro- and prebiotics in dairy products. In Proceedings of the Fourth International FFNet Meeting on Functional Foods, 26–27 March, Budapest, Hungary.

Ozdemir, S., Gocmen, D. and Kumral, A.Y. (2007). A traditional Turkish fermented cereal food: Tarhana. *Food Review International*, 23, 107–121.

Palma, A.S., Feizi, T., Zhang, Y. *et al.* (2006). Ligands for the beta-glucan receptor, Dectin-1, assigned using 'designer' microarrays of oligosaccharide probes (neoglycolipids) generated from glucan polysaccharides. *Journal of Biological Chemistry*, 281, 5771–5779.

Patel, H.M., Wang, R., Chandrashekar, O., Pandiella, S.S. and Webb, C. (2004). Proliferation of *Lactobacillus plantarum* in solid-state fermentation of oats. *Biotechnology Progress*, 20, 110–116.

Pierre, F., Perrin, P., Champ, M. *et al.* (1997). Shortchain fructo-oligosaccharides reduce the occurrence of colon tumors and develop gut-associated lymphoid tissue in Min mice. *Cancer Research*, 57, 225–228.

Phipps, W.R., Martini, M.C., Lampe, J.W., Slavin, J.L. and Kurzer, M.S. (1993). Effect of flax seed ingestion on the menstrual cycle. *Journal of Clinical Endocrinology and Metabolism*, 77, 1215–1219.

Potter, D. (1990). Functional foods – a major opportunity for the dairy industry? *Dairy Industries International*, 55 (6), 16–17.

Qiang, X., YongLie, C. and QianBing, W. (2009). Health benefit application of functional oligosaccharides. *Carbohydrate Polymers*, 77, 435–441.

Reisman, J., Schachter, H.M., Dales, R.E. *et al.* (2006). Treating asthma with omega-3 fatty acids: Where is the evidence? A systematic review. *BMC Complementary and Alternative Medicine*, 6, 26.

Riebroy, S., Banjakul, S., Visessanguan, W. and Tanaka, M. (2007). Effect of iced storage of big-eye snapper (*Priacanthus tayenus*) on the chemical composition, properties and acceptability of Som-fug, a fermented Thai fish mince. *Food Chemistry*, 102, 270–280.

Rivera-Espinoza, Y. and Gallardo-Navarro, Y. (2010). Non-dairy probiotic products. *Food Microbiology*, 27, 1–11.

Roberfroid, M.B., Bornet, F., Bouley, C. and Cummings, J.H. (1995). Colonic microflora: Nutrition and health. *Nutrition Reviews*, 53, 127–130.

Saad, C., Delattre, N., Urdaci, M., Schmitter, J.M. and Bressollier, P. (2013). An overview of the last advances in probiotic and prebiotic field. *LWT – Food Science and Technology*, 50 (1), 1–16.

Sanders, M.E., Kondo, J.K. and Willrett. D.L. (1991). Lactic acid bacteria applications, in *Biotechnologically Derived Ingredients For Food Products* (eds I. Goldberg and R. Williams). Van Nostrand Reinhold, New York, pp. 433-459.

Sheela, C.G., Kumud, K. and Augusti, K.T. (1995). Anti-diabetic effects of onion and garlic sulfoxide amino acids in rats. *Planta Medica*, 61, 356–357.

Siró, I., Kápolna, E., Kápolna, B. and Lugasi, A. (2008). Functional food. Product development, marketing and consumer acceptance – A review. *Appetite*, 51, 456–467.

Soni, S.K., Sandhu, D.K., Vilkhu, K.S. and Kamra, N. (1986). Microbiological studies on Dosa fermentation. *Food Microbiology*, 3, 45–53.

Steinmetz, K.A. and Potter, J.D. (1991). Vegetable, fruits, and cancer. I. Epidemiology. *Cancer Causes Control*, 2, 325–57.

Steer, T., Carpenter, H., Tuohy, K. and Gibson, G.R. (2000). Perspectives on the role of the human gut microbiota and its modulation by pro- and prebiotics. *Nutrition Research Reviews*, 13, 229–254.

Tamime, A.Y. and McNulty, D. (1999). Kishkda dried fermented milk/cereal mixture. 4. Microbiological quality. *Lait*, 79, 449–456.

Thapa, N., Pal, J. and Tamang, J.P. (2004). Microbial diversity in ngari, hentak and tungtap, fermented fish products of North-East India. *World Journal of Microbiology & Biotechnology*, 20, 599–607.

Todorov, S.D., Botes, M., Guigas, C. *et al.* (2008). Boza, a natural source of probiotic lactic acid bacteria. *Journal of Applied Microbiology*, 104, 465–477.

Tou, E.H., Guyot, J.P., Mouquet-Rivier, C. *et al.* (2006). Study through surveys and fermentation kinetics of the traditional processing of pearl millet (*Pennisetum glaucum*) into bensaalga, a fermented gruel from Burkina Faso. *International Journal of Food Microbiology*, 106, 52–60.

Verghese, M., Rao, D.R., Chawan, C.B., Williams, L.L. and Shackelford, L. (2002). Dietary inulin suppresses azoxymethane-induced aberrant crypt foci and colon tumors at the promotion stage inyoung Fisher 344 rats. *Journal of Nutrition*, 132, 2809–2813.

Wood, P.J. and Beer, M.U. (1998). Functional oat products, in *Functional Foods: Biochemical and Processing Aspect* (ed. G. Mazza). Technomic Publishing Co., Lankaster, pp. 1–29.

Williams, C.M. and Jackson, K.G. (2002). Inulin and oligofructose: effects on lipid metabolism from human studies. *British Journal Nutrition*, 87, 261–264.

Zeisel, S.H. (1999). Regulation of "nutraceuticals". *Science*, 285 (5435), 1853–1855.

2

Bioactive Components in Foods

Anil Kumar Anal, Kishore K. Kumaree and Mridula Thapa
Food Engineering and Bioprocess Technology, Asian Institute of Technology, Pathum Thani, Thailand

Functional components in food can be divided in to the following categories: proteins, carbohydrates, lipids, phenols, flavonoids, anthocyanins and glucosinolates. Many academic, scientific and regulatory bodies have developed, or are developing, guidelines to establish the scientific evidence base needed to support and further validate claims for functional components or the foods containing them. The Food Development Agency (FDA) regulates food products according to their intended use and the nature of claims made on the package. Five types of health-related statements or claims are allowed on food and dietary supplement labels:

(1) Nutrient content claims indicate the presence of a specific nutrient at a certain level.
(2) Structure and function claims describe the effect of dietary components on the normal structure or function of the body.
(3) Dietary guidance claims describe the health benefits of broad categories of foods or diets and do not refer to a disease or a health related condition.
(4) Qualified health claims convey a developing relationship between components in the diet and reduced risk of disease, as reviewed by the FDA and supported by the weight of credible scientific evidence available
(5) Health claims confirm a relationship between components in the diet and reduced risk of disease or health condition, as approved by FDA and supported by significant scientific agreement.

2.1 Proteins

The presence of protein in complex food systems as an active component for physiological activities is being increasingly acknowledged. Many of the proteins

Functional Foods and Dietary Supplements: Processing Effects and Health Benefits, First Edition.
Edited by Athapol Noomhorm, Imran Ahmad and Anil Kumar Anal.

occurring in raw food materials show their action indirectly or directly on the hydrolysis of enzymes *in vitro* or *in vivo*. In recent studies, it has been proved that proteins act as a rich source of biologically active peptides. The term 'bioactive peptides' can be explained as the part of protein that has a beneficial effect on the body's metabolic functions or the conditions that ultimately influence health (Kitts and Weiler, 2003). Many peptides that come from either a plant or animal protein source show their regulatory functions in humans beyond normal and satisfactory nutrition. Proteins may have several roles in foods. The main purpose of available protein is to provide and/or stabilize the characteristic structure of individual foods. For example, in a piece of meat, the structure of the muscle is due to the fine arrangement of connective tissues and myofibril. Other than this, in the context of food, this structure also determines the texture of cooked meat.

2.1.1 Food sources of peptides

Many bioactive peptides have been identified from both plant and animal sources, but the most abundant sources are milk-based products. Milk protein is currently considered to be the most valuable source of bioactive peptides and many oher types of peptides have been identified in fermented milk products and cheese (Schanbacher *et al.*, 1998; Meisel, 1998, 2001, 2004; Clare and Swaisgood, 2000; Korhonen and Pihlanto-Leppala, 2001; Kilara and Panyam, 2003; Korhonen and Pihlanto, 2003; Matar *et al.*, 2003; FitzGerald, Murray and Walsh, 2004; Korhonen and Pihlanto-Leppala, 2004; Silva and Malcata, 2005). Table 2.1 gives the details of the bioavailability of proteins and peptides from natural sources.

2.1.2 Health benefits of proteins and peptides

A wide range of activities has been described for proteins and peptides including antimicrobial properties, blood pressure-lowering (acetyl cholinesterase (ACE)-inhibitory) effects, cholesterol-lowering ability, antithrombotic and antioxidant activities, enhancement of mineral absorption/bioavailability, cyto- or immune-modulatory effects, and opioid activities. Moreover, some peptides are multifunctional and can exert more than one of these effects (Meisel, 2004). Figure 2.1 briefly describes the beneficial effects of biopeptides.

2.1.3 Functional product development containing proteins and peptides

Dietary proteins are conventionally known to provide energy and the essential amino acids for growth and for the maintenance of various physiological activities. They also contribute to the sensory properties of foods. In the past decade functional foods containing proteins and peptides have gained popularity because of their positive effect on physiological activity. Many peptides are available in milk. They become activated inside the body, e.g. during gastrointestinal digestion or milk fermentation. Once activation happens, these peptides hold the key to regulate many processes in living system.

In Table 2.2 lists some of the biopeptides in milk and other food products.

Table 2.1 Examples of bioactive peptides derived from food

Effect	Origin	Encrypting protein(s)	Name/remarks/sequence	Reference
ACE inhibitory/	Soy	Soy protein	NWGPLV	Kodera and Nio, 2006
hypotensive	Fish	Fish muscle	LKP, IKP, LRP (derived	Nagai *et al.*, 2006
	Meat	protein	from sardine, bonito,	Vercruysse *et al.*,
	protein	Meat muscle	tuna, squid)	2005
	Milk	α-LA, β-LG	IKW, LKP	Murray and
	Egg	α-, β-, k-CN	Lactokinins (e.g. WLAHK,	FitzGerald, 2006
	Wheat	Ovotransferrin	LRP, LKP	Mizushima *et al.*,
	Broccoli	Ovalbumin	Casokinins (e.g. FFVAP,	2004
		Wheat gliadin	FALPQY, VPP)	Lee *et al.*, 2006b
		Plant protein	KVREGTTY	Miguel and
			Ovokinin (FRADHPPL	Aleixandre, 2006
			Ovokinin (2–7)	Motoi and Kodama,
			(KVREGTTY)	2003
			IAP	Lee *et al.*, 2006a
			YPK	
Immuno-	Rice	Rice albumin	Oryzatensin (GYPMYPLR)	Takahashi *et al.*, 1994
modulatory	Egg	Ovalbumin	Peptides not specified	Mine and
	Milk	α-, β-, k-CN,	Immunopeptides (e.g.	Kovacs-Nolan, 2006
	Wheat	α-LA	α_{s1}-immunocasokinin)	Meisel, 2005
		Wheat gluten	(TTMPLW)	Horiguchi *et al.*, 2005
			Immunopeptides	
Cyto-	Milk	α-, β-CN	α-Casomorphin	Kampa *et al.*, 1997
modulatory	Wheat	Wheat gluten	(HIQKED(V)),	Takahashi *et al.*,
Opioid agonist	Milk	α-LA, β-LG	β-casomorphin-7	2000; Fukudome
		α-, β-CN	(YPFPGPI)	and Yoshikawa,
			Gluten-exorphins A4, A5	1993
			(GYYPT), B4, B5, and C	Silva and Malcata,
			(YPISL)	2005
			α-Lactorphins,	
			β-lactorphins	
			Casomorphins	
Opioid agonist	Milk	Lactoferrin	Lactoferroxins	Clare and Swaisgood,
		k-CN	Casoxins	2000
Antimicrobial	Egg	Ovotransferrin	OTAP-92 (f109–200)[a]	Mine and
	Milk	Lysozyme	Peptides not specified	Kovacs-Nolan, 2006
		Lactoferrin	Lactoferricin	McCann *et al.*, 2006
		α-, β-, k-CN	Casecidins, isracidin,	Hayes *et al.*, 2006
			kappacin	
Anti-thrombotic	Milk	k-CN (glyco-	k-CN (f106–116)[a],	Chabance *et al.*, 1995
		macropeptide)	casoplatelin	
Mineral binding,	Milk	α-, β-CN	Caseinophosphopeptides	Walker *et al.*, 2006
anticariogenic				
Hypo-	Soy	Glycinin	LPYPR	Wang and de Mejia,
cholesterolemic	Milk	β-LG	IIAEK	2005
				Nagaoka *et al.*, 2001
Antioxidant	Fish	Sardine muscle	MY	Erdmann *et al.*, 2006
	Wheat	Wheat germ	Peptides not specified	Zhu *et al.*, 2006
	Milk	protein	MHIRL, YVEEL,	Hernandez-Ledesma
		α-LA, β-LG	YSLAMAASDI	*et al.*, 2005

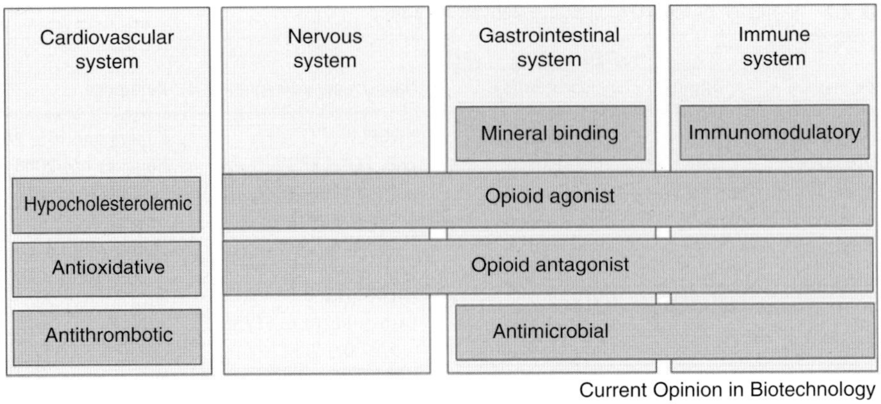

Figure 2.1 Overview of the beneficial effects ascribed to bioactive peptides derived from food proteins. *Source:* Hartmann & Meisel, 2007. Reproduced with permission from Elsevier

2.1.4 Processing techniques of proteins and peptides

In most studies, bioactive peptides are obtained through conventional enzymatic hydrolysis, but some researchers have found other methods with potentially higher yields. Microbial enzymes such as alcalase (an endopeptidase from *Bacillus licheniformis*) and flavourzyme (a protease complex from *Aspergillus oryzae*) are frequently used (Barbana and Boye, 2010). Enzymatic hydrolysis can be performed through conventional batch hydrolysis or continuous hydrolysis (Huang *et al.*, 2011). At the industrial level, most hydrolysis reactions are carried out in a classical batch reactor with controlled temperature and pH. At the end of the reaction, enzymes are inactivated before recovery of the final products. Though this conventional batch-type protein hydrolysis is simple and easy to control, it has high enzyme and labour costs. Perhaps in an effort to reduce these costs, an enzymatic membrane reactor consisting of a membrane separation device coupled to a tank reactor has been developed. The membrane creates a selective barrier so that permeable products can be separated from the reaction mixture while the enzyme is retained in the reaction tank. Huang *et al.* (2011) used ultrafiltration membranes for continuous hydrolysis and found that utilization of the enzymatic ultrafiltration membrane reactor improved the yield and product quality compared to the batch process. On the other hand, Jia *et al.* (2009) enhanced the process of enzymatic hydrolysis with the use of ultrasound. There was an increase in surface hydrophobicity of defatted wheat germ proteins (DWGP) and loosening of the protein tissues under ultrasonic pretreatment, which facilitated the release of hydrophobic amino acids during enzymatic hydrolysis. Since most of the studies discussed here involve extracting bioactive peptides from rarely eaten plants and by-products which are not edible at all, the use of the peptides as nutraceuticals or functional food ingredients are the obvious applications.

The physiological effects of bioactive peptides depend mainly on their ability to reach the target organs in their active form. To determine the resistance of the bioactive peptides to digestion, they are sequentially hydrolysed with pepsin and pancreatic extracts, simulating the gastrointestinal conditions. *In vitro* studies with epithelial intestinal cells have also been carried out for this purpose (Hernandez-Ledesma

Table 2.2 Bioactive peptides identified in fermented milk products

Product	Examples of identified bioactive peptides[a]	Bioactivity	References
Cheese type			
Parmigiano–Reggiano	β-cn *f*(8–16), *f*(58–77),α_{s2}-cn *f*(83–33)	Phosphopeptides, precursor of β-casomorphin	Addeo *et al.*, 1992
Cheddar	α_{s1}- and β-casein fragments	Several phosphopeptides	Singh *et al.*, 1997
Italian varieties: Mozzarella, Crescenza, Italico, Gorgonzola	β-cn *f*(58–72)	ACE inhibitory	Smacchi and Gobbetti, 1998
Gouda	α_{s1}-cn *f*(1–9), β-cn *f*(60–68)	ACE inhibitory	Saito *et al.*, 2000
Festivo	α_{s1}-cn *f*(1–9), *f*(1–7), *f*(1–6)	ACE inhibitory	Ryhänen *et al.*, 2001
Emmental	α_{s1}- and β-casein fragments	Immunostimulatory, several phosphopeptides, antimicrobial	Gagnaire *et al.*, 2001
Manchego	Ovine α_{s1}-, α_{s2}- and β-casein fragments	ACE inhibitory	Gomez-Ruiz *et al.*, 2002
Emmental	Active peptides not identified	ACE inhibitory	Parrot *et al.*, 2003
Fermented milks			
Sour milk	β-cn *f*(74–76, *f*(84–86), κ-cn *f*(108–111)	Antihypertensive	Nakamura *et al.*, 1995
Yoghurt	Active peptides not identified	Weak ACE-inhibitory	Meisel *et al.*, 1997
Dahi	Ser-Lys-Val-Tyr-Pro	ACE inhibitory	Ashar and Chand, 2004
Evolus	VPP, IPP from β- and κ-CN	Hypotensive	Valio, Finland http://www.valio.com/
ProDiet F200	α_{s1}-CN (f91–100)[a]: YLGYLEQLLR	Reduces stress	Ingredia, France
Others			
BioZate	Whey peptides	Hypotensive	Davisco, USA http://www.daviscofoods.com/
BioPURE-GMP	Whey protein hydrolysate	Anticariogenic, antimicrobial, antithrombotic	Davisco, USA http://www.daviscofoods.com/
Tekkotsu Inryou	CPP	Helps mineral absorption	Suntory, Japan http://www.suntory.com/business/food/
Kotsu Kotsu calcium	CPP	Helps mineral absorption	Asahi, Japan Hieny (1994)

Abbreviations: α_{s1}-cn, α_{s1}-casein; β-cn, β-casein; κ-cn, κ-casein.

et al., 2011). *In vitro* studies have demonstrated that several peptides are actually resistant to physiological processes and can reach the circulation. The gastrointestinal resistance tests conducted by Rayaprolu *et al.* (2012) showed that peptide fractions derived from high oleic acid soybean can remain active when consumed. Foltz *et al.* (2009) pointed out that most *in vitro* studies for bioactive peptides are neither realistic nor physiologically relevant. Unlike *in vitro* tests, the human digestive system is capable of handling a wide range of protein sources. Further investigations to assess *in vivo* and clinical hypertensive effects will be critical to confirm observed findings. Functional or novel foods are created by fortifying or adding enriched fractions of the bioactive peptide to the product. Also, genetically modified proteins, such as the soybean proglycin A1aB1b, can be designed to carry multiple copies of the bioactive sequence.

2.2 Carbohydrate

Back in the 1960s when scientists were unveiling the chemical formula and the shape of polysaccharide chains, the term 'functionality' was synonymous with their ability to structure processed food products. Thus a pioneering statement was made that the stability of a seaweed jelly was the outcome of the close bonding of thread-like macromolecules of carrageenan forming a double helix. Today, however, the term 'functional carbohydrates' means so much more!

Carbohydrate holds more than 50% of the energy source present in most human diets. Carbohydrate is the abundant component in most dietary foods like cereals, vegetable, fruits and legumes. It also acts as main source of energy for the human body. From the chemical point of view and using the degree of polymerization, carbohydrates are categorized into mono-, di-, oligo- and polysaccharides. From the nutrition point of view, carbohydrates can be divided into sugars and sugar alcohols, basically mono- and disaccharides and their derivatives, starch polysaccharides, and dietary fibre. Figure 2.2 gives a general idea of carbohydrate classification.

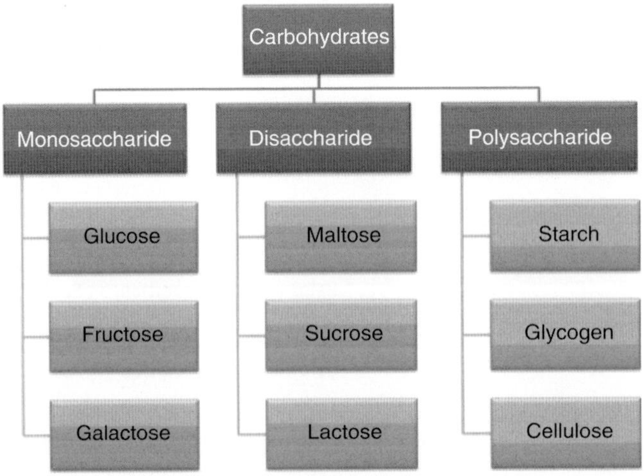

Figure 2.2 Classification of carbohydrates

2.2.1 Classification of carbohydrates

Polysaccharides can be broken down mainly to starch, which is further composed of linear amylase and braced amylopectin. These two branched and non-branched structures are the homo-polymers of glucose. Polysaccharides can also be broken down to non-starch polysaccharides (NSPs), which include cellulose. Plant based foods are the best source for dietary NSPs, because plant cell walls mainly consist of NSPs. The different forms of glucose are shown in Figure 2.3. NSPs can be further differentiated by their attached sugar residue as neutral (containing mainly neutral sugar residues), acidic (containing mainly uranic acid residues, also referred to as pectic substances) and hemicellulose A, B and C, depending on their solubility at different pH. A few polysaccharide food additives are taken in their natural form from plants, for example gums and mucilages. The relative proportions of main monomeric residues (i.e. rhamnose, xylose, arabinose, galactose, glucose, mannose and uranic acids), is another common way to characterize and name food polysaccharides, for example rabinoxylans, galactans, galactomannans and hamnogalacturonans.

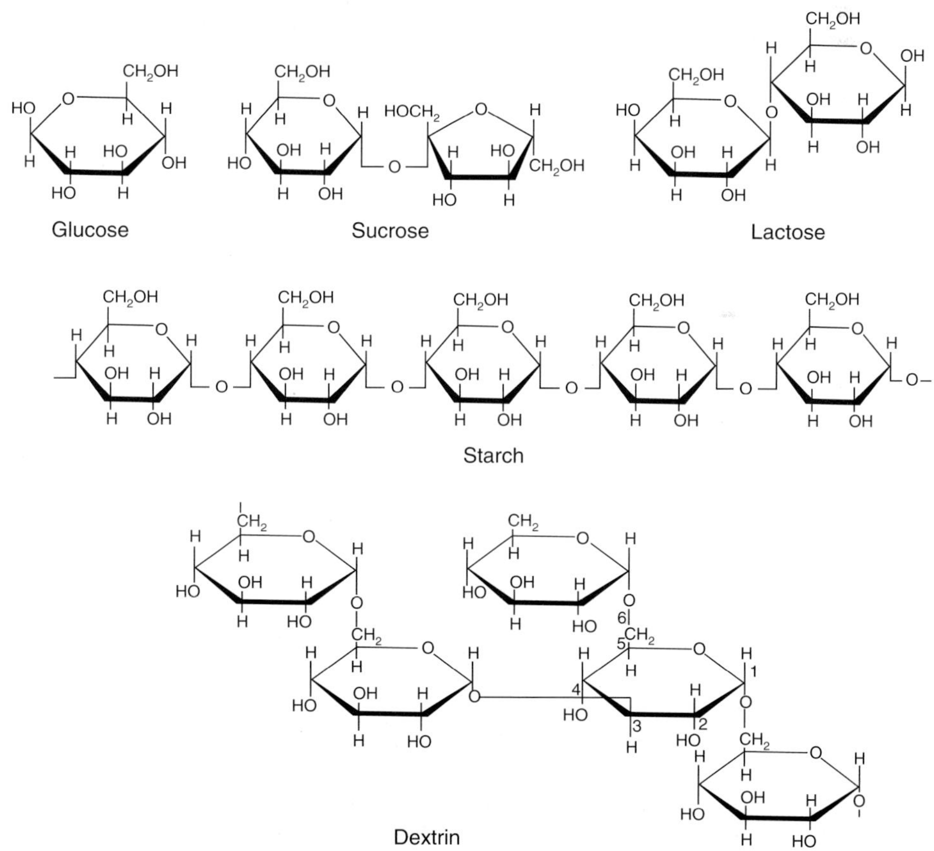

Figure 2.3 Structures of different forms of glucose

Table 2.3 Benefits of carbohydrate on physiology of human health

	Functional carbohydrates	Physiological effects
1	Dietary fibres (general)	Carbohydrate and lipid metabolism modulation
2	Intermediate type of fibres (e.g. β-glucan from oat and barley brans)	Cholesterol lowering
3	Resistant starch	Colon nutrition, reduced risk of cancer
4	Non-digestible oligosaccharides (e.g. inulin and fructo-oligosaccharides)	Prebiotic effect: enrichment of bifidobacteria

2.2.2 Functional carbohydrates and their health benefits

There has been a myth about carbohydrates for many years. Research suggests that for a healthy diet, carbohydrate is an essential requirement. Carbohydrates have a positive effect on the physiology of human health as described in Table 2.3. The main contributions of carbohydrates to health are as follows:

- energy fuel for physical activity,
- the nutrition needed for optimum health, and
- the nutrients necessary for good brain function.

And most beneficial carbohydrates are high fibre foods that help you to:

- lose weight,
- lower cholesterol,
- prevent constipation,
- reduce triglyceride levels,
- carry toxins out of your body,
- avoid or even reverse diabetes,
- maintain stable blood sugar levels,
- decrease your risk of heart disease, and
- have much better sustained energy.

Recent recommendations for the proper control of type 2 diabetes and obesity, suggest that a high intake of dietary fibre is beneficial (Singh, 2007). The chemical structure of fibre helps to control the release of glucose into the blood as it is fibrous and viscous and this helps prevent diabetes mellitus and obesity (Bennett *et al.*, 2006; Huang *et al.*, 2006). Functional oligosaccharides are often thought to be as important dietary fibre in the context of some disorders associated with metabolic syndromes (Roth *et al.*, 2003; Kim and Rajapakse, 2005; de Alcântara *et al.*, 2006). In the market, commercially available oligosaccharides include fructo-oligosaccharides (FOS), isomalto-oligosaccharides, malto-oligosaccharides, arabinoxylan oligosaccharides, glucose-oligosaccharides and galacto-oligosaccharides. Research conducted on animals and humans indicates that the intake of functional oligosaccharides which undergo fermentation in the caeco-colon could be an appealing way to modulate satiety, glucose, lipid metabolism and hypertension (Nesselhut *et al.*, 1993). Low glycaemic index food, such as food high in functional oligosaccharides, has been proven

Table 2.4 Functional oligosaccharides

Type	Monosaccharides	Number of monosaccharides	Bonds indicative of functions
IMOS (isomaltooligosaccharides)	Glucose	2–5	α-1,4
SBOS (soybean oligosaccharides)	Fructose, galactose, glucose	2–4	α-1,6
FOS (fructo-oligosaccharides)	Sucrose, fructose	2–5	β-1,2
XOS (xylo-oligosaccharides)	Xylose	2–7	α-1,4
MOS (malto-oligosaccharides)	Mannitose, glucose	2–10	α-1,2, α-1,4
Gentio-oligosaccharides	Glucose	2–10	β-1,6
Glucose-oligosaccharides	Glucose	2–10	α-1,2, β-1,3, β-1,6
Palatinose	Glucose, fructose	2	β-1,6
Malto-oligosaccharides	Glucose	2–8	α-l,2
Lactosucrose	Galactose, fructose	2–3	β-1,4
Clycosylsucrose	Glucose, fructose	3	α-l,2, β-l,4
Galato-oligosaccharides	Galactose	2–5	β-1,2, α-1,4
Lactulose	Galactose, fructose	2	β-1,4
Raffinose	Galactose, fructose, glucose	3	β-l,2, α-l,4
Stachyose	Galactose, fructose, glucose	4	α-1,4

to decrease the postprandial blood glucose levels and insulin response, hence improving the overall blood glucose and lipid concentration in normal people and in patients with diabetes mellitus (Kawamori *et al.*, 2007). In one study, rats were fed with short-chain FOS at a dose of 10% in their diet. After a few weeks the results showed:

- postprandial glycaemia and triglyceridaemia in normal rats,
- lessened hepatic steatosis and fat mass development in obese Wistar rats fed a high fat diet (this phenomenon could be partly explained by a satietogenic effect of FOS; Delmée *et al.*, 2006; Li, Fang and Zhang, 2007),
- that in streptozotocin (a naturally occurring chemical that is particularly toxic to the insulin-producing beta cells of the pancreas in mammals) treated diabetic rats, FOS feeding during 4–6 weeks improves glucose tolerance, decreases glycaemia and partially restores insulin secretion (Giacco *et al.*, 2004),
- an improvement of glucose/insulin ratio in rats receiving FOS added in a high fructose diet (Giacco *et al.*, 2004).

Details of a few oligosaccharides is given in Table 2.4.

2.2.3 Functional foods containing good carbohydrates

The best sources for healthy carbohydrates are:

- raw and lightly steamed vegetables,
- legumes, beans, nuts and seeds,
- high fibre 100% whole grains,
- raw, whole, fresh fruits, and
- most low fat dairy products.

Table 2.5 Commercial products available with functional carbohydrate

Product	Manufacturer
Dietary fibre	
Oat meal	Quaker
Muesli	Vitalis
Muesli	Kellog's
Functional yoghurt	Vilkyškiai
Dietary fibre supplement	Tony Ferguson
Dietary fibre supplement	UNIQ
Essential Fibre Crispibread	Orgran
Resistant starch	
Hi-Maize	Sternlife
Orange flavoured containing psyllium husk powder and Starmax® resistant starch	Nucolox®
Glycaemic control resistant starch supplement	Durk Pearson and Sandy Shaw'™
Pre-biotic carbohydrates	
Coffee with inulin	Nescafé Protect ProSlim
Fast Max Tea with inulin and guarana	Mokate, DietaFit
Chicory root fibre (containing inulin and oligofructose) Granola Bars	Kashi
LiveActive line, inulin-containing drink	Kraft Foods
Junior Prebiotic Supplement	Nutricia Neocate
Probiotic beverages	Froose

Table 2.5 shows a few of the beneficial carbohydrate foods.

2.3 Lipids

Dietary fats, oils and specifically vegetable oil have gained widespread attention among consumers, clinicians, researchers, food producers and food processors in the past two decades because of their effects on human health. When considering fats and lipids in the diet, it is important to discuss saturated and unsaturated fats as they are considered the most important dietary risk factors in coronary heart disease.

Food oils have both nutritional and functional characteristics. The highest energy (calorie) source per gram of food can be obtained from the consumption of fats and oils. The different properties of saturated and unsaturated fats relates to the different physical behaviour of food during processing; for example, saturated fatty acids gives stability, texture and flavour to foods.

2.3.1 Classification of lipids

Lipids have been divided into eight categories: fatty acyls, glycerolipids, glycerophospholipids, sphingolipids, saccharolipids and polyketides (derived from condensation of ketoacyl subunits); and sterol lipids and prenol lipids (derived from condensation of isoprene subunits). Figure 2.4 gives an overall classification of lipids.

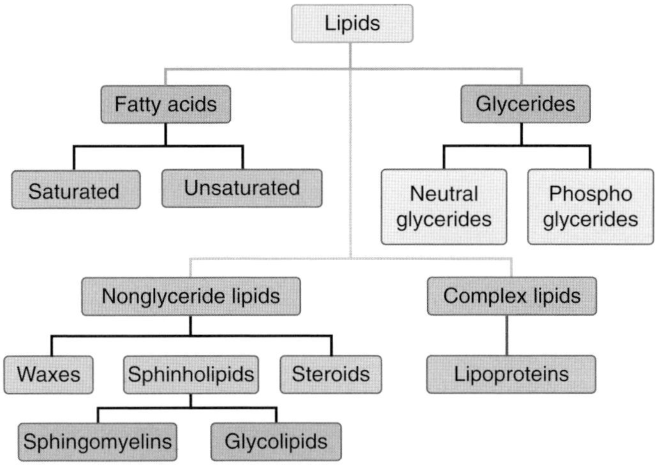

Figure 2.4 Classification of lipids

Polyunsaturated fatty acid (PUFA) has high nutritional value. Fish are the most important dietary source of the *n*-3 highly unsaturated fatty acids (HUFA), eicosapentaenoic (EPA) and docosahexaenoic acid (DHA), which are particularly important in human nutrition reflecting their roles in critical physiological processes. No vertebrate species can synthesize PUFAs *de novo*, as they lack the fatty acid desaturase enzymes required for the production of linoleate (18:2*n*-6) and linolenate (18:3*n*-3) from oleic acid (18:1*n*-9) (Wallis *et al.*, 2002). However, many vertebrates can convert dietary 18:2*n*-6 and 18:3*n*-3 to long-chain HUFA such as arachidonic acid (20:4*n*-6, AA), eicosapentaenoic acid (EPA, 20:5*n*-3) and docosahexaenoic acid (22:6*n*-3, DHA) via a pathway involving a series of microsomal fatty acid desaturation and elongation steps (Cook, 1996). The production of EPA requires D6 and D5 desaturases, and the production of DHA from EPA requires a further desaturation originally thought to be effected by a D4 desaturase acting on a C22 fatty acid intermediate, although evidence now suggests it may actually be effected by a D6 desaturase acting on a C24 intermediate (Sprecher, 2000; De Antueno *et al.*, 2001; D'Andrea *et al.*, 2002). Fish lipids are particularly rich in PUFA. The classification of PUFAs is shown in Figure 2.5.

2.3.2 Functional lipids

Naturally, the human body cannot synthesize essential fatty acids (EFAs), and types include linoleic acid (LA) and alpha linoleic acids (ALA) (Innis, 1996). Arachidonic acid can be synthesized from LA, so it's not taken as EFA. Two more types of PUFAs are EPA and DHA and they are not EFAs either as they are also synthesized from ALA, but they are still considered to be important FAs.

Diets deficient in EFA can cause the following symptoms: dry, scaly skin; skin lesions; hair loss; improper collagen formation; infertility; painful, swollen joints; liver damage/degeneration; lethargy and irritability; and growth retardation.

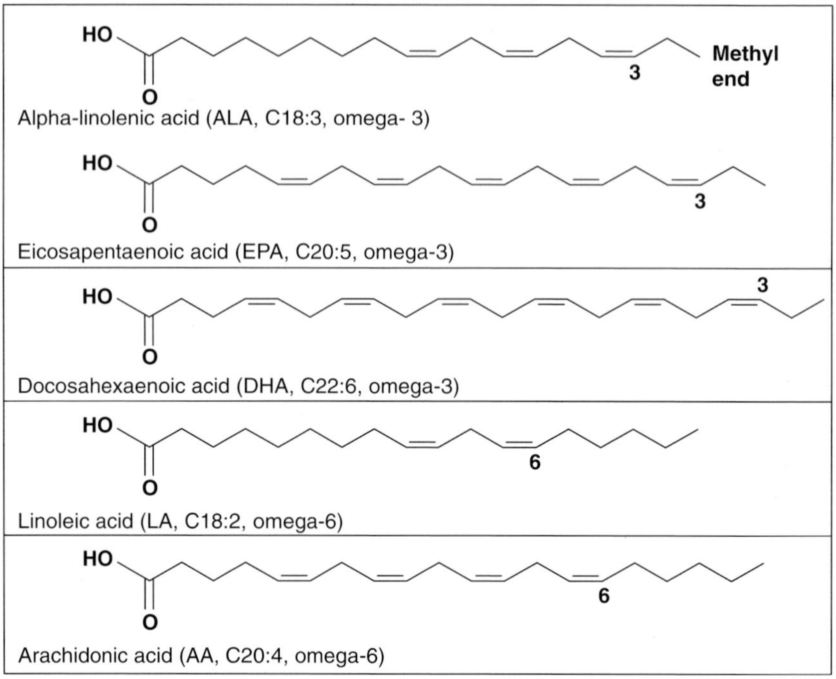

Figure 2.5 Classification of polyunsaturated fatty acids (PUFA)

Vegetable seeds are an natural source of fats and fat-soluble vitamins, both important in the human diet. Certain vegetable fats, solid at room temperature, are called butters. Most natural vegetable oils contain partly saturated fatty acids with an even number of carbon atoms (in its triacylglycerol structure) and partly unsaturated fatty acids with isolated double bounds, particularly in cis-configuration. Some trans-fatty acids are also known to occur naturally, for example within oils of some genera of the Compositae plant family (Tsevegsüren *et al.,* 2000). Fatty acid parts of triacylglycerols convert into their geometrical and positional isomers due to the operating conditions for various processes, such as refining, deodorization and hydrogenation. The trans-fatty acids formed were noted in the early 1970s as nutritionally undesirable. Trans-fatty acids may raise the blood levels of low-density lipoprotein (LDL) to a similar extent to that caused by saturated fatty acids. In addition, recent studies indicate that trans-fatty acids intake is associated with the incidence of heart disease, and that the type, not the amount, of fat in the diet contributes to the risk of this disease (Mensink and Katan, 1990; Katan *et al.*, 1995).

2.3.3 Health benefits

ALA health benefits These are that it:

- protects against heart disease and heart attacks,
- lowers blood pressure,

- lowers blood cholesterol levels,
- improves immune function, and
- may correct deficiency of DHA in the sperm cells of subfertile men.

Functions and roles of EFA These include (Simopoulos, 1999; Kline, 2008):

- being structural components of phospholipids in cell membranes,
- influencing cell fluidity and flexibility, and
- being precursors for eicosanoids, which regulate or influence the following:
  - contraction of smooth muscles,
  - blood pressure,
  - platelet aggregation or 'clumping',
  - cell adhesions,
  - leukocyte chemotaxis,
  - dilation and constriction of blood vessels,
  - body temperature,
  - inflammation,
  - intensity and duration of pain and fever,
  - immune responses,
  - gastric acid secretion.

Eicosanoids and their functions These include (Ursin, 2003: Kline, 2008):

- prostaglandins (PG)
  - contraction of smooth muscle,
  - lower blood pressure,
  - regulation of gastric acid secretion,
  - regulation of body temperature,
  - regulation of platelet aggregation,
  - control of inflammation, vascular permeability;
- prostacyclins (PGI)
  - anti-aggregation of cells,
  - vasodilation,
  - lower blood pressure;
- thromboxanes (TX)
  - pro-aggregation of cells,
  - vasoconstriction,
  - increase blood pressure;
- leukotrienes (LT)
  - leukocyte chemotaxis,
  - cell adhesions.

Table 2.6 gives a list of commercial functional food products.

2.4 Phenols

Polyphenols are major functional components of food that contribute to various properties of food and have a major role as antioxidants (Manach *et al.*, 2004). They also take an active role in other biological activities such as cell signalling (Wheeler

Table 2.6 List of commercial functional food products

Product	Manufacturer
Product with omega-3 fatty acids	
Efekt milk	'Z bregov
UHT omega-3 milk	Dukat
Omega 3-6-9 vegan supplement shake, with blackberry	NutraOrigin
Protein shake	Detour
Oragnic hemp protein shake, chocolate	Nutiva
Omega-3 fatty acids from fruit seeds and then refortifies the dried fruit	Fruit Essentials®
Omega-3 fortified eggs	Organic Valley
Fibre an omega-3 chocolate bar	Quaker
Chocolate	Coromega omega-3
Chocolate chips	Omega Cookie
EFA supplement with omega-3 (EPA, DHA) and omega-6 (LA, GLA).	Xtendlife®
Coconut oil is an excellent source of MCTs (medium-chain triglycerides)	Healthy Delights

et al., 2004) and cell adhesion (Williams *et al.*, 2004). The growing interest on the effects of polyphenols has caused an increase in research. Polyphenols determine the quality of plant-based foods such as the colour of the food, its juices and wines; in development of flavours; antioxidant properties for the browning reaction; and antibacterial/antifungal properties. Researchers have suggested intake amounts for various polyphenols such as flavonols (Crozier *et al.*, 2000), flavanones (Manach *et al.*, 2003), catechins (Higdon and Frei, 2003) and phenolic acids (Scalbert and Williamson, 2000). The estimated amount of intake of polyphenols in our daily diet ranged between 2590 and 3016 mg/day. Of the total polyphenol intake in the daily diet, 48% gets absorbed in the small intestine, 42% is accessible in the large intestine and 10% remains unabsorbed.

Classification of polyphenols are shown in Figure 2.6.

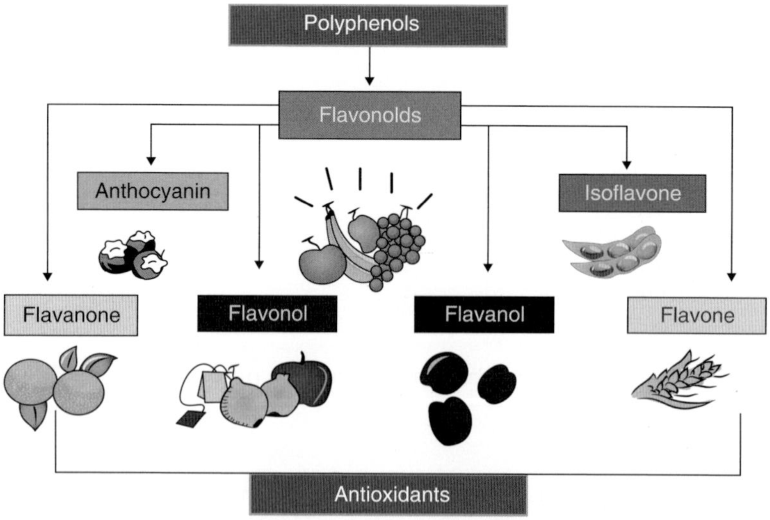

Figure 2.6 Classification of polyphenols

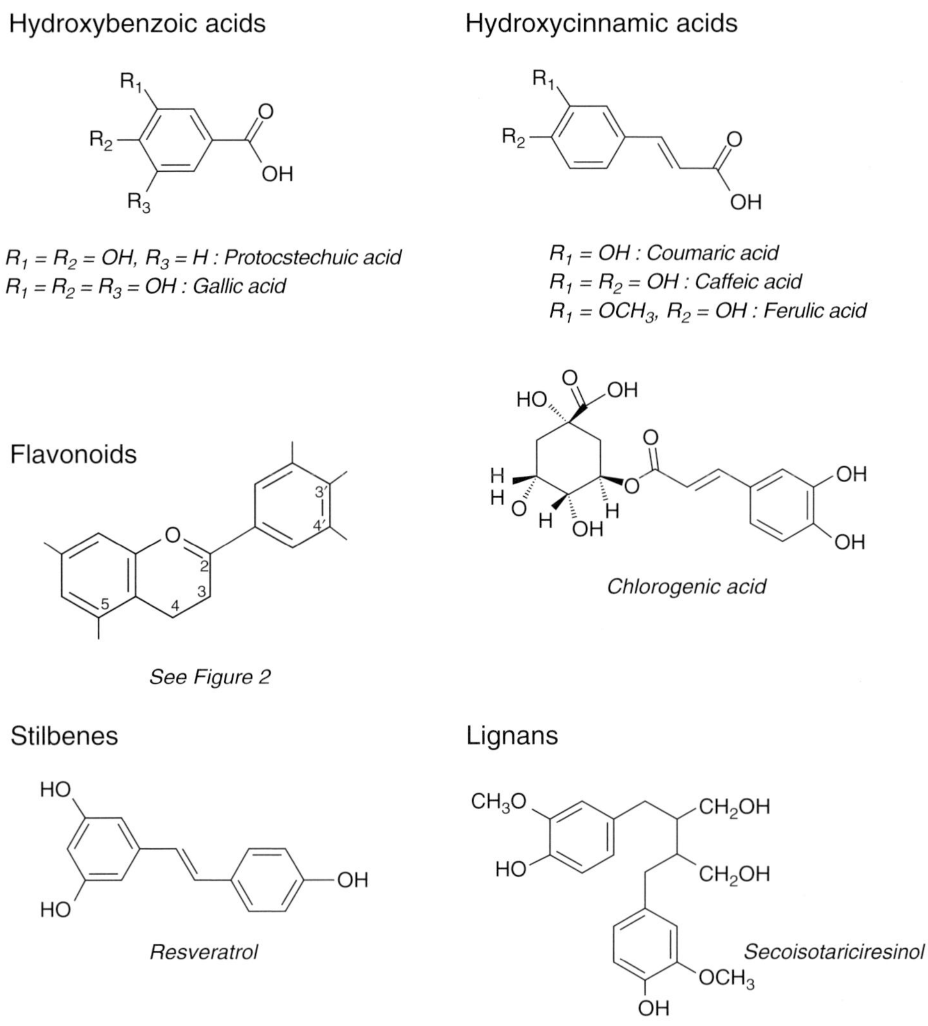

Figure 2.7 Chemical structure of polyphenols

Polyphenols are needed by plants for growth and maintenance, but when ingested by humans they take part in various physiological activities. Thousands of polyphenols have been identified, but they are broadly classified into flavonoids or isoflavonoids. Polyphenol classification is based on the number of phenolic rings present and the structural element bound to these rings. Polyphenols are the secondary metabolites of plants, and are responsible for their metabolic activity. Figure 2.7 shows the structure of polyphenols.

2.4.1 Content of polyphenols in food

Table 2.7 gives the polyphenol content in dietary food.

Table 2.7 Polyphenols content in dietary food

	Polyphenol content		
Source (serving size)	By weight or volume	By serving	
		mg/kg fresh wt (or mg/l)	*mg/serving*
Hydroxybenzoic acids (2, 6)	Blackberry (100 g)	80–270	8–27
Protocatechuic acid	Raspberry (100 g)	60–100	6–10
Gallic acid	Black currant (100 g)	40–130	4–13
p-Hydroxybenzoic acid	Strawberry (200 g)	20–90	4–18
Hydroxycinnamic acids (2, 5–7)	Blueberry (100 g)	2000–2200	200–220
Caffeic acid	Kiwi (100 g)	600–1000	60–100
Chlorogenic acid	Cherry (200 g)	180–1150	36–230
Coumaric acid	Plum (200 g)	140–1150	28–230
Ferulic acid	Aubergine (200 g)	600–660	120–132
Sinapic acid	Apple (200 g)	50–600	10–120
	Pear (200 g)	15–600	3–120
	Chicory (200 g)	200–500	40–100
	Artichoke (100 g)	450	45
	Potato (200 g)	100–190	20–38
	Corn flour (75 g)	310	23
	Flour: wheat, rice, oat (75 g)	70–90	5–7
	Cider (200 ml)	10–500	2–100
	Coffee (200 ml)	350–1750	70–350
Anthocyanins (8–10)	Aubergine (200 g)	7500	1500
Cyanidin	Blackberry (100 g)	1000–4000	100–400
Pelargonidin	Black currant (100 g)	1300–4000	130–400
Peonidin	Blueberry (100 g)	250–5000	25–500
Delphinidin	Black grape (200 g)	300–7500	60–1500
Malvidin	Cherry (200 g)	350–4500	70–900
	Rhubarb (100 g)	2000	200
	Strawberry (200 g)	150–750	30–150
	Red wine (100 ml)	200–350	20–35
	Plum (200 g)	20–250	4–50
	Red cabbage (200 g)	250	50
Flavonols (11–18)	Yellow onion (100 g)	350–1200	35–120
Quercetin	Curly kale (200 g)	300–600	60–120
Kaempferol	Leek (200 g)	30–225	6–45
Myricetin	Cherry tomato (200 g)	15–200	3–40
	Broccoli (200 g)	40–100	8–20
	Blueberry (100 g)	30–160	3–16
	Black currant (100 g)	30–70	3–7
	Apricot (200 g)	25–50	5–10
	Apple (200 g)	20–40	4–8
	Beans, green or white (200 g)	10–50	2–10
	Black grape (200 g)	15–40	3–8
	Tomato (200 g)	2–15	0.4–3.0
	Black tea infusion (200 ml)	30–45	6–9
	Green tea infusion (200 ml)	20–35	4–7
	Red wine (100 ml)	2–30	0.2–3

Table 2.7 *(Continued)*

	Polyphenol content		
Source (serving size)	By weight or volume	By serving	
Flavones (11–12, 14, 18)	Parsley (5 g)	240–1850	1.2–9.2
Apigenin	Celery (200 g)	20–140	4–28
Luteolin			
	Capsicum pepper (100 g)	5–10	0.5–1
Flavanones (19–21)	Orange juice (200 ml)	215–685	40–140
Hesperetin	Grapefruit juice (200 ml)	100–650	20–130
Naringenin			
Eriodictyol			
	Lemon juice (200 ml)	50–300	10–60
Isoflavones (22–25)	Soy flour (75 g)	800–1800	60–135
Daidzein	Soybeans, boiled (200 g)	200–900	40–180
Genistein			
Glycitein			
	Miso (100 g)	250–900	25–90
	Tofu (100 g)	80–700	8–70
	Tempeh (100 g)	430–530	43–53
	Soy milk (200 ml)	30–175	6–35
Monomeric flavanols (6, 17, 26, 27)	Chocolate (50 g)	460–610	23–30
Catechin	Beans (200 g)	350–550	70–110
Epicatechin			
	Apricot (200 g)	100–250	20–50
	Cherry (200 g)	50–220	10–44
	Grape (200 g)	30–175	6–35
	Peach (200 g)	50–140	10–28
	Blackberry (100 g)	130	13
	Apple (200 g)	20–120	4–24
	Green tea (200 ml)	100–800	20–160
	Black tea (200 ml)	60–500	12–100
	Red wine (100 ml)	80–300	8–30
	Cider (200 ml)	40	8

2.4.2 Health benefits of the polyphenolic foods

Growing research proves that polyphenols found in nature have many beneficial effects on lethal diseases such as cancer or metastasis. Recent research shows that many polypenols are present in natural food such as green tea (epicatechin, epigallocatechin, epicatechin-3-gallate, and epigallocatechin-gallate), and in red wine (resveratrol).

Polyphenols may play a major role in the prevention of cancer.

***In vitro* study** The evidence from the medicinal point of view indicates that diets with a high content of antioxidant-containing fruits and vegetables decreases the chance of cancers. This suggests that the antioxidant acts as an active agent for the prevention of tumour formation. The identification of these compounds became a major area of research in the early 2000s. Extracts from many plant sources have been studied on different cancer cell lines in the search for cancer treatments; for example, polyphenol extraction from berries of blackberry, raspberry, blueberry and strawberry yielded anthocyanins, kaempferol, quercetin, esters of coumaric acid and ellagic acid, which showed inhibition against various cell lines namely KB, CAL-27, MCF-7, HT-29, HCT-116, LNCaP, DU-145 of human oral, breast, colon and prostrate cancers, respectively (Seeram *et al.*, 2006; Zhang *et al.*, 2008). Similarly, another phenolic compound studied from soy, the isoflavone genistein, also restricted the growth of different cancer cell lines of leukaemia, lymphoma, prostrate, breast, or lung cancer. Isoflavone from citrus fruit also strongly inhibits cancerous cell lines (HL-60) (Manthey *et al.*, 2001).

***In vivo* effects of polyphenols** Lala *et al.* (2006) revealed that the effects on chemotherapeutic drugs can be prevented by the activity of the anthocyanin-rich extracts (AREs) isolated from the bilberry, chokeberry and grapes. The research was conducted on 344 male rats with colon carcinogens, which were treated with the ARE diets for 14 weeks and a positive significant result was seen. The rats had fewer 'colonic aberrant crypt foci' as compared with the control. Ding *et al.* (2006) conducted research on one of the components of anthocyanin – cyanidin-3-glucoside (C3G) – which was used to inhibit the activity of 7,12-dimethylbenz[a]anthracene-12-*O*-tetradecanolyphorbol-13-acetate, a compound responsible for the induction of skin papillomas in animal skin. The treatment with C3G decreased the number of tumours per mouse. The authors summarized that C3G exhibits chemoprevention and chemotherapeutic activities by inhibiting tumour promoter-induced carcinogenesis and tumour metastasis *in vivo* (Ding *et al.*, 2006).

2.4.3 Processing techniques of polyphenols

Phenolics are more susceptible to loss during processing, especially by leaching from plant tissues into processing water. For instance, artichoke is a rich source of bioactive phenolic compounds, inulin, minerals and fibre, which have therapeutic properties. Artichoke by-products such as leaves, external bracts and stems that are produced by the artichoke processing industry, represent a huge amount of discarded material (about 80–85% of the total biomass of the plant), which could be used as a source of inulin but also of phenolics, and should be considered as a raw material for the production of food additives and nutraceuticals. During food processing and storage, plant phenolics are converted to a variety of derived compounds. While methods to analyse lower molecular weight phenolic compounds are well developed, analysis of polymeric compounds remains a challenge. Indeed, the strong interactions of polymeric phenolics with plant cell wall material limit their extraction resulting in poor resolution and detection, especially of derived structures such as oxidation products. However, recent advances in analytical techniques have allowed some progress in their structural characterization. It is important to know how to analyse polyphnenols

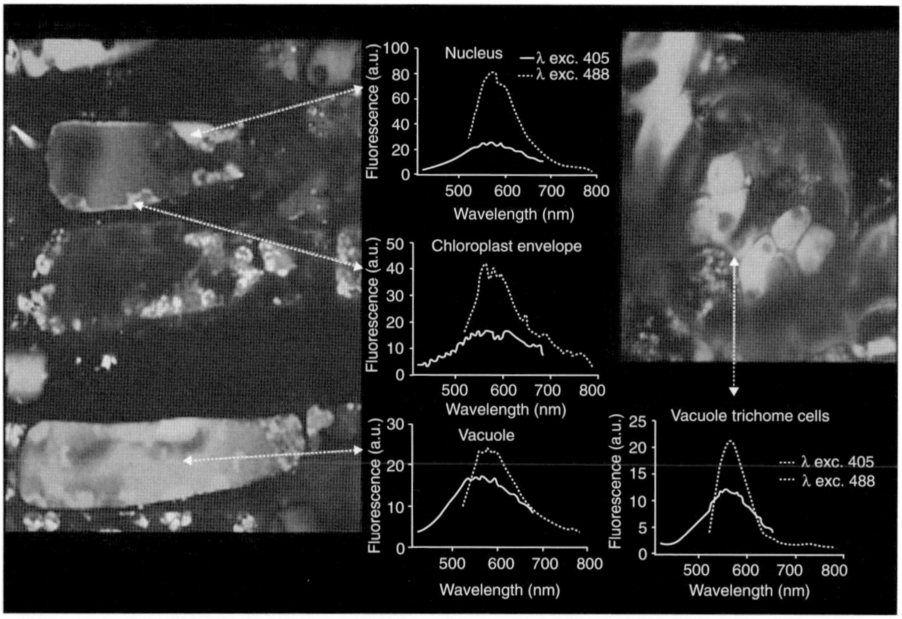

Figure 2.8 Fluorescence micro-imaging of *P. latifolia* leaves showing the subcellular distribution of dihydroxy-substituted phenyl-propanoids. Cross-section, 100 μm-thick, were stained with Naturstoff Reagent and fluorescence recorded with confocal. Views refer to the second layer of palisade parenchyma (at 100 μm depth from the adaxial epidermis) and the glandular trichome cells. The nucleus, the chloroplast envelope and the vacuole of glandular trichome cells are compartments of exclusive accumulation of dihydroxy B-ring-substituted flavonoid glycosides. Indeed, the peak of maximal mission, at approx. 575 nm, did not differ depending on the excitation wavelength. By contrast, in the vacuole of palisade cells which emits at 545 or 575 under 405 or 488 nm excitation, respectively both caffeic acid derivatives (λ_{em} = 525 nm) and di-hydroxy B-ring-substituted flavonoid glycosides are present. Please, note that the light-blue colour associated with the nucleus originates from the dark-blue fluorescence of 4′-6-diamidino-2-phenylindole and the green-fluorescence attributed to flavonoids. *Source:* Agati *et al.*, 2012. Reproduced with permission from Elsevier. For colour details, see the colour plates section

as consumption of fruits and vegetables containing phenolic compounds is thought to be beneficial to health.

2.5 Flavonoids

In the group of flavonoids the most prominent chemicals are flavonols, and from them the main representatives are quercetin and kaempferol. Flavonoids are a broad class of secondary metabolites with low molecular weight produced by plants and found mainly in the leaves, bark and flowers. To date, more than 10 000 flavonoids have been identified. Plants synthesise these chemicals for defence against pathogens and herbivores and also for protection from ultraviolet radiation (Harborne and Williams, 2000). A large array of flavonoids are present in cells and different cell organelles. Figure 2.8 shows a recent study on the presence of flavonoids in plants and Figure 2.9 describes the different classifications of flavonoids.

Class	General structure	Flavonoid	Substitution Pattern	Dietary Sources	TEAC (mM)
Flavanol	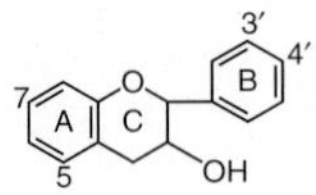	(+)-catechin	3,5,7,3',4'-OH	Tea (camellia sinensis)[6]	2.4
		(-)-epicatechin	3,5,7,3',4'-OH	Tea[6]	2.5
		Epigallocatechin gallate	3,5,7,3',4',5'-OH,3-gallate	Tea[6]	4.75
Flavone	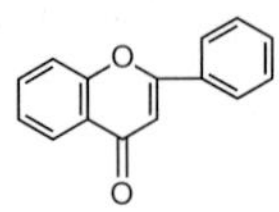	Chrysin	5,7-OH	Fruit skins	1.43
		apigenin	5,7,4'-OH	parsley, celery	1.45
		rutin	5,7,3',4'-OH,3-rutinose	Red wine[5] , buckwheat[7]	2.4
				citrus, tomato skin[8]	2.1
		luteolin	5,7,3',4'-OH	Red pepper[11]	1.74
		luteolin glucosides	5,7,3'-OH, 4'-glucose 5,4'-OH, 4',7-glucose		0.79
Flavonol	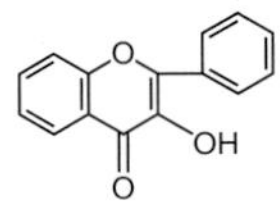	kaempferol	3,5,7,4'-OH	Leek, broccoli, endives grapefruit,black tea	1.34
		quercetin	3,5,7,3',4'-OH	Onion, lettuce, broccoli tomato, tea, red wine berries, olive oil, appleskin	4.7
		myricetin	3,5,7,3',4',5'-OH	Cranberry grapes, red wine	3.1
		tamarixetin	3,5,7,3'-OH,4'-OMe		
Flavanone (dihydroflavon	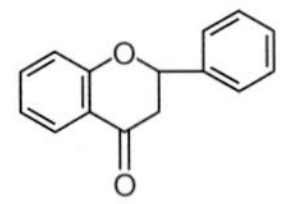	naringin	5,4'-OH,7-rhamnoglucose	Citrus, grapefruit	0.24
		naringenin	5,7,4'-OH	Citrus fruits	1.53
		taxifolin	3,5,7,3',4'-OH	Citrus fruits	1.9
		eriodictyol	5,7,3',4'-OH	Lemons[64]	1.8
		hesperidin	3,5,3'-OH,4'-OMe, 7-rutinose	Oranges[9]	1.08
Isoflavone	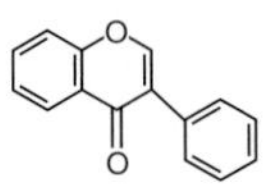	genistin	5,4'-OH,7-glucose	Soybean[10]	1.24
		genistein	5,7,4'-OH	Soybean[10]	2.9
		daidzin	4'-OH, 7-glucose	Soybean[10]	1.15
		daidzein	7,4'-OH	Soybean[10]	1.25
Anthocyanidin	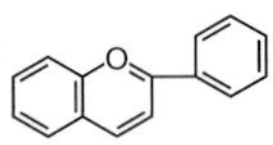	apigenidin	5,7,4'-OH	Colored fruits	2.35
		cyanidin	3,5,7,4'-OH,3,5-OMe	Cherry, raspberry, strawberry	4.42

Figure 2.9 Classification, structure, food sources, and Trolox equivalent antioxidant activities (TEAC) of dietary flavonoids. Higher TEAC values reflect greater antioxidant capability. A free 3-hydroxyl group and 3′, 4′-catechol (dihydroxy) structure, a 2–3 double bond, and a 4-oxo group endow the flavonoid with activity superior to isoforms lacking these features. Glycosidic substitution decreases TEAC. *Source:* Rice-Evans *et al.*, 1995. Reproduced with permission of Elsevier

2.5.1 Health benefits

Most flavonoid health benefits derive from their antioxidant and chelating qualities. Because of their ability to inhibit LDL oxidation, flavonoids have proved themselves to be good cardioprotective agents (Kondo *et al.*, 1996; Mazur *et al.*, 1999). A diet rich in flavonoids has shown to greatly reduce myocardial post-ischaemic damage in rats (Facino *et al.*, 1999). Dietary flavonoids have also been shown to lower mortality due to coronary heart disease and lower the occurrence of myocardial infarction in older men (Hertog *et al.*, 1993). A survey of postmenopausal women also showed that the rate of heart disease decreased by 38% when flavonoids were included in the diet (Yochum *et al.*, 1999). Research showed that consumption of the flavonoid (catechin) in tea acted inversely with the mortality of heart disease in a group of 806 men (Arts *et al.*, 2001).

2.5.2 Flavonoid-containing dietary foods

Table 2.8 gives a rough idea of the distribution of flavonoids in dietary foods.

Table 2.8 Sources of flavonoids

Source	Flavanone	Flavone	Flavanol	Iso-flavonoid	Anthocyanins	Flavins
Beverages		P	P		P	P
Eggs and meat						
Fats and oils						
Fruit	P		P		P	P
Grains		P	P		P	P
Herbs		P	P			
Legumes			P	P	P	
Milk						
Nuts and seeds		P		P		
Sugar and sweets						
Vegetables			P		P	

P, present.
Source: Peterson & Dwyer, 1998. Reproduced with permission from Elsevier.

Beverages Flavans give an astringent taste to many beverages like beer, wine and tea. It's more abundantly found in tea.

Eggs, meat, poultry The reported flavonoid in animal tissues is methoxyflavan. This is found basically from plant origin, and may be found in animals because of its dietary origin.

Fruits and vegetables In citrus fruits the predominant flavonoids are flavanones and flavones. They are the main cause of bitterness in grapes. Flavans are found in almost all fruits. Flavonols are predominant in vegetables. Leafy vegetables, celery and hot peppers contain flavones. Anthocyanins are also often present.

2.5.3 Processing techniques of flavonoids

Flavonoids are sensitive to heat and to the physicochemical environment; thus the steps of processing (heating, mechanical and domestic processes), of formulation (food matrix) and the storage period and conditions may lead to a degradation of the flavonoids and an alteration of their antioxidant properties. Considerable loss of flavonoids have been observed when fruits and vegetables are processed into juice because substantial amounts of the bioactive compounds are left in the discarded skin and pulp, with these losses often surpassing those of heat treatment (Gerard and Roberts, 2004).

To summarise, we can distinguish the processing effects on the degradation of the phenolic compounds such as flavonoids and their antioxidant activity, into different categories:

(i) **The thermal processes** such as pasteurization, baking, cooling and freezing. Most thermal processes lead to a degradation of phenolic compounds, except in some cases such as apple juice processing where an increase of temperature from 40 to 70 °C allows an increase in flavonoid content (50%) (Gerard and Roberts, 2004).

(ii) **The non-thermal processes** such as high pressure, pulsed electric fields and filtration. Certain authors have shown that phenolic antioxidants in food are degraded less by innovative processes (microwave, infrared, high pressure processing) than by thermal processes (Ioannou and Ghoul, 2012).

(iii) **The mechanical processes** such as peeling, cutting or mixing. Major losses of flavonoids took place during the pre-processing step when parts of the product were removed and this processing is expected to affect content, activity and availability of bioactive compounds. However, cutting increased flavonol content in fresh-cut potatoes (Tudela *et al.*, 2002) and fresh-cut onions (Pérez-Gregorio *et al.*, 2011). In fact, wounding enhances flavonol biosynthesis through the induction of phenylalanine ammonialyase enzyme which is related to the wound-healing process for fighting pathogen attack after tissue wounding (Tudela *et al.,* 2002).

2.6 Anthocyanins

Anthocyanins have gained huge interest due to their bright attractive colours and their soluble nature, which makes it convenient for incorporating them into aqueous systems (Timberlake and Henry, 1988; Lauro, 1991; Henry, 1996; Cao *et al.*, 1997; Wang *et al.*, 1997). Anthocyanins have become popular as natural food colourants. The presence of different amounts of anthocyanin causes the species variation in the colour of fruits and vegetables. According to Simmonds (1962), the variation in bract colour in banana flower is correlated with the composition of the anthocyanins present, which is distinctive of species and subspecies. This characteristic of anthocyanin chemistry has become a taxonomic tool for species differentiation (Simmonds, 1962; Horry and Jay, 1988).

2.6.1 Chemical structure

The term anthocyan includes anthocyanin for the glycoside and anthocyanidin for the aglycon. The variation of anthocyanidins found in higher plants are: cyanidin, delphinidin, malvidin, pelargonidin, peonidin and petunidin, which have a distribution in nature of 50%, 12%, 12%, 12%, 7% and 7%, respectively. They occur almost exclusively as anthocyanins. Figure 2.10 gives the structure of anthocyanin.

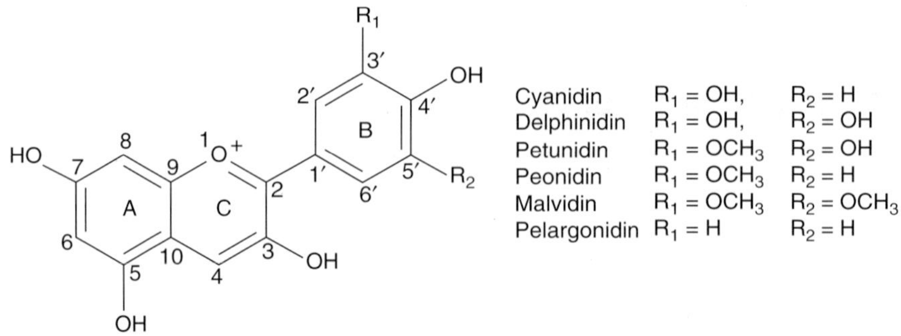

Figure 2.10 Chemical structure of anthocyanin

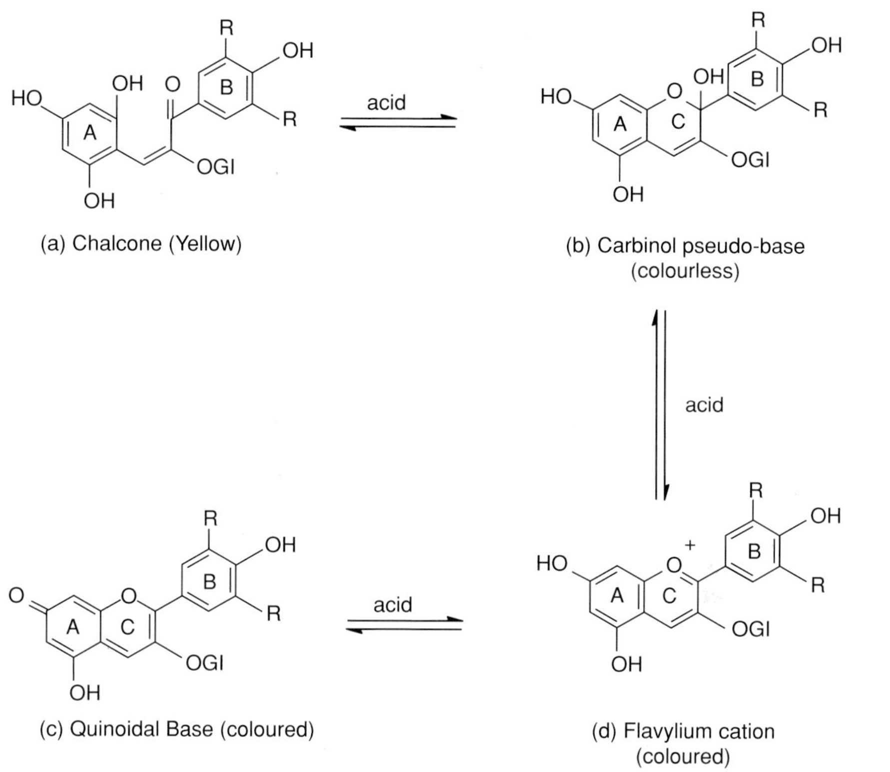

Figure 2.11 pH-dependent conformational rearrangement of the anthocyan molecule, shown here for anthocyanins bearing a sugar (Gl′) on C3. Which conformer predominates depends upon pH. (a) At neutral pH anthocyans occur as chalcones with an open C ring. (b) Under mildly acidic conditions the ring is closed to form a carbinol pseudo base. (c) In strong acid (pH 2), ring C acquires aromaticity involving a flavylium cation, which imparts intense colour on the molecule. (d) In alkali, oxidation of ring A generates a quinoid structure with elimination of the positive charge, this species is also coloured. The ring-opened chalcone can be reformed at neutral pH

Anthocyanins are extremely water soluble and depending on pH conditions, their colour intensity varies. Figure 2.11 gives the pH-dependent conformational rearrangements of the anthocyan molecule.

2.6.2 Health benefits

In a comparative investigation in the Apc ^{Min} mouse, animals received either a mixture of anthocyanins at 800 mg/l or pure cyanidin at 200 mg/l with the drinking water or tart cherries added to the diet (200 g/kg diet). Anthocyanin extracts from berries, grapes or chokeberries at a concentration of 25–75 μg/ml can inhibit the growth of human malignant cell line (HT29) colon cancer cells but not of the non-malignant colon cancer cells (NCM460) (Zhao *et al.*, 2004). Anthocyanins can interfere with activities that help in the promotion of malignancies such as those mediated by cyclooxygenase (COX) enzymes, tyrosine kinases and phosphodiesterases. Table 2.9

Table 2.9 Summary of growth inhibitory effects of anthocyans and anthocyanin-rich extracts

Agent	Cell line	Effect	Reference
Anthocyanidin	CaCo-2	Growth inhibition (20%),	Lazze *et al.*, 2004
Delphinidin	HeLa S3	200 μM	Lazze *et al.*, 2004
	Human embryonic	IC50 200μM	Lazze *et al.*, 2004
	fibroblasts	Growth inhibition (10%),	Meiers *et al.*, 2001
	LXFL529L	200 μM	Meiers *et al.*, 2001;
	A431	IC50 33 μM	Marko *et al.*, 2004
	HT29	IC50 18 μM	Zhang *et al.*, 2005
	MCF-7	IC50 35 μM	Katsube *et al.*, 2003
	HL60	Growth inhibition (66%),	
		662 μM	
		Growth inhibition (88%),	
		100 μM	
		↑Apoptosis, 200 μM	
Peonidin	HT29	IC50 90 μM	Marko *et al.*, 2004
	HL60	Growth inhibition (80%),	Katsube *et al.*, 2003
		400 μM	
Petunidin	MCF-7	Growth inhibition (53%),	Zhang *et al.*, 2005
		633 μM	
Anthocyanin			
Delphinidin-3-	HCT116	Growth inhibition (~85%),	Katsube *et al.*, 2003
glucoside	HT29	863 μM	Olsson *et al.*, 2004
	MCF-7	Growth inhibition (87%),	Olsson *et al.*, 2004;
	HL60	431 μM	Katsube *et al.*, 2003
	HCT116	Growth inhibition (82%),	Katsube *et al.*, 2003
		431 μM	
		Growth inhibition (~75%),	
		216 μM	
		Growth inhibition (~80%),	
		431 μM	
Cyanidin-3-glucoside	HT29	Growth inhibition (88%),	Olsson *et al.*, 2004
	MCF-7	446 μM	Olsson *et al.*, 2004;
	Jurkat	Growth inhibition (85%),	Fimognari *et al.*, 2004
	HL60	446 μM	Fimognari *et al.*, 2004
		IC50 391 μM	
		Growth inhibition (37%),	
		446 μM	
Anthocyanin-rich extract			
Chokeberry extract	NCM 460	IC50 25 μg/ml[b]	Zhao *et al.*, 2004
	HT29	IC50 10 μg/ml[b]	Zhao *et al.*, 2004
		Growth inhibition (37%),	Olsson *et al.*, 2004
		5 mg/ml	Magnuson *et al.*, 2003
		Growth inhibition (69%),	
		10 mg/ml	
Grape extract	MCF-7 [39]	Growth inhibition (19%),	Olsson *et al.*, 2004
	HT29	5 mg/ml	Zhao *et al.*, 2004
	NCM 460	IC50 25 μg/ml[b]	Zhao *et al.*, 2004
	RBA	IC50 75 μg/ml[b]	Singletary *et al.*, 2003
		IC50 ~14 μg/ml	
Black currant	MCF-7	Growth inhibition (45%),	Olsson *et al.*, 2004
		5 mg/ml	

Table 2.9 (*Continued*)

Agent	Cell line	Effect	Reference
Cranberry anthocyanins	CAL27	Growth inhibition (~20%)[c]	Seeram *et al.*, 2004
	KB	Growth inhibition (~20%)[c]	Seeram *et al.*, 2004
	HCT116	Growth inhibition (~15%)[c]	Seeram *et al.*, 2004
	SW620	Growth inhibition (~15%)[c]	Seeram *et al.*, 2004
	RWPE-1	Growth inhibition (~55%)[c]	Seeram *et al.*, 2004
	RWPE-2	Growth inhibition (~60%)[c]	Seeram *et al.*, 2004
	22Rv1	Growth inhibition (~70%)[c]	Seeram *et al.*, 2004

Note:
JB6, mouse skin epidermal cell; U937, human monocytic leukaemia cell; A431, human vulva carcinoma cell; Jurkat, human T-lymphoblastoid cell; HL-60, human promyelocytic leukaemia cell; RBA, rat mammary adenocarcinoma cell; HT-29 and CaCo-2, human colon adenocarcinoma cells; HeLa S3, human uterine carcinoma cell; and Raw264, mouse macrophage cell. *Abbreviations*. TPA, tetradecanoylphorbol acetate; EGFR, epidermal growth factor receptor; PDE, phosphodiesterases; LPS, lipopolysaccharide; COX-2, cyclooxygenase-2 and eNOS, endothelial nitric oxide synthase.
[a]Aglycon formed by alcoholic acid hydrolysis of pigmented rice.
[b]IC50 estimated after 72 h exposure to extracts.
[c]Concentrations equivalent to content of anthocyanins in 200 lg/ml total cranberry extract.

gives a summary of growth inhibitory effects of anthocyans and anthocyanin-rich extracts.

2.6.3 Processing techniques of anthocyanin

Anthocyanins are relatively unstable and reactive molecules and their colours are dependent on pH, temperature, light and the presence of metals. They play the dual role of being natural pigments and bioactive compounds. They impart red, blue and purple hues to fruits and vegetables. These pigments readily degrade under common food-processing conditions and also during storage, resulting in a dramatic impact on colour quality and their nutritional properties. Anthocyanins in blueberries, blackberries and black raspberries are susceptible to degradation during processing, with juices showing the greatest losses due to the physical removal of skins and seeds. This degradation involves cleavage (loss of colour) or polymerization (browning). Anthocyanins are also degraded in processed products stored at ambient temperature with losses accompanied by increased polymeric pigments (PPs).

Total anthocyanin pigment content and indices for polymeric colour and browning are easily measured with simple spectrophotometric methods and by high-performance liquid chromatography (HPLC) and their changes can be monitored. Analytical techniques such as capillary electrophoresis (CE) and liquid chromatography–mass spectrometry (LC–MS) are also used to identify anthocyanins. Processing methods varying in the number of processing steps, heating temperature, and duration can markedly affect anthocyanin content and the antioxidant capacity of fruit and vegetables. In alkaline or acid media or in the presence of the enzyme β-glucosidase, anthocyanin is hydrolysed, removing the sugar moiety and releasing the anthocyanidin, which is more easily degraded than the anthocyanin glycoside. Degradation commences with the opening of the middle ring followed by cleavage at this midpoint of the molecule, forming colourless products. With their reactivity and solubility in water, folates can suffer large losses during food processing and preparation.

Aside from considerable leaching into the water used in washing, blanching, canning or cooking, oxidative degradation can occur.

Processing blueberries into various forms resulted in significant losses of monomeric anthocyanins and antioxidant capacity. Anthocyanin also extensively degraded during storage in all thermally processed products (canned, juices, and purees), with less than 40% of the original total anthocyanins present in the processed products. In canned products, significant amounts of monomeric anthocyanins leached out of the berries into the liquid canning medium (Brownmiller *et al.*, 2008). Freezing and subsequent frozen storage have been shown to have minimal effects on red raspberry anthocyanins (de Ancos *et al.,* 2000; Mullen *et al.,* 2002). In another study involving commercial blueberry products, the researchers reported that semipurified extracts obtained from thermally processed products retained most of the antioxidant activity and total phenolics found in unprocessed whole fruit, but the antiproliferation activities of thermally processed products were lacking or greatly diminished (Schmidt *et al.,* 2005).

Many peer-viewed publications have demonstrated that a high dietary intake of foods rich in anthocyanins is related to a low prevalence of some cardiovascular diseases and to diverse protective effects (Cooke *et al.,* 2005). This also includes antioxidant, anti-allergic, anti-inflammatory, antiviral, antiproliferative, antimutagenic, antimicrobial and anticarcinogenic effects, protection from allergy, microcirculation improvement, peripheral capillary fragility prevention, diabetes prevention and vision improvement.

2.7 Glucosinolates

Glucosinolates were first described by the scientists Robiquet and Boutron, when they both isolated sinalbin from the seeds of white mustard in the year 1832. Since then, a series of studies have been conducted and more than 120 different glucosinolates have been identified. Glucosinolates (S-β-thioglucoside *N* hydroxysulfate) are naturally occurring thioglucosides; the structure is shown in Figure 2.12.

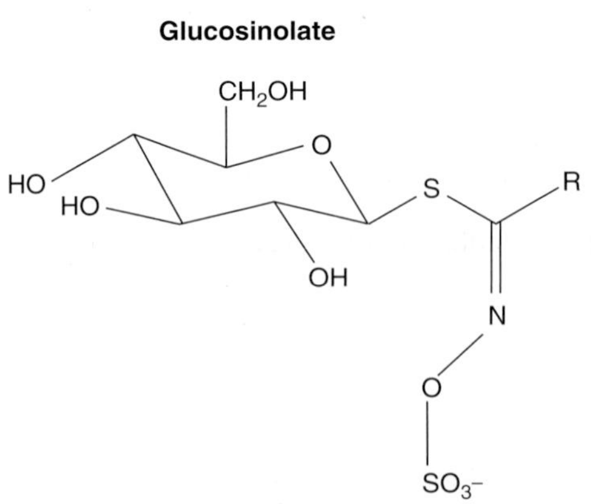

Figure 2.12 Chemical structure of glucosinolate

Table 2.10 Sixteen families of glucosinolate-containing angiosperms

Family	Chemical class	Glucosinolates[a]
Bataceae	I	28, 43
Brassicaceae	A–J	1, 5–20, 22–26, 28–48, 50, 51, 53–69, 72–84, 86–89, 91–95, 99–107, 111, 112, 114
Bretschneideraceae	E, G	14, 31
Capparaceae	A, B, C, D, E, F, G, I	12, 13, 23, 24, 28, 29, 43, 47, 48, 51, 52, 54, 56, 73, 96–98, 107, 108
Caricaceae	G	11
Euphorbiaceae	C, E	26, 29, 56
Gyrostemonaceae	C	61, 62
Limnanthaceae	E, G	31, 45
Moringaceae	C, E, G, J	3, 11, 23, 31, 56, 61, 62, 110
Pentadiplandraceae	G	11, 49
Phytolaccaceae	C, E, G	11, 22, 23, 29, 61
Pittosporaceae	G	23
Resedaceae	E, G, I, J	4, 11, 21–23, 31, 40, 43, 47, 105, 109
Salvadoraceae	C, G	11, 23, 56
Tovariaceae	C	2, 11, 43, 47, 56
Tropaeolaceae	B, C, E, G	11, 16, 23, 31, 46, 56, 61, 62

[a]Each number is a code for a specific glucosinolate.

Glucosinolates are a natural occurring secondary product of plants and are found in almost 500 different species belonging to 16 families of dicotyledonous (Magnoliophyta) higher plants (Fahey *et al.*, 2001) (Table 2.10). They are widely present in the family Cruciferae (Brassicaceae), which belongs amongst the 10 most economically important plant families in the world. It includes vegetables such as cabbage, cauliflower, bok choy, kale, radish, rutabaga, turnip, broccoli and Brussels sprouts. Glucosinolates and/or their breakdown products have mixed effects. The glucosinolates found in some agricultural crops like rapeseed oil (*Brassica napus*) and *Brassica* vegetables are considered to be detrimental because of the toxicological effects of their breakdown products, which include isothiocyanates, thiocyanates, epithionitrile, nitriles and vinyl oxazolidinethiones. On the other hand, other types of glucosinolates found in broccoli show an anticarcinogenic effect. These glucosinolates have also been known for their fungicidal, bacteriocidal, nematocidal and allelopathic properties.

2.7.1 Chemistry of glucosinolates

The main enzyme responsible for the hydrolysis of the glucosinolates is myrosinase (thioglucohydrolase), and different compounds evolved include isothiocyanates, nitriles, thiocyanates, epithionitriles and oxazolidines. Figure 2.13 shows some myrosinase reaction products.

2.7.2 Health benefits

Fungicidal activities Angus (1994), Chan and Close (1987), Gamliel and Stapleton (1993) and Vierheilig and Ocampo (1990) demonstrated that members of the

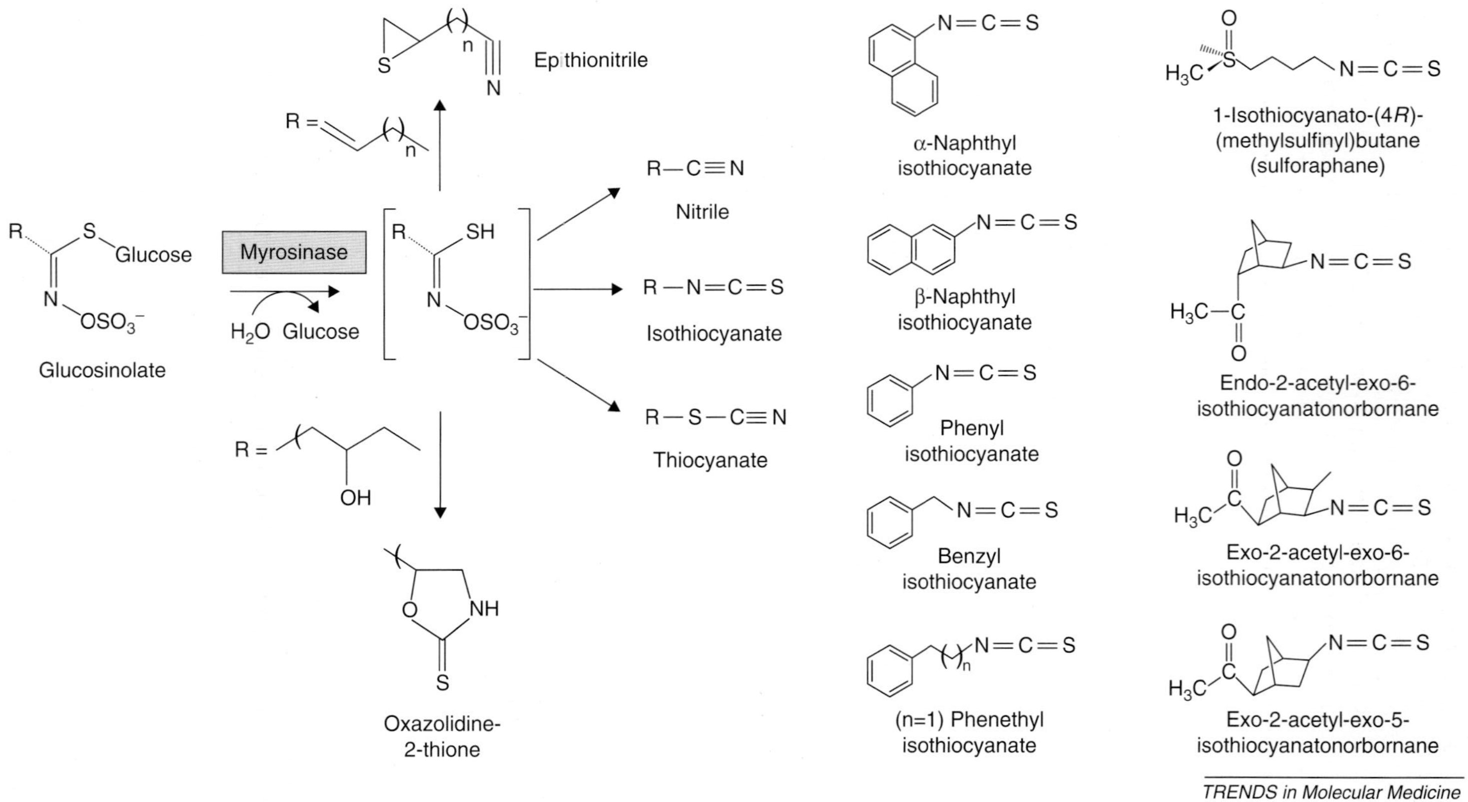

Figure 2.13 Myrosinase reaction products. (a) Possible reaction products of glucosinolate hydrolysis. The hydrolysis of glucosinolates is catalyzed by myrosinase to give unstable aglucones and liberate glucose. Depending on the reaction conditions and the structure of the glucosinolate side chain (R), a series of products can be formed, including nitriles, thiocyanites, epithionitriles, oxazolidine-2-thiones and isothiocyanites. (b) Chemical structures of anticarcinogenic aromatic isothiocyanates. (c) Chemical structures of the naturally occurring isothiocyanate sulforaphane and its synthetic norbornyl analogues. *Source:* Dinkova-Kostova & Kostov, 2012. Reproduced with permission of Elsevier

family Brassicaceae have the ability to control the growth of phytopathogenic fungi. Walker *et al.* (1937) observed the antifungal activity of mustard oils and of cruciferous plant extracts containing allyl and phenethyl isothiocyanates, which was confirmed by Hooker *et al.* (1943). In addition, Greenhalgh and Mitchell (1976) and Gamliel and Stapleton (1993) reported that isothiocyanates released from cabbage tissues are toxic towards *Peronospora parasitica*, *Pythium ultimum* and *Sclerotium rolfsii*. Later in 1994, Angus reported that volatile compounds from macerated *Brassica* root tissue inhibited the fungal pathogen of wheat, *Gaeumannomyces graminis*. Mari *et al.* (1993, 1996) reported the protective effect of enzymatic hydrolysis products during the shelf life of fruits against some postharvest pathogenic fungi.

Bioherbicidal potential Glucosinolates may represent a viable source of allelochemical control for a variety of weeds. Germination bioassays were conducted by Brown and Morra (1995) with *Lactuca sativa* seeds in the presence of defatted meal of *B. napus*. Only tissues containing glucosinolates produced volatiles which inhibited germination. The results suggested that this type of control could contribute to a reduction in synthetic pesticide usage, if weed seeds are targeted. This effect recently had been referred to as biofumigation. The biofumigation potential of *Brassica* spp. in terms of effect of environment and ontogeny on glucosinolate production, and *in vitro* toxicity of isothiocyanates (ITCs) to soil-borne fungal pathogen have been described by Sarwar and Kirkegaard (1998) and Sarwar *et al.* (1998).

Antioxidant activity Vitamin C, vitamin E and carotenoids are direct antioxidants as they neutralize free radicals before they can harm cells. Glucosinolates and their hydrolysis products are indirect antioxidants, as they do not neutralize free radicals directly, but rather by modulating the activity of xenobiotic metabolizing enzymes (phase I and phase II enzymes), that trigger the long-lasting antioxidant activity. Phase I enzymes (cytochrome P450 enzymes) generally increase the reactivity of fat soluble compounds and as a consequence of this process, some reactive molecules are produced which may be more toxic than the parent molecule. While phase II enzymes (glutathione-*S*-transferase, aldehyde reductase *S*-methyl transferase, *N*-acetyltransferase, etc.) increase water solubility and promote the excretion of these metabolites from the body.

2.7.3 Processing techniques of glucosinolates

Glucosinolates are unique class of secondary plant metabolites containing β-D-thioglucose and sulfonated oxime moieties. Glucosinolates are mostly found in *Brassica* vegetables like green cabbage, broccoli and cauliflower, Brussels sprouts, or turnips. Epidemiological studies infer that glucosinolate breakdown products derived from *Brassica* vegetables may protect against cancer in the gastrointestinal tract, breast, colorectal and lungs. This preventive and health-promoting characteristic is not caused by glucosinolates themselves, but by their breakdown products, in particular isothiocyanates, thiocyanates and indoles. Isothiocyanates also inhibit mitosis and stimulate apoptosis in human tumour cells, *in vitro* and *in vivo*.

Glucosinolates can be degraded or leached during culinary processing or during digestion. When the vegetables are cut or chewed, these substrates come in contact with the endogenous enzyme myrosinase which hydrolyses them. But after ingestion, any remaining intact glucosinolates are broken down by plant myrosinase in the small intestine or by bacterial myrosinase in the gut. The moisture content affects both the rate of glucosinolate degradation and myrosinase activity during thermal treatments of broccoli, affecting the formation of the breakdown products and thus their intake. Cooking at high temperatures denatures myrosinase in vegetable material, resulting in a lower conversion of glucosinolates to isothiocyanates when chewed. Therefore, the level of glucosinolates can vary greatly based on the method of cooking, time–temperature profile and the vegetable–water ratio.

The glucosinolate content of *Brassica* vegetables may also be influenced by storage. Studies showed that there was no significant or minimal loss of glucosinolate content when stored at ambient temperature. Rodrigues and Rosa (1999) reported that refrigeration at 4 °C and freezing were the best preservation processes for maintaining a high level of glucosinolates in broccoli. The frozen vegetables had, however, been blanched by steaming prior to freezing (Rodrigues and Rosa, 1999). Glucosinolates can also be preserved by thermal inactivation of myrosinase when the vegetables are cooked by steaming, microwaving or stir-frying. Also, broccoli glucosinolates can be broken down during drying by heat or oxidation, myrosinase activity can be inhibited and cellular structures can be altered.

Different processing mechanisms have an influence on the presence of isothiocyanates in our foods as discussed earlier: thermal degradation of glucosinolates, enzymatic hydrolysis (endogenous enzyme myrosinase) of glucosinolates and leaching of glucosinolates into the cooking water. All these modifications might reduce the formation of target compounds such as bioactive isothiocyanates from the glucosinolates and therefore compromises the health-protective effects of these cruciferous vegetables. The bioavailability of isothiocyanates can be preserved or increased by avoiding boiling vegetables and using moderate process conditions while drying the plant products.

Earlier studies and the literature on the chemoprevention of cancer by dietary compounds has shown an inverse relationships between cancer risk and the intake of *Brassica* vegetables (Thornalley, 2002; Thornalley and IARC Workgroup, 2004), especially raw vegetables, which are more effective than cooked vegetables (Link and Potter, 2004;Conaway *et al.*, 2001; Rouzaud *et al.*, 2004). Studies also focused on lowering the glucosinolate content from the plant tissues because of their characteristic property of imparting a bitter taste and a pungent odour. But plants use substances derived from glucosinolates as natural pesticides and for defence against herbivores. Here we have emphasized on the potential benefits emerging from the bioactivities of glucosinolates such as their antifungal, antibacterial, bioherbicidal, antioxidant, antimutagenic and anticarcinogenic properties.

References

Addeo, F., Chianes, L., Salzano, A. *et al.* (1992). Characterization of the 12% trichloroacetic acid-insoluble oligopeptides of Parmigiano–Reggiano cheese. *Journal of Dairy Research*, 59, 401–411.

de Ancos, B., Ibanez, E., Reglero, G. and Cano, M.P. (2000). Frozen storage effects on anthocyanins and volatile compounds of raspberry fruit. *Journal of Agricultural Food Chemistry*, 48, 873–879.

Agati, G., Azzarello, E., Pollastri, S. and Tattini, M. (2012). Flavonoids as antioxidants in plants: Location and functional significance, *Plant Science*, 196, 67–76.

Angus, J. F. (1994). Biofumigation: isothiocyanates released from Brassica roots inhibit the growth of the take-all fungus. *Plant and Soil*, 162, 107–112.

de Antueno, R.J., Knickle, L.C., Smith, H. *et al.* (2001). Activity of human Δ^5 and Δ^6 desaturases on multiple *n-3* and *n-6* polyunsaturated fatty acids. *FEBS Letters*, 509, 77–80.

Arts, I.C., Hollman, P.C., Feskens, E.J., Bueno de Mesquita, H.B. and Kromhout, D. (2001). Catechin intake and associated dietary and lifestyle factors in a representative sample of Dutch men and women. *European Journal of Clinical Nutrition*, 55 (2), 76–81.

Ashar, M.N. and Chand, R. (2004). Fermented milk containing ACE-inhibitory peptides reduces blood pressure in middle aged hypertensive subjects. *Milchwissenschaft*, 59, 363–366.

Barbana, C. and Boye, J.I. (2010). Angiotensin I-converting enzyme inhibitory activity of chickpea and pea protein hydrolysates. *Food Research International*, 43, 1642–1649.

Bennett, N., Greco, D.S., Peterson, M.E. *et al.* (2006). Comparison of a low carbohydrate-low fiber diet and a moderate carbohydrate high fiber diet in the management of feline diabetes mellitus. *Journal of Feline Medicine and Surgery*, 8, 73–84.

Brown, P.D. and Morra, M.J. (1995). Hydrolysis products of glucosinolates in *Brassica napus* tissues as inhibitors of seed germination. *Plant and Soil*, 181, 307–316.

Brownmiller, C., Howard, L.R. and Prior, R.L. (2008). Processing and storage effects on monomeric anthocyanins, percent polymeric colour, and antioxidant capacity of processed blueberry products. *Journal of Food Science*, 73 (5), H72–H79.

Cao, G., Sofic, E. and Prior, R.L. (1997). Antioxidant and proxidant behaviour of flavonoids: structure–activity relationships. *Biology & Medicine*, 22 (5), 749–760.

Clare, D.A. and Swaisgood, H.E. (2000). Bioactive milk peptides: A prospectus. *Journal of Dairy Science*, 83 (6), 1187–1195.

Chabance, B., Jolles, P., Izquierdo, C. *et al.* (1995). Characterization of an antithrombotic peptide from kappa-casein in newborn plasma after milk ingestion. *British Journal of Nutrition*, 73, 583–590.

Chan, M.K.Y. and Close, R. C. (1987). Aphanomyces root rot of peas control by the use of cruciferous amendments. *New Zealand Journal of Agricultural Research*, 30, 225–233.

Chandrasekara, N. and Shahidi, F. (2011). Effect of roasting on phenolic content and antioxidant activities of whole cashew nuts, kernels, and testa. *Journal of Agricultural and Food Chemistry*, 59, 5006–5014.

Choi, Y., Lee, S.M., Chun, J., Lee, H.B. and Lee, J. (2006). Influence of heat treatment on antioxidant activities and polyphenolic compounds of Shiitake (*Lentinus edodes*) mushroom. *Food Chemistry*, 99, 381–387.

Conaway, C.C., Getahun, S.M., Liebes, L. *et al.* (2001). Disposition of glucosinolates and sulforaphane in humans after ingestion of steamed and fresh broccoli. *Nutrition and Cancer*, 38, 168–178.

Cook, H.W. (1996). Fatty acid desaturation and chain elongation in eukaryote, in *Biochemistry of Lipids, Lipoproteins and Membranes* (eds D.E. Vance and J.E. Vance). Elsevier, Amsterdam, pp. 129–152.

Cooke, D., Steward, W.P., Gescher, A.J. and Marczylo, T. (2005). Anthocyans from fruits and vegetables – Does bright colour signal cancer chemopreventive activity? *European Journal of Cancer*, 41, 1931–1940.

D'andrea, S., Guillou, H., Jan, S. *et al.* (2002). The same rat Δ^6-desaturase not only acts on 18- but also on 24-carbon fatty acids in very-long-chain polyunsaturated fatty acid biosynthesis. *The Biochemical Journal*, 364, 49–55

de Alcântara, P.H.N., Martim, L., Silva, C.O., Dietrich, S.M.C. and Buckeridge, M.S. (2006). Purification of a b-galactosidase from cotyledons of *Hymenaea courbaril* L. (Leguminosae). Enzyme properties and biological function. *Plant Physiology and Biochemistry*, 44, 619–627.

Delmée, E., Cani, P. D., Gual, G. *et al.* (2006). Relation between colonic proglucagon expression and metabolic response to oligofructose in high fat diet-fed mice. *Life Sciences*, 79, 1007–1013.

Ding, M., Feng, R., Wang, S.Y. *et al.* (2006). Cyanidin-3-glucoside, a natural product derived from blackberry, exhibits chemopreventive and chemotherapeutic activity. *The Journal of Biological Chemistry*, 281 (25), 17359–68.

Dinkova-Kostova, A.T. and Kostov, R.V. (2012). Glucosinolates and isothiocyanates in health and disease. *Trends in Molecular Medicine*, 18 (6), 337–347.

Dong, J., Ma, X., Fu, Z. and Guo, Y. (2011). Effects of microwave drying on the contents of functional constituents of *Eucommia ulmoides* flower tea. *Industrial Crops and Products*, 34 (1), 1102–1110.

Erdmann, K., Grosser, N., Schipporeit, K. and Schroder, H. (2006). The ACE inhibitory dipeptide Met-Tyr diminishes free radical formation in human endothelial cells via induction of heme oxygenase-1 and ferritin. *The Journal of Nutrition*, 136, 2148–2152.

Facino, R.M., Carini, M., Aldini, G. *et al.* (1999). Diet enriched with procyanidins enhances antioxidant activity and reduces myocardial post-ischaemic damage in rats. *Life Sciences*, 64 (8), 627–42.

Fahey, J.W., Zalcmann, A.T. and Talaly, P. (2001). The chemical diversity and distribution of glucosinolates and isothiocyanantes among plants. *Phytochemistry*, 56, 5–51.

Fimognari, C., Berti, F., Nusse, M. *et al.* (2004). Induction of apoptosis in two human leukemia cell lines as well as differentiation in human promyelocytic cells by cyanidin-3-*O*-beta-glucopyranoside. *Biochemical Pharmacology*, 67, 2047–2056.

FitzGerald, R.J., Murray, B.A., and Walsh, D.J. (2004). Hypotensive peptides from milk proteins. *The Journal of Nutrition*, 134 (4), 980S–988S.

Foltz, M., van der Pijl, P.C. and Duchateau, G.S. (2009). Current *in vitro* testing of bioactive peptides is not valuable. *The Journal of Nutrition*, 140 (1), 117–118.

Fukudome, S. and Yoshikawa, M. (1993). Gluten exorphin-C – a novel opioid peptide derived from wheat gluten. *FEBS Letters*, 316, 17–19.

Gagnaire, V., Molle, D., Herrouin, M. and Leonil, J. (2001). Peptides identified during Emmental cheese ripening: Origin and proteolytic systems involved. *Journal of Agricultural and Food Chemistry*, 49, 4402–4413.

Gamliel, A. and Stapleton, J.J. (1993). Characterization of antifungal volatile compounds evolved from solarized soil amended with cabbage residues *Phytopathology*, 83, 899–905.

Gerard, K.A. and Roberts, J.S. (2004). Microwave heating of apple mash to improve juice yield and quality. *Lebensmittel-Wissenschaft und Technologie*, 37 (5), 551–557.

Giacco, R., Clemente, G., Luongo, D. *et al.* (2004). Effects of short-chain fructo-oligosaccharides on glucose and lipid metabolism in mild hypercholesterolaemic individuals. *Clinical Nutrition*, 23, 331–340.

Gomez-Ruiz, J.A., Ramos, M. and Recio, I. (2002). Angiotensin converting enzyme-inhibitory peptides in Manchego cheeses manufactured with different starter cultures. *International Dairy Journal*, 12, 697–706.

Greenhalgh, J.R. and Mitchell, N.D. (1976). The involvement of flavour volatiles in the resistance to downy mildew of wild and cultivated forms of *Brassica oleracea*. *New Phytologist*, 77, 391–398.

Harborne, J.B. and Williams, C.A. (2000). Advances in flavonoid research since 1992. *Phytochemistry*, 55, 481–504.

Hartmann, R. and Meisel, H. (2007). Food-derived peptides with biological activity: From research to food applications. *Current Opinion in Biotechnology*, 18, 163–169.

Hartmann, A., Patz, C.-D., Andlauer, W., Dietrich, H. and Ludwig, M. (2008). Influence of processing on quality parameters of strawberries. *Journal of Agricultural and Food Chemistry*, 56 (20), 9484–9489.

Hayes, A., Ross, R.P., Fitzgerald, G.F., Hill, C. and Stanton, C. (2006). Casein-derived antimicrobial peptides generated by Lactobacillus acidophilus DPC6026. *Appl Environ Microbiol*, 72, 2260–2264.

Henry, B.S. (1996). Natural food colours, in *Natural Food Colourants,* 2nd edn (eds G.A.F. Hendry and J.D. Houghton). Champman & Hall, London.

Hernandez-Ledesma, B., Davalos, A., Bartolome, B. and Amigo, L. (2005). Preparation of antioxidant enzymatic hydrolysates from alpha-lactalbumin and beta-lactoglobulin. Identification of active peptides by HPLC-MS/MS. *Journal of Agricutural and Food Chemistry*, 53, 588–593.

Hernández-Ledesma, B., Hsieh, C.-C. and de Lumen, B.O. (2011). Relationship between lunasin's sequence and its inhibitory activity of histones H3 and H4 acetylation. *Molecular Nutrition and Food Research*, 55 (7), 989–998.

Higdon, J. V. and Frei, B. (2003). Tea catechins and polyphenols: Health effects, metabolism, and antioxidant functions. *Critical Reviews in Food Science and Nutrition*, 43, 89–143.

Hertog, M.G., Feskens, E.J., Hollman, P.C., Katan, M.B. and Kromhout, D. (1993). Dietary antioxidant flavonoids and risk of coronary heart disease: the Zutphen Elderly Study. *Lancet*, 342 (8878), 1007–1011.

Hooker, W.J., Walker, J.C. and Smith, F.G. (1943). Toxicity of beta-phenethyl isothiocyanate to certain fungi. *American Journal of Botany*, 30, 632–637.

Horiguchi, N., Horiguchi, H. and Suzuki, Y. (2005). Effect of wheat gluten hydrolysate on the immune system in healthy human subjects. *Bioscience, Biotechnology and Biochemistry*, 69, 2445–2449.

Horry, J.P. and Jay, M. (1988). Distribution of anthocyanins in wild and cultivated banana varieties. *Phytochemistry*, 27, 2667–2672.

Huang, G., Ren, Z. and Jiang, J. (2011). Separation of iron-binding peptides from shrimp processing by products hydrolysates. *Food Bioprocessing Technology*, 4 (8), 1527–1532.

Huang, Q.L., Zhang, L.N., Cheung, P.C.K. and Tan, X.T. (2006). Evaluation of sulfated a glucans from *Poria cocos* mycelia as potential antitumour agent. *Carbohydrate Polymers*, 64, 337–344.

Huanga, W.H., Lee, A.R. and Yang, C.H. (2006). Antioxidative and anti-inflammatory activities of polyhydroxyflavonoids of *Scutellaria baicalensis* GEORGI. *Bioscience, Biotechnology and Biochemistry*, 70, 2371–2380.

Hyun, J.W. and Chung, H.S. (2004). Cyanidin and malvidin from *Oryza sativa* cv. Heugjinjubyeo mediate cytotoxicity against human monocytic leukemia cells by arrest of G(2)/M phase and induction of apoptosis. *Journal of Agricultural and Food Chemistry*, 52, 2213–2217.

Innis, S.M. (1996). *Present Knowledge in Nutrition: Essential Dietary Lipids. Publications of the International Life Science Institute, Chapter 7.* International Life Science Institute, pp. 58–66.

Institute of Medicine (2002–2005). Dietary reference intakes for energy, carbohydrate, fibre, fat, fatty acids, cholesterol, protein, and amino acids (2002/2005). Food and Nutrition Board, Institute of Medicine, National Academies. www.nap.ed [reports accessed 16 July 2013].

Ioannou, I. and Ghoul, M. (2012). Biological activities and effects of food processing on flavonoids as phenolic antioxidants, in *Advances in Applied Biotechnology* (ed. M. Petre). DOI: 10.5772/30690. http://www.intechopen.com/books/advances-in-applied-biotechnology/biological-activities-and-effects-of-food-processing-on-flavonoids-as-phenolic-antioxidants [accessed 16 July 2013].

Jia, J., Ma, H., Zhao, W. *et al.* (2009). Effect of ultrasound treatment on physicochemical and functional properties of wheat germ globulin. *Nongye Jixie uebao/Transactions of the Chinese Society of Agricultural Machinery*, 40 (8), 105–110.

Kampa, M., Bakogeorgou, E., Hatzoglou, A. *et al.* (1997). Opioid alkaloids and casomorphin peptides decrease the proliferation of prostatic cancer cell lines (LNCaP, PC3 and DU145) through a partial interaction with opioid receptors. *European Journal of Pharmacology*, 335, 255–265.

Kang, S.Y., Seeram, N.P., Nair, M.G. *et al.* (2003). Tart cherry anthocyanins inhibit tumour development in Apc (Min) mice and reduce proliferation of human colon cancer cells. *Cancer Letters*, 194, 13–19.

Kawamori, R., Kadowaki, T., Onji, M., Seino, Y. and Akanuma, Y. (2007). Hepatic safety profile and glycemic control of pioglitazone in more than 20,000 patients with type 2 diabetes mellitus: Postmarketing surveillance study in Japan. *Diabetes Research and Clinical Practice*, 76, 229–235.

Katan, M.B., Zock, P.L. and Mensink, R.P. (1995). Trans fatty acids and their effects on lipoproteins in humas. *Annual Review of Nutrition*, 15, 473–493.

Katsube, N., Iwashita, K., Tsushida, T. *et al.* (2003). Induction of apoptosis in cancer cells by bilberry (*Vaccinium myrtillus*) and the anthocyanins. *Journal of Agricultural and Food Chemistry*, 51, 68–75.

Kilara, A. and Panyam, D. (2003). Peptides from milk proteins and their properties. *Critical Reviews in Food Science and Nutrition*, 43, 607–633.

Kim, S.-K. and Rajapakse, N. (2005). Enzymatic production and biological activities of chitosan oligosaccharides (COS): A review. *Carbohydrate Polymers*, 62, 357–368.

Kitts, D.D. and Weiler, K. (2003) Bioactive proteins and peptides from food sources. Applications of bioprocesses used in isolation and recovery. *Current Pharmaceutical Design*, 9, 1309–1323.

Kline, D.A. (2008). *Nutrition for Women Part I: Immune Components & Nutrients*, 6th edn. Nutrition Dimension, Ashland, OR.

Kodera, T. and Nio, N. (2006). Identification of an angiotensin I-converting enzyme inhibitory peptides from protein hydrolysates by a soybean protease and the antihypertensive effects of hydrolysates in spontaneously hypertensive model rats. *Journal of Food Science*, 71, C164–C173.

Kondo, K., Hirano, R., Matsumoto, A., Igarashi, O. and Itakura, H. (1996). Inhibition of LDL oxidation by cocoa. *Lancet*, 348, 1514.

Korhonen, H. and Pihlanto-Leppala, A. (2001). Milk protein-derived bioactive peptides novel opportunities for health promotion. *IDF Bulletin*, 363, 17–26.

Korhonen, H. and Pihlanto, A. (2003). Food-derived bioactive peptides – opportunities for designing future foods. *Current Pharmaceutical Design*, 9, 1297–1308.

Korhonen, H. and Pihlanto-Leppala, A. (2004). Milk-derived bioactive peptides: Formation and prospects for health promotion, in *Handbook of Functional Dairy Products. Functional Foods and Nutraceuticals Series 6.0* (Eds C. Shortt and J. O'Brien). CRC Press, FL, pp. 109–124.

Lala, G., Malik, M., Zhao, C. *et al.* (2006): Anthocyanin-rich extracts inhibit multiple biomarkers of colon cancer in rats. *Nutrition and Cancer*, 54, 84–93.

Lauro, G.J (1991). A primer on natural colours. *American Association of Cereal Chemists*, 36 (11), 949–953.

Lazze, M.C., Savio, M., Pizzala, R. *et al.* (2004). Anthocyanins induce cell cycle perturbations and apoptosis in different human cell lines. *Carcinogenesis*, 25, 1427–1433.

Lee, J.E., Bae, I.Y., Lee, H.G. and Yang, C.B. (2006). Tyr-Pro-Lys, an angiotensin I-converting enzyme inhibitory peptide derived from broccoli (*Brassica oleracea* Italica). *Food Chemistry*, 99, 143–148.

Lee, N.Y., Cheng, J.T., Enomoto, T. and Nakano, Y. (2006). One peptide derived from hen ovotransferrin as pro-drug to inhibit angiotensin converting enzyme. *Journal of Food and Drug Analysis*, 14, 31–35.

Li, Y.-Q., Fang, L. and Zhang, K.-C. (2007). Structure and bioactivities of a galactose rich extracellular polysaccharide from submergedly cultured *Ganoderma lucidum*. *Carbohydrate Polymers*, 68, 323–328.

Link, L.B. and Potter, J.D. (2004). Raw versus cooked vegetables and cancer risk. *Cancer Epidemiology, Biomarkers and Prevention*, 13, 1422–1435.

Magnuson, B.A., Lala, G., Kwon, Y.J. *et al.* (2003). Anthocyanin-rich extracts inhibit growth of human colon cancer cells and azoxymethane-induced colon aberrant crypts in rats: Implications for colon cancer chemoprevention. *Cancer Epidemiology, Biomarkers and Prevention*, 12, 1323S–1324S.

Manach, C., Morand, C., Gil-Izquierdo, A., Bouteloup-Demange, C. and Remesy, C. (2003). Bioavailability in humans of the flavanones hesperidin and narirutin after the ingestion of two doses of orange juice. *European Journal of Clinical Nutrition*, 57, 235–242.

Manach, C., Scalbert, A., Morand, C., Remesy, C. and Jimenez, L. (2004). Polyphenols: food sources and bioavailability. *American Journal of Clinical Nutrition*, 79, 727–747.

Manthey, J.A., Grohmann, K. and Guthrie, N. (2001). Biological properties of citrus bioflavonoids pertaining to cancer and inflammation. *Current Medicinal Chemistry*, 8 (2), 135–153.

Mari, M., Iori, R., Leoni, O. and Marchi, A. (1993). *In vitro* activity of glucosinolate-derived isothiocyanatcs against postharvest pear pathogens. *Annals of Applied Biology*, 123, 155–161.

Marko, D., Puppel, N., Tjaden, Z. *et al.* (2004). The substitution pattern of anthocyanidins affects different cellular signaling cascades regulating cell proliferation. *Molecular Nutritoim anfd Food Research*, 48, 318–325.

Matar, C., LeBlanc, J.G., Martin, L. and Perdigón, G. (2003). Biologically active peptides released in fermented milk: Role and functions, in *Handbook of Fermented Functional Foods. Functional Foods and Nutraceuticals series* (ed. E.R. Farnworth). CRC Press, FL, pp. 177–201.

Mazur, A., Bayle, D., Lab, C., Rock, E. and Rayssiguier, Y. (1999). Inhibitory effect of procyanidin-rich extracts on LDL oxidation *in vitro*. *Atherosclerosis*, 145 (2), 421–422.

Meiers, S., Kemeny, M., Weyand, U. *et al.* (2001). The anthocyanidins cyanidin and delphinidin are potent inhibitors of the epidermal growth-factor receptor. *Journal of Agricultural and Food Chemistry*, 49, 958–962.

Meisel, H. (1998). Overview on milk protein-derived peptides. *International Dairy Journal*, 8, 363–373.

Meisel, H. (2001). Bioactive peptides from milk proteins: A perspective for consumers and producers. *Australian Journal of Dairy Technology*, 56, 83–92.

Meisel, H. (2004). Multifunctional peptides encrypted in milk proteins. *Biofactors*, 21, 55–61.

Meisel, H. (2005), Biochemical properties o f peptides encrypted in bovine milk proteins. *Current Medicinal Chemistry*, 12, 1905–1919.

Meisel, H., Goepfert, A. and Gunther, S. (1997). ACE-inhibitory activities in milk products. *Milchwissenschaft*, 52, 307–311.

Mensink, R.P. and Katan, M.B. (1990). Effect of dietary trans fatty acids on high density and low-density lipoprotein cholesterol levels in healthy subjects. *New England Journal of Medicine*, 323, 439–445.

McCann, K.B., Shiell, B.J., Michalski, W.P. *et al.* (2006). Isolation and characterisation of a novel antibacterial peptide from bovine aS1-casein. *International Dairy Journal*, 16, 316–323

Miguel, M. and Aleixandre, A. (2006). Antihypertensive peptides derived from egg proteins. *The Journal of Nutrition*, 136, 1457–1460.

Mine, Y. and Kovacs-Nolan, J. (2006). New insights in biologically active proteins and peptides derived from hen egg. *Worlds Poultry Science Journal*, 62, 87–95.

Mizushima, S., Ohshige, K., Watanabe, J. *et al.* (2004). Randomized controlled trial of sour milk on blood pressure in borderline hypertensive men. *American Journal of Hypertension*, 17, 701–706.

Motoi, H. and Kodama, T. (2003). Isolation and characterization of angiotensin I-converting enzyme inhibitory peptides from wheat gliadin hydrolysate. *Nahrung/Food*, 47, 354–358.

Mullen, W., Stewart, A.J., Lean, M.E.J. *et al.* (2002). Effect of freezing and storage on the phenolics, ellagitannins, flavonoids, and antioxidant capacity of red raspberries. *Journal of Agricultural and Food Chemistry*, 50, 5197–5201.

Murray, B.A. and FitzGerald, R.J. (2006). Angiotensin converting enzyme inhibitory peptides derived from food proteins: biochemistry, bioactivity and production. *Current Pharmaceutical Design*, 13, 733–791.

Nagaoka, S., Futamura, Y., Miwa, K. *et al.* (2001). Identification of novel hypocholesterolemic peptides derived from bovine milk beta-lactoglobulin. *Biochemical and Biophysical Research Communications*, 281, 11–17.

Nakamura, Y., Yamamoto, M., Sakai, K. *et al.* (1995). Purification and characterization of angiotensin I-converting enzyme inhibitors from sour milk. *Journal of Dairy Science*, 78, 777–783.

Nagai, T., Suzuki, N. and Nagashima, T. (2006). Antioxidative activities and angiotensin I-converting enzyme inhibitory activities of enzymatic hydrolysates from commercially available Kamaboko species. *Food Science Technology*, 12, 335–346.

Nesselhut, T., Rath, W., Grunow, E. *et al.* (1993).The relationship between urinary Tamm–Horsfall glycoprotein excretion and urinary activity of glycosidases in normal pregnancy and pre-eclampsia. *European Journal of Obstetrics, Gynecology and Reproductive Biology*, 48, 23–31.

Olsson, M.E., Gustavsson, K.E., Andersson, S. *et al.* (2004). Inhibition of cancer cell proliferation *in vitro* by fruit and berry extracts and correlations with antioxidant levels. *Journal of Agricultural and Food Chemistry*, 52, 7264–7271.

Parrot, S., Degraeve, P., Curia, C. and Martial-Gros, A. (2003). *In vitro* study on digestion of peptides in Emmental cheese: *Nahrung*, 47 (2), 87–94.

Pérez-Gregorio, M.R., Garcia-Falcon, M.S. and Simal-Gandara, J. (2011). Flavonoids changes in fresh-cut onions during storage in different packaging systems. *Food Chemistry*, 124, 652–658.

Peterson, J. and Dwyer, J. (1998). Flavonoids: Dietary occurrences and biochemical activity. *Nutrition Research*, 18 (12), 1995–2018.

Rayaprolu, S.J., Hettiarachchy, N.S., Chen, P., Kannan, A. and Mauromostakos, A. (2013). Peptides derived from high oleic acid soybean meals inhibit colon, liver and lung cancer cell growth. *Food Research International*, 50 (1), 282–288.

Rice-Evans, C.A., Miller, N.J., Bolwell, P.G., Bramley, P.M. and Pridham, J.B. (1995). The relative antioxidant activities of plant-derived polyphenolic flavonoids. *Free Radical Research*, 22, 375–383.

Rodrigues, A.S. and Rosa, E.A.S. (1999). Effect of post-harvest treatments on the level of glucosinolates in broccoli. *Journal of the Science of Food and Agriculture*, 79, 1028–1032.

Roth, J., Ziak, M. and Zuber, C. (2003). The role of glucosidase II and endomannosidase in glucose trimming of asparagine-linked oligosaccharides. *Biochimie*, 85, 287–294.

Rouzaud, G., Young, S.A. and Duncan, A.J. (2004). Hydrolysis of glucosinolates to isothiocyanates after ingestion of raw or microwaved cabbage by human volunteers. *Cancer Epidemiology, Biomarkers and Prevention*, 13, 125–131.

Ryhanen, E.L., Pihlanto-Leppala, A. and Pahkala, E. (2001). A new type of ripened, low-fat cheese with bioactive properties. *International Dairy Journal*, 11, 441–447.

Saito, T., Nakamura, T., Kitazawa, H., Kawai, Y. and Itoh, T. (2000). Isolation and structural analysis of antihypertensive peptides that exist naturally in Gouda cheese. *Journal of Dairy Science*, 83, 1434–1440.

Sarwar, M. and Kirkegaard, J. A. (1998). Biofumigation potential of brassicas. *Plant and Soil*, 201, 91–101.

Sarwar, M., Kirkegaard, J. A., Wong, P.T.W. and Desmarchelier, J. M. (1998). Biofumigation potential of brassicas. III *In-vitro* toxicity of isothiocyanates to soil-borne fungal pathogens. *Plant and Soil*, 201, 103–112.

Scalbert, A. and Williamson, G. (2000). Dietary intake and bioavailability of polyphenols. *The Journal of Nutrition*, 130, 2073S–2085S.

Schanbacher, E.L., Talhouk, R.S., Murray, EA. Gherman. L.I. and Willett, L.B. (1998). Milk-borne bioactive peptides. *International Dairy Journal*, 8, 393–403.

Schmidt, B.M., Erdman, J.W. and Lila, M.A. (2005). Effects of food processing on blueberry antiproliferation and antioxidant activity. *Journal of Food Science*, 70, S389–S394.

Seeram, N.P., Adams, L.S., Hardy, M.L. *et al.* (2004). Total cranberry extract versus its phytochemical constituents: antiproliferative and synergistic effects against human tumour cell lines. *Journal of Agricultural and Food Chemistry*, 52, 2512–2517.

Seeram, N.P., Adams, L.S., Zhang, Y. *et al.* (2006). Blackberry, black raspberry, blueberry, cranberry, red raspberry, and strawberry extracts inhibit growth and stimulate apoptosis of human cancer cells *in vitro*. *Journal of Agricultural and Food Chemistry*, 54 (25), 9329–9339.

Sharma, P. and Gujral, H.S. (2011). Effect of sand roasting and microwave cooking on antioxidant activity of barley. *Food Research International*, 44, 235–240.

Smacchi, E. and Gobbetti, M. (1998). Peptides from several Italian cheeses inhibitory to proteolytic enzymes of lactic acid bacteria; *Pseudomonas fluorescens* ATCC 948 and to the angiotensin I-converting enzyme. *Enzyme Microbiology and Technology*, 22, 687–694.

Silva, S.V. and Malcata, F.X. (2005). Caseins as source of bioactive peptides. *International Dairy Journal*, 15, 1–15.

Simmonds, N.W. (1962). Anthocyanins in wild bananas, in *The Evolution of Bananas*. Longmans, London, pp. 23–25.

Simopoulos, A.P. (1999). Essential fatty acids in health and chronic disease. *American Journal of Clinical Nutrition*, 70 (suppl), 560S–569S.

Singh, B. (2007). *Psyllium* as therapeutic and drug delivery agent. *International Journal of Pharmaceutics*, 334, 1–14.

Singh, T.K., Fox, P.F. and Healy, A. (1997). Isolation and identification of further peptides in the diafiltration retentate of the water-soluble fraction of Cheddar cheese. *Journal of Dairy Research*, 64, 433–443.

Singletary, K.W., Stansbury, M.J., Giusti, M. *et al.* (2003). Inhibition of rat mammary tumourigenesis by concord grape juice constituents. *Journal of Agricultural and Food Chemistry*, 51, 7280–7286.

Sprecher, H. (2000). Metabolism of highly unsaturated $n-3$ and $n-6$ fatty acids. *Biochimica et Biophysica Acta*, 1486, 219–231.

Takahashi, M., Fukunaga, H., Kaneto, H., Fukudome, S.I. and Yoshikawa, M. (2000). Behavioral and pharmacological studies on gluten exorphin A5, a newly isolated bioactive food protein fragment, in mice. *Japanese Journal of Pharmacology*, 84, 259–265.

Takahashi, M., Moriguchi, S., Yoshikawa, M. and Sasaki, R. (1994). Isolation and characterization of oryzatensin a novel bioactive peptide with ileum-contracting and immune-modulating activities derived from rice albumin. *Biochemical and Molecular Biology International*, 33, 1151–1158.

Thornalley, P.J. (2002). Isothiocyanates: mechanism of cancer chemopreventive action. *Anti-Cancer Drugs*, 13, 331–338.

Thornalley, P.J. and IARC Workgroup (2004). Cruciferous vegetables, isothiocyanates and indoles, in *IARC Handbook on Chemoprevention of Cancer*. IARC Press, pp. 1–261.

Timberlake, C.F. and Henry, B.S. (1988). Anthocyanins as natural food colorants. *Progress in Clinical and Biological Research*, 280, 107–121.

Tsevegsüren, N., Aitzetmüller, K., Brühl, L. and Werner, G. (2000). Seed oil fatty acids of Mongolian compositae: The trans-fatty acids of *Heteropappus hispidus*, *Asterothamnus centrali-asiaticus* and *Artemisia palustris*. *Journal of High Resolution Chromatography*, 23 (5), 360–366.

Tudela, J.A., Cantos, E., Espin, J.C. *et al.* (2002). Induction of antioxidant flavonol biosynthesis in fresh-cut potatoes. effect of domestic cooking. *Journal of Agricultural and Food Chemistry*, 50, 5925–5931.

Ursin, V.M. (2003). Modification of plant lipids for human health: development of functional land-based 1–3 fatty acids. *The Journal of Nutrition*, 133, 4271–4274.

Vierheilig, H. and Ocampo, J.A. (1990). Effect of isothiocyanates on germination of spores of *G. mosseae*. *Soil Biology and Biochemistry*, 22, 1161–1163.

Viña, S.Z. & Chaves, A.R. (2008). Effect of heat treatment and refrigerated storage on antioxidant properties of pre-cut celery (*Apium graveolens* L.). *International Journal of Food Science and Technology*, 43, 44–51.

Viña, S.Z., Olivera, D.F., Marani, C.M. *et al.* (2007). Quality of Brussels sprouts (*Brassica oleracea* L. gemmifera DC) as affected by blanching method. *Journal of Food Engineering*, 80, 218–225.

Walker, J.C., Morell, S. and Foster, H.H. (1937). Toxicity of mustard oils and related sulfur compounds to certain fungi. *American Journal of Botany*, 24, 536–541.

Walker, G., Cai, F., Shen, P. *et al.* (2006). Increased remineralization of tooth enamel by milk containing added casein phosphopeptide-amorphous calcium phosphate. *Journal of Dairy Research*, 73, 74–78.

Wallis, J.G., Watts, J.L. and Browse, J. (2002). Polyunsaturated fatty acid synthesis: What will they think of next? *Trends in Biochemical Science*, 27, 467–473.

Wang, H., Cao, G. and Prior, R.L. (1997). Oxygen radical absorbing capacity of anthocyanins. *Journal of Agricultural and Food Chemistry*, 45, 304–309.

Wang, W. and de Mejia, E.G. (2005). A new frontier in soy bioactive peptides that may prevent age-related diseases. *Comprehensive Reviews in Food Science and Food Safety*, 4, 63–78.

Wheeler, D.S., Catravas, J.D., Odoms, K. *et al.* (2004). Epigallocatechin-3-gallate, a green tea-derived polyphenol, inhibits IL-1 b-dependent proinflammatory signal transduction in cultured respiratory epithelial cells. *The Journal of Nutrition*, 134, 1039–1044.

Williams, M.J., Sutherland, W.H., Whelan, A.P., McCormick, M.P. and de Jong, S.A. (2004). Acute effect of drinking red and white wines on circulating levels of inflammation-sensitive molecules in men with coronary artery disease. *Metabolism*, 53, 318–323.

Vercruysse, L., Van Camp, J. and Smagghe, G. (2005). ACE inhibitory peptides derived from enzymatic hydrolysates of animal muscle protein: a review. *Journal of Agricultural and Food Chemistry*, 53, 8106–8115.

Yochum, L., Kushi, L.H., Meyer, K. and Folsom, A.R. (1999). Dietary flavonoid intake and risk of cardiovascular disease in postmenopausal women. *American Journal of Epidemiology*, 149 (10), 943–949.

Yu, J., Ahmedna, M. and Goktepe, I. (2005). Effects of processing methods and extraction solvents on concentration and antioxidant activity of peanut skin phenolics. *Food Chemistry*, 90, 199–206.

Zainol, M.M., Abdul-Hamid, A., Bakar, F.A. and Dek, S.P. (2009). Effect of different drying methods on the degradation of selected flavonoids in *Centella asiatica*. *International Food Research Journal*, 16 (4), 531–537.

Zhang, M., Chen, H., Li, J., Pei, Y. and Liang, Y. (2010). Antioxidant properties of tartary buckwheat extracts as affected by different thermal processing methods. *LWT – Food Science and Technology*, 43, 181–185.

Zhang, Y., Seeram, N.P., Lee, R., Feng, L. and Heber, D. (2008). Isolation and identification of strawberry phenolics with antioxidant and human cancer cell antiproliferative properties. *Journal of Agricultural and Food Chemistry*, 56, 670–675.

Zhang, Y., Vareed, S.K. and Nair, M.G. (2005). Human tumour cell growth inhibition by nontoxic anthocyanidins, the pigments in fruits and vegetables. *Life Science*, 76, 1465–1472.

Zhao, C., Giusti, M.M., Malik, M. *et al.* (2004). Effects of commercial anthocyanin-rich extracts on colonic cancer and non-tumorigenic colonic cell growth. *Journal of Agricultural and Food Chemistry*, 52, 6122–6128.

Zhu, K.X., Zhou, H.M. and Qian, H.F. (2006). Antioxidant and free radical-scavenging activities of wheat germ protein hydrolysates (WGPH) prepared with alcalase. *Process Biochemistry*, 41, 1296–1302.

Zielinski, H., Mishalska, A., Amigo-Benavent, M., Del Castillo, M. D. and Piskula, M. K. (2009). Changes in protein quality and antioxidant properties of buckwheat seeds and groats induced by roasting. *Journal of Agricultural and Food Chemistry*, 57, 4771–4777.

II
Major Sources of Functional Foods

3

Processing Effects on Functional Components in Cereals and Grains

Binod K. Yadav and J. Jerish Joyner
Indian Institute of Crop Processing Technology, Thanjavur, Tamilnadu, India

3.1 Introduction

Food not only satisfies hunger, it provides necessary nutrients, prevent nutrition-related diseases and improve physical and mental well-being (Nothlings *et al.*, 2007; Takachi *et al.*, 2008). Awareness of the functionality of certain foods and their benefits to human health is growing daily.

Foods or food components beneficial to human health and wellbeing are known as functional foods or functional components. The term functional food was first introduced in Japan in the mid-1980s and refers to processed food containing ingredients that aid specific bodily functions in addition to being nutritious. To date, Japan is the only country that has formulated a specific regulatory approval process for functional food. The Institute of Medicine's Food and Nutrition Board (IOM/FNB) defined functional food as 'any food or food ingredient that may provide a health benefit beyond the traditional nutrients it contains' (Hasler, 2002). Health Canada defines functional food as a product that resembles traditional food but possesses demonstrated physiological benefits (Shahidi, 2009).

Functional food comprises:

- conventional food containing naturally occurring bioactive substances (e.g., dietary fibre),
- food enriched with bioactive substances (e.g., probiotics, antioxidants),
- synthesized food ingredients introduced to traditional food (e.g. prebiotics).

Functional food and components are thought to provide benefits beyond basic nutrition and may play a role in reducing or minimizing the risk of certain diseases.

Functional Foods and Dietary Supplements: Processing Effects and Health Benefits, First Edition.
Edited by Athapol Noomhorm, Imran Ahmad and Anil Kumar Anal.

Examples of these foods include fruits and vegetables, whole cereal grains, fortified foods and beverages and some dietary supplements. Functional characteristics of many traditional foods are being discovered and studied, while new food products are being developed to include beneficial components. Most important functional foods are made with cereals and grains as the base and have been modified to provide health benefits over and above basic nutrition, keeping a similar appearance to conventional foods that are intended to be consumed as part of a normal diet (Roberfroid, 2000).

Among all the sources of functional foods, cereals, grains and legumes are important economic commodities worldwide. Cereals are grown in over 73% of the total harvested area of the world. They contribute over 60% of the world's food production providing the dietary fibre, proteins, energy, minerals and vitamins required for human health as well as functional components such as phytoestrogens of the lignan family and several phenolic acids with antioxidant properties (Charalampopoulos *et al.* 2002). In recent years, cereals have been investigated for their potential use in developing functional foods. Cereals contain dietary fibres (β-glucan and arabinoxylan) and carbohydrates (resistant starch and oligosaccharides – galacto- and fructo-oligosaccharides) can also be used as fermentable substrates for the growth of probiotic microorganisms (Charalampopoulos *et al.* 2002). The contents of some cereals exhibit protective effects such as preventing cancer and cardiovascular disease and reducing tumor incidence; lowering blood pressure, the risk of heart disease, cholesterol and the rate of fat absorption; delaying gastric emptying and supplying gastrointestinal health (Chaturvedi *et al.*, 2011).

Several studies have reported the effects of storage and processing of raw materials on the nutrient content and bioprotective components of functional foods. Normally, processing operations reduce the content of these nutrients and bioprotective substances (Truswell, 2002).

Functional foods are commonly made from rice, corn, soybean and legumes. Functional foods based on cereal and grains are increasingly pouring in to stores despite their ambiguous health benefits. Understanding the nature of the functional components of cereals and legumes is essential for the development of functional food products. Therefore, in this chapter we attempt to provide collective information on the nutrients and bioactive substances in rice, corn, soybean and legumes.The effects of different processing conditions on functional components are also discussed.

3.2 Functional components in cereals and grains

The major cereals considered in the discussion are rice, corn, soybean and legumes in general.

3.2.1 Functional components in rice and their health benefits

Rice is an important source of energy, protein and components with versatile functional properties (Mazza, 1998). Rice proteins are considered valuable because they are colourless, bland, hypoallergenic and hypocholesterolaemic (Ju *et al.*, 2001). The rice kernel comprises 20% hull, 8–12% bran and embryo and 70–72% endosperm or milled rice based on the degree of milling. Rice kernel bran has often been reported for its functional components.

Rice bran Bran is one of the most abundant co-products produced in the rice milling industry. It contains a high concentration of nutritional compounds, including edible lipids and other phytochemicals that exhibit health benefits (Khuwijitjaru *et al.*, 2007). It is evident from Table 3.1 that rice bran and various co-products make it a valuable ingredient in developing functional food formulations. Major components of bran used for developing functional foods are rice bran oil, defatted rice bran and rice bran enzymatic extract (RBEE).

Table 3.1 Functional components present in rice bran and their health benefits

Sl. no	Functional component	Functional effects/health benefits	Reference
1	Dietary fibres – beta-glucan – pectin – gum	Removes the toxics and at optimum pH improves digestive function	Saikia and Deka, 2011
		Adds bulk to gastrointestinal track and prevents colon cancer Lowers LDL and increases HDL cholesterol, hence aiding cardio vascular health	Wells, 1993
2	Lutein and Zeaxanthin	Improves eyesight, reduces the chance of cataracts	Saikia *et al.*, 2011
3	n3, n6, n9 fatty acid and folic acid, PUFA	Promote eye health	
4	Vit. K and Inositol hexaphosphate	Prevent kidney stones	
5	Inositol, phospholipid and Vit. B	Detoxifies liver, contol liver cirrhosis, improve cell regeneration	
6	α-lipoic acid	Lowers glycemic index and controls body weight	
7	Magnesium	Improves glycemic control and helps prevent insulin resistance	
8	Tocopherol, tocotrienol and oryzanol and beta-sitosterol	Can replace synthetic antioxidants like BHA/BHT	Hettiarachchy *et al.*, 1993
		Used in the cure of nerve imbalance and disorders of menopause	Rogers *et al.*, 1993
		Tends to lessen gallstone formation	Babcock, 1987
		Anticancer activity	Komiyama *et al.*, 1992
		Antioxidant activity	Qureshi *et al.*, 2001; Chiang An-Na *et al.*, 2006; Fan *et al.*, 2000
		Decreases hepatic cholesterol biosynthesis and plasma cholesterol	Rong *et al.*, 1997
9	Rice bran enzymatic extract-Protein	High bio-absorbable protein enriched diet formulation	Hamada *et al.*, 1998; Matthews, 1977
10	Rice bran enzymatic extract-sulfur amino acids (cysteine + methionine)	Anti-proliferative tumor cell growth	Parrado *et al.*, 2006

Rice bran oil The rice bran contains almost 12–18.5% oil. It contains a range of fats, of which 47% are monounsaturated, 33% polyunsaturated, and 20% saturated. Also it contains highly unsaponifiable components of around 4.3%. This fraction contains functional components like tocotrienols (a form of vitamin E), gamma oryzanol, and beta-sitosterol. These components are very powerful antioxidants (Godber and Wells, 1994). Rice bran oil has a higher tocol concentration (196–219 mg/kg) compared to brown rice (46.4–65.0 mg/kg) (Aguilar-Garcia *et al.*, 2007).

Rice bran enzymatic extract (RBEE) RBEE is a water-soluble compound which contains proteins, carbohydrates, fat, vitamins and minerals (Parrado *et al.,* 2006). The main component of RBEE is protein (38.1%) in the form of peptide. This high bioabsorbable protein can be used for making protein-enriched diet formulations. RBEE also contains free amino acids of which 6% are sulfur amino acids which contribute to its antiproliferative activity (Parrado *et al.*, 2006).

Defatted rice bran Rice bran, due to its lipid content, is prone to oxidation resulting in losses of its nutrients and phytochemicals.The deterioration and decrease of nutritional value is a major threat due to rapid oxidation, especially when raw bran is stored in large quantities and used in small amounts. Therefore, rice bran is defatted and dried in order to preserve and store it for a long period without maintaining a low temperature. After heat treatment to remove the oil, rice bran is designated as heat-stabilized defatted rice bran (HSDRB) (Tang *et al.*, 2003). The defatted residues of bran contain 15.4% protein (Hamada, 2000). This protein can be used as a nutraceutical and functional food ingredient (Tang *et al.*, 2003).

The stabilized rice bran may be used directly or the functional components extracted from the bran can be used for functional food formulations. The use of rice for developing functional food has already been explained by several researchers (Prakash and Ramaswamy, 1996; Ye Xudong *et al.*, 2000, Jiamyangyuen *et al.*, 2005; Parrado *et al.*, 2006).

3.2.2 Functional components in corn and their health benefits

Corn (*Zea mays*), also called maize, is a good source of many nutrients including thiamine (vitamin B_1), pantothenic acid (vitamin B_5), vitamin C, folate, phosphorus and manganese. Apart from these it also possesses several functional components like carotenoids, phenolic acids, dietary fibres, phytosterols and phytostanols which contribute to its abundant functional and health benefits (Table 3.2).

Corn controls the level of homocysteine, an intermediate product in an important metabolic process called the methylation cycle in the human body. Homocysteine is directly responsible for damage of blood vessels, heart attack, and stroke or peripheral vascular disease. Corn is also a good source of folate. It has been estimated that consumption of 100% of the daily value (DV) of folate would, by itself, reduce the incidence heart attacks by 10% (Bazzano *et al.*, 2002). It has been found that cryptoxanthin, a natural carotenoid pigment from corn, can reduce the risk of lung cancer by 27% when consumed daily (Yuan and Burkin, 2003). The content of insoluble-bound

Table 3.2 Functional components present in corn and their health benefits

Sl. no	Functional component	Functional effects/health benefits	Reference
1	Dietary fibre	Prevent diseases like bowel disease, Crohn's disease, colon cancer, constipation, diabetes, diverticulosis, gallstones, heart disease, high cholesterol, hyperlipidemia, and obesity	Singh *et al.*, 2012
2	Carotenoids xanthophylls, lutein and zeaxanthin	Promote eye health	Mozaffarieh *et al.*, 2003
3	Phenolic acids p-coumaric acid (CA), ferulic acid (FA)	Anti-inflammatory activity naturally occurring antioxidants Act as antimutagens to reduce the risk of cancer	Kim *et al.*, 2012 Graf, 1992; Cuvelier *et al.*, 1992 Karoon *et al.*, 1997; Ferguson *et al.*, 2003
4	Phenolic amides di feruloyl putrescine (DFP), p-coumaroyl feruloyl putrescine (CFP) and p-dicoumaroyl putrescine (DCP)	Antidiabetic Inhibition of aflatoxin biosynthesis Antioxidant and anti-melanogenic activities	Niwa *et al.*, 2003 Mellon and Moreau, 2004 Choi *et al.*, 2007
5	Arabinoxylan and lutein	Anti-inflammatory activity	Ogawa *et al.*, 2005; Rafi and Shafaia, 2007
6	Hemicellulose	Antioxidative activity	Ohta *et al.*, 1994
7	Phytosterols – 4-desmethylsterols – 4-monomethylsterols – 4, 4-dimethylsterols	Recognized as cancer preventive biologically active substances	Canabate-Díaz *et al.*, 2007
8	Phytostanols	Reduce serum cholesterol levels	Santos *et al.*, 2007; Hicks and Moreau, 2001

phenolic compound in corn is significantly higher (0.411 mg/g of grain) compared to rice (0.407 mg/g of grain), wheat (0.368 mg/g of grain) and oats (0.343 mg/g of grain) (Adom and Liu, 2002). Phenolic compounds of corn may exert their effects via antioxidation and relief from oxidative stress and its consequences.

Corn is one of the most important sources of tocols – tocopherols (TP) and tocotrienols (TT) – containing between 7.24 and 85.62 mg/kg (Kurilich and Juvik, 1999). The most prominent tocols in corn are γ-TP, followed by α-TP and γ-TT (Moreau and Hicks, 2006).

Major components of corn used for functional food development are corn bran, corn kernel oil, corn fibre, cellulosic fibre gel, corn fibre gum, corn fibre oil and corn protein hydrolysates.

Corn bran Corn bran, a by-product in the corn milling industry, has traditionally been used in animal feed. However, corn bran has a high dietary fibre content (76–90%) and can be used for human consumption (Burge and Duensing, 1989). These dietary fibres provide enormous health benefits and have the potential to be incorporated into cakes and other foods (Singh *et al.*, 2012).

Corn kernel oil Corn oil extracted from whole kernel is very rich in phytosterols (Verleyen *et al.*, 2002; Ferrari *et al.*, 1996) and it also contains phytostanols, 4-desmethylsterols, 4-monomethylsterols and 4,4-dimethylsterols (Harrabi *et al.*, 2007). These compounds are known to reduce the absorption of cholesterol in the gut and thereby lower blood cholesterol levels (Santos *et al.*, 2007).

The average dietary consumption of phytosterols and phytostanols among different populations is approximately 250 and 25 mg/day, respectively (Nair *et al.*, 2006). Corn oil can be served as a good supplement to meet the nutritional requirements for phytosterols and phytostanols.

Corn fibre Corn fibre (CF) is the most abundant low-valued coproduct of the industrial wet-milling process. It contains a large percentage of valuable hemicelluloses which are reported to have antioxidant activity (Ohta *et al.*, 1994; Yadav *et al.*, 2012). Both corn bran and corn fibre are mainly composed of the pericarp; however, corn fibre contains cell wall material from the endosperm, which is not contained in corn bran (Singh *et al.*, 2000).

Cellulosic fibre gel Corn bran contains about 200 g cellulose/kg (Rose *et al.*, 2010). Cellulose exhibits undesirable characteristics in foods besides having few desirable functional properties (Harris *et al.*, 2006). It is modified by disrupting the native structure of cellulose in a two-stage high-shear process to yield a cellulosic fibre gel (Inglett, 1997, 1998). Cellulosic fibre gel from corn bran exhibits high hydration capacity, high viscosity, a gel-like structure and can be used as a good fat replacer (Inglett and Carriere, 2001).

Cellulosic fibre gel has found commercial success. For example, Z-Trim (Z Trim Holdings, Inc., Mundelein) is promoted as a fat mimetic or flour substitute used in baked goods, condiments, dairy foods and processed meats (http://www.ztrim.com). Furthermore, in the United States, Z-Trim has applications in school lunches to help meet the strict nutritional guidelines outlined in the National School Lunch Program set forth by the Food and Nutrition Service of the US Department of Agriculture (Lapp and Hansen, 2013).

Corn fibre gum The fibre fractions from the kernel's pericarp and endosperm produced by the corn-wet milling industry are called 'coarse' and 'fine' fibres, respectively and collectively they are called 'white fibre'. The extraction of this white fibre using a mild alkaline hydrogen peroxide process yields a hemicellulose (arabinoxylan)-enriched fraction called corn fibre gum (CFG) (Yadav *et al.*, 2012). The CFG, with its low solution viscosity, can be used as a stabilizer for oil-in-water emulsions. CFGs isolated from both coarse and fine corn fibre contain functional protein, lipid and also nutraceutical phenolic compounds (Yadav *et al.*, 2007). The presence of these phenolic acids, lipids and proteins in CFG may contribute to its excellent emulsifying properties and combine to give improved physicochemical and nutritional properties (Rose *et al.*, 2010). Hence, new applications could explore the application of CFG in expanded snacks, baked goods, beverages, specialty foods, edible coatings, supplements and the development of functional foods to make use of its functional components and their benefits.

Corn fibre oil Corn oil from fibre has been of recent interest because of its ability to lower cholesterol in animal studies probably due to high levels of ferulate phytosterol esters, the most predominant being sitostanyl ferulate (Norton *et al.*, 1995; Moreau *et al.*, 1999; Wilson *et al.*, 2000; Ramjiganesh *et al.*, 2002; Jain *et al.*, 2008). Corn fibre contains three to six times more of these components than corn bran (Inglett *et al.*, 2009). Unfortunately, the amounts are still quite low compared to the levels of similar compounds in other bran-derived oils such as rice bran oil (Norton, 1995). Therefore, before corn fibre oil can be used commercially, ways to increase its oil yield and phytosterol content must be examined.

Corn protein hydrolysates Corn protein is a complex mixture of highly diversified protein components including albumins, gluobulins and zein fractions (Paulis *et al.*, 1975). The protein hydrolysates prepared from corn are antioxidative in nature and they can effectively inhibit lipid oxidation in foods (Zhou *et al.*, 2012). They can also be used for making edible coatings and packaging films (Park *et al.*, 1994; Hernandez-Izquierdo and Krochta, 2008).

3.2.3 Functional components in soybean and their health benefits

Soybeans (*Glycine max* L. Merr.) are unique among the legumes because they are low in saturated fat and high in protein, complex carbohydrates, fibre and oil. Besides their excellent nutritional profile, they are also good sources of functional components such as isoflavones, soyasaponins and tocopherols (Messina, 1999). Due to the presence of these bioactive compounds, soybeans are widely used in the food industry for developing functional foods that have several health benefits (Table 3.3). Soyabeans in the form of soybean carbohydrates, soybean oil, soy proteins and soy germ are widely used in a range of food products for their functional benefits.

Soybean carbohydrates Soybean contains around 35% carbohydrates, most of which are non-starch polysaccharides. These constituents move the food through the digestive system, absorb water and make defecation easier, preventing many associated diseases.

Soybean also contains galacto-oligosaccharides (GOS) such as stachyose (4%) and raffinose (1.1%) (Grieshop *et al.*, 2003). These GOS are non-digestible carbohydrates. Humans do not possess the enzyme α-galactosidase required to digest these oligosaccharides. Hence the intact oligosaccharides reach the colon, where they are preferentially fermented by beneficial bifidogenic microorganisms that contain the enzyme (Liu, 1999). This results in production of gases such as carbon dioxide, hydrogen, methane, etc. and short-chain fatty acids, which are interesting because of their prebiotic activity and associated health benefits (Tomomatsu, 1994; Gibson and Roberfroid, 1995). Hence these GOS can be used as potential ingredients for making functional foods.

Table 3.3 Functional components present in soybean and their health benefits

Sl. no	Functional component	Functional effects/health benefits	Reference
1	Insoluble dietary fibre	Adds bulk to stool and improves bowel function	Písaříková and Zralý, 2010
2	Linoleic acid (n-6 PUFA)	Has favorable effects on platelet reactivity	De Lorgeril *et al.*, 1994
3	α-linolenic acid (n-3 PUFA)	Possess cardioprotective effect	Harper and Jacobson, 2001; Holguin *et al.*, 2005
		Beneficial effects on obesity, insulin resistance	Moreno-Aliaga *et al.*, 2010
		Secretion of bioactive adipokines including leptin, adiponectin and visfatin	
		Modulate the anti-inflammatory process inside the blood vessels	Tull *et al.*, 2009
4	Stearic acid	Trans-free, oxidatively stable, non-LDL-cholesterol-raising	Hunter *et al.*, 2010
5	Phospholipids	Contribute to the structure of cell membrane, used as a natural food emulsifier	Dixit *et al.*, 2011
6	Tocopherols	Possess strong antioxidant activity-prevents disorders of the skin, eye, lungs, and other lipid-rich body constituents	Niki and Noguchi, 2004
7	Phytosterols-(β-sitosterol, campesterol and stigmasterol)	Cholesterol-lowering activity and decreases lipid peroxidation of platelet membranes *in vitro*	Law, 2000; Van Rensburg *et al.*, 2000
8	Isoflavones	Estrogenic, hypocholesterolaemic, improves digestive tract function, prevents breast, prostate, and colon cancer, bone health, improve lipid metabolism	Sugano, 2006
		Potent α-glucosidase inhibitor i.e. reducing blood sugar	Chen *et al.*, 2007; Lee and Lee, 2001
9	Soyasaponins	Hypocholesterolaemic, anticarcinogenic activities	Gurfinkel and Rao, 2003
		Beneficial effect against liver injury	Kuzuhara *et al.*, 2000
10	Ferritin	Highly bioavailable iron from soybean ferritin helps recover from anaemia	Lönnerdal, 2009

Soybean oil Soybean contains roughly 19% oil characterized by relatively large amounts of polyunsaturated fatty acids (PUFA), namely 55% linoleic acid and 8% α-linolenic acid (Messina, 1999). These PUFAs have several well-known health benefits (Table 3.3).

Soy proteins The use of soy proteins as functional ingredients in foods continues to gain increased acceptance due to their low cost, and their nutritional and potential health benefits such as the prevention of hypercholesterolaemia, atherosclerosis and cancer (Oakenfull *et al.*, 1984; Fournier *et al.*, 1998; Messina, 1999).

Soy germ Soy germ, which accounts for only 2% of the total seed weight, is naturally 6- to 10-fold higher concentration of total isoflavones than cotyledons (Dayde *et al.*, 2002). Isoflavones possess antioxidant activity and α-glucosidase inhibitory activity, which has proved effective in the treatment of type 2 diabetes mellitus.

There are very high concentrations of total soyasaponins in soy germ (Hubert *et al.*, 2005). The oil extracted from the germ is also a rich source of phytosterols and tocopherols than the oil extracted from the cotyledons. The functional components in soy germ and their associated health benefits are shown in Table 3.3.

3.2.4 Functional components in legumes and their health benefits

Legumes are high in protein and dietary fibres, low in saturated fat and cholesterol-free. To achieve nutritional balance, cereals and legumes need to be consumed in the approximate ratio of 65 (cereal) to 35 (legume). In addition to their nutritive value, legumes contain significant quantities of functional components like phenolic and polyphenolic compounds including phenolic acids, flavonoids, lignins, tocopherols, dietary fibres and phytochemicals (Dabrowski and Sosulski, 1984; Sosulski and Dabrowski, 1984). These functional components provide valuable health benefits such as antiatherosclerotic, antihypertensive, antilipemic, antithrombotic, lipase inhibitory, lipid peroxidation inhibitory, lipoxygenase inhibitory and platelet aggregation inhibitory activities (Table 3.4). As per the Traditional Chinese Medicine Database (TCMD), legumes, apart from having these functions, are also associated with ameliorating type 2 diabetes (Zhang *et al.*, 2008).

3.3 Processing of cereals and grains and its effect on the functional components

3.3.1 Rice

Rice processing involves primary processing activities such as cleaning and grading and secondary processing activities such as parboiling, dehusking/shelling and polishing. Germination is a vital process which also makes important nutritional changes in the grain.

In general, primary processing does not affect the functional components. However, processes such as germination, parboiling, milling and cooking have marked effects on the functional components in rice.

Germination Germination is a process in which some seed reserves are degraded and used for respiration and synthesis of new cell constituents for the developing embryo, thereby causing significant changes in the biochemical, nutritional and sensory characteristics of the cereal (López-Amorós *et al.*, 2006).

Apart from changing the level of nutrients, the biochemical activities occurring during germination can also generate bioactive components including antioxidants – such as ascorbic acid, tocopherols, tocotrienols and phenolic compounds – thus resulting in an increase of antioxidant activity (Frias *et al.*, 2005; Fernandez-Orozco *et al.*,

Table 3.4 Functional components present in legumes and their health benefits

Sl. no.	Functional component	Functional effects/health benefits	Reference
1	Phytochemicals Hydrophilic phytochemicals	Enhancement of the immune system functionality; reduced cancer risk	Cho *et al.*, 2007; Dillard and German, 2000
	Lipophilic phytochemicals	Prevent the risk of cardiovascular diseases and some eye pathologies	
2	Polyphenols flavonoid compounds	Enhances the antioxidant capacity of erythrocytes	Koren *et al.*, 2010
	– anthocyanins, quercetin glycosides and protoanthocyanidins	High antioxidant capacity	Beninger and Hosfield, 2003; Wu *et al.*, 2004
3	Lectins	Resistant to proteolysis in the gastrointestinal tract Agglutinating erythrocytes of some blood types in vitro	Sharon, 1998
		Anti-carcinogenic	González de Mejía and Prisecaru, 2005
4	Tocopherols α-TP	Main contributor to the vitamin E activity	Bramley *et al.*, 2000
	γ-TP	Highest antioxidant activity in food	Bramley *et al.*, 2000
		Decreasing platelet aggregation and delaying arterial thrombogenesis Functions in the detoxification of nitrogen dioxide and other reactive nitrogen species Protect against cardiovascular disease	Amarowicz and Pegg, 2008
5	Resistant starch (RS)	Produces an enhanced butyric acid, which is a very active biomolecule of therapeutic significance in preventing colon cancer Increases fecal bulking and lowers fecal ph preventing colon cancer	Phillips *et al.*, 1995; Scheppach *et al.*, 1988
6	Dietary fibre Insoluble fibre (cellulose, hemicelluloses and lignin)	Improves laxation, facilitates a low glycemic response, low serum cholesterol levels, and a decrease of colon cancer risk factors	Rodríguez *et al.*, 2006; Serrano and Goni, 2004
	Soluble fibre (oligosaccharides, pectins, b-glucans and galactomanan gums)	Helps to lower blood cholesterol and regulate blood glucose levels	

2008). New compounds, such as γ-amino butyric acid (GABA), γ-oryzanol and useful amino acids are synthesized during germination (Ang, 1991).

GABA in rice grains is synthesized from glutamic acid by glutamate decarboxylase (GAD), which shows high correlation with the germination ratio (Bautista *et al.*, 1964). Thus, GABA is an important biofunctional component responsible for decreasing blood pressure *in vivo* without affecting electrolyte metabolism or the activity of angiotensin-I-converting enzyme (Kohama *et al.*, 1987; Tsuji *et al.*, 1992;

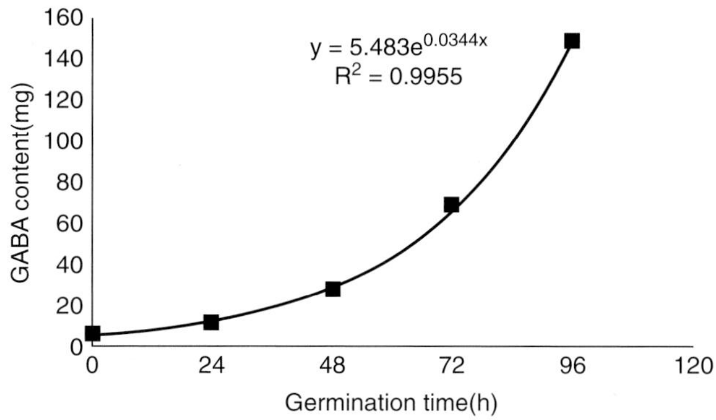

Figure 3.1 Variation of GABA content in brown rice with increasing germination time. *Source:* Data from Ohtsubo *et al.*, 2005. Reproduced with permission from Elsevier

Kushiro *et al.*, 1996). It can also lower hypertension and promote sleepiness (Okada *et al.*, 2000).

It has been reported that GABA content of brown rice increased during germination from an initial level of 6.04 mg to as high as 149.03 mg after 96 h (Ohtsubo *et al.*, 2005). The GABA content in brown rice showed an exponential growth with increasing germination time (Figure 3.1).

Germinated brown rice contains more insoluble dietary fibre (150%), total dietary fibre (145%), total ferulic acid (126%), soluble dietary fibre (120%) and inositol (112%) compared to the brown rice (Ohtsubo *et al.*, 2005). Also, there is an increase in the amount of crude protein (8%), linoleic acid (4.6%), GABA (107%) and vitamin E (22.4%) after germination, whereas there is a decrease in phytic acid (39%), oleic acid (7.8%) and palmitic acid (2.13%) after germination (Kim *et al.*, 2012).

Parboiling The parboiling process involves hydrothermal treatment steps consisting of soaking, steaming and drying the paddy before milling. The important functional components which are affected during parboiling are vitamin E and γ-oryzanol which suffer a loss of about 60 and 20%, respectively, compared to the initial level. Among the homologues of vitamin E, α-tocopherol was the most sensitive to parboiling and showed a loss of 93%, followed by γ-tocotrienol which reduced by approximately 60% (Pascual *et al.*, 2011).

Storage and cooking Storage of brown rice at room temperature ($25 \pm 5\,^{\circ}C$) causes a loss of 70% of tocols while parboiled rice showed a loss of 85%. Cooking causes a further loss of tocols and the final amounts were irrelevant in both cooked non-parboiled and parboiled rice (Pascual *et al.*, 2011). It has also been reported that different cooking conditions (different rice–water ratios) influence the retention of tocols in rice bran. A variable retention of total tocols from 1 to 59% was noted depending on the rice–water ratio used for cooking (Kumar *et al.*, 2006). The combined treatments, parboiling, a 6-month storage period and cooking, lead to a significant loss in the concentrations of total tocols in brown rice while only just over 10% of the original γ-tocotrienol content remained (Pascual *et al.*, 2011).

Storage of parboiled rice resulted in a loss of about 40% of γ-oryzanol content, whereas cooking caused almost no change in its level. Overall, vitamin E was far more affected than γ-oryzanol during parboiling, storage and cooking (Pascual *et al.*, 2011).

In contrast, it has been reported that cooking rice in excess water increased the level of tocols due to leaching of soluble dry matter (23%) during cooking. This was to loss of soluble solids as well as a release of bound tocols (Qureshi *et al.*, 2000; Finocchiaro *et al.*, 2007).

Milling Milling of cereal grains generally removes the bran and germ layers that are rich in fibre and phytochemicals, causing significant loss of these in the form of by-products including hulls and polish waste. These low-value fractions may be potential sources of functional components.

The tocol content of the fractions obtained from milling of cereal grains is important for determining the nutritional value of food products. Tocol content also depends on the level of supplementation as well as on the type of milling fraction of cereal grain used in product development. During milling, the tocol content of whole grain becomes concentrated in certain milling fractions such as bran and germ (Bramley *et al.*, 2000). The tocopherols (α-, β-, γ-, δ-) are concentrated mostly on the bran layer while the tocotrienols (α-, γ-) except β- are concentrated mostly on the germ layer (Tiwari and Cummins, 2009). During polishing of dehulled rice, a 71% reduction in tocol levels was reported, indicating the greater loss of tocopherols (Finocchiaro *et al.*, 2007). The loss of tocols increases with an increase in the degree of milling (Ha *et al.*, 2006).

3.3.2 Corn

The processing of corn for food is carried out at industrial as well as domestic levels. Industrial processing of corn involves one of the two milling techniques: dry-milling or wet-milling. Corn dry-milling involves milling clean, tempered grain (moisture content 200 g/kg) to separate components such as endosperm for use as corn grits, meals and flours, germ and bran for oil recovery (Burge and Duensing, 1989; Duensing *et al.*, 2003). Wet-milling of corn involves first steeping the grain in water to increase the moisture content up to about 450 g/kg followed by steeping in sulfur dioxide to soften the kernels and to help separate the components such as starch, gluten, fibre and germ (Johnson *et al.*, 2003). The products of wet-milling are the starch (endosperm) and oil (germ) from the corn kernel and the co-products are corn fibre, corn gluten and steeping solids (Johnson *et al.*, 2003).

In households, corn is processed in different ways around the world. Corn cobs with or without husks are boiled in water, steamed or cooked over a fire, flavoured with salt, cream, butter, margarine and sauces. A common feature of all these methods is cooking the grain by boiling, baking or frying. The temperatures and duration of cooking vary considerably. Corn grain is also steeped in alkaline (nixtamalization) or other aqueous environments and can be fermented for production of other foods (Rooney and Serna-Saldivar, 2003).

Though corn is consumed worldwide, white maize is generally preferred for foods in Asia, Latin America and Africa, while yellow maize is preferred in Brazil, China and Argentina and used in many traditional cuisines. In Latin America, corn is processed into tortillas, arepas, couscous, polenta, porridges and various meals and gruels. These are the basis for many traditional foods. In Africa and Asia, corn is generally milled into grits, meals and flours for production of flat breads, that is *roti*, corn bread, unfermented and fermented porridges, steamed foods (couscous, rice-like corn grits), snacks, popcorn and alcoholic and non-alcoholic beverages (Rooney and Serna-Saldivar, 2003).

To prepare traditional foods, corn kernel undergoes many processes such as milling, thermal processing, nixtamalization, baking and frying.

Milling During milling, the main functional components affected are the tocols. In cereal grains like corn, wheat, oats and barley, the tocols are mainly concentrated in the outer aleurone, subaleurone layer and germ (Ko *et al.*, 2003). Therefore, removal of the hulls, aleurone layer and germ during the milling process influences the level of tocols in the final milling products, including starchy endosperm and flour. The tocopherol and tocotrienol contents in the germ fraction of corn are respectively, 446.7 and 16.7 mg/kg. The tocopherol and tocotrienol contents in the hull fraction of corn are respectively, 5.9 and 44.4 mg/kg (Tiwari *et al.*, 2009).

Thermal processing Sweetcorn is generally processed by heat to increase its palatability. Thermal processing at 115 °C for 25 min significantly elevated the total antioxidant activity of sweetcorn by 44% and increased phytochemical content such as ferulic acid by 55% and total phenolics by 54%, although a 25% vitamin C loss was observed. Processed sweetcorn has an increased antioxidant activity equivalent to 210 mg of vitamin C/100 g of corn (Dewanto *et al.*, 2002).

Nixtamalization Food products such as tortillas, tortilla chips and corn chips are made from corn by nixtamalization (Serna-Saldivar *et al.*, 1990). This process involves alkaline/lime cooking, steeping, washing and stone-grinding of the kernels to produce masa/flour (Gomez *et al.*, 1992). Nixtamalization increases the calcium content, improves niacin bioavailability, removes most of the pericarp, and significantly reduces mycotoxins present in raw kernels (Serna-Saldivar *et al.*, 1990). The cooking liquor, called *nejayote*, is rich in solids including important phytochemicals. But these phytochemicals are lost during cooking due to leaching (Velazco-Martinez *et al.*, 1997). It has been reported that most anthocyanins and 50% of carotenoids were lost during lime-cooking by leaching into the steep solution or nejayote. Lime-cooking also significantly decreased the lutein content in high-carotenoid corns (de la Parra *et al.*, 2007).

Nixtamalized grains have a high concentration of free phenolics and soluble conjugated ferulic acid. The hydrophilic antioxidant activity of phenolics in the bound form, however, decreases after lime-cooking. The activity decreases approximately 30% in masa. High-carotenoid corn contained the highest antioxidant capacity (de la Parra *et al.*, 2007).

Baking and frying Table tortillas and fried tortilla chips are obtained from fresh masa or dry masa/flour. Corn masa is kneaded and moulded, then baked on a hot griddle to produce table tortillas. It is baked and fried again for making tortilla chips.

The main effects of tortilla baking and chip frying were on the bound phenolic content. Bound phenolics of tortillas and chips were approximately half of the total phenolic compound in the raw corn. The content of bound phenolics of chips was statistically lower ($p < 0.05$) than the bound phenolic content of the other nixtamalized products, masa and tortillas. The antioxidant activity for raw grains ranged from 41.5 ± 2.9 to 49.6 ± 4.40 μmol of vitamin C equiv/100 g. The values for masa, tortillas and chips varied from 68.0 to 114.1 μmol of vitamin C equiv/100 g. The hydrophilic antioxidant activity in the bound form decreased approximately 50% in tortilla chips, when compared to raw corn. This indicates that deep fat frying has the largest detrimental effect on antioxidant activity. Tortilla baking and tortilla chip frying also increase the amount of free and soluble conjugated ferulic acid in corn (de la Parra *et al.*, 2007).

3.3.3 Soybeans

Soybeans are processed to extract edible oil and the meal/cake by-products are used for animal feed. The process involves cleaning, drying the soybeans to 10–11% moisture at temperatures ranging from 71 to 79 °C, cracking and aspiration for hull removal followed by pulverizing. The pulverized pieces are then flaked using smooth rolls to increase surface area and facilitate solvent extraction of soybean oil. The solvent is removed from the soybean flakes by steaming, which toasts the defatted meal to inactivate trypsin inhibitors and lectin antinutrients and to denature other soy proteins (Hettiarachchy and Kalapathy, 1999). After oil extraction, the defatted soy flakes can be further processed into soybean meal for animal feed, ground to produce soy flour, sized to produce soy grits or texturized to produce textured vegetable protein (TVP) for human food uses. Further processing can produce high protein food ingredients such as soy protein concentrates and isolated soy protein. These ingredients have functional and nutritional applications in various types of bakery, dairy and meat products, infant formulas and other soy foods (Hammond and Jez, 2011).

In Asian countries, soybeans are processed into fermented (soy sauce, miso, natto, yogurts and sufu) and non-fermented products (kinako, edamame, soy sprouts, protein crisp, desserts, baby food, and soy milk which is further processed into tofu, aburage, yuba, etc.). Roasted whole soybeans and their flour are used as ingredients for traditional confectionery products and snacks in China, Japan, Korea and Indonesia. These soy products are used in soy and tofu burgers, soy sausages and chicken nuggets, soy ice cream, yoghurt and numerous other products (Liu, 2004a, 2004b; Golbitz, 1995).

To produce these products, soybeans undergo various processing operations such as thermal treatment, drying, fermentation and hydrogenation.

Thermal processing Thermal processing and cooking conditions affect the content and profile of phenolic compounds in soy foods (Bressani and Elias, 1980; Davies *et al.*, 1998; Xu and Chang, 2008a). On average, about 30–60% of phenolic compounds are eliminated during soybean cooking depending on the seed colour. Heating decreases the total content of phenolic acids to 32.1–67.3% in yellow soybeans seeds and to 24.9–64.5% in black soybeans seeds (Bressani and Elias, 1980; Xu and Chang, 2008a).

During soy food production, isoflavone profiles are altered by thermal processing conditions, but the total isoflavone content does not change if there was no mass loss (Wang and Murphy, 1996). It has ben reported that baking or frying of TVP made of soy at 190 °C and baking of soy flour in cookies did not alter the total isoflavone content (Coward *et al.*, 1998).

Steaming converts more malonyl-β-glucosides in soy to β-glucosides than dry heat treatment methods, which convert only limited amounts of malonyl-β-glucosides to acetyl-β-glucosides (Coward *et al.*, 1998; Mathias *et al.*, 2006). These β-glucosides are required to hydrolyse isoflavones in soy and increase their bioavailability. Continuous steaming helps to diminish the characteristic beany flavour of raw soy products due to the volatilization of monocarbonyl compounds resulting from oxidation of fatty acids by the enzyme lipoxygenase. However, excessive heating destroys certain amino acids that are sensitive to heat such as lysine, with possible losses of more than 50% (Winarno and Karyadi, 1976).

Drying Drying soybeans at temperatures ranging from 50 to 150 °C decreases the total isoflavones (TI) in all cases. Higher drying temperatures (130 and 150 °C) lead to a significant decrease of TI in soybean (from 8.186 to 7.544 μmol/g dry soybean). However, lower drying temperatures (50 and 70 °C) do not significantly decrease TI (from 8.186 to 8.009 μmol/g dry soybean). The content of aglycones increases with increasing drying temperature from 50 to 130 °C (Niamnuy *et al.*, 2011).

Drying of soybean at temperatures ranging from 50 °C to 150 °C increases the 1,1-diphenyl-2-picrylhydrazyl radicals (DPPH) radical scavenging capacity from 11.67 to 17.02 lM Trolox/g dry sample and ferric reducing antioxidant power (FRAP) from 66.70 to 113.54 lM FeSO4/g dry sample. Thus, the antioxidant activity increases with an increase in the drying temperature (Niamnuy *et al.*, 2011).

It is known that inhibition of α-glucosidase helps delay the process of carbohydrate digestion and blocks the uptake of postprandial blood glucose (Shinde *et al.*, 2008). Isoflavones in the form of aglycones have been recommended for diabetic patients as these compounds have been identified as a potent α-glucosidase inhibitors (Chen *et al.*, 2007). Raw soybean and soybean dried at lower drying temperatures (50 and 70 °C) do not show α-glucosidase inhibitory ability because of an inadequate amount of α-glucosidase inhibitor. Soybean dried at 130 °C possesses the highest α-glucosidase inhibitory activity (7.73 mg acarbose/g dry sample), followed by beans dried at 150 °C (3.68 mg acarbose/g dry sample) (Niamnuy *et al.*, 2011).

Fermentation Fermented soybean products include miso (in Japan), sufu (in China), and tempeh (in Indonesia) (Chang *et al.*, 2007). During the fermentation of soybean by fungi, isoflavone glycosides are hydrolysed to release free isoflavone aglycone by fungal-β-glucosidase and therefore adding health benefits to fermented soybean products (Chiou and Cheng, 2001). Many studies have revealed that isoflavone aglycones are far superior to isoflavone glycosides in various bioactivities due to their effective absorption (Izumi *et al.*, 2000; Kawakami *et al.*, 2005; Nielsen and Williamson, 2007; Walsh *et al.*, 2007).

Fermented soy germ extracts exhibit a higher inhibition effect against the superoxide anion radical and lesser but significant ferric-reducing and DPPH radical scavenging effects compared to raw soy germ (Hubert *et al.*, 2008). When compared to the traditional whole seed-based products, fermented soy germ exhibits higher levels of phytochemicals like isoflavones, saponins, phytosterols and tocopherols which contribute to the antioxidant capacity of soy germ thereby providing a good scope for fermented soy to be used as a functional food.

Hydrogenation Hydrogenation is generally applied to solidify the oil. The partial selective hydrogenation of soybean oil reduces the linolenic acid content of the oil while leaving a high concentration of linoleic acid. Linolenic acid content was reduced because it causes many organoleptic problems. The hydrogenation process and particularly the formation of trans fatty acids has led to an increase in serum cholesterol concentrations whereas linoleic acid in its regular state in oil is associated with a reduced serum cholesterol concentration (Grundy, 1990; Simopoulos, 2002).

3.3.4 Legumes

Legumes are processed to increase their digestibility, to improve palatability, to enhance aroma, sensory qualities, nutritional attributes and to increase the bioavailability of nutrients (Tharanathan and Mahadevamma, 2003). Legumes are generally processed by various methods such as milling to produce *dhal*, heat processing methods to produce snack foods, dehydration and grinding to produce flour to be used in different food preparations, or as germinated grains by soaking (Kurien, 1981).

Germination Germination causes changes in the nutrients, including functional components, through aerobic respiration and biochemical metabolism. Sprouting also removes antinutrients such as enzyme inhibitors in the seeds, thus making sprouts safe for the diet (Mwikya *et al.*, 2001). It has also been reported that the vitamin content of legumes increases considerably when they germinate (Vijayaraghavan, 1981 cited by Tharanathan and Mahadevamma, 2003).

Antioxidative compounds, such as total phenolics and total flavonoids of legumes with have dark seed coats significantly decrease after short-term germination at 25 °C for 1 day. This is because the seed coats lose pigments when the seeds are soaked and germinated. However, antioxidative compounds increase after long-term germination at 25 °C for 4 days (Lin and Lai, 2006).

Soaking Soaking selected legumes for 24 hours in water reduces the total phenolic content by about 2–12% in pea and chickpea and about 9–38% in lentil. DPPH free-radical scavenging capacities are reduced by about 9–18% in green pea, 6–14% in yellow pea, 10–35% in chickpea and about 8–10% in lentil after soaking by removing soaking water. Oxygen radical absorbance capacity is decreased by 43–59% in green pea, 18–52% in yellow pea, 4–33% in chickpea and about 24–70% in lentil (Xu and Chang, 2008b).

The soaking process also has marked effects on total dietary fibre. However, the effect on the insoluble and soluble fractions varies significantly (Aguilera *et al.*, 2009). Soaking caused a 10% reduction in the insoluble dietary fibre (IDF) fraction in pink mottled cream beans when compared to raw samples. The soluble fraction of total dietary fibre in all soaked legumes increased compared to raw forms, by 33% in chickpea, 18% in pink-mottled cream bean and 13% in white bean (Xu and Chang, 2008b).

Thermal processing Many legumes contain toxic and antinutritional factors such as protease inhibitors, haemagglutinins and growth inhibitors, which are either partially or completely eliminated by different methods of heat processing (Swaminathan, 1974). This also improves flavour, nutritional quality and overall acceptability of the foods prepared using the legumes. Roasting, parching, toasting and frying are some of the dry heat processing methods used for whole legume seeds while boiling, cooking and steaming are the common wet heat processing methods. Legumes processed by dry heat processing are eaten as snack foods, for example fried ground nuts, roasted chickpeas, bengal gram dhal and green gram dhal deep-fat-fried with mixtures of spice and salt added, and fried bean cakes made from fried ground legume paste. (Tharanathan and Mahadevamma, 2003).

Boiling Boiling reduces the free radical scavenging capacities of food legumes to about 60–70% in green pea, 50–60% in yellow pea, 85–95% in chickpea and 9–30% in lentil. Pressure boiling causes more loss in free radical scavenging capacities (about 26–30%) than regular boiling (8– 10%) in lentil. Oxygen radical absorbance capacities of regular boiled legumes are reduced by 58–77% in green pea, 53–58% in yellow pea, 56–69% in chickpea and 54–62% in lentil (Xu and Chang, 2008b). The oxygen radical absorbance capacities of pressure boiled (34.47 to 103.42 kPa) legumes are increased by about 27–114% in green pea, 12–67% in yellow pea, 25–40% in chickpea as compared to respective raw legume after. However, oxygen radical absorbance capacities are decreased by about 11–16% in lentil after pressure boiling (Xu and Chang, 2008b).

Soaking and cooking During cooking, about 30–40% of phenolics are removed from common beans (Bressani and Elias, 1980), 40–50% from green pea, yellow pea and chickpea, and 50–68% from lentil by leaching into the cooking water. Pressure cooking leads to more loss of the total phenolic content (about 68%) than regular cooking (about 50–56%) in lentil (Xu and Chang, 2008b).

Cooking of selected legumes after soaking causes a significant increase of total dietary fibre, that is 17% in chickpea, 12% in pink mottled cream bean and 10% in white bean (Aguilera *et al.*, 2009). The formation of resistant starch from amylose–lipid complexes and Maillard-reaction products during cooking has been described as a factor contributing to observed increase in dietary fibre (Su and Chang, 1995).

Cooking of legume seeds causes a significant decrease in ash contents (by 11–48%), polyphenols (by 10–70%) and protein (to 19%) in the flours made from legumes. Cooking also causes losses of resistant starch (by 61–71%) and slowly digestible starch (by 56–84%) in legume flours (Piecyk *et al.*, 2012).

Steaming After steaming in an atmospheric steam cooker for 15 min, the free radical scavenging capacities of food legumes were reduced by 51–67% in green pea,

49–67% in yellow pea, 33–83% in chickpea and 14–26% in lentil. The loss of DPPH was partly due to soluble antioxidants in leached water and the heat effect (Xu and Chang, 2008b).

Similarly, oxygen radical absorbance capacity of regular steamed legumes was reduced by 2.7% in green pea, 8.9% in yellow pea, 7.3% in chickpea and 1.4% in lentil by removing soaking and steaming water. But after pressure steaming (34.47 to 103.42 kPa), oxygen radical absorbance capacities were increased by 69–175% in green pea, 99–153% in yellow pea, 84–122% in chickpea and 5–13% in lentil compared to respective original unprocessed legumes (Xu and Chang, 2008b).

Dehydration Raffinose family oligosaccharides are the main compounds in legumes causing flatulence. Dehydration at 75 $\pm$ 3 °C for 6 h in a forced-air tunnel produces significant reductions of these soluble compounds: 76% for white bean, 57% for chickpea and 41% for pink-mottled cream bean. Therefore, dehydration is an efficient process to reduce flatulence compounds, and legume flours can be proposed as functional ingredients for their beneficial health effects (Aguilera *et al.*, 2009).

3.4 Conclusion

A continuously increasing demand for health-promoting food is expected as consumers become more aware and interested in the relationship between dietary intake of beneficial foods and health. Serving functional food in the correct quantities has proven to promote health and reduce the risk of various diseases. In general, cereals and grains often carry the whole complement of functional components. Currently, inclusion of these functional components into specialty food products has been in the forefront of research and development. Further, the optimal dietary intake of functional food components required to provide maximal protection against various diseases needs to be determined, as for other nutrients. Even though some of the raw materials are rich in functional components, part of these components are often lost during processing. However, some functional components are increased during processing to develop palatable functional foods. This warrants a thorough understanding of the effect of processing on the functional components as well as their bioavailability. Currently, knowledge of these topics is limited and so much more research needs to be done. Therefore, the information presented in this chapter will be useful in formulating special diets for preventing particular diseases and promoting health.

Also, different functional components in diets may have similar biological effects or a single compound may elicit different biological responses. The overall effect of these components in a diet composed of different cereals and grains can be additive and may often be synergistic so they need to be taken into account when formulating special diets with cereals and grains. Future research in this area could evaluate the interaction between different functional components in different cereal grains when they are formulated into special diets, their combined action in the diet and ultimately their health implications. Efforts could also be invested in developing processing methods that positively contribute to preserve or enhance the functional components of the foodstuffs.

References

Adom, K.K. and Liu, R.H. (2002). Antioxidant activity of grains, *Journal of Agricultural and Food Chemistry*, 50 (21), 6182–6187.

Aguilar-Garcia, C., Gavino, G., Baragaño-Mosqueda, B., Hevia, P. and Gavino, V.C. (2007). Correlation of tocopherol, tocotrienol, Gamma-oryzanol and total polyphenol content in rice bran with different antioxidant capacity assays. *Food Chemistry*, 102 (4), 1228–1232.

Aguilera, Y., Martin-Cabrejas, M.A., Benıtez, V. *et al.* (2009). Changes in carbohydrate fraction during dehydration process of common legumes. *Journal of Food Composition and Analysis*, 22, 678–683.

Amarowicz, R. and Pegg, R.B. (2008). Legumes as a source of natural antioxidants. *European Journal of Lipid Science and Technology*, 110 (10), 865–878.

Ang, J.F. (1991). Water retention capacity and viscosity effect of powdered cellulose. *Journal of Food Science*, 56, 1682–1684.

Babcock, D. (1987). Rice bran as a source of dietary fibre. *Cereal Foods World*, 32, 538–540.

Bautista, G.M., Lugay, J.C., Lourades, J., Cruz, J. and Juliano, B.O. (1964). Glutamic acid decarboxylase activity as viability of artificially dried and stored rice. *Cereal Chemistry*, 41, 188–191.

Bazzano, L.A., He, J., Ogden, L.G. *et al.* (2002). Fruit and vegetable intake and risk of cardiovascular disease in US adults: The first National Health and Nutrition Examination Survey Epidemiologic Followup Study. *American Journal of Clinical Nutrition*, 76 (1), 93–99.

Beninger, C.W. and Hosfield, G.L. (2003). Antioxidant activity of extracts, condensed tannin fractions, and pure flavonoids from *Phaseolus vulgaris* L. seed coat color genotypes. *Journal of Agricultural and Food Chemistry*, 51 (27), 7879–7883.

Bramley, P.M., Elmadfa, I., Kafatos, A. *et al.* (2000). Vitamin E (review). *Journal of Science and Food Agriculture*, 80, 913–938.

Bressani, A. and Elias, L.G. (1980). The nutritional role of polyphenols in beans. Proceedings of the Symposium on Polyphenols in Cereal and Legumes (ed. J.H. Hulse),10–13 June 1979, St. Louis Missouri, USA. International Development Research Center, Ottawa, Canada, pp. 61–68.

Burge, R.M. and Duensing, W.J. (1989). Processing and dietary fibre ingredient application of cereal bran. *Cereal Foods World*, 34 (535), 537–538.

Canabate-Díaz, B., Segura Carretero, A., Fernández-Gutiérrez, A., Belmonte Vega, A., Garrido Frenich, A., Martínez Vidal, J. L., *et al.* (2007). Separation and determination of sterols in olive oil by HPLC–MS. *Food Chemistry*, 102, 593–598.

Chang, T.-S., Ding, H.-Y., Tai, S. S.-K. and Wu, C.-Y. (2007). Metabolism of the soy isoflavones daidzein and genistein by fungi used in the preparation of various fermented soybean foods. *Bioscience, Biotechnology and Biochemistry*, 71 (5), 1330–1333.

Charalampopoulos, D., Wang, R., Pandiella, S.S. and Webb, C. (2002). Application of cereals and cereal components in functional foods: a review. *International Journal of Food Microbiology*, 79 (1), 131–141.

Chaturvedi, N., Sharma, P., Shukla, K., Singh, R. and Yadav, S. (2011). Cereals nutraceuticals, health ennoblement and diseases obviation: A comprehensive review. *Journal of Applied Pharmaceutical Science*, 1 (7), 6–12.

Chen, J., Cheng, Y.-Q., Yamaki, K. and Li, L.-T. (2007). Anti-a-glucosidase activity of Chinese traditionally fermented soybean (douchi). *Food Chemistry*, 103, 1091–1096.

Chiang, A.N., Wu, H.L., Yeh, H.I. *et al.* (2006). Antioxidant effects of black rice extract through the induction of superoxide dismutase and catalase activities. *Lipids*, 41 (8), 797–803.

Chiou, R.Y. and Cheng, S.L. (2001). Isoflavone transformation during soybean koji preparation and subsequent miso fermentation supplemented with ethanol and NaCl. *Journal of Agricultural and Food Chemistry*, 49 (8), 3656–3660.

Hubert, J., Berger, M. and Dayde, J. (2005). Use of a simplified HPLC-UV analysis for Soyasaponin B determination: Study of saponin and isoflavone variability in soybean cultivars and in soy-based health food products. *Journal of Agricultural and Food Chemistry*, 53 (10), 3923–3930.

Hubert, J., Berger, M., Nepveu, F., Paul, F. and Daydé, J. (2008). Effects of fermentation on the phytochemical composition and antioxidant properties of soy germ. *Food Chemistry*, 109 (4), 709–721.

Hunter, J.E., Zhang, J. and Kris-Etherton, P.M. (2010). Cardiovascular disease risk of dietary stearic acid compared with trans, other saturated, and unsaturated fatty acids: a systematic review. *The American Journal of Clinical Nutrition*, 91 (1), 46–63.

Inglett, G.E. and Carriere, C.J. (2001). Cellulosic fibre gels prepared from cell walls of maize hulls. *Cereal Chemistry*, 78, 471–475.

Inglett, G.E. (1997). Development of a dietary fibre gel for calorie-reduced foods. *Cereal Foods World* 42, 382–384.

Inglett, G.E. (1998). Dietary fibre gels for calorie reduced foods and method for preparing the same. US Patent 5766662.

Izumi, T., Piskula, M.K., Osawa, S. *et al.* (2000). Soy isoflavone aglycones are absorbed faster and in higher amounts than their glucosides in humans. *The Journal of Nutrition*, 130 (7), 1695–1699.

Jain, D., Ebine, N., Jia, X. *et al.* (2008). Corn fibre oil and sitostanol decrease cholesterol absorption independently of intestinal sterol transporters in hamsters. *Journal of Nutritional Biochemistry*, 19, 229–236.

Jiamyangyuen, S., Srijesdaruk, V. and Harper, W.J. (2005). Extraction of rice bran protein concentrate and its application in bread. *Songklanakarin Journal of Science and Technology*, 27 (1), 55–64.

Johnson, L.A., May, J.B. and White, P.J. (2003).Wet milling: the basis for corn biorefineries, in *Corn: Chemistry and Technology*, 2nd edn (eds P.L. White and L.A. Johnson). American Association of Cereal Chemists, St Paul, MN, pp. 449–494.

Ju, Z.Y., Hettiartachchy, N.S. and Bath, N. (2001). Extraction, denaturation and hydrophobic properties of rice flour proteins. *Journal of Food Science*, 66, 229–232.

Karoon, P.A., Faulds, C.B., Ryden, P., Robertson, J.S. and Williamson, G. (1997). Release of covalently bound ferulic acid from fibre in human colon. *Journal of Agricultural and Food Chemistry*, 45, 661–667.

Kawakami, Y., Tsurugasaki, W., Nakamura, S. and Osada, K. (2005). Comparison of regulative functions between dietary soy isoflavones aglycone and glucoside on lipid metabolism in rats fed cholesterol. *The Journal of Nutritional Biochemistry*, 16 (4), 205–212.

Khuwijitjaru, P., Nualchan, P. and Adachi, S. (2007). Foaming and emulsifying properties of rice bran extracts obtained by subcritical water treatment. *Silpakorn University Science and Technology Journal*, 1 (1), 7–12.

Kim, H.Y., Hwang, I.G., Kim, T.M. *et al.* (2012). Chemical and functional components in different parts of rough rice (*Oryza sativa* L.) before and after germination. *Food Chemistry*, 134, 288–293.

Ko, S.-N., Kim, C.-J., Kim, H. *et al.* (2003). Tocol levels in milling fractions of some cereal grains and soybean. *Journal of the American Oil Chemists' Society*, 80 (6), 585–589.

Kohama, Y., Matsumoto, S., Mimura, T. *et al.* (1987). Isolation and identification of hypotensive principles in red-mold rice. *Chemical and Pharmaceutical Bulletin*, 35, 2484–2489.

Komiyama, K., Hayashi, M., Cha, S. and Yamaoka, M. (1992). Antitumor and antioxidant activity of tocotrienols, in *Lipid Soluble Antioxidants: Biochemistry and Clinical Applications* (eds S.H. Ong and L. Packer). BirkhauserVerlag, Basel, Switzerland, pp. 1159–1542.

Koren, E., Kohen, R., Ginsburg, I. (2010). Polyphenols enhance total oxidant scavenging capacities of human blood by binding to RBC. *Experimental Biology and Medicine*, 235, 689–699.

Kumar, H.G.A., Khatoon, S., Prabhakar, D.S. and Krishna, A.G.G. (2006). Effect of cooking of rice bran on the quality of extracted oil. *Journal of Food Lipids*, 13, 341–353.

Kurien, P.P. (1981). Processing of pulses. *Proceedings of the Workshop on Grain Legumes* (eds A.S. Aiyer and K.R. Iyer). Protein Foods and Nutrition Development Association of India, Bombay, pp. 68–77.

Kurilich, A.C. and Juvik, J.A. (1999). Quantification of carotenoids and tocopherol antioxidants in *Zea mays*. *Journal of Agricultural and Food Chemistry*, 47 (5), 1948–1955.

Kushiro, T., Hashida, J., Kawamura, H. *et al.* (1996). Clinical effects of beni-koji in mild essential hypertension-a multi-center double-blind comparison with placebo. *Nippon Jinzo Gakkai Shi*, 38, 625–633.

Kuzuhara, H., Nishiyama, S., Minowa, N., Sasaki, K. and Omoto, S. (2000). Protective effects of soyasapogenol A on liver injury mediated by immune response in a concanavalin A-induced hepatitis model. *European Journal of Pharmacology*, 391 (1–2), 175–181.

Lapp, J. and Hansen, B. (2013). 'Who Benefits From the Mystery Fat Substitute Z Trim?' http://www.aaanet.org/press/an/0507/lapp-hansen.html [accessed 19 July 2013].

Law, M.R. (2000). Plant sterol and stanol margarines and health. *British Medical Journal.*, 320 (7238), 861–864.

Lee, D.S. and Lee, S.H. (2001). Genistin, a soy isoflavone, is a potent a-glucosidase inhibitor. *FEBS Letters*, 501, 84–86.

Lin, P.Y. and Lai, H.M. (2006). Bioactive compounds in legumes and their germinated products. *Journal of Agricultural and Food Chemistry*, 54 (11), 3807–3814.

Liu, K. (2004a). Edible soybean products in the current market, in *Soybeans as Functional Foods and Ingredients* (ed. K. Liu). AOCS Press, pp. 23–51.

Liu, K. (2004b). Soy sauce as natural seasoning. In *Soybeans as Functional Foods and Ingredients* (ed. K. Liu). AOCS Press, pp. 248–263.

Liu, K.S. (1999). Chemistry and nutritional value of soybean components. In *Soybeans: Chemistry, Technology and Utilization*. Aspen Publ. Inc., Gaithersburg, MD, pp. 25–113.

Lönnerdal, B. (2009). Soybean ferritin: implications for iron status of vegetarians. *The American Journal of Clinical Nutrition*, 89 (5), 1680S–1685S.

López-Amorós, M.L., Hernandez, T. and Estrella, I. (2006). Effect of germination on legume phenolic compounds and their antioxidant activity. *Journal of Food Composition and Analysis*, 19, 277–283.

Mathias, K., Ismail, B., Corvalan, C.M. and Hayes, K.D. (2006). Heat and pH effects on the conjugated forms of genistin and daidzin isoflavones. *Journal of Agricultural and Food Chemistry*, 54, 7495–7502.

Matthews, D.M. (1977). Memorial lecture: protein absorption – then and now. *Gastroenterology*, 73 (6), 1267.

Mazza, G. (1998). *Functional Foods: Biochemical and Processing Aspects*. Technomic Publishing Company, Inc., Lancaster, PA, pp. 71–89.

Mellon, J.E. and Moreau, R.A. (2004). Inhibition of aflatoxin biosynthesis in *Aspergillus flavus* by diferuloylputrescine and *p*-coumaroylferuloylputrescine. *Journal of Agricultural and Food Chemistry*, 52, 6660–6663.

Messina, M.J. (1999). Legumes and soybeans: overview of their nutritional profiles and health effects. *American Journal of Clinical Nutrition*, 70 (3), 439s–450s.

Moreau, R.A. and Hicks, K.B. (2006). Reinvestigation of the effect of heat pretreatment of corn fibre and corn germ on the levels of extractable tocopherols and tocotrienols. *Journal of Agricultural and Food Chemistry*, 54 (21), 8093–8102.

Moreau, R.A., Singh, V., Eckhoff, S.R. *et al.* (1999). Comparison of yield and composition of oil extracted from corn fibre and corn bran. *Cereal Chemistry*, 76, 449–451.

Moreno-Aliaga, M.J., Lorente-Cebrián, S. and Martínez, J.A. (2010). Regulation of adipokine secretion by *n*-3 fatty acids. *The Proceedings of the Nutrition Society*, 69 (3), 324–332.

Mozaffarieh, M., Sacu, S. and Wedrich, A. (2003). The role of the carotenoids, lutein and zeaxanthin, in protecting against age-related macular degeneration: a review based on controversial evidence. *Nutrition Journal*, 2 (1), 20–28.

Mwikya, S.M., Camp, J.V., Rodriguez, R. and Huyghebaert, A. (2001). Effects of sprouting on nutrient and antinutrient composition of kidney beans (*Phaseolus vulgaris* var. Rose coco). *European Food Research and Technology*, 212 (2), 188–191.

Nair, V.D.P., Kanfer, I. and Hoogmartens, J. (2006). Determination of stigmasterol, bsitosterol and stigmastanol in oral dosage forms using high performance liquid chromatography with evaporative light scattering detection. *Journal Pharmaceutical and Biomedical Analysis*, 41, 731–737.

Niamnuy, C., Nachaisin, M., Laohavanich, J. and Devahastin, S. (2011). Evaluation of bioactive compounds and bioactivities of soybean dried by different methods and conditions. *Food Chemistry*, 129 (3), 899–906.

Niki, E. and Noguchi, N. (2004). Dynamics of antioxidant action of vitamin E. *Accounts of Chemical Research*, 37 (1), 45–51.

Nielsen, I.L.F. and Williamson, G. (2007). Review of the factors affecting bioavailability of soy isoflavones in humans. *Nutrition and Cancer*, 57 (1), 1–10.

Niwa, T., Doi, U. and Osawa, T., (2003). Inhibitory activity of corn-derived bisamide compounds against a-glucosidase. *Journal of Agricultural and Food Chemistry*, 51, 90–94.

Norton, R. (1995). Quantitation of steryl ferulate and *p*-coumarate esters from corn and rice. *Lipids* 30, 269–274.

Nothlings, U., Murphy, S.P., Wilkens, L.R., Henderson, B.E. and Kolonel, L.N. (2007). Flavonols and pancreatic cancer risk the multiethnic cohort study. *American Journal of Epidemiology*, 166 (8), 924–931.

Oakenfull, D.G., Topping, D.L., Illman, R.J. and Fenwick, D.E. (1984). Prevention of dietary hypercholesterolemia in the rat by soya bean and Quillaja saponins. *Nutrition Reports International*, 29, 1039–1046.

Ogawa, K., Takeuchi, M. and Nakamura, N., (2005). Immonological effects of partially hydrolyzed arabinoxylan from corn husk in mice. *Bioscience, Biotechnology and Biochemistry*, 69, 19–25.

Ohta, T., Yamasaki, S., Egashira, Y. and Sanada, H. (1994). Antioxidative activity of corn bran hemicellulose fragments. *Journal of Agricultural and Food Chemistry*, 42, 653–656.

Ohtsubo, K., Suzuki, K., Yasui, Y. and Kasumi, T. (2005). Bio-functional components in the processed pre-germinated brown rice by a twin-screw extruder. *Journal of Food Composition and Analysis*, 18, 303–316.

Okada, T., Sugishita, T., Murakami, T. *et al.* (2000). Effect of the defatted rice germ enriched with GABA for sleeplessness, depression, autonomic disorder by oral administration. *Nippon Shokuhin Kagaku Kogaku Kaishi=Journal of the Japanese Society for Food Science and Technology*, 47 (8), 596–603.

Park, H.J., Chinnan, M.S. and Shewfelt, R.L. (1994). Edible corn-zein film coating to extend storage life of tomatoes. *Journal of Food Processing and Preservation*, 18 (4), 317–331.

de la Parra, C., Saldivar, S.O.S. and Liu, R.H. (2007). Effect of processing on the phytochemical profiles and antioxidant activity of corn for production of masa, tortillas, and tortilla chips. *Journal of Agricultural and Food Chemistry*, 55 (10), 4177–4183.

Parrado, J., Miramontes, E., Jover, M. *et al.* (2006). Preparation of a rice bran enzymatic extract with potential use as functional food. *Food Chemistry*, 98, 742–748.

Pascual, C.D.S.C.I., Massaretto, I.L., Kawassaki, F. *et al.* (2011). Effects of parboiling, storage and cooking on the levels of tocopherols, tocotrienols and γ-oryzanol in brown rice (*Oryza sativa* L.). *Food Research International*. doi:10.1016/j.foodres.2011.07.013.

Paulis, J.W., Bietz, J.A. and Wall, J.S. (1975). Corn protein subunits. Molecular weights determined by sodium dodecyl sulfate-polyacrylamide gel electrophoresis. *Journal of Agricultural and Food Chemistry*, 23 (2), 197–201.

Phillips, J., Muir, J.G., Birkett, A. *et al.* (1995). Effect of resistant starch on faecal bulk and fermentation dependent events in humans. *American Journal of Clinical Nutrition*, 62, 121–130.

Piecyk, M., Wołosiak, R., Druzynska, B. and Worobiej, E. (2012). Chemical composition and starch digestibility in flours from Polish processed legume seeds. *Food Chemistry*, 135, 1057–1064.

Písaříková, B. and Zralý, Z. (2010). Dietary fibre content in lupine (*Lupinus albus* L.) and soya (*Glycine max* L.) seeds. *Acta Veterinaria Brno*, 79 (2), 211–216.

Prakash, J. and Ramaswamy, H.S. (1996). Rice bran proteins: properties and food uses. *Critical Reviews in Food Science and Nutrition*, 36 (6), 537–552.

Qureshi, A.A., Huanbiao, M., Packer, L. and Peterson, D.M. (2000). Isolation and identification of novel tocotrienols from rice bran with hypocholesterolemic, antioxidant, and antitumor properties. *Journal of Agricultural and Food Chemistry*, 48 (8), 3130–3140.

Qureshi, A.A., Sami, S.A., Salser, W.A. and Khan, F.A. (2001). Synergistic effect of tocotrienol-rich fraction (TRF25) of rice bran and lovastatin on lipid parameters in hypercholesterolemic humans. *Journal of Nutritional Biochemistry*, 12, 318–329.

Rafi, M.M., Shafaia, Y. (2007). Dietary lutein modulates inducible nitric oxide synthase (iNOS) gene and protein expression in mouse macrophage cells (RAW 264.7). *Molecular Nutrition & Food Research*, 51, 333–340.

Ramjiganesh, R.S.T., Freake, H.C., McIntyre, J.C. and Fernandez, M.L. (2002). Corn fibre oil lowers plasma cholesterol by altering hepatic cholesterol metabolism and up-regulating LDL receptors in guinea pigs. The *Journal of Nutrition*, 132, 335–340.

Roberfroid, M.B. (2000). Global view on functional foods: European perspectives. *British Journal of Nutrition*, 88 (2), S133–S138.

Rodríguez, R., Jiménez, A., Fernández-Bolaños, J., Guillén, R. and Heredia, A. (2006). Dietary fibre from vegetable products as a source of functional ingredients. *Trends in Food Science and Technology*, 17, 3–15.

Rogers, E.J., Rice, S.M., Nicolosi, R.J. *et al.* (1993). Identification and quantitation of γ-oryzanol components and simultaneous assessment of tocols in rice bran oil. *Journal of the American Oil Chemists' Society*, 70 (3), 301–307.

Rong, N., Ausman, L.M. and Nicolosi, R.J. (1997). Oryzanol decreases cholesterol absorption and aortic fatty streaks in hamsters. *Lipids*, 32, 303–309.

Rooney, L.W. and Serna-Saldivar, S.O. (2003). Food use of whole corn and dry-milled fractions, in *Corn Chemistry and Technology*, 2nd edn, Chapter 13 (eds P.J. While and L.A. Johnson). American Association of Cereal Chemists, Inc., St. Paul, MN, pp. 495–535.

Rose, D.J., Inglett, G.E. and Liu, S.X. (2010). Utilisation of corn (*Zea mays*) bran and corn fiber in the production of food components. *Journal of the Science of Food and Agriculture*, 90 (6), 915–924.

Saikia, D. and Deka, S.C. (2011).Cereals: from staple food to nutraceuticals. *International Food Research Journal*, 18: 21–30

Santos, R., Limas, E., Sousa, M., *et al.* (2007). Optimization of analytical procedures for GC–MS determination of phytosterols and phytostanols in enriched milk and yoghurt. *Food Chemistry*, 102, 113–117.

Sosulski, F.W. and Dabrowski, K.J. (1984). Composition of free andhydrolyzable phenolic acids in the flours and hulls of 10 legume species. *Journal of Agricultural and Food Chemistry*, 32 (1), 131–133.

Scheppach, W., Fabian, C., Sachs, M. and Kasper, H. (1988). The effect of starch malabsorption on faecal short chain fatty acids excretion in man. *Scandinavian Journal of Gasteroenterology*, 23, 755–759.

Serna-Saldivar, S.O., Gomez, M.H. and Rooney, L.W. (1990). Technology, chemistry and nutritive value of alkaline cooked corn products, in *Advances in Cereal Science and Technology*, Vol. 10 (ed. Y. Pomeranz). American Association of Cereal Chemists, St. Paul, MN, pp. 243–295.

Serrano, J. and Goni, I. (2004). Role of black bean *Phaseolus vulgaris* on the nutritional status of Guatemalan population. *Archivos latinoamericanos de nutrición*, 54 (1), 36–44.

Shahidi, F. (2009). Nutraceuticals and functional foods: whole versus processed foods. *Trends in Food Science and Technology*, 20 (9), 376–387.

Sharon, N. (1998). Glycoproteins now and then: A personal account. *Acta Anatomica Basel*, 161 (1–4), 7–17.

Shinde, J., Taldone, T., Barletta, M. *et al.* (2008). α-Glucosidase inhibitory activity of *Syzygium cumini* (Linn.) Skeels seed kernel *in vitro* and in Goto-Kakizaki (GK) rats. *Carbohydrate Research*, 343, 1278–1281.

Simopoulos, A.P. (2002). The importance of the ratio of omega-6/omega-3 essential fatty acids. *Biomedicine and Pharmacotherapy*, 56 (8), 365–379.

Singh, V., Doner, L.W., Johnston, D.B., Hicks, K.B. and Eckhoff, S.R. (2000). Comparison of coarse and fine corn fiber gum yields and sugar profiles. *Cereal Chemistry*, 77 (5), 560–561.

Singh, M., Liu, S.X. and Vaughn, S.F. (2012). Effect of corn bran as dietary fiber addition on baking and sensory quality. *Biocatalysis and Agricultural Biotechnology*, 1 (4), 348–352.

Su, H.L. and Chang, K.C., (1995). Physicochemical and sensory properties of dehydrated bean paste products as related to bean varieties. *Journal of Food Science*, 60, 764–794.

Sugano, M., Ed., (2006). *Soy in Health and Disease Prevention.* CRC Press, FL, USA.

Swaminathan, M. (1974). *Pulses – Essentials of Food and Nutrition*. Madras: Ganesh and Co., pp. 355–356.

Takachi, R., Manami, I., Junko, I. *et al.* (2008). Fruit and vegetable intake and risk of total cancer and cardiovascular diseasee Japan public health center-based prospective study. *American Journal of Epidemiology*, 167 (1), 59–70.

Tang, S., Hettiarachchy, N.S., Horax, R. and Eswaranandam, S. (2003). Physicochemical properties and functionality of rice bran protein hydrolyzate prepared from heat-stabilized defatted rice bran with the aid of enzymes. *Journal of Food Science*, 68, 152–157.

Tharanathan, R.N., Mahadevamma, S. (2003). Grain legumes-a boon to human nutrition. *Trends in Food Science and Technology*, 14, 507–518.

Tiwari, U., Cummins, E. (2009).Nutritional importance and effect of processing on tocols in cereals. *Trends in Food Science and Technology*, 20, 511–520.

Tomomatsu, H. (1994). Health effects of oligosaccharides. *Food Technology*, Oct, 61–65.

Truswell, A.S. (2002). Cereal grains and coronary heart disease. *European Journal of Clinical Nutrition*, 56 (1), 1–14.

Tsuji, K., Ichikawa, T., Tanabe, N. *et al.* (1992). Effects of two kinds of koji on blood pressure in spontaneously hypertensive rats. *Nippon Nogeikagaku Kaishi*, 66, 1241–1246.

Tull, S.P., Yates, C.M., Maskrey, B.H. *et al.* (2009). Omega-3 fatty acids and inflammation: Novel interactions reveal a new step in neutrophil recruitment. *PLoS Biology*, 7 (8). DOI: 10.1371/journal.pbio.1000177.

Van Rensburg, S.J., Daniels, W.M., van Zyl, J.M. and Taljaard, J.J. (2000). A comparative study of the effects of cholesterol, beta-sitosterol, beta-sitosterol glucoside, dehydroepiandrosterone sulphate and melatonin on *in vitro* lipid peroxidation. *Metabolic Brain Disease*, 15, 257–265.

Velasco-Martinez, M., Angulo, O., Vazquez-Couturier, D.L., Arroyo-Lara, A., & Monroy-Rivera, J.A. (1997). Effect of dried solids of nejayote on broiler growth. *Poultry science*, 76 (11), 1531–1534.

Verleyen, T., Forcades, M., Verhe, R. *et al.* (2002). Analysis of free and esterified sterols in vegetable oils. *Journal of American Oil Chemist's Society*, 79, 117–122.

Walsh, K.R., Haak, S.J., Bohn, T. *et al.* (2007). Isoflavonoid glucosides are deconjugated and absorbed in the small intestine of human subjects with ileostomies. *The American Journal of Clinical Nutrition*, 85 (4), 1050–1056.

Wang, H.J. and Murphy, P.A. (1996). Mass balance study of isoflavones during soybean processing. *Journal of Agricultural and Food Chemistry*, 44, 2377–2383.

Wells, J.H. (1993). Utilization of rice bran and oil in human diets. *Louisiana Agriculture*, 36 (3), 5–8.

Wilson, T.A., DeSimone, A.P., Romano, C.A. and Nicolosi, R.J. (2000). Corn fibre oil lowers plasma cholesterol levels and increases cholesterol excretion greater than corn oil and similar to diets containing soy sterols and soy stanols in hamsters. *Journal of Nutritional Biochemistry*, 11, 443–449.

Winarno, F.G. and Karyadi, D. (1976). Nutrition and processing of soybeans. *INTSOY Series No. 10: Expanding the Use of Soybeans* (ed. R.M. Goodman). College of Agriculture, University of Illinois at Urbana-Champaign, pp. 137–142.

Wu, X.L., Beecher, G.R., Holden, J.M. *et al.* (2004). Lipophilic and hydrophilic antioxidant capacities of common foods in the United States. *Journal of Agricultural and Food Chemistry*, 52, 4026–4037.

Xu, B. and Chang, K.C. (2008a). Total phenolics, phenolic acids, isoflavones, and anthocyanins and antioxidant properties of yellow and black soybeans as affected by thermal processing. *Journal of Agricultural and Food Chemistry*, 56, 7165–7175.

Xu, B. and Chang, K.C. (2008b). Effect of soaking, boiling, and steaming on total phenolic content and antioxidant activities of cool season food legumes. *Food Chemistry*, 110, 1–13.

Yadav, M.P., Moreau, R.A. and Hicks, K.B. (2007). Phenolic acids, lipids, and proteins associated with purified corn fibre arabinoxylans. *Journal of Agricultural and Food Chemistry*, 55, 943–947.

Yadav, M.P., Moreau, R.A., Hotchkiss, A.T. and Hicks, K.B. (2012). A new corn fibre gum polysaccharide isolation process that preserves functional components. *Carbohydrate Polymers*, 87, 1169– 1175.

Ye, X., Al-Babili, S., Klöti, A. *et al.* (2000). Engineering the provitamin A (β-carotene) biosynthetic pathway into (carotenoid-free) rice endosperm. *Science*, 287 (5451), 303–305.

Yuan, B.Z., Durkin, M. E. and Nicholas, C. P. (2003). Promoter hypermethylation of DLC-1, candidate tumor suppressor gene, in several common human cancers. *Cancer Genetics and Cytogenetics*, 140 (2), 113–117.

Zhang, H.Y., Tang, G.Y., and Li, X.J. (2008). Antidiabetic components contained in vegetables and legumes. *Molecules*, 13, 1189–1194.

Zhou, K., Sun, S. and Canning, C. (2012). Production and functional characterisation of antioxidative hydrolysates from corn protein via enzymatic hydrolysis and ultrafiltration. *Food Chemistry*, 135, 1192–1197.

4 Tropical Fruits

Mandeep Kaur[2] and H. K. Sharma[1]
[1]Food Engineering and Technology Department, Sant Longowal Institute of Engineering and Technology (Deemed-to-be-University), Punjab, India
[2]Amity Institute of Food Technology, Amity University, Noida, India

4.1 Introduction

Tropical fruits are produced in countries with warm climates. The most common tropical fruits of Asian origin are: mango *(Mangifera indica)*, guava *(Psidium guajava)*, banana *(Musa acuminate)*, bael fruit *(Aegle marmelos)*, pomegranate (*Punica granatum*), jackfruit *(Artocarpus heterophyllus)*, lychee *(Litchi chinensis)*, papaya *(Carica papaya)*, Coconut (*Cocos nucifera*), kiwi *(Actinidia chinensis)*, passion fruit *(Passiflora edulis)* and, phalsa (*Grewia subinaequalis*). Many tropical fruits have been used by humans for centuries, and some fruits are in high demand globally because an increased consumption of tropical fruits is considered beneficial to health.

Tropical fruits are a potentially valuable source of antioxidants because they are rich in functional bioactive compounds. Antioxidants delay or inhibit the oxidation process caused by reactive oxygen species, thus enhancing the shelf life and quality of the products as well as protecting biological systems (Duthie *et al.*, 1996). Antioxidant compounds found in fruits play therapeutic and preventive roles against several diseases, for example many chronic diseases, including type 2 diabetes (Carter *et al.*, 2010), dementia (Hughes *et al.*, 2010), inflammation and certain cancers, and cardiovascular diseases (Ajila *et al.*, 2010, Vivekananthan *et al.*, 2003). Antioxidant vitamins as well as various phytochemicals present in fruits and vegetables may provide protection against several of these age-related pathological conditions because the diseases may involve free oxygen radicals (Knekt *et al.*, 2002). This chapter presents an overview of the functional properties of some tropical fruits and the effect of processing on their functional value.

Functional Foods and Dietary Supplements: Processing Effects and Health Benefits, First Edition.
Edited by Athapol Noomhorm, Imran Ahmad and Anil Kumar Anal.

4.2 Mango

Mango (*Mangifera indica*), an ancient fruit of Indian origin, is of great importance throughout the tropics. India is the leading producer of mango in the world, with 41% of the world's production (10 800 000 MT) provided by India, followed by China, Thailand, Mexico, Pakistan, Indonesia, the Philippines, Nigeria and Brazil (FAO, 2004). Mango is a good source of nutrients and energy (carbohydrates, fatty acids, amino acids, minerals, proteins, organic acids, vitamins A, C, and D, etc.) and has different medicinal virtues (USDA, 2010).

Mango is allowed to ripen for market; therefore it is harvested at a physiologically mature-green stage. The chemical composition of mango varies with variety, cultivar, maturity, etc. (Ajila *et al.*, 2007; Ribeiro *et al.*, 2008; Manthey and Perkins-Veazie, 2009). During the ripening process, textural softening of mango pulp occurs due to enzymatic action on the cell wall carbohydrates (pectin and hemicellulose). Polygalacturonase (PG) and β-D-galacturonase are responsible for tissue softening, as enzyme levels increase simultaneously with pectin depolymerization (Ali *et al.*, 1995; Muda *et al.*, 1995). Mango contains bioactive compounds with antioxidative, antiatherosclerotic, antimutagenic, anticarcinogenic and angiogenesis inhibitory activities (Cao and Cao, 1999) that are beneficial to health. Phenolic compounds found in mango can prevent DNA oxidative damage, quench lipid peroxidation, scavenge free radicals (Cao and Cao, 1999; Schieber *et al.*, 2000; Ajila *et al.*, 2008, 2010) and prevent inhibition of cell communication (Sigler and Ruch, 1993).

4.2.1 Polyphenolic constituents of mango

The main parts of mango fruit are pulp, peel and seed kernel. The major polyphenol present in mango pulp is gallic acid (6.9 mg/kg) followed by mangiferin (4.4 mg/kg) (Schieber *et al.*, 2000). Other polyphenolic compounds found in pulp are six hydrolysable tannins and four minor compounds, *p*-OH-benzoic acid, *m*-coumaric acid, *p*- coumaric acid, and ferulic acid (Kim *et al.*, 2007). Mango peel is also a good source of polyphenols (Singh *et al.*, 2004; Mahattanatawee *et al.*, 2006). The polyphenolic constituents of mango peel include mangiferin, quercetin, rhamnetin, ellagic acid, kaempferol and their related conjugates. The total phenols have been found to be higher in the peel than in the flesh at all stages of fruit development (Lakshminarayana *et al.*, 1970). Total polyphenol content of mango peel was found to be 4066 mg Gallic Acid Equivalents (GAE)/kg (dry matter) (Berardini *et al.*, 2005). Polyphenolic constituents of mango peel are shown in Table 4.1.

Mango seed kernels are usually discarded as waste during processing and consumption. Various studies indicate that mango seed kernels contain different phenolic compounds and stable fat rich in saturated fatty acids, making it a good source of natural antioxidants (Nunez-Selles, 2005). Polyphenolic compounds found in mango seed kernel are tannin, gallic acid, coumarin, caffeic acid, vanillin, mangiferin, ferulic acid, cinnamic acid and unknown compounds. The total polyphenolic content of the mango seed kernel extract was estimated to be 112 mg (GAE)/100 g (Ahmed *et al.*, 2007). The amount of phenolic compounds present in mango increases during ripening (Palafox-Carlos *et al.*, 2012). Since polyphenolics are natural antioxidants in quenching and neutralizing free radicals, changes to these compounds following postharvest

Table 4.1 Phenolic compounds in mango peel

Constituent	Amount (mg/kg on dry matter basis)
Kaempferol 3-*O*-glucoside	36.1
Quercetin 3-*O*-arabinopyranoside	101.5
Quercetin	65.3
Isomangiferin gallate	82.0
Quercetin 3-*O*-galactoside	651.2
Quercetin 3-*O*-glucoside	557.7
Quercetin 3-*O*-xylooside	207.3
Mangiferrin Gallate	321.9
Quercetin 3-*O*-arabinofuranoside	103.6
Quercetin 3-*O*-rhamnoside	20.1
Mangiferin	1690.4
Rhamnetin 3-*O* galactoside/glucoside	94.4
Isomangiferin	134.5

Source: Masibo & He, 2008. Reproduced with permission from Wiley-Blackwell.

treatment and ripening is an important link to the potential health benefits of mangoes.

4.2.2 Functional properties of mango

The first compounds defined as major polyphenolics present in mango were gallic acid and gallotannins (Saleh and El-Ansari, 1975). Other polyphenols such as mangiferin, quercetin, kaempferol, *p*-OH-benzoic acid, *m*-coumaric acid, *p*-coumaric acid and ferulic acid have also been identified (Schieber *et al.*, 2000; Singh *et al.*, 2004; Mahattanatawee *et al.*, 2006; Ajila *et al.*, 2008). Phenolic compounds present in mango, including gallic acid and gallotannins, were found to naturally decrease during storage, due to ripening, resulting in loss of astringency, which is a characteristic of mango (Saleh and El-Ansari, 1975). Fruit phenolic phytochemicals are capable of reducing the risks of cardiovascular disease, stroke and atherosclerosis (Hertog *et al.*, 1992; Kelly *et al.*, 2001), through the prevention of cellular oxidative damage. Their antioxidant activities inhibit oxidative damage to cellular DNA, preventing mutagenesis and tumorigenesis (Kelly *et al.*, 2001). Acting as antioxidants on low-density lipoprotein (LDL) free radicals, polyphenolic compounds can lower the amount of oxidized LDL cholesterol, which in turn can reduce the risk of coronary atherosclerosis (De Whalley *et al.*, 1990; Vinson and Hontz, 1995). Some phenolic compounds, such as ellagic acid, tannic acid and quercetin, act as potent tyrosinase inhibitors (Rompel *et al.*, 1999; Shimogaki *et al.*, 2000). Tyrosinase catalyses melanin biosynthesis in human skin and epidermal hyperpigmentation may cause various dermatological disorders, such as freckles, melasma and age spots (Karioti *et al.*, 2007). Recently, safe and effective tyrosinase inhibitors have become important for their potential applications in improving food quality and preventing pigmentation disorders and other melanin-related health problems in humans (Miyazawa *et al.*, 2003). The bioactivity of the main mango polyphenolics is given as follows:

Mangiferin The nutraceutical importance of mangiferin, an important polyphenol in mango (Andreu *et al.*, 2005), has been extensively demonstrated and continues to invite attention, since it provides health benefits. Mangiferin has a number of biological effects, for example it acts as an antidiabetic (Muruganandan *et al.*, 2005), has antitumour (Noratto *et al.*, 2010; Rajendran *et al.*, 2008) and antioxidant effects (Barreto *et al.*, 2008; Dar *et al.*, 2005) and prevents diseases related to blood vessels (Daud *et al.*, 2010) and many others. Mangiferin is able to scavenge reactive oxygen species and inhibit all those processes leading to red blood cell damage and membrane destabilization, as well as aiding in protection against sickness induced by radiation and it is reported to inhibit glucose absorption from the intestine, hence reducing blood glucose levels in the body. It protects mitochondrial membranes against lipid peroxidation (Lemus-Molina *et al.*, 2009) and possesses an iron-complexing ability which is considered a primary mechanism for the protection of liver mitochondria against Fe^{2+} citrate-induced lipid peroxidation (Halliwell and Gutteridge, 1986). It also acts as an antibacterial and antifungal agent. The antifungal effect of mangiferin has been demonstrated for *Thermoascus aurantiacus, Saccharomyces cerevisiae, Trichoderma reesei* and *Aspergillus flavus* (Chakrabarti and Ghosal, 1985). Both Gram-positive and Gram-negative bacteria are sensitive to mangiferin. *Bacillus pumilus* is reported as the most sensitive species to mangiferin among the Gram-positive microorganisms, whereas *Salmonella agona* is most sensitive among the Gram-negative species (Stoilova *et al.*, 2005).

Flavonoids Flavanoids are the major contributors to the total antioxidant capacity of mango (Ma *et al.*, 2011) and possess important biological activities including antifungal and antibacterial activity (Galeotti *et al.*, 2008; Sathiamoorthy *et al.*, 2007). Catechin, quercetin, epicatechin, isoquercetin (quercetin-3-glucoside), fisetin and astragalin (kaempferol-3-glucoside) are the important flavonoids of mango. A reddish tint in some mango varieties may be attributed to the presence of anthocyanins (Rice-Evans *et al.*, 1997). Quercetin (Figure 4.1a) identified in unripe mango fruits (El-Ansari *et al.*, 1969) works mainly as an antioxidant. At high doses it inhibits cell proliferation in colon carcinoma cell lines and in mammary adenocarcinoma cell lines, but at low doses it is reported to increase cell proliferation in colon and breast cancer cells (Woude *et al.*, 2003). Quercetin has also been found to exhibit antihistamine and anti-inflammatory effects associated with various forms of arthritis (Appleton, 2010).

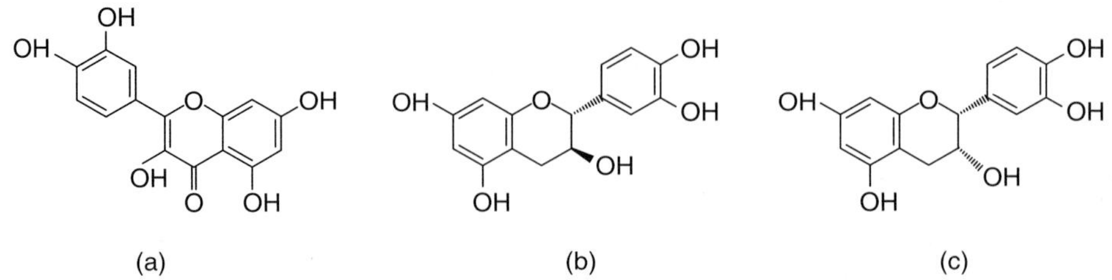

Figure 4.1 Chemical structure of (a) quercetin; (b) (+)-catechin; (c) (−)-epicatechin. *Source:* Adapted from Medić-Šarić *et al.*, 2009 and Qurecetin chemical structure, 2013

(+)-Catechin (Figure 4.1b) is a flavonoid from the group of catechins including (–)-epicatechin, (–)-epigallocatechin, (–)-epicatechingallate and (+)-gallocatechin. Catechins exhibit antioxidant and free radical scavenging activities (Augustyniak *et al.*, 2005), which enable them to act against cancer (Yamanaka *et al.*, 1997) and several other diseases. Both (+)-catechin and (–)-epicatechin (Figure 4.1b and c) have been reported in mango stem bark extract as an antioxidant with great medicinal use (Rastraelli *et al.*, 2002).

Gallic acid (GA) and gallotannin (GT) GA and GT are reported as the major polyphenolic compounds in mango. Chemical changes taking place decrease the content of phenolic compounds mainly GA and GTs along with total soluble phenolics (Kim *et al.*, 2009). Mango contains numerous high molecular weight GTs that can be broken down into smaller GTs (Berardini *et al.*, 2004). It is also possible that the biosynthesis of GTs occurred via galloyltransferases present in mangoes (El Ansari *et al.*, 1971), at an optimum reaction temperature of 45 °C (Niemetz and Gross, 2001).

GA possesses antifungal activity and has been associated with phytotoxicity. It has been of great interest for protection against atherosclerosis (Abella, 1997). *In vitro* studies have shown that it has anticancer activities against leukaemia HL-60RG and against certain prostate, colon and lung cancer cells (Yoshioka *et al.*, 2000). Both GA and GT are reported to act as free radical scavengers. GA donates hydrogen ions and stabilizes free radicals, hence acts as an antioxidant. GA, however, has also been reported as a pro-oxidant, while GT has been reported as effective antioxidant (Sakagami *et al.*, 1997) which contradicts radical scavenging properties demonstrated by antioxidant assays.

4.2.3 Processing effects

Since polyphenolics are natural antioxidants that quench and neutralize free radicals, changes to these compounds following postharvest treatment and ripening affects the potential health benefits of mangoes. Mangoes may host *Ceratitis capitata* (Mediterranean fruit fly) and *Anastrepha* spp. (Mexican fruit fly), thereby posing a risk of infestation from adults, larvae and eggs (Jacobi *et al.*, 2001). Therefore mangoes are subjected to quarantine treatment, such as hot water treatment (HWT), hot vapour treatment, or irradiation, to eradicate invasive pests and insect species. HWT has also been reported to decrease the severity of skin disorders. Chemical changes taking place during thermal treatments include a decrease in the content of phenolic compounds (Kim *et al.*, 2009). Prolonged heat treatment times were a significant factor in lowering the two predominant phenolic compounds present in mangoes (Berardini *et al.*, 2004).

Mango is commonly processed to prepare pickle, juice, candies, jam and other products, during which physical and chemical changes take place. The greatest hurdle to the commercial marketing of minimally processed fruits is their limited shelf life due to cut-surface browning and tissue softening (Soliva-Fortuny and Martín-Belloso, 2003). Browning reactions can be inhibited by adding antioxidants, excluding oxygen, or inhibiting the activity of the enzyme responsible, polyphenol oxidase (Saltveit, 2003). Browning inhibition by antioxidants is due to an indirect effect on polyphenol oxidase (PPO) activity where vitamin C reduces the *o*-quinones formed from diphenols. This is a major benefit of dipping treatments containing antioxidants (such as ascorbic acid, citric acid and CaCl2 to reduce browning) and has also been reported for various fruits such as pineapple, banana as well as mango (González-Aguilar *et al.*, 2004, 2008). Deterioration of fresh cut mango can also be delayed by dipping treatments containing calcium (González-Aguilar *et al.*, 2008). Browning in mangoes can also be inhibited by applying an alginate edible coating in conjunction with antibrowning agents (ascorbic and citric acid) to mango cubes. Mango consumption could provide significant amounts of bioactive compounds with antioxidant activity to the human diet (Robles-Sánchez *et al.*, 2013).

4.3 Guava

Guava (*Psidium guajava* L.) is an important fruit crop of tropical regions. Fully ripened guava fruits are very soft and therefore difficult to handle and transport to market. Fruits are ready for harvest 120–150 days after flowering and should be harvested only when the green colour of the skin starts to fade, as this indicates the onset of ripening. Its delicate nature, short postharvest life and susceptibility to chilling injury and diseases, limit the potential for commercialization of guava fruit (Brown and Wills, 1983). Because of its commercial and nutritional value, guava is considered a common man's fruit and can be rightly termed as the 'apple of the tropics.' Guava is of commercial importance in about 58 countries, but the leading countries are India, Brazil, Egypt, South Africa, Colombia, United States, Puerto Rico, Jamaica, Taiwan, Sudan, Kenya, Israel, Philippines, Pakistan, Malaysia, Australia and West Indies (Eipeson and Bhowmik, 1992).

4.3.1 Composition of guava

The main parts of guava fruit are peel, flesh and seeds of which flesh makes up about 50% of the total fruit, peel 20% and seeds 30%. The moisture content of the fruit varies between 74–83%, dry matter is 13–26%, protein content 1%, calorific value 275 kJ/100 g and fat 0.9–1.5% (Mukherjee and Datta, 1967). The amount of total soluble solids increases from 10.5 to 12.75% and ascorbic acid increases from 118.53 to 199.26 mg/100 g during ripening, while acidity decreases from 0.72 to 0.55% during this period (Agrawal *et al.*, 2002). Guava is a good source of many vitamins such as ascorbic acid, pantothenic acid, thiamine, niacin, riboflavin and vitamin A. Guava fruit is one of the richest sources of pectin ranging from 0.5 to 1.8% and this is affected by various factors such as variety, stage of maturity and crop season (Dhingra *et al.*, 1983). Guava fruit is not only rich in dietary fibre but also a good source of natural antioxidant compounds such as polyphenols. The presence of polyphenols gives an astringent taste to fruits. As the fruit matures, the polyphenols decrease considerably and so does the astringency.

4.3.2 Functional properties of guava

Guava is a rich source of various constituents beneficial to health such as antioxidants and fibre. Antioxidants are substances that can prevent or delay oxidative damage of lipids, proteins and nucleic acids by reactive oxygen species, which include reactive free radicals such as superoxide, hydroxyl, peroxyl, alkoxyl and non-radicals such as hydrogen peroxide, hypochlorous, etc. Antioxidants scavenge radicals by inhibiting initiation and breaking chain propagation. Antioxidants are also reported to suppress formation of free radicals by binding to the metal ions and quenching superoxide and singlet oxygen (Shi *et al.*, 2001). Antioxidants help lower the incidence of degenerative diseases such as cancer, arthritis, arteriosclerosis, heart disease, inflammation, brain dysfunction and acceleration of the ageing process (Gordon, 1996). Similarly dietary fibre also plays a very important role in protection against several diseases.

Ascorbic acid, total phenolic and total carotenoid Ascorbic acid content in guava shows a tremendous variation depending on the cultivar, season and flesh colour. Sachan and Ram (1970) reported 37–1000 mg of vitamin C per 100 g in guava fruits. Pink-flesh guava contained more ascorbic acid than the white-fleshed ones (Kumar and Hoda, 1974). The vitamin C content varies with climatic conditions. Vitamin C reaches a maximum in green guava but decreases as the fruit ripens. The vitamin C content is generally highest in skin and decreases towards the central core. The amount of ascorbic acid (AA), total phenolics (TPH), and total carotenoids expressed as β-carotene (BET) are significantly different (Thaipong *et al.*, 2006) among guava clones. Luximon-Ramma *et al.* (2003) reported that white pulp guavas had higher AA and TPH than pink pulp guavas. The AA, TPH and BET contents in guavas were found to be higher than other fruit crops.

Guava and papaya are the only fruits which have higher ascorbic acid levels than orange (67 ± 9 mg/100 g). Guava's ascorbic acid content (50–300 mg/100 g) is three to six times higher than oranges (Taipong *et al.*, 2006). The antioxidant content is always higher in guava fruit with skin than fruit with the skin peeled off (Lim *et al.*, 2007). Red-fleshed Brazilian guava contains several carotenoids such as β-carotene, phytofluene, β-cryptoxanthin, γ-carotene, lycopene, cryptoflavin, rubixanthin and lutein (Mercadante *et al.*, 1999; Taipong *et al.*, 2006). Guava is also a rich source of phenolic compounds, for example apigenin and myricetin (Miean and Mohamed, 2001).

Free radicals are constantly formed in the body by normal metabolic actions. These actions are resisted by a balanced system of antioxidant defences, including antioxidants and enzymes. A disturbance in this balanced system causes oxidative stress that can lead to cell injury and death (Halliwell and Gutteridge, 1986). Therefore, much attention has been focussed on the use of antioxidants, especially natural antioxidants, to inhibit lipid peroxidation, or to protect against the damage of free radicals (Vendemiale *et al.*, 1999). Current research into free radicals has confirmed that foods rich in antioxidants play an essential role in the prevention of several debilitating diseases.

Oxidative stress imposed by reactive oxygen species (ROS) plays an important role in many chronic and degenerative diseases, such as cardiovascular diseases, cancer, diabetes mellitus, ageing and neurodegenerative diseases (Young and Woodside, 2001). ROS scavenging is effective in depressing the level of oxidative stress in humans for the prevention and treatment of some chronic and degenerative diseases. It has been reported that intake of guava is inversely associated with the risk of many chronic diseases, such as cardiovascular diseases and cancer. Natural antioxidants in guava, such as vitamins and polyphenols, are considered to be responsible for these health benefits (Leja, *et al.*, 2003). Phenolic compounds are important phytochemicals that exist universally in plants and have high antioxidant abilities and free radical scavenging capacities. They work by inhibiting the enzymes responsible for ROS production and reducing highly oxidized ROS (Robards *et al.*, 1999).

There has been renewed interest in the use of natural compounds as anticoagulant and antithrombotic compounds for diabetes patients. Based on the observations mentioned here, it appears that glycation, hypercoagulability and platelet dysfunctions contribute to the development of cardiovascular pathogenesis in diabetes. Therefore, the agents with antiglycation, anticoagulant and antiplatelet properties would have priority in the search to alleviate diabetic complications. Guava is also used as a hypoglycaemic in folk medicine. Cheng and Yang (1983) demonstrated the hypoglycaemic effects of guava juice in mice. The potent antioxidant activity in guava leaf extracts has been reported and attributed to their phenolic compounds (Chen and Yen, 2007).

Lycopene Recently, lycopene has gained attention among nutritionists. This constituent normally occurs in red fruits such as guava, tomato, papaya and watermelon. The consumption of lycopene-rich guava is inversely associated with the risk of atherosclerosis, cardiovascular disease (Ito *et al.*, 2006), prostate cancer (Zhang *et al.*, 2007) and other diseases. Pink guava (*Psidium guajava* L.) is also high in ellagic acid, anthocyanin, vitamin C, dietary fibre and carotenoids, especially lycopene (Wilberg and Rodriguez-Amaya, 1995). Its extract is reported to be a good source of antioxidants (Thaipong *et al.*, 2006). Pink guava has also been reported as a good source of pro-vitamin A (Setiawan *et al.*, 2001). The comparison of lycopene content and lipophilic antioxidant capacity was explored by Kong and Ismail (2011) among pink guava fruit and by-products of its puree production industry namely refiner, siever and decanter. Lycopene content and antioxidant capacity were in the order of fruits > decanter > siever > refiner. Decanter exhibited the highest lycopene content and antioxidant among the studied by-products could be a potential source of lycopene and antioxidant compounds (Kong and Ismail, 2011).

There is increasing evidence that oxidative stress, particularly stress caused by reactive oxygen species and reactive nitrogen species, can lead to numerous inflammatory and degenerative diseases (MacDonald-Wicks *et al.*, 2006). Meanwhile, antioxidants such as lycopene have been reported to have health benefits in preventing oxidative stress and carcinogenesis (Basu and Imrhan, 2007). Lycopene exhibits a physical quenching ability up to two times higher than β-carotene and ten times higher than α-tocopherol (Di Mascio *et al.*, 1989), making it the most popular antioxidant for use in human health.

Dietry fibre Raw ripe fresh guava is also an excellent source of dietary fibre (12.72 g/100 g) among the commonly consumed foods (Li *et al.*, 2002). Dietary fibres may protect against cardiovascular disease, provide improvements in gastrointestinal health, in glucose tolerance and in the insulin response, reduce the risk of developing some cancers and influence lipid digestion, hence contributing to some degree to weight management (Kaur *et al.*, 2012; Ayala-Zavala *et al.*, 2011). Fibre-rich co-products may be incorporated into food products as inexpensive, non-caloric bulking agents for the partial replacement of flour, fat or sugar, as enhancers of water and oil retention and to improve emulsion or oxidative stability (Elleuch *et al.*, 2011).

4.3.3 Processing effects

Guava is low in fats, carbohydrates and proteins but has a high vitamin C (more than 10 mg/100 g fruit) and fibre content (2.8–5.5 g/100 g fruit) and contains extractable polyphenols (Gutiérrez *et al.*, 2008). In addition to its nutritious properties, this fruit is very appetizing due to its sensory (flavour and colour) properties (Jiménez-Escrig *et al.*, 2001). There are various processed guava products (e.g. jams, juices marmalades, jellies, and other soft drinks), but this fruit is usually consumed fresh. Export of fresh guavas has been restricted because it is highly perishable and susceptible to tropical fruit fly attack. Also, pectin degradation during processing softens its texture, which causes loss of market value. Ascorbic acid degradation is susceptible to environmental conditions such as temperature and water activity and so it takes place during thermal processing operations.

During thermal processing, the phenol–pectin interaction is beneficial in texture maintenance. This may be because of the cross-linking between hydroxycinnamic acid, such as ferulic acid, and cell wall polysaccharide, such as pectin, through the formation of esterified phenolic compounds. Therefore it has been found that cross-linking may reduce cell detachment during thermal processing of the fruit and increase rigidity of the plant cell walls (Parker *et al.*, 2003). Phenolic infiltration might improve the texture and antioxidant capacity of processed guava slices through phenol–pectin interaction (Tsai *et al.*, 2010). Carbonation and sonication are also effective tools for maintaining a high-quality guava product. Ascorbic acid content is reported to be significantly higher in samples treated with carbonation and sonication than the control samples (Cheng *et al.*, 2007). The carbonation provides more nuclei for cavitations that permit the elimination of dissolved oxygen in the juice.

Some nutrients are also lost as waste during guava processing. Pink guava (*Psidium guajava*) has a high lycopene content, making up more than 80% of its total carotenoids (Padula and Rodriguez-Amaya, 1986). The lycopene content in pink guava is 4–6 mg/100 g of edible portion (Wilberg and Rodriguez-Amaya, 1995). During production of pink guava puree, by-products are created that make up 25% of the total loading weight and have been reported to have a high lycopene content (Padula and Rodriguez-Amaya, 1986).

4.4 Pomegranate

Pomegranate (*Punica granatum L.*) is an important tropical fruit highly appreciated for its delicacy, is becoming more popular because of its beneficial health properties (antiatherogenic, antioxidant, antihypertensive, etc.). This fruit is cultivated in India, Iran, Afghanistan, Mediterranean basin (Morocco, Spain, Turkey, Tunisia, and Egypt), and Middle East countries are the world's leading producers (Melgarejo *et al.*, 2009).

4.4.1 Chemical composition of pomegranate

The pomegranate fruit has several functional constituents in its different parts which can be divided mainly into peel, seeds and arils (Figure 4.2). The edible part of the

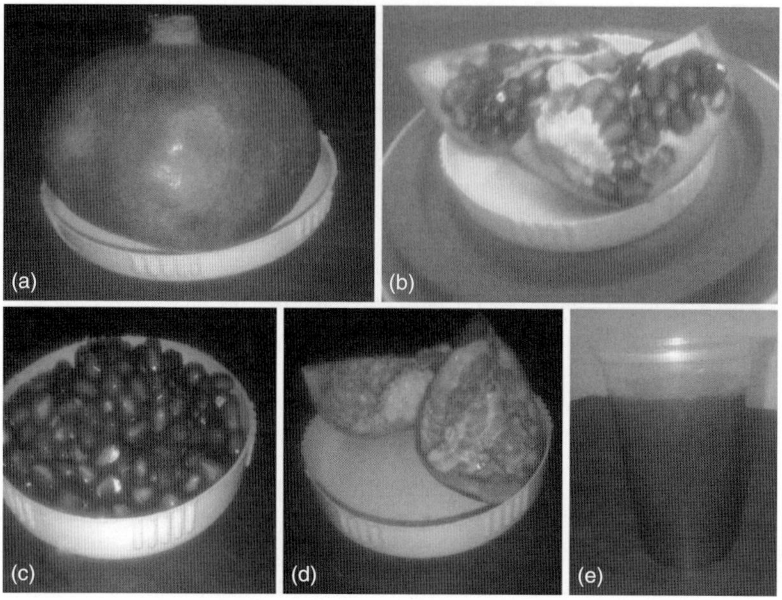

Figure 4.2 (a) Pomegranate fruit; (b) pomegranate internal part; (c) pomegranate arils; (d) pomegranate peel; (e) pomegranate juice (Kaur & Sharma, 2013). For colour details, see the colour plates section

pomegranate fruit (50%) consists of 40% arils and 10% seeds. Arils contain 85% water, 10% total sugars (mainly fructose and glucose), 1.5% pectin, organic acid such as ascorbic acid, citric acid and malic acid, and bioactive compounds such as phenolics and flavonoids, principally anthocyanins (Tezcan *et al.*, 2009). The seeds are a rich source of total lipids; pomegranate seed oil makes up 12–20% of the total seed weight. About 50% of the total fruit weight corresponds to the peel, which is an important source of bioactive compounds such as phenolics, flavonoids, ellagitannins (ETs) and proanthocyanidin compounds (Li *et al.*, 2006) and of minerals, mainly potassium, nitrogen, calcium, phosphorus, magnesium and sodium (Mirdehghan and Rahemi, 2007).

The main constituents of pomegranate seed oil and juice reported by various researchers are given in Table 4.2. The chemical composition of pomegranate may vary depending upon the type of cultivar, region, climate, maturity, cultivation, etc. Significant variations in phenolic compounds, organic acids, sugars, minerals and water-soluble vitamins of pomegranates have been reported by various researchers (Mirdehghan and Rahemi, 2007; Tezcan *et al.*, 2009).

4.4.2 Functional properties of pomegranate

The different compounds in different parts of the pomegranate fruit, have different functional properties (Tehranifar *et al.*, 2010). These compounds act as antioxidant (Çam *et al.*, 2009), antimicrobial (Reddy *et al.*, 2007), anticarcinogenic (Bell and Hawthorne, 2008), and antitumoural agents (Hamad and Al-Momene, 2009). Many researchers have shown that preparations containing pomegranate juice and

Table 4.2 Constituents of pomegranate seed oil and juice

Component	Main constituents	Reference
Seed oil	Linoleic acid, eleostearic acid, Conjugated linolenic acid, oleic acid, stearic acid, punicic acid, catalpic acid	Sassano *et al.*, 2009; El-Nemr *et al.*, 2006; Ozgul-Yucel, 2005; Fadavi *et al.*, 2006
Juice	Gallic acid, caffeic acid, Anthocyanins, glucose, organic acid, ascorbic acid, ellagic acid, ellagitannins, catechin, minerals, quercetin, rutin, tannins	Jaiswal *et al.*, 2010; Lansky & Newman, 2007; Ignarro *et al.*, 2006; Mousavinejad *et al.*, 2009; Poyrazoglu *et al.*, 2002; Heber *et al.*, 2007; Aviram and Dornfeld, 2001; Passamonti *et al.*, 2003

Source: Viuda-Martos *et al.*, 2010. Reproduced with permission from Wiley-Blackwell.

peel extract can be used to reduce blood pressure, are antiatherosclerotic and significantly reduce LDL oxidation and prevent and/or cure atherosclerosis, diarrhoea, gastric ulcer, venereal disease and oestrogen-related diseases (Reddy *et al.*, 2007).

Tannins Hydrolysable tannins (HTs) are dominant polyphenols in pomegranate juice and account for 92% of its antioxidant activity (Passamonti *et al.*, 2003). The antiatherogenic effects of pomegranate juice on lipoproteins, macrophages and platelets may be linked to its potent antioxidative capacity juice against lipid peroxidation. Aviram and Dornfeld (2001) reported that pomegranate juice, which is rich in tannins, antiatherosclerotic properties that could be related to its potent antioxidative characteristics. Four hydrolysable tannins (punicalagin, punicalin, strictinin A and granatin B) from pomegranate displayed a dose-dependent and inhibitory effect on nitric oxide production in *in vitro* studies (Lee *et al.*, 2010).

Flavonoids Flavonoids are low-molecular-weight compounds and their structure mainly consists of two aromatic rings joined by a 3-carbon bridge, usually in the form of a heterocyclic ring (Balasundram *et al.*, 2006). Anthocyanins are the largest and most important group of flavonoids present in pomegranate arils, which are used to obtain the juice. These pigments impart colour to the fruit and juice (Afaq *et al.*, 2005). There is a great variety of anthocyanins present in pomegranate juice, principally cyanidin-3-*O*-glucoside, cyanidin-3,5-di-*O*-glucoside, delphinidin-3-*O*-glucoside, delphinidin-3,5-di-*O*-glucoside, pelargonidin-3-*O*-glucoside, and pelargonidin-3,5-di-*O*-glucoside (Lansky and Newman 2007; Jaiswal *et al.*, 2010). Pomegranate juice and extract are more potent inhibitors for cell growth than isolated individual polyphenols in cell lines, indicating synergistic or/and additive effects of several phytochemicals present including proanthocyanidins, anthocyanins and flavonoid glycosides (Hong *et al.*, 2008).

Phenolic acids The naturally occurring antioxidant properties of pomegranate components and their derivatives are being given greater importance by researchers over synthetic antioxidants. The use of synthetic antioxidants is increasingly restricted due to the secondary effects they may cause. The different activities may be due to the presence of diverse phenolic compounds in pomegranate. The phenolic acids present in pomegranate juice can be divided into two groups: (1) hydroxybenzoic acids, mainly gallic acid and ellagic acid (Amakura *et al.*, 2000); and (2) hydroxycinnamic acids, principally caffeic acid, chlorogenic acid and *p*-coumaric acid (Poyrazoglu *et al.*, 2002). Diabetes is becoming more widespread due to life style and the various other factors causing cardiovascular and oncological disorders. Different researchers have explored the antidiabetic activity of phenolic acids (Li *et al.*, 2008). The hypoglycaemic activity of pomegranate seeds, juice and flowers has also been reported (Katz *et al.*, 2007). The mechanisms for these functional effects are still unknown; however, recent research suggests that prevention of diabetic sequelae is via peroxisome proliferator-activated receptor-γ (PPARγ) binding and nitric oxide production. The polyphenols are the major compounds – possessing antidiabetic properties – that may affect glycaemia by different mechanisms, including glucose absorption inhibition in the gut or its uptake by peripheral tissues (Scalbert *et al.*, 2005).

Madrigal-Carballo *et al.* (2009) indicated that polyphenolic molecules in pomegranate undergo redox reactions because phenolic hydroxyl groups readily donate hydrogen ions to reducing agents. A significant increase in the reducing power of pomegranate peel extracts has been reported when the concentration is increased from 50 to 400 ppm (Negi and Jayaprakasha, 2003). Pin-Der (1998) noted that reducing properties are generally associated with the presence of reductones. The antioxidative action of reductones is based on the mechanism of breaking the free radical chain by donating a hydrogen atom (Gordon, 1990). The reductones also react with some precursors of peroxides, thus inhibiting peroxide formation (Naveena *et al.*, 2008). However, the antioxidant activity of phenolic compounds is suggested to be mainly due to their ability to scavenge free radicals or chelate metal cations (Amarowicz *et al.*, 2004).

4.4.3 Processing effects

Pomegranates are commonly consumed as fresh fruit, beverages (juice and wine) and other food products (jams and jellies). The production process for concentrated pomegranate juice involves various steps and is considered a difficult fruit to process because of the difficulty of separating the arils from the peels. Incorrect technology may also contaminate the juice with tannic elements, which greatly damages juice quality.

Anthocyanin is an important compound present in pomegranate that gives the juice an appealing colour. During processing, degradation of anthocyanins takes place (Kırca and Cemeroglu, 2003; Wang and Xu, 2007); therefore, it is difficult to maintain the colour of pomegranate juice. The effect of processing temperature and storage on the physical and chemical characteristics of raw pomegranate juice has been studied (Miguel *et al.*, 2004; Alighourchi and Barzegar, 2009). There is a need to study the effect of food additives and preservatives on the colour of pomegranate juice. The effect of different processing techniques on the functional properties of various products obtained from pomegranate is another area for study.

4.5 Summary and future trends

Tropical fruits have been used by humans for centuries and some fruits are in high demand worldwide. There is a long list of tropical fruits of Asian origin but this chapter has focused on mango, guava and pomegranate. Functional compounds present in these fruits such as ascorbic acid, β-carotene, phenolics, flavonoids, tannins, ascorbic acid and anthocyanins are receiving recognition since they play therapeutic and preventive roles against ageing and obesity and several diseases such as diabetes, inflammation, cardiovascular diseases, chronic diseases and cancers of the lung, oesophagus, stomach, mouth, pharynx, pancreas, breast, bladder and colon. Antioxidants have the ability to scavenge free radicals and other reactive species. Therefore consumption of these fruits is recommended by scientific research carried out globally by various health organizations. The health effects of different bioactive compounds depend on both their bioavailability and respective intakes, which can vary greatly. Numerous environmental and technologic factors may affect the bioactive compounds in fruits, for example variety, stage of maturity and crop season.

The effects of processing on bioactive compounds present in mango, guava and pomegranate are also briefly summarized. Recent research indicates that thermal processing of fruits can affect bioactive compounds in tropical fruits. There are numerous mechanisms by which bioactive compounds degrade. To meet the demand for safe, nutritious foods (without deterioration of bioactive compounds), requires the application of non-thermal novel techniques and the development of new techniques. Several novel techniques for improving the nutritient values of processed fruits have been developed during the past few years. Therefore such novel technologies (e.g. high pressure processing, microwave heating, ohmic heating) should be chosen to minimize the destruction of nutrients. Future studies need to evaluate the entire farm-to-fork supply chain including the time of plantation, time of harvest and postharvest handling prior to the application. Research studies should be focused on developing and comparing technologies to traditional thermal processing methods. From that data, new methods of processing and preserving fruits can be developed to minimize the loss of nutrients.

References

Abella, A., Chalas, J., Claise, C. *et al.* (1997). Interest of ethyl esters of polyphenolic acids in prevention of atherosclerosis. *Atherosclerosis*, 3, 199.

Afaq, F., Saleem, M., Krueger, C.G., Reed, J.D. and Mukhtar, H. (2005). Anthocyanin and hydrolyzable tannin-rich pomegranate fruit extract modulates MAPK and NF-kappa B pathways and inhibits skin tumorigenesis in CD-1 mice. *International Journal of Cancer*, 113, 423–433.

Agrawal, R., Parihar, P., Mandhyan, B.L. and Jain, D.K. (2002). Physico-chemical changes during ripening of guava fruit (*Psidium guajava* L.). *Journal of Food Science and Technology*, 39 (1), 94–95.

Ahmed, A., Saeid, D., Eman, A. and Reham, E. (2007). Egyptian mango by-product 1. Compositional quality of mango seed kernel. *Food Chemistry*, 103, 1141–1152.

Ajila, C.M., Aalami, M., Leelavathi, K. and Rao, U.J.S.P. (2010). Mango peel powder: A potential source of antioxidant and dietary fibre in macaroni preparations. *Innovative Food Science & Emerging Technologies*, 11 (1), 219–224.

Ajila, C.M., Bhat, S.G. and Rao, U.J.S.P. (2007). Valuable components of raw and ripe peels from two Indian mango varieties. *Food Chemistry*, 102, 1006–1011.

Ajila, C.M. (2008). Protection against hydrogen peroxide induced oxidative damage in rat erythrocytes by *Mangifera indica* L. peel extract. *Food Chemistry and Toxicology*, 46 (1), 303–309.

Alighourchi, H. and Barzegar, M. (2009). Some physicochemical characteristics and degradation kinetic of anthocyanin of reconstituted pomegranate juice during storage. *Journal of Food Engineering*, 90, 179–185.

Ali, Z.M., Armugam, S. and Lazan, H. (1995). Beta-Galactosidase and its significance in ripening mango fruit. *Phytochemistry*, 38, 1109–1114.

Amakura, Y., Okada, M., Tsuji, S. and Tonogai, Y. (2000). High-performance liquid chromatographic determination with photodiode array detection of ellagic acid in fresh and processed fruits. *Journal of Chromatography A*, 896, 87–93.

Amarowicz, R., Pegg, R.B., Rahimi-Moghaddam, P., Barl, B. and Weil, J.A. (2004). Free-radical scavenging capacity and antioxidant activity of selected plant species from the Canadian prairies. *Food Chemistry*, 84, 551–562.

Appleton, J. (2010). Evaluating the bioavailability of quercetin. *Natural Medicine Journal*, 2(1), 1–6.

Andreu, G.L., Delgado, R., Velho, J.A., Curti, C. and Vercesi, A.E. (2005). Mangiferin, a natural occurring glucosyl xanthone, increases susceptibility of rat liver mitochondria to calcium-induced permeability transition. *Archives of Biochemistry and Biophysics*, 439 (2), 184–193.

Augustyniak, A., Waszkiewicz, E. and Skrzydlewska, E. (2005). Preventive action of green tea from changes in the liver antioxidant abilities of different aged rats intoxicated with ethanol. *Nutrition*, 21, 925–932.

Aviram, M. and Dornfeld, L. (2001). Pomegranate juice consumption inhibits serum angiotensin-converting enzyme activity and reduces systolic blood pressure. *Atherosclerosis*, 158 (1), 195–198.

Ayala-Zavala, J.F., Vega-Vega, V., Rosas-Domínguez, C. *et al.* (2011). Agro-industrial potential of exotic fruit byproducts as a source of food additives. *Food Research International*, 44 (7), 1866–1874.

Balasundram, N., Sundram, K. and Samman, S. (2006). Phenolic compounds in plants and agri-industrial by-products: antioxidant activity, occurrence, and potential uses. *Food Chemistry*, 99, 191–203.

Barreto, J.C., Trevisan, M.T., Hull, W.E. *et al.* (2008). Characterization and quantitation of polyphenolic compounds in bark, kernel, leaves, and peel of mango (*Mangifera indica* L.). *Journal of Agriculture and Food Chemistry*, 56, 5599–5610.

Basu, A. and Imrhan, V. (2007). Tomatoes versus lycopene in oxidative stress and carcinogenesis: Conclusions from clinical trials. *European Journal of Clinical Nutrition*, 61 (3), 295–303.

Bell, C. and Hawthorne, S. (2008). Ellagic acid, pomegranate and prostate cancer – a mini review. *Journal of Pharmacy and Pharmacology*, 60, 130–144.

Berardini, N., Carle, R. and Schieber, A. (2004). Characterization of gallotannins and benzophenone derivatives from mango (*Mangifera indica* L. cv. Tommy Atkins) peels, pulp and kernels by high performance liquid chromatography/electrospray ionization mass spectrometry. *Rapid Communications in Mass Spectrometry*, 18, 2208–2216.

Berardini, N., Schieber, A., Klaiber, I. *et al.* (2005). 7-*O*-methylcyanidin 3-*O*-β-D-galactopyranoside, a novel anthocyanin from mango (*Mangifera indica* L.) cv. 'Tommy Atkins' peels. *Chemical Science*, 60 (7), 801–804.

Brown, B.I. and Wills, R.B.H. (1983). Post harvest changes in guava fruits of different maturity. *Scientia Horticulturae*, 19, 237–243.

Çam, M., Jisil, Y. and Durmaz, G. (2009). Classification of eight pomegranate juices based on antioxidant capacity measured by four methods. *Food Chemistry*, 112, 721–726.

Cao, Y.H. and Cao, R.H. (1999). Angiogenesis inhibited by drinking tea. *Nature*, 6726, 381–398.

Carter, P., Gray, L.J., Troughton, J., Khunti, K. and Davis, M.J. (2010). Fruit and vegetable intake and incidence of type 2 diabetes mellitus: systematic review and meta-analysis. *British Medical Journal*, 341, 4229.

Chakrabarti, D. and Ghosal, S. (1985). Effect of *Fusarium moniliforme* var. *subglutinans* infection on mangiferin production in the twigs of *Mangifera indica*. *Phytopathologische Zeitschrift-Journal of Phytopathology*, 113, 47–50.

Chen, H.Y. and Yen, G.C. (2007). Antioxidant activity and free radical-scavenging capacity of extracts from guava (*Psidium guajava* L.) leaves. *Food Chemistry*, 101, 686–694.

Cheng, L.H., Soh, C.Y., Liew, S.C. and The, F.F. (2007). Effects of sonication and carbonation on guava juice quality. *Food Chemistry*, 104, 1396–1401.

Cheng, J.T. and Yang, R.S. (1983). Hypoglycemic effect of guava juice in mice and human subjects. *The American Journal of Chinese Medicine*, 11 (1–4), 74–76.

Dar, A., Faizi, S., Naqvi, S. *et al.* (2005). Analgesic and antioxidant activity of mangiferin and its derivatives: The structure activity relationship. *Biological Pharmaceutical. Bulletin*, 28, 596–600.

Daud, N.H., Aung, C.S., Hewavitharana, A.K. *et al.* (2010). Mango extracts and the mango component mangiferin promote endothelial cell migration. *Journal of Agriculture and Food Chemistry*, 58, 5181–5186.

De Whalley, C., Rankin, S., Hoult, J., Jessup, W. and Leake, D. (1990). Flavonoids inhibit the oxidative modification of low density lipoproteins by macrophages. *Biochemical Pharmacology*, 39, 1743–1750.

Dhingra, M.K., Gupta,O.P. and Chundawant, B.S. (1983). Studies on pectin yield and quality of some guava cultivars in relation to cropping season and fruit maturity. *Journal of Food Science and Technology*, 20, 10–14.

Di Mascio, P., Kaiser, S. and Sies, H. (1989). Lycopene as the most efficient biological carotenoid singlet oxygen quencher. *Archives of Biochemistry and Biophysics*, 274 (2), 532–538.

Duthie, S.J., Ma, A., Ross, M.A. and Collins, A.R. (1996). Antioxidant supplementation decreases oxidative DNA damage in human lymphocytes. *Cancer Research*, 56, 1291–1295.

Eipeson, W.E. and Bhowmik, S.R. (1992). Indian fruit and vegetable processing industry-Potential and challenges. *Indian Food Packer*, 46 (5), 7–12.

El-Ansari, M., Reddy, K., Sastry, K. and Nayudamma, Y. (1969). Polyphenolic components of mango (*Mangifera indica*) fruit. *Leather Science*, 16, 13–14.

El-Ansari, M.A., Reddy, K.K., Sastry, K.N.S. and Nayudamma, Y. (1971). Polyphenols of *Mangifera indica*. *Phytochemistry*, 10, 2239–2241.

Elleuch, M., Bedigian, D., Roiseux, O. *et al.* (2011). Dietary fibre and fibre-rich by-products of food processing: Characterisation, technological, functionality and commercial applications: A review. *Food Chemistry*, 124 (2), 411–421.

El-Nemr, S.E., Ismail, I.A. and Ragab, M. (2006). Chemical composition of juice and seeds of pomegranate fruit. *Die Nahrung*, 34 (7), 601–606.

Fadavi, A., Barzegar, M. and Azizi, H.M. (2006). Determination of fatty acids and total lipid content in oilseed of 25 pomegranates varieties grown in Iran. *Journal Food Composition Analysis*, 19, 676–680.

FAO (2004). Products Year Report. Food and Agriculture Organization, Rome.

Galeotti, F., Barile, E., Curir, P., Dolci, M. and Lanzotti, V. (2008). Flavanoids from carnation (*Dianathus caryophyllus*) and their antifungal activity. *Phytochemistry Letters*, 1, 44–48.

González-Aguilar, G.A., Celis, J., Sotelo-Mundo, R.R. *et al.* (2008). Physiological and biochemical changes of different fresh cut mango cultivars stored at 5 °C. *International Journal of Food Science and Technology*, 43, 91–101.

González-Aguilar, G.A., Ruiz Cruz, S., Cruz Valenzuela, R., Rodríguez Félix, A. and Wang, C.Y. (2004). Physiological and quality changes of fresh-cut pineapple treated with antibrowning agents. *Labensmittel-Wissenschaft und-Technologie,* 37, 369–376.

Gordon, M.F. (1990). The mechanism of antioxidant action *in vitro*, in *Food Antioxidants* (ed. B.J.F. Hudson), Elsevier Applied Science, London, pp. 1–18.

phenolic profiles of five commercial varieties of mango (*Mangifera indica* L.). *Journal of Agriculture and Food Chemistry*, 57, 10825–10830.

Masibo, M. and He, Q. (2008). Major Mango polyphenols and their potential significance to human health, *Comprehensive Reviews in Food Science and Food Safety,* 7, 309–319.

Medić-Šarić, M., Rastija, V., Bojić1, M. and Maleš, Z. P. (2009). From functional food to medicinal product: Systematic approach in analysis of polyphenolics from propolis and wine. *Nutrition Journal*, 33 (8), 1–18.

Melgarejo, P., Martínez, J.J., Hernández, F. *et al.* (2009). Cultivar identification using 18S-18S rDNA intergenic spacer- RFLP in pomegranate (*Punica granatum* L.). *Scientia Horticulture*, 120, 500–503.

Mercadante, A.Z., Steck, A. and Pfander, H. (1999). Carotenoids from guava (*Psidium guajava* L.): Isolation and structure elucidation. *Journal of Agricultural and Food Chemistry*, 47 (1), 145–151.

Miean, K.H. and Mohamed, S. (2001). Flavonoid (myricetin, quercetin, kaempferol, luteolin, and apigenin) content of edible tropical plants. *Journal of Agricultural and Food Chemistry*, 49, 3106–3112.

Miguel, G., Dundlen, S., Antunes, D., Neves, A. and Martins, D. (2004). The effect of two methods of pomegranate juice extraction on quality during storage at 4°C. *Journal of Biomedicine and Biotechnology*, 5, 332–337.

Mirdehghan, S.H. and Rahemi, M. (2007). Seasonal changes of mineral nutrients and phenolics in pomegranate (*Punica granatum* L.) fruit. *Science Horticulture*, 111 (2), 120– 127.

Miyazawa, M., Oshima, T., Koshio, K., Itsuzaki, Y. and Anzai, J. (2003). Tyrosinase inhibitor from black rice bran. *Journal of Agricultural and Food Chemistry*, 51, 6953–6956.

Mousavinejad, G., Emam-Djomeh, Z., Rezaei, K. and Khodaparast, M.H.H. (2009). Identification and quantification of phenolic compounds and their effects on antioxidant activity in pomegranate juices of eight Iranian cultivars. *Food Chemistry*, 115, 1274–1278.

Muda, P., Seymour, G., Errington, N. and Tucker, G. (1995). Compositional changes in cell wall polymers during mango fruit ripening. *Carbohydrate Polymers*, 26, 255–260.

Mukherjee, S.K. and Datta, M.N. (1967). Physico-chemical changes in Indian guava during fruit development. *Current Science*, 36, 674–676.

Muruganandan, S., Srinivasan, K., Gupta, S., Gupta, P.K. and Lal, J. (2005). Effect of mangiferin on hyperglycemia and atherogenicity in streptozotocin diabetic rats. *Journal of Ethnopharmacology*, 97, 497–501.

Naveena, B.M., Sen, A.R., Kingsly, R.P., Singh, D.B. and Kondaiah, N. (2008). Antioxidant activity of pomegranate rind powder extract in cooked chicken patties. *International Journal of Food Science and Technology*, 43, 1807–1812.

Negi, P.S. and Jayaprakasha, G.K. (2003). Antioxidant and antibacterial activities of *Punica granatum* peel extracts. *Journal of Food Science*, 68, 1473–1477.

Niemetz, R. and Gross, G.G. (2001). Gallotannin biosynthesis: b-Glucogallin: hexagalloyl 3-*O*-galloyltransferase from *Rhus typhinia* leaves. *Phytochemistry*, 58, 657–661.

Noratto, G.D., Bertoldi, M.C., Krenek, K. *et al.* (2010). Anticarcinogenic effects of polyphenolics from mango (*Mangifera indica*) varieties. *Journal of Agriculture and Food Chemistry*, 58, 4104–4112.

Nunez-Selles, A.J. (2005). Antioxidant therapy: myth or reality. *Journal of Brazilian Chemist Society*, 16 (4), 699–710.

Ozgul-Yucel, S. (2005). Determination of conjugated linolenic acid content of selected oil seeds grown in Turkey. *Journal of American Oil Chemist Society*, 82 (12), 893–897.

Padula, M. and Rodriguez-Amaya, D.B. (1986). Characterisation of the carotenoids and assessment of the vitamin A value of Brasilian guavas (*Psidium guajava* L.). *Food Chemistry*, 20 (1), 11–19.

Palafox-Carlos, H., Yahia, E., Islas-Osuna, M.A. *et al.* (2012). Effect of ripeness stage of mango fruit (*Mangifera indica* L., cv. Ataulfo) on physiological parameters and antioxidant activity. *Scientia Horticulturae*, 135, 7–13.

Parker, C.C., Parker, M.L., Smith, A.C. and Waldron, K.W. (2003). Thermal stability of texture in Chinese water chestnut may be dependent on 8,80-diferulic acid. *Journal of Agricultural and Food Chemistry*, 51, 2034–2039.

Passamonti, S., Vrhovsek, U., Vanzo, A. and Mattivi, F. (2003). The stomach as a site for and anthocyanins absorption from food. *FEBS Letters*, 544 (1), 210–213.

Pin-Der, D. (1998). Antioxidant activity of burdock (*Arctium lappa* L.): its scavenging effects on free radical and active oxygen. *Journal of American Oil Chemist Society*, 75, 455–461.

Poyrazoglu, E, Gökmen, V. and Artιk, N. (2002). Organic acids and phenolic compounds in pomegranates (*Punica granatum* L.) grown in Turkey. *Journal of Food Composition and Analysis*, 15, 567–575.

Ask.About. Chemistry (2013). Qurecetin chemical structure. http://chemistry.about.com/od/factsstructures/ig/Chemical-Structures—Q/Quercetin.htm [accessed 12 July 2013].

Rajendran, P., Ekambaram, G. and Sakthisekaran, D. (2008). Effect of mangiferin on benzo(a)pyrene induced lung carcinogenesis in experimental Swiss albino mice. *Natural Product Research*, 22, 672–680.

Rastraelli, L., Selles, A.J.N., Castro, H.T.V. *et al.* (2002). Isolation and quantitative analysis of phenolic antioxidants, free sugars, and polyols from mango (*Mangifera indica* L.) stem bark aqueous decoction used in Cuba as a nutritional supplement. *Journal of Agriculture and Food Chemistry*, 50, 762–766.

Reddy, M.K., Gupta, S.K., Jacob, M.R., Khan, S.I. and Ferreira, D. (2007). Antioxidant, antimalarial and antimicrobial activities of tannin-rich fractions, ellagitannins and phenolics acids from *Punica granatum* L. *Planta Medica*, 73, 461–467.

Ribeiro, S.M.R., Barbosa, L.C.A., Queiroz, J.H., Knodler, M. and Schieber, A. (2008). Phenolic compounds and antioxidant capacity of Brazilian mango (*Mangifera indica* L.) varieties. *Food Chemistry,* 110, 620–626.

Rice-Evans, C.A., Miller, N.J. and Paganga, G. (1997). Antioxidant properties of phenolic compounds. *Tropical Plant Science*, 2, 152–159.

Robards, K., Prenzler, P.D., Tucker, G., Swatsitang, P. and Glover, W. (1999). Phenolic compounds and their roles in oxidative process in fruits. *Food Chemistry,* 66, 401–436.

Robles-Sánchez, R.M., Rojas-Graü, M.A., Odriozola-Serrano, I., González-Aguilar, G. and Martin-Belloso, O. (2013). Influence of alginate-based edible coating as carrier of antibrowning agents on bioactive compounds and antioxidant activity in fresh-cut Kent mangoes. *LWT – Food Science and Technology,* 50, 240–246.

Rompel, A., Fischer, H., Meiwes, D. *et al.* (1999). Substrate specificity of catechol oxidase from *Lycopus europaeus* and characterization of the bioproducts of enzymic caffeic acid oxidation. *FEBS Letters*, 445 (1), 103–110.

Sachan, B.P. and Ram, K. (1970). Ascorbic acid content of different varieties of guava (*Psidium guajava* L.) in Allahabad region. *Indian Food Packer*, 24, 6–10.

Sakagami, H., Satoh, K., Hatano, T., Yoshida, T. and Okuda, T. (1997). Possible role of radical intensity and oxidation potential for gallic acid-induced apoptosis. *Anticancer Research*, 17, 377–380.

Saleh, N.A.M. and El-Ansari, M.A.I. (1975). Polyphenolics of twenty local varieties of *Mangifera indica. Planta Medica*, 28, 124–130.

Saltveit, M. (2003). Fresh-cut vegetables, in *Postharvest Physiology and Pathology of Vegetables* (eds J.A. Bartz and J.K. Brecht), CRC Press, New York, pp. 691–697.

Sassano, G., Sanderson, P., Franx, J. *et al.* (2009). Analysis of pomegranate seed oil for the presence of jacaric acid. *Journal of the Science of Food and Agriculture*, 89, 1046–1052.

Sathiamoorthy, B., Gupta, P., Kumar, M. *et al.* (2007). New antifungal flavonoid glycoside from *Vitex negundo. Bioorganic and Medical Chemistry Letters*, 17, 239–242.

Scalbert, A., Manach, C., Morand, C., Rémésy, C. and Jiménez, L. (2005). Dietary polyphenols and the prevention of diseases. *Critcal Reviews in Food Science and Nutrition*, 45, 287–306.

Schieber, A., Ullrich, W. and Carle, R. (2000). Characterization of polyphenols in mango puree concentration by HPLC with diode array and mass spectrometric detection. *Innovative Food Science Emerging Technology*, 1, 161–166.

Setiawan, B., Sulaeman, A., Giraud, D.W. and Driskell, J.A. (2001). Carotenoid content of selected Indonesian fruits. *Journal of Food Composition and Analysis*, 14 (2), 169–176.

Shi, H.L., Noguchi, N. and Niki, E. (2001). Introducing natural antioxidants, in *Antioxidants in Food: Practical Applications* (ed. J. Pokorny), Woodhead Publishing Ltd. and CRC Press.

Shimogaki, H., Tanaka, Y., Tamai, H. and Masuda, M. (2000). *In vitro* and *in vivo* evaluation of ellagic acid on melanogenesis inhibition. *International Journal of Cosmetic Science*, 22, 291–303.

Sigler, K. and Ruch, R.J. (1993). Enhancement of gap junctional intercellular communication in tumor promoter-treated cells by components of green tea. *Cancer Letters*, 69, 1, 15–19.

Singh, U.P., Singh, D.P. and Singh, M. (2004). Characterization of phenolic compounds in some Indian mango cultivars. *International Journal of Food Science and Nutrition*, 55 (2), 163–169.

Soliva-Fortuny, R.C. and Martín-Belloso, O. (2003). New advances in extending the shelf-life of fresh-cut fruits: A review. *Trends in Food Science and Technology*, 14, 341–353.

Stoilova, I., Gargova, S., Stoyanova, A. and Ho, L. (2005). Antimicrobial and antioxidant activity of the polyphenol mangiferin. *Herbal Polonica*, 51, 37–44.

Tehranifar, A., Zarei, M., Nemati, Z., Esfandiyari, B. and Vasifeshenas, M.R. (2010). Investigation of physico-chemical properties and antioxidant activity of twenty Iranian pomegranate (*Punica granatum* L.) cultivars. *Scientia Horticulturae*, 126, 180–185.

Tezcan, F., Gültekin-Özgüven, M., Diken, T., Özçelik, B. and Erim, F.B. (2009). Antioxidant activity and total phenolic, organic acid and sugar content in commercial pomegranate juices. *Food Chemistry*, 115 (3), 873–877.

Thaipong, K., Boonprakob, U., Crosby, K., Cisneros-Zevallos, L. and Byrne, D.H. (2006). Comparison of ABTS, DPPH, FRAP, and ORAC assays for estimating antioxidant activity from guava fruit extracts. *Journal of Food Composition and Analysis*, 19, 669–675.

Tsai, P.J., Sun, Y.F. and Hsiao, S.M. (2010). Strengthening the texture of dried guava slice by infiltration of phenolic compounds. *Food Research International*, 43, 825–830.

USDA (2010). National Nutrient Database for Standard Reference, SR-23, Fruit Reports-09, Mango, raw. United States Department for Agriculture, p. 449.

Vendemiale, G., Grattagliano, I. and Altomare, E. (1999). An update on the role of free radicals and antioxidant defense in human disease. *International Journal of Clinical and Laboratory Research*, 29, 49–55.

Vinson, J. and Hontz, B. (1995). Phenol antioxidant index: comparative antioxidant effectiveness of red and white wines. *Journal of Agriculture and. Food Chemistry,* 43, 401–403.

Viuda-Martos, M., Fernández-López, J. and Pérez-Álvarez, J.A. (2010). Pomegranate and its many functional components as related to human health: A review. *Comprehensive Reviews in Food Science and Food Safety*, 9, 635–654.

Vivekananthan, D.P., Penn, M.S., Hsu, A. and Topol, E.J. (2003). Use of antioxidant vitamins for the prevention of cardiovascular disease: Meta-analysis of randomised trials. *Lancet*, 361, 2017–2023.

Wang, W.D. and Xu, S.Y. (2007). Degradation kinetics of anthocyanins in blackberry juice and concentrate. *Journal of Food Engineering*, 82, 271–275.

Wilberg, V.C. and Rodriguez-Amaya, D.B. (1995). HPLC quantitation of major carotenoids of fresh and processed guava, mango and papaya. *LWT – Food Science and Technology*, 28 (5), 474–480.

Woude, H.V.D., Gliszcynska-Swiglo, A., Struijs, K. *et al.* (2003). Biphasic modulation of cell proliferation by quercetin at concentrations physiologically relevant in humans. *Cancer Letters*, 200, 41–7.

Yamanaka, N., Oda, O. and Nagao, S. (1997). Green tea catechins such as (+)-epicatechin and (–)-epigallocatechin accelerate Cu^{2+}-induced low-density lipoprotein oxidation in propagation phase. *FEBS Letters*, 401, 230–234.

Yoshioka, K., Kataoka, T., Hayashi, T. *et al.* (2000). Induction of apoptosis by gallic acid in human stomach cancer KATO III and colon adenocarcinoma COLO 205 cell lines.*Oncology Reports*, 7 (6), 1221–1223.

Young, I.S. and Woodside, J.V. (2001). Antioxidants in health and disease. *Journal of Clinical Pathology*, 54, 176–186.

Zhang, J., Dhakal, I., Stone, A. *et al.* (2007). Plasma carotenoids and prostate cancer: a population-based case–control study in Arkansas. *Nutrition and Cancer*, 59 (1), 46–53.

5

Bioactive Compounds in Meat and their Functions

Punchira Vongsawasdi[1] and Athapol Noomhorm[2]
[1]Department of Microbiology, King Mongkut's University of Technology Thonburi, Bangkok, Thailand
[2]Food Engineering and Bioprocess Technology, Asian Institute of Technology, Pathum Thani, Thailand

5.1 Introduction

Meat and meat products are generally recognized as being important sources of nutrition. They are necessary for growth, maintenance and repair of the body. Red meat is not only a good source of high biological value protein, vitamins (vitamin B_2, vitamin B_6, vitamin B_{12}, pantothenic acid and niacin) and minerals (iron, zinc, phosphorus and selenium) but also a source of endogenous antioxidants (such as coenzyme Q10, glutathione, lipoic acid, etc.) and other bioactive substances (such as conjugated linoleic acid and essential omega-3 polyunsaturated fats) (Williams, 2007). Conversely, some substances in meat and meat products, especially saturated fatty acids and cholesterol, are harmful to consumer health, contributing to cardiovascular disease, hypertension, obesity and some types of cancer. Total fat and cholesterol profiles in beef and lamb are similar. The total fat and cholesterol for beef is about 1.7–12.7 g/100 g red meat and 35–99 mg/100 g red meat, respectively while that for lambs are 3.2–10.2 g/100 g and 54–96 mg/100 g, respectively. Lower amounts are found in veal, which contains 1.1–2.0 g fat/100 g red meat and 35–85 mg cholesterol/100 g red meat (Williams *et al.*, 2007). Appropriate technology is used to improve the functionality of meat and meat products. Enzymatic hydrolysis, lactic acid fermentation and physical methods of extraction such as supercritical fluid extraction, pressurized liquid extraction and ultrasound-assisted extraction have been used to isolate functional compounds (Lahl and Braun, 1994; Ryam *et al.*, 2011; Ibañez *et al.*, 2012). In this chapter, the active components that can promote health and/or complement the effect of nutrients from meat such as bioactive peptides, L-carnitine, coenzyme Q10, carnosine, taurine,

Functional Foods and Dietary Supplements: Processing Effects and Health Benefits, First Edition.
Edited by Athapol Noomhorm, Imran Ahmad and Anil Kumar Anal.

(ESI-MS) with quadrupole mass spectrometers are not only useful for obtaining peptide profiles of protein hydrolysates or semi-purified fractions, but also for accurately measuring masses of proteins up to 100 kDa or more (Careri and Mangia, 2003). As reported by Rajapakse *et al.* (2005), MALDI-TOF mass spectroscopic and sodium dodecylsulfate–polyacrylamide gel electrophoresis (SDS-PAGE) analysis were successful in identification of the purified protein of yellowfin sole which possessed anticoagulant activity. In 2012, Nazeer *et al.* investigated the antioxidant activity of hydrolysate from croaker (*Otolithes ruber*). The researchers fractionated the hydrolysate by passage through fast protein liquid chromatography on a diethylaminoethyl (DEAE) anion exchange column then purified it by loading onto a Sephadex G-25 gel filtration column. Identification of peptides was conducted by electrospray ionization tandem mass spectrometry (ESI-MS/MS).

Functional properties of bioactive peptides Bioactive peptides have many potential applications in foods, health-care products and pharmaceuticals. Their functionality depends upon the sequence and number of amino acids. Many sequences of bioactive substances show similar effects whereas some of them exhibit multifunctional effects.

Antihypertensive properties Hypertension or high blood pressure is a chronic medical condition in which the cardiovascular blood pressure in the arteries is elevated. It is one of the major risk factors for many diseases including cardiovascular disease and coronary heart disease (Yokoyama *et al.*, 1992; Arihara, 2006). ACE or kininase II or dipeptidyl carboxy metalopeptidase (EC 3.4.15.1) plays an important role by promoting the conversion of angiotensin-I (Ang I, inactive decapeptide), to the potent octapeptide vasoconstrictor (angiotensin-II, Ang II) in the rennin–angiotensin system and deactivating the catalytic activity of the hypotensive peptide, bradykinin (Ondetti *et al.*, 1977). Ang II is a documented potent vasoconstrictor that acts directly on vascular smooth muscle cells. The function of Ang II is expanding vascular volume through sodium retention and fluid retention (Padfield and Morton, 1977) while the function of bradykinin is regulating uterine and ileal smooth muscle contraction, enhancing vascular permeability, activating peripheral and C fibres and increasing mucus secretion (Proud and Kaplan, 1988). The role of ACE inhibitors is to maintain the balance between the associated vasoconstrictive and salt-retentive attributes of Ang II with the vasodilatory effect of bradykinin (Brown *et al.*, 1998). ACE-inhibitory peptides function by reacting with ACE, resulting in unavailable ACE to cleave Ang I, hence preventing the production of the vasoconstrictor Ang II (Ahhmed and Muguruma, 2010). The mechanisms of the interaction between the peptides and ACE have been explained by Wijesekara and Kim (2010). The first mechanism is the binding of peptides to the active site of the ACE. The second is the binding of peptides to an inhibitor site located on the ACE. Both mechanisms can lead to modification of the protein conformation, thus preventing Ang I from binding to the ACE active site.

Bioactive peptides from fish sauces are found to have antihypertensive properties. ACE-inhibitory peptides from each fish species are different. Fish sauce from fermented anchovy contains AP (Ala-Pro), KP (Lys-Pro), RP (Arg-Pro), GP (Gly-Pro), EP (Glu-Pro), TP (Thr-Pro), VP (Val-Pro), GI (Gly-Ile), and DF (Asp-Phe). The ACE-inhibitory peptides of AP (Ala-Pro), GP (Gly-Pro), TP (Thr-Pro), VP (Val-Pro), NP (Asn-Pro), DM (Asp-Met), DL (Asp-Leu), AV (Ala-Val), and GV

(Gly-Val) were isolated from fermented sardine sauce while AP (Ala-Pro), RP (Arg-Pro), GP (Gly-Pro) and AGP (Ala-Gly-Pro) were isolated from fermented bonito sauce (Ichimura *et al.*, 2003). AP (Ala-Pro), KP (Lys-Pro) and RP (Arg-Pro) have high inhibitory activity since they have IC50 of 21–29 μM whereas IC50 of other peptides ranges from 290 to 2000 μM.

ACE-inhibitory peptides and their activities experimentally generated from porcine skeletal muscle protein (Arihara and Ohata, 2008) and from extracts of several fermented meat products (Sentandreu and Toldrá, 2007; Arihara and Ohata, 2008) have been reported. Digestion of porcine myosin by thermolysin resulted in myopentapeptide A and myopentapeptide B. The amino acid sequences of myopentapeptide A and B are MNPPK (Met-Asn-Pro-Pro-Lys) and ITTNP (Ile-Thr-Thr-Asn-Pro), respectively (Arihara *et al.*, 2001). Those two pentapeptides were proven to be potent antihypertensive peptides *in vivo* (Nakashima *et al.*, 2002). Crude myosin B in porcine skeletal muscle was a source of antihypertensive peptides when it was hydrolysed with pepsin. The peptide sequence was KRVITY (Lys-Arg-Val-Ile-Thr-Tyr) corresponding to positions 191–196 on the myosin heavy chain (Muguruma *et al.*, 2009). Octapeptide VKKVLGNP (Val-Lys-Lys-Val-Leu-Gly-Asn-Pro) corresponding to positions 47–54 on the myosin light chain was generated by digesting crude myosin light chain with pepsin (Katayama *et al.*, 2007). Troponin from porcine skeletal muscle was a source of active ACE-inhibitory peptides. A bioactive nanopeptide sequence RMLGQTPTK (Arg-Met-Leu-Gly-Gln-Thr-Pro-Thr-Lys) was categorized as a non-competitive inhibitor (Katayama *et al.*, 2004) while a peptide of seven amino acid sequence KRQHYDI (Lys-Arg-Gln-His-Tyr-Asp-Ile) was a substrate type inhibitor and it inhibited ACE activity *in vivo* in the short term (Katayama *et al.*, 2008).

ACE-inhibitory hydrolysates and peptides can be produced by digestion of collagenous materials such as porcine skin, bovine skin, fish cartilage, fish scales, squid tunics and sea cucumbers with proteases such as trypsin, chymotrypsin, pepsin, alcalase, pronase E, collagenase, bromelain and papain (Gómez-Guillén *et al.*, 2011). The ACE-inhibitory activity from collagen and gelatin hydrolysates and peptides was presumably related to the high concentration of hydrophobic amino acids, as well as high Pro levels (Ryan *et al.*, 2011). Kim *et al.* (2001) isolated ACE-inhibitory peptide from bovine skin gelatin hydrolysate using sequential protease treatments (alcalase, pronase E and collagenase) and a three-step ultrafiltration membrane reactor. The results showed that two peptides with amino acid sequences of GPV (Gly-Pro-Val) and GPL (Gly-Pro-Leu) were responsible for ACE-inhibitory activity. Peptides from fish skin gelatin contained a repetition of tripeptide GPHyp (Gly-Pro-Hyp) with high ACE-inhibitory effects in their structure (Kimand Mendis, 2006). Saiga *et al.* (2003a) reported that the most potent ACE-inhibitory activity peptides from chicken breast hydrolysate contained an amino acid sequence of GFHypGYHypGLHypGF (Gly-Phe-Hyp-Gly-Thr-Hyp-GlyLeu-Hyp-Gly-Phe) which was similar with that of collagen.

Many studies have shown that C-terminal end of ACE-inhibitory peptides is the controlling factor for ACE-inhibitory activity. The C-terminal amino acid residues of ACE-inhibitory peptides with potent activity are usually tryptophan, phenylalanine, tyrosine and proline (Cheung *et al.*, 1980; Maruyama and Suzuki, 1982). This is possibly because those hydrophobic amino acid residues have high affinity to achieve the subsites of ACE (Ryan *et al.*, 2011).

Anticoagulant Anticoagulant is a compound used to prevent the formation of blood clots. Enzymatically hydrolysed fish muscle peptides have shown anticoagulant and antiplatelet properties when tested *in vitro*. Rajapakse *et al.* (2005) reported that bioactive peptides from yellowfin sole (*Limanda aspera*) inhibited the activated coagulation factor XII (FXIIa) by forming an inactive complex regardless of Zn^{2+} mediation. The protein also acted to antagonize platelet membrane glycoprotein integrin, to arrest platelet aggregation. The experiment *in vitro* revealed that thrombosis inhibition occurred when the peptides bound with FXIIa and platelet membrane integrins.

Antioxidative activities Lipid oxidation results in secondary by-products which are potential carcinogens. Mostly they are reactive oxygen/nitrogen species (ROS/RNS) such as peroxyl radical (ROO·), alkoxyl radical (RO·), iron-oxygen complexes (ferryl and perferryl radicals), and nitric oxide (·NO). Those ROS/RNS can attack membrane lipids, damage DNA and have some effect on cellular signal transduction. Therefore, inhibition of oxidative processes is very important for cell survival. Lipid oxidation is an undesired process in food products as well. The formation of free radicals results in deterioration of nutrition values and shortens product shelf life (Ladikos and Lougovois, 1990). Consumption of these lipid-oxidized products may cause diseases due to a toxic reaction (Je *et al.*, 2007; Jung *et al.*, 2007).

The function of an antioxidant is either scavenging ROS/RNS to stop radical chain reactions, or inhibiting the reactive oxidants from being formed in the first place (preventive process) (Huang *et al.*, 2005). Antioxidants in the diet can be radical chain reaction inhibitors, metal chelators, oxidative enzyme inhibitors as well as antioxidant enzyme cofactors. The method to determine the antioxidant activity of a bioactive substance is usually based on its ability to scavenge ROS and free radicals or to prevent oxidation in model systems. Many antioxidant peptides derived from meat protein hydrolysates show potent antioxidant activity. They are effective against both enzymatic and non-enzymatic peroxidation. Je *et al.* (2007) found that tuna backbone protein hydrolysate could inhibit lipid peroxidation in a linoleic acid emulsion system and also quench free radicals (diphenylpicrylhydrazyl (DPPH), hydroxyl and superoxide) in a dose-dependent manner. The authors reported that peptic hydrolysate with the amino acid sequence VKAGFAWTANQQLS (Val-Lys-Ala-Gly-Phe-Ala-Trp-Thr-Ala-Asn-Gln-Gln-Leu-Ser) showed the highest antioxidant activity compared to other hydrolysates obtained by alcalase, α-chymotrypsin, neutrase, papain and trypsin. Sardinelle (*Sardinella aurita*) protein by-products from fish manufacturing are also a good source of antioxidant peptides. According to Bougatef *et al.* (2010), the industrial wastes from sardine processing were hydrolysed by crude enzyme extracted from sardine and then fractionated by size exclusion chromatography. Seven antioxidant peptides including LHY (Leu-His-Tyr), LARL (Leu-Ala-Arg-Leu), GGE (Gly-Gly-Glu), GAH (Gly-Ala-His), GAWA (Gly-Ala-Trp-Ala), PHYL (Pro-His-Tyr-Leu) and GALAAH (Gly-Ala-Leu-Ala-Ala-His) were discovered. Among those peptides, LHY (Leu-His-Tyr) exhibited the highest DPPH radical scavenging activity. Wu *et al.* (2003) found antioxidant activity in peptides derived from hydrolysate of mackerel. The antioxidant properties of those peptides included inhibiting the autoxidation of linoleic acid, quenching the free radical α,α-diphenyl-β-picrylhydrazyl (DPPH) and reducing ferric ions. Hydrolysis of fish skin gelatin with trypsin provided hydrolysate peptides with the amino acid sequence HGPLGPL

(His-Gly-Pro-Leu-Gly-Pro-Leu). The peptide acted as a strong DPPH radical scavenger and antioxidant against linoleic acid peroxidation. Its activity was closer to the highly active synthetic antioxidant butylated hydroxytoluene (BHT) but more effective than α-tocopherol in inhibiting lipid peroxidation (Mendis *et al.*, 2005).

Saiga *et al.* (2003b) reported that peptides obtained from porcine myofibrillar proteins hydrolysed with papain and actinase E could inhibit peroxidation of linoleic acid, DPPH scavenging and metal chelating activities. The peptides were identified as DSGVT (Asp-Ser-Gly-Val-Thr, actin), IEAEGE (Ile-Glu-Ala-Glu-Gly-Glu, unknown), DAQEKLE (Asp-Ala-Gln-Glu-Lys-Leu-Glu, tropomyosin), EELDNALN (Glu-Glu-Leu-Asp-Asn-Ala-Leu-Asn, tropomyosin) and PSIDDQEELM (Pro-Ser-Ile-Asp-Asp-Gln-Glu-Glu-Leu-Met, myosin heavy chain). Liu *et al.* (2010) discovered that hydrolysate from porcine plasma also contained active antioxidant. The most active fraction was less than 3 kDa with the amino acid sequence HNGN (His-Asn-Gly-His). The peptide showed effective inhibition of lipid oxidation, DPPH scavenging, metal chelating and reducing agent properties. Similar properties of antioxidant activities from chicken essence hydrolysates were reported by Wu *et al.* (2005). The peptide sequences were HVTEE (His-Val-Thr-Glu-Glu) and PVPVEGV (Pro-Val-Pro-Val-Glu-Gly-Val).

Metal binding activity Metal ions are important in many metabolic processes, for example, triggering mechanisms, stabilizing structure and controlling redox reactions in the body. The reaction between the metals and the metal-binding compounds makes soluble forms of the metals that are readily available for organisms (Jung *et al.*, 2006; Kovacs-Nolan and Mine, 2006). Peptides can function as metal-binding compounds. It is believed that side chains of amino acid residues interact with ions. Metal-binding peptides are believed to play a significant role in metal homeostasis and aid detoxification of some heavy ions (Walther and Sieber, 2011).

The calcium cation has many significant roles such as providing rigidity to the skeleton and acting as a secondary messenger in regulating numerous intracellular events by taking advantage of its large membranous concentration gradient. Calcium deficiency is associated with a number of common and chronic diseases such as osteoporosis, osteoarthritis, cardiovascular disease (hypertension and stroke), diabetes, obesity and cancer (Anderson and Garner, 1996). To enhance the bioavailability of calcium, the amount of calcium ingested and the substances coexisting with it should be considered. Huang *et al.* (2011) purified peptides from protein hydrolysates of shrimp processing by-products and found that TCH (Thr-Cys-His) was responsible for higher calcium binding properties. The authors postulated that high calcium binding ability might be due to the presence of the sequence of His residue. Fouchereau-Peron *et al.* (1999) reported that fish protein hydrolysates also involved calcium metabolism by accelerating calcium absorption and decreasing the number of osteoclasts.

Antimicrobial activity Bioactive peptides can inhibit microbial growth. Their action modes are disrupting membranes, interfering with metabolism and targeting cytoplasmic components which result in inhibition of cell wall synthesis, alteration of the cytoplasmic membrane, activation of autolysin, inhibition of DNA, RNA and protein synthesis, and inhibition of certain enzymes (Huang *et al.*, 2011). Many researchers have investigated the antimicrobial activity of bioactive peptides from various foods. Lactoferrin from whey protein demonstrates high bacteriostatic and bactericidal properties attributed to its ability to chelate iron or to bind to bacterial surfaces (Sharma *et al.*, 2011). For meat and meat products, Di Bernardini *et al.* (2011) found that hydrolysates from bovine heart myofibrillar proteins showed some potential to be used as antimicrobial agents, whereas myofibrillar proteins actin and myosin extracted from bovine skeletal muscle and their hydrolysates exhibited no antimicrobial and antithrombotic activity. Different results were discovered by Jang *et al.* (2008) who investigated antimicrobial activity of extracted previously identified ACE-inhibitory peptides from a bovine meat source. The authors found that the octapeptides GLSDGEWQ (Gly-Leu-Ser-Asp-Gly-Glu-Trp-Gln) inhibited the growth of both Gram-positive (*Bacillus cereus* and *Listeria monocytogenes*) and Gram-negative (*Salmonella typhimurium* and *Escherichia coli*) microorganisms, whereas GFHI (Gly-Phe-His-Ile) as well as FHG (Phe-His-Gly) inhibited the growth of *Pseudomonas aeruginosa.*

Antiproliferative activity Antiproliferative peptides have been less documented in meat and meat products. Jang *et al.* (2008) studied the cytotoxic effect of previously identified ACE-inhibitory peptides by using the cell lines breast adenocarcinoma (MCF-7), stomach adenocarcinoma (AGS) and lung carcinoma (A549) cells. The results showed that the peptide GFHI (Gly-Phe-His-Ile) exhibited the strongest cytotoxic effect on MCF-7 cells while the peptide GLSDGEWQ (Gly-Leu-Ser-Asp-Gly-Glu-Trp-Gln) potently inhibited AGS cell proliferation. Peptide fractions from tuna dark muscle by-product hydrolysis also demonstrated potential antiproliferative activity when they were exposed to human breast cell line MCF-7 (Hsu *et al.*, 2010). The strongest antiproliferative activities were found in the peptides LPHVLTPEAGAT (Leu-Pro-His-Val-Leu-Thr-Pro-Glu-Ala-Gly-Ala-Thr) from papain hydrolysate and PTAEGVYMVT (Pro-Thr-Ala-Glu-Gly-Val-Tyr-Met-Val-Tre) from protease XXIII.

5.2.2 Fermentation

With the concept of probiotics, traditional fermented meat products can be considered functional food. Probiotics are defined as live microorganisms that offer benefits to the host when ingested (FAO/WHO, 2001). The examples of probiotic strains are *Lactobacillus acidophilus, Lactobacillus rhamnosus, Lactobacillus casei, Lactobacillus salivarius, Lactobacillus plantarum, Lactobacillus paracasei, Lactobacillus brevis, Bifidobacterium bifidum, Bifidobacterium infantis, Bifidobacterium longum, Bifidobacerium breve, Streptococcus thermophilus, Lactobacillus bulgaricus, Lactobacillus gasseri, Bifidobacterium lactis* and *Saccharomyces boulardii* (Agrawal, 2005; Tanasupawat, 2009). The functions of probiotics are well documented. Their duties consist of preventing diarrhoea, ameliorating constipation, lowering faucal enzyme activities, lowering blood cholesterol level, modulation of immune responses, preventing of food allergies, preventing cancer and acting as an adjuvant in *Helicobacter pylori* treatment (Agrawal, 2005; Lesbros-Pantoflickova *et al.*, 2007). Probiotics are often used in dairy products. However, their application in meat products is still being explored. Traditional styles of fermented sausages from Europe are uncooked meat products. They consist of coarse mixtures of lean meats and fatty tissues combined with non-food ingredients such as salt, nitrite, sugar and spices (Heinz and

Hautzinger, 2007). The typical flavour and texture of the fermented sausages are usually developed during the ripening phase. Examples of European fermented sausages include salami, mettwurst and summer sausage. In Asia, sucuk is a fermented sausage made in Turkey. The sausage mix consists of beef, spices (with garlic and pepper) and filled in an inedible casing. In Thailand, there are many varieties of fermented sausage which are specialities of a specific region. Nham is one of the most popular dishes. It is made with coarsely ground pork, sliced pork skins, cooked sticky rice (gelatinous), salt, nitrite and spices. The sausage is wrapped in banana leaves or a plastic bag and fermented for 3–5 days at room temperature. The fermentation process enables the growth of lactic acid bacteria derived from the raw materials, which accounts for the sourness of the sausage. Lactic acid bacteria found in Thai sausage fermentation are *Lactobacilli* sp., *Pediococci* sp. and *Leuconostoc* sp. The *Lactobacilli* sp. is found during early stage of the fermentation, while the *Pediococci* sp. and the *Leuconostoc* sp. grow successively towards the end of the fermentation process after the pH has reached 4.6. Another example is Sai Krok Isan. This type of sausage uses coarsely cut pork lard instead of pork skin and the entire mixture is stuffed into casings derived from the small intestines of pig or cattle.

Several researchers have intensively investigated probiotics in fermented sausages. In 1998, Arihara *et al.* reported that *Lactobacillus gasseri* showed the greatest fermentation performance in meats as compared with other strains in the *Lactobacillus acidophilus* group (*L. acidophilus, L. crispatus, L. amylovorus, L. gallinarum, L. gasseri, L. johnsonii).* In the same year, Sameshima *et al.* (1998) found that *L. rhamnosus* and *L. paracasei* subsp. *paracasei* inhibited the growth and enterotoxin production of *Staphylococcus aureus* in sausages during fermentation. Erkkilä, *et al.* (2001) found that *Lactobacillus rhamnosus* GG and *Lactobacillus rhamnosus* E-97800 are suitable for use as probiotic starter cultures in fermenting dry sausage.

5.3 L-Carnitine

L-Carnitine (γ-trimethyamino-β-hydroxy butylic acid) is generated from the amino acids lysine and methionine (Schmid, 2010). Since L-carnitine can be synthesized in the human body, it is not considered a dietary essential. However, this bioactive compound is considered a conditionally essential nutrient for people who have genetic or certain disorders where its production does not meet their needs under certain conditions (Rebouche, 1999). L-Carnitine is produced in the liver and kidneys and stored in the skeletal muscle, heart, brain and nearly all tissues. Schmid (2010) reported that only about 25% of the L-carnitine is produced in the human body while about 75% is taken from food. Red meat is a good source of L-carnitine. Beef steak, ground beef and lamb chop have an L-carnitine content of 65, 87.5 and 40.5 mg/100 g fresh weight, respectively. The concentration of L-carnitine in poultry and fish are not as high as in red meat. The concentration in chicken breast without skin and tuna fish are 10.4 and 1.5 mg/100 g fresh weight, respectively (Demarquoy *et al.*, 2004). The major function of L-carnitine is to transport long chain fatty acids across inner mitochondrial membranes where the fatty acids are converted into biological energy by β-oxidation (Arihara and Ohata, 2011). That energy is necessary for muscular and all other activities throughout the body. Vescovo *et al.* (2002) demonstrated that L-carnitine plays a significant role in blocking apoptosis and preventing skeletal muscle myopathy in heart failure. As a food supplement, it is used as an adjunct to standard medical therapy. It has a positive influence on primary and secondary carnitine deficiencies, myocardial infarction and heart failure (Iliceto *et al.*, 1995), intermittent claudication (Hiatt, 2001), end-stage renal disease (Calvani *et al.*, 2004), type 2 diabetes (Mingrone *et al.*, 1999), Alzheimer's disease (Montgomery *et al.*, 2003), HIV infection (Ilias *et al.*, 2004) and male infertility (Ng *et al.*, 2004). L-Carnitine as a food supplement is also believed to enhance athletic performance due to its role in energy production (Schmid, 2010). However, evidence that carnitine supplements can improve exercise or physical performance in healthy subjects are not consistent (Brass, 2000).

5.4 Coenzyme Q10

Coenzyme Q10 or CoQ10 or ubiquinone or 2, 3-dimethoxy-5-methyl-6-multiprenyl-1,4-benzoquinone is an oil soluble, vitamin-like substance. Meat, fish, pulses, nuts, dairy products and various vegetables are good sources of coenzyme Q10 (Kamei *et al.*, 1986). Coenzyme Q10 contents in various diets was exclusively reviewed by Pravst *et al.* (2010). The amount of coenzyme Q10 in beef, chicken and pork meat are 16.1–36.5, 14–21 and 24.3–41.1 mg/kg, respectively. Their internal organs are excellent sources of coenzyme Q10. Beef heart, chicken heart and pork heart contains 113.3, 92.3–192 and 118.1–282 mg/kg, respectively whereas their livers contain 39.2–50.5, 116.2–132.2 and 22.7–54.0 mg/kg, respectively (Mattila and Kumpulainen, 2001). The biosynthesis of coenzyme Q10 begins from tyrosine through a multistage process requiring eight vitamins, namely tetrahydrobiopterin, vitamins B_2, B_6, B_{12}, folic acid, niacin, pantothenic acid and vitamin C (Folkers, 1996). The quinone ring structure is derived from the amino acid tyrosine, the methyl groups on the ring supplied by methionine and the isoprenoid side chain coming from the mevalonate pathway (the same pathway shared by cholesterol) (Pravst *et al.*, 2010).The bioactive compound is localized on the hydrophobic side of phospholipid double layer of cell membrane (Schmid, 2010). It is a naturally occurring antioxidant and acts as a key component of cellular respiration. The functions of coenzyme Q10 in antioxidant protection and cellular energy production are based on the ability to exchange electrons between ubiquinol (reduced coenzyme Q10 or coenzyme QH2 or CoQH2) and ubiquinone (oxidized coenzyme Q10) in a redox cycle (Mellors and Tappel, 1966a, 1966b). Coenzyme Q10 can neutralize free radicals which cause cell damage and/or cell death (Schmid, 2009). In aerobic cellular respiration, it exhibits a significant role in an electron transport chain by carrying electrons from enzyme complex I and II to enzyme complex III within mitochondria (Bentinger *et al.*, 2010) thus preventing oxidative stress – the condition in which large quantities of oxygen radicals occur in an organism (Schmid, 2009). The exceptionally high efficiency of coenzyme Q10 as an antioxidant is exclusively explained by Bentinger *et al.* (2010). Coenzyme Q10 prevents lipid peroxidation by impeding the production of lipid peroxyl radicals ($LOO^{\cdot}$) and CoQH2 reduces the initial perferryl radicals, with concomitant formation of ubisemiquinone (partially reduced form) and H_2O_2. The quenching of the initiating perferryl radicals can protect both lipids and proteins from the oxidation process. This property makes coenzyme Q10 superior to other antioxidants. Moreover, the fully reduced form of coenzyme Q10 (ubiquinol) is capable of regenerating other antioxidants such as tocopherol (vitamin E) and ascorbate (vitamin C) (Frei *et al.*, 1990). According to Bindoli *et al.* (1985), ubiquinol regenerates α-tocopherol from α-tocopherolquinone to α-tocopherolhydroquinone. This important finding confirms the sparing effect of ubiquinol-10 on α-tocopherol (Frei *et al.*, 1990; Ernster and Dallner, 1995).

Coenzyme Q10 can be used as a supplement for heart failure patients. It helps reduce swelling in the legs, fluid in the lungs and makes breathing easier (Khatta *et al.*, 2000; Rosenfeldt *et al.*, 2003). The reduced form of the bioactive compound may be involved in the ageing process since it has been found that aged people have reduced coenzyme Q10 biosynthesis and have lost the ability to convert ubiquinone to ubiquinol (Wada *et al.*, 2007). Other possible health benefits of coenzyme Q10 is healing people with periodontal disease (gum disease). The cause of inflammation is the excess generation of reactive oxygen species (ROS). Coenzyme Q10 intake may lead to faster healing and tissue repair. Coenzyme Q10 is also associated with neurodegenerative illness. It can be used as part of the treatment for Parkinson's disease (Dhanasekaran and Ren, 2005).

5.5 Carnosine

Carnosine (β-alanyl-L-histidine) is a natural imidazole-containing compound only found in meat, poultry and some fish. Purchas *et al.* (2004) found carnosine quantities of 400 mg/100 g in lamb. Its content in pasture-finished cattle displays a comparable value of 453 mg/100 g (Purchas and Zou, 2008). Mora *et al.* (2008a) reported that there were quantities of between 211–419 mg/100 g in pork muscles. The histidyl dipeptide is synthesized in muscle and brain. It acts as proton buffering neutropeptide with high buffer capacity in the muscle (Artioli *et al.*, 2010). Therefore, it can stabilize intramuscular pH, resulting in an enlarged capacity for anaerobic performance and tolerance for oxygen deficit conditions (Abe, 2000). Hipkiss (2010) found that carnosine may play an important role in ageing protection by helping advanced glycation end-products (AGE) scavenging macrophages to better recognize the AGE molecules thus facilitating the AGE elimination process. Moreover, it can react with methylglyoxal and possibly other deleterious carbonyl compounds. Methylglyoxal is postulated to be involved in the formation of AGEs. It is considered to be a risk marker for pathophysiological conditions in age-related diseases such as diabetes, arteriosclerosis and Alzheimer's disease (Schimd, 2010). Preston *et al.* (1998) reported that carnosine inactivated and blocked β amyloid, a substance that interacted with certain RAGE receptors, thus causing damage to the nerves and arteries of the brain in Alzheimer's disease patients. Carnosine's other ability is as an antioxidant that stabilizes and protects cell membranes. It has been proven to scavenge ROS (Yoshikawa *et al.*, 1991). The review by Guiotto *et al.* (2005), showed that carnosine could act as a natural scavenger of dangerous reactive aldehydes such as malondialdehyde (MDA), which occurred from the degradative oxidative pathway of endogenous molecules. MDA can cause harm to health by damaging lipids and DNA (Marnett, 1999). Some studies have proposed that carnosine can form a complex with various transition metals and display different biological functions. Decker *et al.* (2001) discovered that carnosine can inhibit low density lipoprotein (LDL) oxidation, the early events in the production of atherosclerosis, through copper chelation. In pharmacological activity, Polaprezinc or the Zn(II) complex of carnosine is effective against *Helicobacter pylori,* a causative agent for stomach ulcers (Baran, 2000). Carnosine could potentially be used as a natural antioxidant in meat products. It could reduce oxidative processes and metmyoglobin formation in ground beef and beef patties after irradiation and during storage (Bard, 2007).

5.6 Taurine

Taurine (2-aminoethanesulfonic acid) is an amino sulfonic acid. It is abundant in meat, poultry, fish, clams and shellfish. The taurine contents in beef and pork are 43.1–46.3 mg/100 g and 50.1–61.2 mg/100 g, respectively. (Pasantes-Morales *et al.*, 1989; Laidlaw *et al.*,1990). In bivalves, the tuarine contents in mussels, oysters and clams display between 97.4 and 655.4 mg/100 g (Laidlaw *et al.*, 1990). Offal is also a rich source of taurine. Zhao Xi-he (1994) reported that liver, kidney and heart of pig contain 42, 120 and 200 mg of taurine/100 g, respectively. Taurine is a major constituent of bile and a small amount can be synthesized in human liver from methionine and cysteine (Wójcik *et al.*, 2010). The component has multiple functions and plays a significant role in many physiological processes, such as osmoregulation, immunomodulation and bile salt formation (Bouckenooghe *et al.*, 2006). It regulates serum cholesterol levels by conjugation of cholesterol to form bile salts. The amino terminal group of taurine reacts with chenodeoxycholic acid and cholic acid which alters cholesterol solubility and enables cholesterol excretion (Wójcik *et al.*, 2010). It may also lower cholesterol levels via an upregulation of the hepatic low density lipoprotein receptor (LDLR) and/or via an improvement in the binding of LDL to LDLR (Wójcik *et al.*, 2010). Taurine controls blood pressure by decreasing Ang II signals, or enhancing the kinin–kallikrein system in kidney that causes vasodilation. In addition, it involves osmoregulation by aiding the movement of potassium and magnesium into the cell membranes while helping the movement of excessive sodium out (Bouckenooghe *et al.*, 2006). The other approach to lowering blood pressure is by enhancing endorphin production (Khosh and Khosh, 2001). Taurine also acts as an antioxidant and anti-inflammatory since it can react with a powerful oxidant such as hypochlorous acid and form taurine chloramine which is more stable (Wójcik *et al.*, 2010). The research data of Militante and Lombardini (2002) revealed that taurine was an important neurochemical factor in the visual system. It is considered a conditionally essential compound in infant nutrition since it cannot be synthesized in sufficient quantities. The functions of taurine in the newborn infant are fat absorption, prevention of granulation of the retina and electroencephalographic changes and improving maturation of auditory-evoked responses (Chesney *et al.*, 1998).

5.7 Creatine

Creatine (3-methylguanidinoacetic acid or *N*-(aminoiminomethyl)-*N*-methylglycine) is a nitrogenous organic acid. It is found in red meat and fish. High amounts of creatine (401 mg/100 g) are present in fresh beef. Lower concentrations are found in beef heart, beef cheek and beef liver (Purchas *et al.*, 2004). Creatine can be synthesized in human liver, kidney and pancreas from L-arginine, L-glycine and L-methionine (Edison, 2007; Gualano *et al.*, 2011). Processing has significant effects on creatine. Mora *et al.* (2008b) reported that creatine continuously decreased during cooking. At high pH, creatine efflorescence could be formed on the surface of sausage (Kroeckel, 2004). The main function of creatine is energy provision in muscle contraction (Schmid, 2010). Creatine and its phosphorylated form exert a vital role in energy metabolism by maintaining ATP homeostasis at specific sites of high energy turnover at the onset of steady state contraction or during non-steady state contraction. Other functions are as an energy carrier and maintaining the ATP/ADP ratio in subcellular locations where creatine kinase is coupled to ATP-consuming and ATP-producing pathways (Greenhalff, 2001). Creatine exhibits antioxidant activity by scavenging radical species in a cellular setting (Sestil *et al.*, 2011). It is believed to strengthen muscle and is suggested as a complementary treatment for conditions in which muscle weakness occurs, such as muscular dystrophy, congestive heart failure, Huntington's disease, McArdle's disease (myophosphorylase deficiency or glycogen storage disease type V), amyotrophic lateral sclerosis, myasthenia gravis, Parkinson's disease and after injury or surgery (Tarnopolsky, 2008; Schmid, 2010; Gualano *et al.*, 2011).

5.8 Glutathione

Glutathione or γ-glutamyl-L-cysteinylglycine is composed of cysteine, glutamic acid and glyceine. It is found in two forms: a reduced glutathione (GSH) and an oxidized glutathione (GSSG) (Meister and Anderson, 1983). Dietary glutathione occurs in high amounts in fresh (uncooked) meat due to its cysteine content. However, hormones and toxins can virtually neutralize GSH, unless the meat is truly organic. The loss of GSH from foods is significant when foods are processed, especially by canning, drying and curing (Jones, 2011). Beef steak and pork chop are good sources of glutathione. Beef steak has GSH and GSSG of 12.3 mg/100 g and 13.4 mg/100 g, respectively whereas 18.9 mg/100 g and 23.6 mg/100 g, respectively are detected in pork chop (Jones *et al.*, 1992). Glutathione plays vital roles in the body. It is not only a blood booster but also an excellent antioxidant as well as a cell detoxifier. As food for blood, glutathione enables the body to produce more white blood cells and helps them to function properly (Fidelus and Tsan, 1987). Glutathione possesses antioxidant properties because the thiol group in its cysteine moiety is a reducing agent. A thiol group in the reduced state can donate a reducing equivalent to reactive oxygen species, thereby protecting against oxidative damage to DNA and protein. Glutathione becomes reactive after donating an electron but it promptly reacts with another reactive glutathione to form glutathione disulfide (GSSG). The oxidized glutathione can be broken down to the single active molecule again by NAPPH-dependent glutathione reductase (Jones, 2011). This bioactive compound is considered an excellent antioxidant (Schafer and Buettner, 2001; Bray and Taylor, 1994.). It protects cells throughout the body including all organ tissues. Glutathione also functions as a detoxifier of heavy metals and may protect against radiation poisoning as well as the detrimental effects of cigarette smoke and alcohol abuse (Meister and Anderson, 1983; Rahman and MacNee, 1999; James *et al.*, 2005). Glutathione in the liver is crucial to the liver's ability to detoxify. High levels of glutathione in the liver results in a high capacity of the liver to detoxify harmful chemicals such as heavy metals, alcohol and acetaminophen. There are three phases in detoxification process, namely: phase I toxin modification, phase II toxin conjugation and phase III excretion. Glutathione enhances phase II of the process by binding to or conjugating directly to toxic metabolites thus making them unable to diffuse across membranes. The conjugated substances are afterward removed from the body in phase III. The bioactive compound has been involved skin lightening. Various depigment mechanisms were proposed by Villarama and Maibach (2005). There were: (i) direct inactivation of the enzyme tyrosinase by binding with the copper-containing active site of the enzyme; (ii) mediating the switch mechanism from eumelanin to phaeomelanin production; (iii) quenching of free radicals and peroxides that contribute to tyrosinase activation and melanin formation; and (iv) modulation of the depigmenting abilities of melanocytotoxic agents. Glutathione is used to reduce symptoms associated with Parkinson's disease (Offen *et al.*, 1996). It neutralizes reactive oxygen species that cause the depletion of dopaminergic cells, the neurons found in the substantia nigra in the central nervous system. The dopaminergic cells release the essential neurotransmitter dopamine, which assists the body in controlling movement and coordination. Therefore, inadequacy in dopamine results in the development of Parkinson's disease symptoms (Offen *et al.*, 1996). In addition, dopamine is crucial for efficient information processing; deficiencies, perhaps, relate to Alzheimer's disease. Glutathione is also associated with the prevention and treatment of other diseases such as cardiovascular disease (Stamler and Slivka, 1996), cancer and tumour (Saydam *et al.*, 1997; Perquin *et al.*, 2000), pulmonary disease (Morris and Bernard, 1994) and autoimmune disease, that is rheumatoid arthritis and systemic lupus erythematosus (Fidelus and Tsan, 1987).

5.9 Lipoic acid

Lipoic acid or thioctic acid or (*R*)-5-(1,2-dithiolan-3-yl) pentanoic acid is a sulfur-containing coenzyme. It is derived from octanoic acid (caprylic acid) and sulfur amino acid (cysteine). Within the eight-carbon chain, there are two sulfur atoms attached at position six and eight. Lipoic acid can be found in dark green leafy vegetables like spinach, collard green and broccoli. Animals provide a small amount of this bioactive compound and their internal organs (liver, kidney and heart) have a slightly higher content compared to muscle (Mattulat and Baltes, 1992). Lipoic acid involves the conversion of nutrient energy into adenosine triphosphate (ATP). It is part of several multienzyme complexes in mitochondria such as pyruvate dehydrogenase (PDH), alpha-ketoglutarate dehydrogenase (alpha-KGDH) and branched-chain keto-acid dehydrogenase (BCKADH). PDH and alpha-KGDH are required in the Krebs cycle whereas BCKADH involves deriving energy from branched-chain amino acids including leucine, isoleucine and valine (Jacob *et al.*, 1995). Lipoic acid is also classified as an antioxidant (Packer *et al.*, 1995). Lipoic acid, or its reduced form, dihydrolipoic acid (DHLA), maintains the antioxidant defence system in the body by binding with reactive oxygen species such as superoxide radicals, hydroxyl radicals, hypochlorous acid, peroxyl radicals and singlet oxygen. The unique feature of lipoic acid is its ability to function equally well both in water-based and fat-based environments. Therefore, it helps regenerate vitamin C and vitamin E in the body. In addition, it can extend the activity of glutathione (Packer *et al.*, 1995; Biewenga *et al.*, 1997; Golbidi *et al.*, 2011). Lipoic acid is a powerful chelator of divalent metal ions *in vitro*. It can form stable complexes with Mn^{2+}, Cu^{2+}, Fe^{2+}, Pb^{2+} and Zn^{2+} (Ou *et al.*, 1995). DHLA can prevent low density lipoprotein (LDL) peroxidation in humans by either reductive inactivating Cu^{2+} when Cu^{2+} is excessive, or effective chelating of Cu^{2+} when DHLA is excessive. It, therefore, has both pro- and antioxidant properties depending upon the ratio of Cu^{2+} : DHLA (Bustamante *et al.*, 1998). In people with diabetes, hyperglycaemia leads to the formation of AGEs by increase of ·OH radicals resulting from glucose autoxidation. Lipoic acid can slow down the AGE formation by quenching those reactive oxygen species as well as increasing the conversion and storage of glucose through the stimulation of glucose transporter-1 (GLUT-1) and glucose transporter-4 (GLUT-4) (Golbidi *et al.*, 2011). The bioactive compound is also renoprotective. The progression of diabetic renal complications is prevented by decreasing oxidative stress, particularly, by reducing NADPH-induced generation of superoxide anion ($O^{\bullet -2}$) and regulating the expression of NADPH oxidase subunits (Bhatti *et al.*, 2005). Lipoic acid indirectly heals oxidized proteins in vital tissues such as brain, heart and liver by increasing the level of GSH and /or GSH/GSSG (the key components in maintaining protein thiols in a reduced form) in those tissues (Golbidi *et al.*, 2011). It is believed to help with cataracts, Parkinson's disease and Alzheimer's disease.

5.10 Opioids

Opioids are peptides with morphine-like activity. They have an affinity for an opiate receptor which is a transmembrane protein found in the dorsal horn of the spinal cord and in the brain regions. They function as hormone and neuromodulators. Therefore, their roles vary from regulating gastrointestinal motility as well as gastric and pancreatic secretions to increasing the amount produced in response to stress and relieving pain (Froehlich, 1997; Walther and Sieber, 2011). Opioid peptides can be produced by the body or absorbed from partially digested food. The endogenous peptides are formed in the central nervous system (CNS) and in various glands throughout the body (Froehlich, 1997) The opioid food peptides, also called exorphins, are found in milk (casomorphin), gluten (gluten exorphin and gliadorphin/gluteomorphin) and spinach (rubiscolin). Two exorphins from meat and poultry are those released from the digestion of serum albumin into serorphin and bovine haemoglobin into haemorphin (Walther and Sieber, 2011).

Haemorphins were first isolated from enzymatically treated bovine blood. Later, these peptides were found in the brain, plasma, and cerebrospinal fluid (Nyberg *et al.*, 1997). Investigation of bovine blood haemoglobin peptic hydrolysate revealed the presence of biologically active peptides with an affinity for opioid receptors (Nyberg *et al.*, 1997; Zhao *et al.*, 1997). Fruiter-Arnaudin *et al.* (2003) reported that hydrolysis of the beta-, kappa-, delta-, or epsilon-chain of the bovine blood protein haemoglobin by cathepsin D resulted in liberating VV-haemorphin 7 (Val-Val-Tyr-Pro-Trp-Thr-Gln-Arg-Phe) and LVV-hemorphin-7 (Leu-Val-Val-Tyr-Pro-Trp-Thr-Gln-Arg-Phe). Haemorphins are probably involved in regulatory functions *in vivo* during pain, physical effort, inflammation and blood pressure variation. Also, a study on quantification of haemorphin in brains from patients with Alzheimer's disease has suggested that these peptides could be candidates for pharmacological prevention of this disease (Poljak *et al.*, 2004). Another study has demonstrated that valorphin (Val-Val-Tyr-Pro-Trp-Thr-Gln), a fragment of haemorphins, could suppress the proliferation of tumour cells (Blishchenko *et al.*, 2002).

5.11 Conjugated linoleic acid (CLA)

Conjugated linoleic acid is a meat-based bioactive substance that has been studied for its potential beneficial effects. It is a mixture of positional and geometric isomers of octadecadienoic acid (linoleic acid (LA), 18:2*n*-6) (Bhattacharya *et al.*, 2006). Two main forms of CLA are cis-9, trans-11–18:2 and trans-10, cis-12–18:2. The former is the most abundant isomer in nature while the latter is found in minor amounts (Wahle *et al.*, 2004; Bhattacharya *et al.*, 2006). CLA is produced directly by bacterial hydrogenation in the rumen. Dhiman *et al.* (2000) elucidated that grass-fed ruminants contained higher CLA than grain-fed animals. CLA concentrations are the highest in lamb with 5.6 mg/g fat while beef contains CLA of 2.9–4.3 mg/g fat (Chin *et al.*, 1992). According to reports by Chin *et al.* (1992) and Parodi (2003), seafood, pork, poultry and vegetable oils are not remarkable sources of CLA. CLA can be produced by delta-9 desaturation of the co-product vaccenic acid (trans-11–18:1) in most mammalian tissues including human tissue (Wahle *et al.*, 2004). CLA has effects on body composition, lipoprotein metabolism, inflammation and carcinogenesis (Roche *et al.*, 2001). Several studies have reported that CLA intake is beneficial against many common diseases, including obesity, atherosclerosis, chronic inflammatory diseases and cancer (Azain, 2003; Wahle *et al.*, 2004; Bhattacharya *et al.*, 2006). However, there are some studies which found detrimental effects on CLA intake. They reported that trans-10, cis-12 CLA could not only elicit a pro-carcinogenic effect in animal models of colon and prostate cancer but could also increase prostaglandin production in cells (Wahle *et al.*, 2004).

5.12 Omega-3 PUFA

Two types of PUFAs, that is eicosapentaenoic acid (EPA, 20:5 (*n*-3), *all-cis*-5,8,11,14,17-eicosapentaenoic acid) and docosahexaenoic acid (DHA, 22:6 (*n*-3), *all-cis*-4,7,10,13,16,19-docosahexaenoic acid) found in fish oil are classified as omega-3 fatty acids. Marine animals, especially cold-water fish species, are good sources of EPA and DHA. Herring contains a high content of 1.7–1.8 g EPA + DHA/g oil. Fresh tuna contains 0.24–1.28 g EPA + DHA/g oil. The quantities of 0.24–1.28, 0.98–1.7, 0.68–1.83, 0.34–1.57, 1.71–1.81, 0.84–0.98 and 0.4–1.0 g EPA + DHA/g oil were observed in tuna, sardines, salmon, mackerel, herring, rainbow trout and halibut, respectively (Kris-Etherton *et al.*, 2002). The key processes of fish oil production are extraction and separation. Approaches to fish oil extraction include high-speed centrifugation (Hirata *et al.*, 1993), low temperature solvent extraction (Moffat *et al.*, 1993) and supercritical fluid extraction (Dunford *et al.*, 1997). Since the extracted oil usually contains a complex mixture of triacylglycerols, a separation process is required. The successful procedures are crystallization, distillation, supercritical fluid extraction and column liquid chromatography. The health-promoting roles of omega-3 fatty acids as protective components that act against certain types of diseases are comprehensively discussed by Kim and Mendis (2006). Omega-3 fatty acids can reduce blood pressure by directly modulating intracellular calcium ion (Ca^{2+}) signalling in vascular smooth muscle cells, thus resulting in a vasodilation effect (Khosh and Khosh, 2001). Adequate intake of the fish oil exerts beneficial effects against atherosclerosis (Schacky, 2000) and arrhythmias (Christensen *et al.*, 1997; Kris-Etherton *et al.*, 2002) which are the causes of cardiovascular disease. Potential mechanisms by which omega-3 fatty acid may reduce risk for this disease are reducing susceptibility of the heart to ventricular arrhythmia, antithrombogenicity, hypotriglyceridaemic activity (fasting and postprandial), retarding growth of atherosclerotic plaque, promoting nitric oxide-induced endothelial relaxation and a mild antihypertensive effects (Kris-Etherton *et al.*, 2002). Omega-3 fatty acids also exhibit beneficial effects against diabetes mellitus (Sheehan *et al.*, 1997), manic-depressive illness (Rondanelli *et al.*, 2011), chronic obstructive pulmonary diseases (Shahar *et al.*, 1994) and relapses in patients with Crohn's disease (Belluzzi *et al.*, 1996). In addition, there are research reports which discovered that fish oil could reduce symptoms in asthma patients (Broughton *et al.*, 1997), reduce blood pressure (Appel *et al.*, 1993; Kris-Etherton *et al.*, 2002), alleviate symptoms of cystic fibrosis (Lawrence and Sorrell, 1993) and improve the survival of cancer patients (Gogos *et al.*, 1998).

5.13 Conclusion

Meat and meat products are promising food sources for both nutrition and bioactive compounds. The significant bioactive compounds are bioactive peptides, L-carnitine, coenzyme Q10, carnosine, taurine, creatine, glutathione, lipoic acid, opioids, conjugated linoleic acid and omega-3 PUFA. Bioactive peptides are derived from meat by either hydrolysis or fermentation whereas others occur in small amounts in meat muscle and offal. Intensive studies have evaluated the beneficial effects of meat bioactive compounds. Many meat bioactive compounds exhibit antihypertensive effects as well as protective effects on cardiovascular disease. Their antioxidant capability to inhibit oxidative processes in the human body is very important since oxidative stress can cause progression of renal complications in diabetes and is also associated with various neurodegenerative illnesses such as cataracts, Parkinson's disease and Alzheimer's disease. Some bioactive compounds from meat are indispensable to cellular energy production and help/improve body functions. Other favourable effects are antithrombotic, antimicrobial and metal binding capacity.

References

Abe, H. (2000). Role of histidine-related compounds as intracellular proton buffering constituents in vertebrate muscle. *Biochemistry (Moscow)*, 65, 757–65.

Agrawal, R. (2005). Probiotics: an emerging food supplement with health benefits. *Food Biotechnology*, 19, 227–246.

Ahmed, A.M. and Muguruma, M. (2010). A review of meat protein hydrolysates and hypertension. *Meat Science*, 86, 110–118.

Anderson, J.J.B. and Garner, S.C. (1996). Calcium and phosphorous nutrition in health and disease: Introduction, in *Calcium and Phosphorous in Health and Disease* (eds J.J.B. Anderson and S.C. Garner). CRC Press, New York, pp. 1–5.

Appel, L.J., Miller, E.R., Seidler, A.J. and Whelton, P.K. (1993). Does supplementation of diet with 'fish oil' reduce blood pressure? A meta-analysis of controlled clinical trials. *Archives of Internal Medicine*, 153, 1429–1438.

Arihara, K., Ota, H., Itoh, M. *et al.* (1998). *Lactobacillus acidophilus* group lactic acid bacteria applied to meat fermentation. *Journal of Food Science*, 63, 544–547.

Arihara, K., Nakashima, Y., Mukai, T., Ishikawa, S. and Itoh, M. (2001). Peptide inhibitors for angiotensin I-converting enzyme from enzymatic hydrolysates of porcine skeletal muscle proteins. *Meat Science*, 57, 319–324.

Arihara, K. (2006). Functional properties of bioactive peptides derived from meat proteins. In Barbosa-Cánovas, G.V. *et al.* (Eds.). *Advanced technologies for meat processing*. (pp. 245–273). New York: CRC press.

Arihara, K. and Ohata, M. (2008). Bioactive compounds in meat, in *Meat Biotechnology* (ed. F. Toldra). Springer, New York, pp. 231–249.

Arihara, K. and Ohata, M. (2011). Functional meat products, in *Functional Foods: Concept to Product*, 2nd edn (ed. V.T.T. Saarela). Woodhead Publishing Ltd, Cambridge, pp. 512–533.

Artioli, G.G., Gualano, B., Smith, A., Stout, J. and Lancha, A.H. Jr (2010). Role of beta-alanine supplementation on muscle carnosine and exercise performance. *Medicine and Science in Sports and Exercise*, 42, 1162–1173.

Azain, M. (2003). Conjugated linoleic acid and its effects on animal products and health in single-stomached animals. *Proceedings of the Nutrition Society*, 62, 319–328.

Baran, E.J. (2000). Metal complexes of carnosine. *Biochemistry (Moscow)*, 65, 789–797.

Bard, H.M. (2007). Antioxidative activity of carnosine in gamma irradiated ground beef and beef patties. *Food Chemistry*, 104, 665–679.

Brass, E.P. (2000). Supplemental carnitine and exercise. *American Journal of Clinical Nutrition*, 72, 618S–623S.

Belluzzi, A., Brignola, C., Campieri, M. *et al.* (1996). Effect of an enteric-coated fish-oil preparation on relapses in Crohn's disease. *The New England Journal of Medicine*, 334, 1557–1560.

Bentinger, M., Tekle, M. and Dallner, G. (2010). Coenzyme Q – Biosynthesis and functions. *Biochemical and Biophysical Research Communications*, 396, 74–79.

Bhattacharya, A., Banu., J., Rahman, M., Causey, J. and Fernandes, G. (2006). Biological effects of conjugated linoleic acids in health and disease. *The Journal of Nutritional Biochemistry*, 17, 789–810.

Bhatti, F., Mankhey, R.W., Asico, L. *et al.* (2005). Mechanisms of antioxidant and pro-oxidant effects of a-lipoic acid in the diabetic and nondiabetic kidney. *Kidney International*, 67, 1371–1380.

Biewenga, G.P., Haenen, G.R. and Bast, A. (1997). The pharmacology of the antioxidant lipoic acid. *General Pharmacology*, 29, 315–331.

Bindoli, A., Valente, M. and Cavallini, L. (1985). Inhibition of lipid peroxidation by alpha-tocopherolquinone and alpha-tocopherolhydroquinone. *Biochemistry International*, 10, 753–761.

Blishchenko, E., Sazonova, O., Surovoy, A. *et al.* (2002). Antiproliferative action of valorphin in cell cultures. *Journal of Peptide Science*, 8, 438–452.

Bouckenooghe, T., Remacle, C. and Reusens, B. (2006). Is taurine a functional nutrient? *Current Opinion in Clinical Nutritionand Metabolic Care*, 9, 728–733.

Bougatef, A., Nedjar-Arroume, N., Manni, L. *et al.* (2010). Purification and identification of novel antioxidant peptides from enzymatic hydrolysates of sardinelle (*Sardinellaaurita*) by-products proteins. *Food Chemistry*, 118, 559–565.

Bray, T.M. and Taylor, C.G. (1994). Enhancement of tissue glutathione for antioxidant and immune functions in malnutrition. *Biochemical Pahrmacology*, 47, 2113–2123.

Broughton, K.S., Johnson, C.S., Pace, B.K., Liebman, M. and Kleppinger, K.M. (1997). Reduced asthma symptoms with ω-3 fatty acid ingestion are related to 5-series leukotriene production. *American Journal of Clinical Nutrition*, 65, 1011–1017.

Brown, N.J., Douglas, E. and Vaughan, D.E. (1998). Angiotensin-converting enzyme inhibitors. *Circulation*, 97, 1411–1420.

Bucci, L.R. and Unlu, L. (2000). Protein and amino acid supplements in exercise and sport, in (eds I. Wolinsky and J.A. Driskell) *Energy Yielding Macronutrients and Energy Metabolism in Sports Nutrition*. CRC Press, FL, pp. 191–212.

Bustamante, J., Lodge, J.K., Marcocci, L. *et al.* (1998). Alpha-lipoic acid in liver metabolism and disease. *Free Radical Biology and Medicine*, 24, 1023–1039.

Calvani, M., Benatti, P., Mancinelli, A. *et al.* (2004). Carnitine replacement in end-stage renal disease and hemodialysis. *Annals of the New York Academy of Sciences*, 1033, 52–66.

Careri, M. and Mangia, A. (2003). Analysis of food proteins and peptides by chromatography and mass spectrometry: a review. *Journal of Chromatography A*, 1000, 609–635.

Chabeaud, A., Vandanjon, L., Bourseau, P., Jaouen, P. and Guérard, F. (2009). Fractionation by ultrafiltration of a saithe protein hydrolysate (*Pollachius virens*): Effect of material and molecular weight cut-off on the membarne performances. *Journal of Food Engineering*, 91, 408–414.

Chesney, R.W., Helms, R.A., Christensen, M. *et al.* (1998). The role of taurine in infant nutrition. *Advances in Experimental Medicine and Biology*, 442:463–476.

Cheung, H.S., Wang, F.L., Ondetti, M.A., Sabe, E.F. and Cushman. D.W. (1980). Binding of peptide substrate and inhibition of angiotensin-converting enzyme: Importance of the COOH-terminal dipeptides sequence. *Journal of Biological Chemistry*, 255, 401–407.

Chin, S.F., Liu, W., Storkson, J.M. *et al.* (1992). Dietary sources of conjugated dienoic isomers of linoleic acid, a newly recognized class of anticarcinogens. *Journal of Food Composition and Analysis*, 5, 185–197.

Christensen, J.H. (2011). Omega-3 polyunsaturated fatty acids and heart rate variability. *Frontiers in Physiology*, 2, 84.

Christensen, J.H., Korup, E., Aaroe, J. *et al.* (1997). Fish consumption, n-3 fatty acids in cell membranes, and heart rate variability in survivors of myocardial infarction with left ventricular dysfunction. *American Journal of Cardiology*, 79, 1670–1673.

Cinq-Mars, C.D. and Li-Chan, E.C.Y. (2007). Optimizing angiotensin I-converting enzyme inhibitory activity of Pacific hake (*Merluccius productus*) fillet hydrolysate using response surface methodology and ultrafiltration. *Journal of Agricultural and Food Chemistry*, 55, 9380–9388.

Decker, E.A., Ivanov, V., Zhu, B.Z. and Frei, B. (2001). Inhibition of low-density lipoprotein oxidation by carnosine and histidine. *Journal of Agricultural and Food Chemistry*, 49, 511–516.

Demarquoy, J., Georges, B., Rigault, C. *et al.* (2004). Radioisotopic determination of L-carnitine content in foods commonly eaten in Western countries. *Food Chemistry*, 86, 137–142.

Dhanasekaran, M. and Ren, J. (2005). The emerging role of coenzyme Q-10 in aging, neurodegeneration, cardiovascular disease, cancer and diabetes mellitus. *Current Neurovascular Research*, 2, 447–459.

Dhiman, T.R., Satter, L.D., Pariza, M.W. *et al.* (2000). Conjugated linoleic acid (CLA) content of milk from cows offered diets rich in linoleic and linolenic acid. *Journal of Dairy Science*, 83, 1016–1027.

Di Bernardini, R., Bolton, D., Harnedy, P. *et al.* (2011). Antioxidant and antimicrobial peptidic hydrolysates from muscle protein sources and by-products. *Food Chemistry*, 124, 1296–1307.

Dunford, N.T., Temmeli, F. and LeBlanc, E. (1997). Supercritical CO_2 extraction of oil and residual proteins from Atlantic mackerel (*Scomber scombrus*) as affected by moisture content. *Journal of Food Science*, 62, 289–294.

Edison, E.E., Brosnan, M.E., Meyer, C. and Brosnan, J.T. (2007). Creatine synthesis: Production of guanidinoacetate by the rat and human kidney *in vivo*. *American Journal of Physiology – Renal Physiology*, 293, F1799– F1804.

Erkkilä, S., Suihko, M.-L., Eerola, S., Petäjä, E. and Mattila-Sandholm, T. (2001). Dry sausages fermented by *Lactobacillus rhamnosus* strains. *International Journal of Food Microbiology*, 64, 205–210.

Ernster, L. and Dallner, G. (1995). Biochemical, physiological and medical aspects of ubiquinone function. *Biochimica et Biophysica Acta*, 271, 195–204.

Fidelus, R.K. and Tsan, M.F. (1987). Glutathione and lymphocyte activation: A function of ageing and auto-immune disease. *Immunology*, 61, 503–508.

Folkers, K. (1996). Relevance of the biosynthesis of coenzyme Q10 and of the four bases of DNA as a rationale for the molecular causes of cancer and a therapy. *Biochemical and Biophysical Research Communications*, 224, 358–361.

FAO/WHO (2001). Health and nutritional properties of probiotics in food including powder milk with live lactic acid bacteria. Report of a Joint FAO/WHO Expert consultation on evaluation of health and nutritional properties of probiotics in food including powder milk with live lactic acid bacteria. Food and Agriculture Organization of the United Nations/World Health Organization. 34 pp.

Fouchereau-Peron, M., Duvail, L., Michel, C. *et al.* (1999). Isolation of an acid fraction from a fish protein hydrolysate with a calcitonin-gene-related-peptide-like biological activity. *Biotechnology and Applied Biochemistry*, 29, 87–92.

Frei, B., Kim, M.C. and Ames, B.N. (1990). Ubiquinol-10 is an effective lipid-soluble antioxidant at physiological concentrations. *Proceedings of the National Academy of Sciences of the United States of America*, 87, 4879–4883.

Froehlich, J.C. (1997). Opioid peptides. *Alcohol Health and Research World*, 21, 132–136.

Fruiter-Arnaudin, I.I., Cohen, M.M., Nervi, S.S. *et al.* (2003). Reduced level of opioid peptides, hemorphin-7 peptides, in serum of diabetic patients. *Diabetes Care*, 26, 2480.

Gogos, C.A., Ginopoulos, P., Salsa, B. *et al.* (1998). Dietary omega-3 polyunsaturated fatty acids plus vitamin E restore immunodeficiency and prolong survival for severely ill patients with generalized malignancy. *Cancer*, 82, 395–402.

Golbidi, S., Badran, M. and Laher, I. (2011). Diabetes and alpha lipoic acid. *Frontiers in Pharmacology*, 2, 69.

Gómez-Guillén, M.C., Giménez, B., López-Caballero, M.E. and Montero, M.P. (2011). Functional and bioactive properties of collagen and gelatin sources: A review. *Food Hydrocolloids*, 25, 1813–1827.

Greenhalff, P. (2001). The creatine–phosphocreatine system: there's more than one song in its repertoire. *The Journal of Physiology*, 537(3), 657.

Gualano, B., Roschel, H., Lancha-Jr, A.H., Brightbil, C.E. and Rawson, E.S. (2011). In sickness and in health: the widespread application of creatine supplementation. *Amino Acids (Wien. Internet)*. 11, 1–11.

Guerard, F. (2006). Enzymatic methods for marine by-product recovery, in *Maximising the Value of Marine By-products* (ed. F. Shahidi). Woodhead Publishing Ltd, Cambridge, pp. 107–143.

Guiotto, A., Calderan, A., Ruzza, P. and Borin, G. (2005). Carnosine and carnosine-related antioxidants: a review. *Current Medicinal Chemistry*, 12, 2293–2315.

Heinz, G. and Hautzinger, P. (2007). Raw fermented sausages. Meat processing technology: For small-to medium-scale producers. Food and Agriculture Organization of the United Nations, Regional Office for Asia and the Pacific. Bangkok.

Hiatt, W.R., Regensteiner, J.G., Creager, M.A. *et al.* (2001). Propionyl-L-carnitine improves exercise performance and functional status in patients with claudication. *American Journal of Medicine*, 110, 616–622.

Hipkiss, A.R. (2010). Aging, proteotoxicity, mitochondria, glycation, NAD^+ and carnosine: Possible inter-relationships and resolution of the oxygen paradox. *Frontiers in Aging Neuroscience*, 2, 10.

Hirata, H., Saeki, H., Nonaka, M. *et al.* (1993). Recovery of fish oil from the manufacturing process of highly nutritional fish meat for foodstuffs from sardine. *Nippon Suisan Gakkaishi*, 59, 111–116.

Hsu, K.C., Li-Chan, E.C.Y. and Jao, C.L. (2010). Antiproliferative activity of peptides prepared from enzymatic hydrolysates of tuna dark muscle on human breast cancer cell line MCF-7. *Food Chemistry*, 126, 617–622.

Huda, H.N., Rosma, A. and Wan Nadiah, WA. (2001). The tuna fishing industry: A new outlook on fish protein hydrolysates. *Comprehensive Reviews in Food Science and Food Safety*, 10, 195–207.

Huang, G., Ren, L. and Jiang, J. (2011). Purification of a histidine-containing peptide with calcium binding activity from shrimp processing byproducts hydrolysate. *European Food Research Technology*, 232, 281–287.

Huang, D., Ou, B. and Prior, R.L. (2005). The chemistry behind antioxidant capacity assays. *Journal of Agricultural and Food Chemistry*, 53, 1841–1856.

Ibañez, E., Herrero, M., Mendiola, J.A. and Castro-Puyana, M. (2012).Extraction and characterization of bioactive compounds with health benefits from marine resources: macro and micro algae, cyanobacteria, and invertebrates, in *Marine Bioactive Compounds: Sources, Characterization and Applications*. (ed. M. Hayes). Springer Science + Business Media, New York, pp. 55–98.

Ichimura, T., Hu, J.N., Aita, D. Q. and Maruyama, S. (2003). Angiotensin I-converting enzyme inhibitory activity and insulin secretion stimulative activity of fermented fish sauce. *Journal of Bioscience and Bioengineering*, 96, 496–499.

Ilias, I., Manoli, I., Blackman, M.R., Gold, P.W. and Slesci, S. (2004). L-Carnitine and acetyl-L-carnitine in the treatment of complications associated with HIV infection and antiretroviral therapy. *Mitochondrion*, 4,163–168.

Iliceto, S., Scrutinio, D., Bruzzi, P. *et al.* (1995). Effects of L-carnitine administration on left ventricular remodeling after acute anterior myocardial infarction: The L-Carnitine Ecocardiografia Digitalizzata Infarto Miocardico (CEDIM). *Journal of the American College of Cardiology*, 26, 380–387.

Jacob, S., Henriksen, E.J., Schiemann, A.L., *et al.*, 1995. Enhancement of glucose disposal in patients with Type 2 diabetes by alpha-lipoic acid. *Arzneimittelforschung*. 45, 872–874.

Jang, A., Jo, C., Kang, K.S. and Lee, M. (2008). Antimicrobial and human cancer cell cytotoxic effect of synthetic angiotensin-converting enzyme (ACE) inhibitory peptides. *Food Chemistry*, 107, 327–336.

James, S.J., Slikker III, W., Melnyk, S. *et al.* (2005). Thimerosal neurotoxicity is associated with glutathione depletion: Protection with glutathione precursors. *Neurotoxicology*, 26, 1–8.

Je, J.Y., Oian, Z.J., Byun, H.G. and Kim, S.K. (2007). Purification and characterization of an antioxidant peptide obtained from tuna backbone protein by enzymatic hydrolysis. *Process Biochemistry*, 42, 840–846.

Jeon, Y., Byun, H. and Kim, S. (1999). Improvement of functional properties of cod frame protein hydrolysates using ultrafiltration membranes. *Process Biochemistry*, 35, 471–478.

Jones, D.P, Coates, R.J., Flagg, E.W. and Eley, J.W. (1992). Glutathione in foods listed in the National Cancer Institute's Health Habits and History Food Frequency Questionnaire. *Nutrition and Cancer*, 17, 57–75.

Jones, D.P. (2011). The health dividend of glutathione. *Natural Medicine Journal* (online). http://www.naturalmedicinejournal.com/article_content.asp?article=18 [accessed 29 July 2013].

Jung, W.K., Lee, B.J. and Kim, S.K. (2006). Fish-bone peptide increases calcium solubility and bioavailability in ovariectomised rats. *British Journal of Nutrition*, 95, 124–128.

Jung, W.K., Oian, Z.J., Lee, S.H. *et al.* (2007). Free radical scavenging activity of a novel antioxidative peptide isolated from *in vitro* gastrointestinal digests of *Mytilus coruscus*. *Journal of Medical Food*, 10, 197–202.

Kamei, M., Fujita, T., Kanbe, T. *et al.* (1986). The distribution and content of ubiquinone in foods. *International Journal for Vitamin and Nutrition Research*, 56, 57–63.

Katayama, K., Tomatsu, M., Kawahara, S. *et al.* (2004). Inhibitory profile of nonapeptide derived from porcine troponin C against angiotensin I-converting enzyme. *Journal of Agricultural and Food Chemistry*, 52, 771–775.

Parodi, P.W. (2003). Conjugated linoleic acid in food, in *Advances in Conjugated Linoleic Acid Research*, Vol. 2 (eds J.-L. Sebedio, W.W. Christie and R. Adlof). AOCS Press, Champaign IL, pp. 101–122.

Pasantes-Morales, H., Quesada, O., Alcocer, L. and Sanchez-Olea, R. (1989). Taurine content in foods. *Nutrition Reports International*, 40, 793–801.

Pasupuleti, V.K. and Braun, S. (2010). State of the art manufacturing of protein hydrolysates, in *Protein Hydrolysates in Biotechnology* (eds V.K. Pasupuleti and A.L. Demain). Springer, New York.

Perquin, M., Oster, T., Maul, A. *et al.* (2000). The glutathione-related detoxification pathway in the human breast: a highly coordinated system disrupted in the tumour tissues. *Cancer Letters*, 158, 7–16.

Preston, J.E., Hipkiss, A.R., Himsworth, D.T., Romero, I.A. and Abbott, J.N. (1998). Toxic effects of beta-amyloid (25–35) on immortalised rat brain endothelial cell: protection by carnosine, homocarnosine and beta-alanine. *Neuroscience Letters*, 242,105–108.

Pravst, I., Zmitek, K. and Zmitek, J. (2010). Coenzyme Q10 contents in foods and fortification strategies. *Critical Reviews in Food Science and Nutrition*, 50, 269–280.

Poljak, A., McLean, C.A., Sachdev, P., Brodaty, H. and Smythe, G.A. (2004). Quantification of hemorphins in Alzheimer's disease brains. *Journal of Neuroscience Research*, 75, 704–714.

Proud, D. and Kaplan, A.P. (1988). Kinin formation: mechanisms and role in inflammatory disorders. *Annual Review of Immunology*, 6, 49–83.

Purchas, R., Rutherfurd, S., Pearce, P., Vather, R. and Wilkinson, B.H. (2004). Concentrations in beef and lamb of taurine, carnosine, coenzyme Q10, and creatine. *Meat Science*, 66, 629–37.

Purchas, R.W. and Zou, M. (2008). Composition and quality differences between the longissimus and infraspinatus muscles for several groups of pasture-finished cattle. *Meat Science*, 80, 470–479.

Rahman, I. and MacNee, W.L. (1999). Glutathione and oxidative stress: Implications in cigarette smoke-induced airway disease. *American Journal of Physiology*, 277, 1067–1088.

Rajapakse, N., Jung, W.K., Mendis, E., Moon, S.H. and Kim, S.K. (2005). A novel anticoagulant purified from fish protein hydrolysate inhibits factor XIIa and platelet aggregation. *Life Science,* 76, 2607–2619.

Rebouche, C.J. (1999). Carnitine, in *Modern Nutrition in Health and Disease*, 9th edn (eds M.E. Shils, J.A. Olson, M. Shike and A.C. Ross). Lippincott Williams and Wilkins, New York, pp. 505–512.

Roche, H.M., Noone, E. and Gibney, A.N. (2001). Conjugated linoleic acid: A novel therapeutic nutrient? *Nutrition Research Reviews*, 14, 173–188.

Rondanelli, M., Giacosa, A., Opizzi, A. *et al.* (2011). Long chain omega 3 polyunsaturated fatty acids supplementation in the treatment of elderly depression: Effects on depressive symptoms, on phospholipids fatty acids profile and on health-related quality of life. *Journal of Nutrition Health and Aging*, 15, 37–44.

Rosenfeldt, F., Hilton, D., Pepe, S. and Krum, H. (2003). Systematic review of effect of coenzyme Q10 in physical exercise, hypertension and heart failure. *Biofactors*, 18, 91–100.

Ryan, J. T., Ross, R. P. Bolton, D., Fitzgerald, G. F. and Stanton, C. (2011). Bioactive peptides from muscle sources: Meat and fish. *Nutrients*, 3, 765–791.

Sharma, S., Singh, R. and Rana, S. (2011). Bioactive peptides: A review. *International Journal of Bioautomation*, 15, 223–250.

Saiga, A., Okumura, T., Makihara, T. *et al.* (2003a). Angiotensin I-converting enzyme inhibitory peptides in a hydrolyzed chicken breast muscle extract. *Journal of Agricultural and Food Chemistry*, 51, 1741–1745.

Saiga, A., Tanabe, S. and Nishimura, T. (2003b). Antioxidant activity of peptides obtained from porcine myofibrillar proteins by protease treatment. *Journal of Agricultural and Food Chemistry*, 51, 3661–3667.

Sameshima, T., Magome, C., Takeshita, K. *et al.* (1998). Effect of intestinal *Lactobacillus* starter cultures on the behaviour of *Staphylococcus aureus* in fermented sausage. *International Journal of Food Microbiology*, 41, 1–7.

Saydam, N., Kirb, A., Demir, Ö. *et al.* (1997). Determination of glutathione, glutathione reductase, glutathioneperoxidase and glutathione S-transferase levels in human lung cancer tissues. *Cancer Letters*, 119, 13–19.

Schacky, C.V. (2000). ω-3 Fatty acids and the prevention of coronary atherosclerosis. *American Journal of Clinical Nutrition*, 71, 224–227.

Schafer, F.Q. and Buettner, G.R. (2001). Redox environment of the cell as viewed through the redox state of the glutathione disulfide/glutathione couple. *Free Radical Biology and Medicine*, 30, 1191–1212.

Schmid, A. (2010). Bioactive substances in meat and meat products. *Fleischwirtschaft International*, 25 (2), 127–133.

Sentandreu, M.A. and Toldrá, F. (2007). Evaluation of ACE inhibitory activity of dipeptides generated by the action of porcine muscle dipeptidyl peptidases. *Food Chemistry*, 102, 511–515

Sestil, P., Martinelli, C., Colombo, E. *et al.* (2011). Creatine as an antioxidant. *Amino Acids*, 40, 1385–96.

Šližyte, R., Daukšas, E., Falch, E. and Storrø, I. (2005). Yield and composition of different fractions obtained after enzymatic hydrolysis of cod (*Gadus morhua*) by-products. *Process Biochemistry*, 40, 1415–1424.

Shahar, E., Folsom, A.R., Melnick, S.L. *et al.* (1994). Dietary ω-3 polyunsaturated fatty acids and smoking-related chronic obstructive pulmonary disease. *New England Journal of Medicine*, 331, 228–233.

Sheehan, J.P., Wei, I.W., Ulchaker, M. and Tserng, K.Y. (1997). Effect of high fibre intake in fish oil-treated patients with non-insulin-dependent diabetes mellitus. *American Journal of Clinical Nutrition*, 66, 1183–1187.

Stamler, J.S. and Slivka, A. (1996). Biological chemistry of thiols in the vasculature and in vascular-related disease. *Nutrition Reviews*, 54, 1–30.

Tanasupawat, S. (2009). Thai lactic acid bacteria: Diversity and applications. *Srinakharinwirot University Science Journal*, 25, 1–13.

Tarnopolsky, M.A. (2008). Clinical use of creatine in neuromuscular and neurometabolic disorders, in *Subcellular Biochemistry Vol. 46: Creatine and Creatine Kinase in Health and Disease* (eds G.S. Salomons and M. Wyss). Springer, New York, pp. 183–204.

Thorkelsson, G. and Kristinsson, H.G. (2009). Bioactive peptides from marine sources. State of art. Report to the NORA fund Matis-Food Research, Innovation and Safety, pp. 5–7.

Thorkelsson, G., Slizyte, R., Gildberg, A. and Kristinsson, H.G. (2009). Fish protein and peptide products: Processing methods, quality and functional properties, in *Marine Functional Food* (ed. J.B. Luten). Wageningen Academic Publisher, Wageningen, pp. 115–133.

Vandanjon, L., Grignon, M., Courois, E., Bourseau, P. and Jaouen, P. (2009). Fractionating white fish fillet hydrolysates by ultrafiltration and nanofiltration. *Journal of Food Engineering*, 95, 36–44.

Vandanjon, L., Johannsson, R., Derouiniot, M., Bourseau, P. and Jaouen, P. (2007). Concentration and purification of blue whiting peptide hydrolysates by membrane processes. *Journal of Food Engineering*, 83, 581–589.

Venugopal, V. (2009). Seafood protein: functional properties and protein supplement, in *Marine Products for Healthcare: Functional and Bioactive Nutraceutical Compounds from the Ocean*. CRC Press, New York, pp. 51–101.

Vescovo, G., Ravara, B., Gobbo, V. *et al.* (2002). L-Carnitine: A potential treatment for blocking apoptosis and preventing skeletal muscle myopathy in heart failure. *American Journal of Physiology*, 283, C802–C810.

Villarama, C.D. and Maibach, H.I. (2005). Glutathione as a depigmenting agent: An overview. *International Journal of Cosmetic Science*, 27, 147–153.

Wada, H., Goto, H., Hagiwara, S. and Yamamoto, Y. (2007). Redox status of coenzyme Q10 is associated with chronological age. *Journal of the American Geriatrics Society*, 55, 1141–1142.

Walther, B. and Sieber, R. (2011). Bioactive proteins and peptides in foods. *International Journal for Vitamin and Nutrition Research*, 81, 181–192.

Wahle, K.W., Heys, S.D. and Rotondo, D. (2004). Conjugated linoleic acids: Are they beneficial or detrimental to health? *Progress in Lipid Research*, 43, 553–587.

Wijesekara, I. and Kim, S.K. (2010). Angiotensin-I-Converting Enzyme (ACE) inhibitors from marine resources: Prospects in the pharmaceutical industry. *Marine Drugs*, 8, 1080–1093.

Williams, P. (2007). Nutritional composition of red meat. *Nutritionand Dietetics*, 64 (Suppl. 4), S113–S119.

Williams, P., Droulez, V., Levy, G. and Stobaus, T. (2007). Composition of Australian red meat (2002). 3. Nutrient profile. *Food Australia*, 59, 331–341.

Wójcik, O.P., Koenig, K.L., Zeleniuch-Jacquotte, A., Costa, M. and Chen, Y. (2010). The potential protective effects of taurine on coronary heart disease. *Atherosclerosis*, 208, 19.

Wu, H.C., Chen, H.M. and Shiau, C.Y. (2003). Free amino acids and peptides as related to antioxidant properties in protein hydrolysates of mackerel (*Scomber austriasicus*). *Food Research International*, 36, 949–957.

Wu, H.C., Pan, B.S., Chang, C.L. and Shiau, C.Y. (2005). Low-molecular-weight peptides as related to antioxidant properties of chicken essence. *Journal of Food and Drug Analysis*, 13, 176–183.

Yokoyama, K., Chiba, H. and Yoshikawa, M. (1992). Peptide inhibitors for angiotensin I-converting enzyme from thermolysin digest of dried bonito. *Bioscience Biotechnology and Biochemistry*, 56, 1541–5.

Yoshikawa, T., Naito, Y., Tanigawa, T., Yoneta, T. and Kondo, M. (1991). The antioxidant properties of a novel zinc-carnosine chelate compound, *N*-(3-aminopropionyl)-L-histidinato zinc. *Biochimica et Biophysica Acta*, 1115, 15–22.

Zhao, Q., Garreau, I., Sannier, F. and Piot, J.M. (1997). Opioid peptides derived from hemoglobin: Hemorphins. *Biopolymers*, 43, 75–98.

Zhao, Xi-he (1994). Dietary protein, amino acids and their relation to health. *Asia Pacific Journal of Clinical Nutrition*, 3, 131–134.

6
Bioactive Materials Derived from Seafood and Seafood Processing By-products

Ratih Pangestuti[1,3] and Se-Kwon Kim[2]

[1]*Marine Bioprocess Research Center, Pukyong National University, Busan, Republic of Korea*
[2]*Marine Biochemistry Laboratory, Department of Chemistry, Pukyong National University, Busan, Republic of Korea*
[3]*Research and Development Center for Marine and Fisheries Product Processing Technology, Ministry of Marine and Fisheries, Petamburan VI, Jakarta, Indonesia*

6.1 Introduction

The ocean covers more than 70% of the Earth's surface and is the richest reservoir of living and non-living resources (Shahidi and Janak Kamil, 2001; Swing, 2003; Shahidi, 2008; Kim and Wijesekara, 2010; Shahidi and Alasalvar, 2011). Due to their phenomenal biodiversity, marine products are attractive not only as nutritious food items, but also as source of biologically active (bioactive) compounds (Pangestuti and Kim, 2011a).

Seafood is an important source of nutrients for humans. There is a particular interest from the food and the pharmaceutical industries for the development of bioactive materials from seafood. The increasing demand for seafood may be due to its health benefits and to a willingness to include seafood into the daily diet. Everyday habits of seafood consumption have made possible a large number of epidemiological studies showing the health benefits linked to seafood consumption. When considered in combination with international diet-related chronic disease incidences, significant diet factors including dietary differences between populations varying in seafood consumption have been revealed (Pangestuti and Kim, 2011b). As an example, the

Functional Foods and Dietary Supplements: Processing Effects and Health Benefits, First Edition.
Edited by Athapol Noomhorm, Imran Ahmad and Anil Kumar Anal.

prevalence of breast and prostate cancer rates in Japan and China are lower than Western countries (Pisani *et al.*, 2002; Yuan and Walsh, 2006). Studies showed that a low incidence of breast and prostate cancer cases in Japan and China is associated with a high consumption of seafood. In East Asian culture, seafood has been used in food diets since ancient times and has always been of particular interest (Khan *et al.*, 2010).

Seafood may represent a valuable source of bioactive compounds, which in association with a proper diet and moderate physical activity can be beneficial to health. The seafood processing industry is mainly concerned with the food and nutritional value of the products. The presence of bioactive materials in seafood such as sulfated polysaccharides, bioactive peptides, phlorotannins, natural pigments, omega-3 polyunsaturated fatty acids (PUFAs), vitamins and minerals has been associated with their dietary health benefits. For example, omega-3 PUFAs in seafood are thought to reduce the incidence of cardiovascular diseases in humans. Soluble polysaccharides in seafood are primarily associated with hypocholesterolaemic and hypoglycaemic effects in our body (Panlasigui *et al.*, 2003; Kim *et al.*, 2011). In addition, carotenoids have been identified as the major antioxidant compounds responsible for antioxidant activity in some marine algal species (Yan *et al.*, 1999; Sachindra *et al.*, 2007).

According to the Food and Agricultural Organization, world seafood production increases annually. In the past few years, consumers' perception of food has changed with a clear leaning towards health-promoting functional foods and nutraceuticals. Seafood has an important role in these areas because of its nutritional value. Several regulatory agencies have advised that seafood should be a component of a healthy diet. Recent increases in consumer interest has encouraged many pharmaceutical companies to engage themselves in the production of nutraceuticals and pharmaceuticals derived from seafood.

Seafood processing also produces a large quantity of by-products. In 2001 it was estimated that seafood processing by-products exceeded 20 million tonnes, equivalent to 25% of the total production of marine capture fisheries (Kim and Mendis, 2006). Therefore, there is a great potential in the marine bioprocess industry to convert and utilize more of these seafood by-products into valuable products. The term by-products is, however, not clearly defined to distinguish from waste and is often identified as leftovers that are not ordinarily saleable, but which can be recycled after treatment.

Initial identification of bioactive materials from seafood processing by-products paved the way for the use of huge amounts of these by-products, which had a considerable effect on environmental pollution. Most fisheries' by-products are presently used to produce fish oil, fishmeal, fertilizer, pet food and fish silage. However, most of the recycled seafood processing by-products possess low economic value. Recent studies have identified a number of bioactive materials from the remaining fish skin, fish internal organ, fish bone, and shellfish and crustacean shells. Generally, a far better profitability is obtained by producing human consumables and the highest profitability is currently expected from bioactive materials derived from seafood processing by-products. These bioactive materials can be extracted and purified with technologies varying from simple to complex, and such materials may include preparation and isolation of bioactive peptides, oligosaccharides, fatty acids, enzymes, water-soluble minerals and biopolymers for biotechnological applications. Seafood processing by-products have now acquired a commercial value as industrial raw materials because it has been recognized that functional materials can be isolated from them.

For many years, identification of bioactive materials from seafood and seafood processing by-products has been a major effort in many research groups. However, to develop these bioactive materials as nutraceuticals and pharmaceuticals, further research and clinical studies are needed. This chapter focuses on the current efforts to isolate bioactive materials derived from seafood and seafood processing by-products and their potential use as nutraceuticals and pharmaceuticals.

6.2 Bioactive materials derived from seafood and seafood processing by-product

6.2.1 Sulfated polysaccharides

Sulfated polysaccharides comprise a complex group of macromolecules with a wide range of health benefits. These polymers are chemically anionic and can be found in marine algae, mammals and invertebrates (Costa *et al.*, 2010). Marine algae are the most important source of non-animal sulfated polysaccharides and the chemical structure of these polymers varies depending on the algal species (Li *et al.*, 2008). The amount of sulfated polysaccharides present in marine algae is found to differ according to class. The major sulfated polysaccharides found in marine algae include fucoidan and laminarans of brown algae, carrageenan of red algae and ulvan of green algae. In recent years, various sulfated polysaccharides isolated from marine algae have attracted much attention in the fields of food, cosmetics and pharmacology. Compared with other sulfated polysaccharides isolated from marine algae, fucoidans are widely available commercially from various cheap sources; hence, more and more fucoidans have been investigated in recent years to develop novel drugs and functional foods (Cui *et al.*, 2010).

Bioactivities of sulfated polysaccharides depend on their chemical structure, molecular weight and chain conformations. As an example, low molecular weight sulfated polysaccharides have shown potent antioxidant activity compared with those of high molecular weight. Sulfated polysaccharides have exhibited various beneficial biological activities such as acting as anticoagulants (Mao *et al.*, 2006), antivirals (Zhu *et al.*, 2006), antioxidants (Rha, 2007), anticancer agents (Kwon and Nam, 2006), and anti-inflammation agents (Leiro *et al.*, 2007). Sulfated polysaccharides are also known to be important free-radical scavengers and antioxidants for the prevention of oxidative damage, which is an important contributor in carcinogenesis. Taken together, marine algae-derived sulfated polysaccharides have proven to be a useful candidates in the search for effective, non-toxic substances with potential health-promoting activity.

6.2.2 Bioactive peptides

Proteins are fundamental and integral food components, functionally and nutritionally. Seafood is an excellent source of functionally active and nutritive protein. For example, fish has been recognized as cheap source of animal proteins. The protein contents of most raw finfish flesh range from 17 to 22%, whereas tuna contains around 30%. Crustaceans and cephalopods contain slightly higher levels of protein. Thus high amounts of protein in seafood means that seafood can be used to obtain bioactive peptides.

Bioactive peptides are specific protein fragments that have a positive impact on a body function or condition and ultimately may influence human health; which expected to be provided by a safe, reliable, and consistent oral delivery system (Ryu *et al.*, 2010). The discovery of the bioregulatory role of different endogenous peptides in the organism as well as an understanding of the molecular mechanisms of action of some bioactive peptides obtained from natural sources on specific cellular targets, has led to peptides being promising lead candidates of bioactive materials in the food and pharmaceutical industries. Marine-derived bioactive peptides have been shown to possess many physiological functions, including antihypertensive or angiotensin-I-converting enzyme (ACE) inhibition, and antioxidant, anticoagulant and antimicrobial activities. Moreover, some of these bioactive peptides may have the potential to promote human health and reduce the risk from disease (Shahidi and Zhong, 2008; Kim and Wijesekara, 2010). Thus, the possible role of marine food-derived bioactive peptides in reducing the risk of cardiovascular disease has been well demonstrated.

Marine bioactive peptides may be produced by several methods such as solvent extraction, enzymatic hydrolysis and microbial fermentation. In the food and pharmaceutical industries the enzymatic hydrolysis method is preferred because the products do not become contaminated with organic solvents, toxic chemicals or microorganisms (Wijesinghe and Jeon, 2011). Production of bioactive peptides can be achieved by *in vitro* hydrolysis of protein sources using appropriate proteolytic enzymes. Proteolytic enzymes from microbes, plants and animals can be used for the hydrolysis process of marine proteins to develop bioactive peptides (Aneiros and Garateix, 2004). The physico-chemical conditions of the reaction media, such as temperature, hydrolysis time, substrate to enzyme ratio and pH of the protein solution, must be adjusted to optimize the activity of the enzyme used to achieve efficient recovery of peptides with the desired biological activity and functional properties. Meanwhile, fermentation as one of the oldest food preservation techniques specifically practiced in Asian countries is believed to enhance the nutraceutical value of fermented foods as well as their storability. The breakdown of food proteins by microbial proteases to produce bioactive peptides may explain the development of these properties during fermentation. Therefore, there is an increasing interest in using enzyme hydrolysis and fermented foods including seafood to identify bioactive peptides.

6.2.3 Phlorotannins

Phlorotannins are polymers of phloroglucinol (1,3,5-trihydroxybenzene), a class of polyphenolic compounds restricted to the brown algae (Phaeophyceae) (Wijesekara *et al.*, 2010). They are secondary metabolites that occur in a wide range of molecular sizes ranging from 126 to 650 000 Da (Fallarero *et al.*, 2003). Based on the means of linkage, phlorotannins can be classified into four subclasses: fuhalols and phlorethols (phlorotannins with an ether linkage), fucols (with a phenyl linkage), fucophloroethols (with an ether and phenyl linkage) and eckols (with a dibenzodioxin linkage).

Ecklonia cava, one of the most popular edible brown algae in the Eastern hemisphere, is the richest source of phlorotannins of all brown algae species (Li *et al.*,

2011). These phlorotannins help to protect brown algae from stress conditions and predators. The biological activities of phlorotannins include being antioxidant (Li *et al.*, 2009), anti-HIV (Artan *et al.*, 2008), anticancer (Kong *et al.*, 2009), anti-inflammatory (Jung *et al.*, 2009), radioprotective (Zhang *et al.*, 2008), antidiabetic (Iwai, 2008), antiallergic (Sailasree *et al.*, 2008), antimicrobial (Nagayama *et al.*, 2002), antihypertensive (Jung *et al.*, 2006a) and neuroprotective (Vidal Novoa *et al.*, 2001). Mounting evidence indicates that phlorotannins from marine algae have a key role as bioactive ingredients and play a vital role in the algae themselves as well as in human health and nutrition. Hence, the possibilities for designing phlorotannins as new functional foods and pharmaceuticals to reduce or regulate diet-related chronic malfunctions are promising.

6.2.4 Natural pigments

Natural pigments are widespread not only in marine algae but also in all living matter such as mammals, fungi and invertebrates (Delgado-Vargas *et al.*, 2000). Seafood, however, is a potential source of marine natural pigments (Khan *et al.*, 2010).

Three basic classes of natural pigments found in seafood are chlorophylls, carotenoids and phycobiliproteins. Chlorophylls are greenish lipid-soluble natural pigments which contain a porphyrin ring and are found in all algae, higher plants and cyanobacteria. Structurally, chlorophyll is a substituted tetrapyrrole with a centrally bound magnesium atom; the porphyrin tetrapyrrole is further esterified to a diterpene alcohol, phytol, to form chlorophyll (Ferruzzi and Blakeslee, 2007). There are four kinds of chlorophyll found in marine algae; the first and most important is chlorophyll *a* (Figure 6.1a) which absorbs most energy from violet blue and orange-red light (Holdt and Kraan, 2011). These natural pigments are essential molecules for photosynthesis, passing energized electrons on to molecules which will manufacture sugars. The second and third chlorophylls are chlorophyll *b* and *c*. The fourth type, chlorophyll *d*, was found in red algae (Larkum and Kühl, 2005). Information on the bioavailability of chlorophyll derivatives is limited partially because of the general assumption that chlorophylls cannot be absorbed by humans. However, considering the natural abundance of chlorophyll in edible marine algae, the diversity of derivatives formed through marine algae processing and preparation, dietary exposure to these natural pigments can be significant. Furthermore, the sensitivity of chlorophylls to extreme pH and temperature allows the formation of several distinct derivatives such as pheophytin *a* (Figure 6.1b) and pheophorbide *a* (Figure 6.1c), through processing of marine algae tissue and human digestion (Ferruzzi and Blakeslee, 2007).

Carotenoids are linear polyenes that function as light energy harvesters and antioxidants that inactivate reactive oxygen species (ROS) formed by exposure to light and air (Larkum and Kühl, 2005; Sousa *et al.*, 2006; Ioannou and Roussis, 2009). Crustacean exoskeleton is a rich source of carotenoproteins. Two complexes (red and blue) have been isolated and characterized from the carapace of American crayfish (*Procrambarus clarkii*). The blue colour in the carapace of the lobster is due to a complex between carotenoid α-crustacyanin and a protein. The ovaries and eggs of fish and shellfish are almost always pigmented. The colours range from yellow, orange and red to green, blue and purple, mainly due to the presence of carotenoids and/or

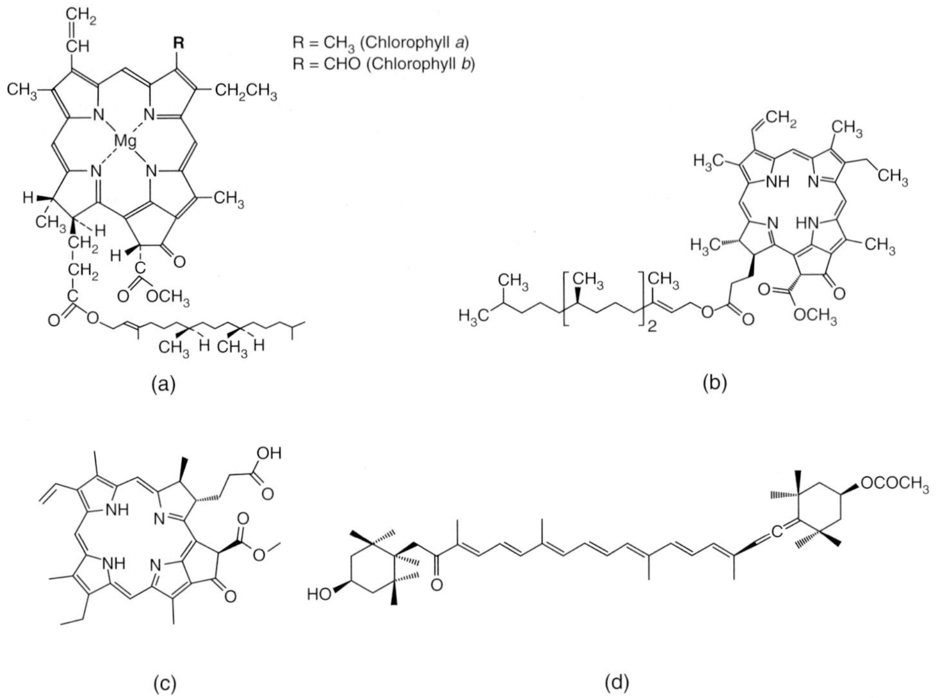

Figure 6.1 Chemical structures of natural pigments derived from marine algae: (a) chlorophyll *a*, *b*; (b) pheophytin *a*; (c) pheophorbide *a*; (d) fucoxanthin. *Source:* Adapted from Gross, 1991 and Jeffrey *et al.*, 1997

carotenoproteins. Major carotenoproteins present in the ovaries of marine invertebrates have been well characterized (Shahidi and Brown, 1998).

One very visible carotenoid in algae is fucoxanthin (Figure 6.1d); the brown pigment which colours kelps and other brown algae as well as diatoms. Fucoxanthin is one of the most abundant carotenoids contributing around 10% of the estimated total production of carotenoids in nature (Matsuno, 2001). It has a unique structure including an unusual allenic bond and a 5,6-monoepoxide in its molecule. Different brown algal strains have different fucoxanthin profiles and compositions (Terasaki *et al.*, 2009). In the human body, fucoxanthin absorption strongly depends on a number of factors which are not entirely understood, for example, the amount and possibly type of dietary lipids consumed, the stability of the matrix to which the carotenoid was bound, and additional dietary factors such dietary fibre (Bohn, 2008). Bioavailability of fucoxanthin seems to be very low; however, there is a scientific controversy about it. Strand *et al.* (1998) found that fucoxanthin metabolites but not fucoxanthin were transferred to the egg yolks of laying hens fed a diet supplemented with 15% *Fucus serratus*. In serial studies, Sugawara *et al.* (2002, 2009) reported that esterification of fucoxanthin in human intestinal caco-2 cells and mice was mediated by enzymatic activity after intestinal absorption. The esterified fucoxanthin was likely to be incorporated into the lipid core in chylomicron and carried into a variety of tissues including the skin. In addition, by esterifying fucoxanthin into highly non-polar products, intestinal cells might be protected from the possible toxic effects of fucoxanthin (Sugawara *et al.*, 2009). Fucoxanthinol was identified as a prime metabolite of fucoxanthin in mice and rats (Asai *et al.*, 2004; Sangeetha *et al.*, 2010). Interestingly, amarouciaxanthin A was found as a major metabolite of fucoxanthin in rat liver, suggesting that liver enzymes may play a role in hydrolysing fucoxanthin into amarouciaxanthin A (Sangeetha *et al.*, 2010). In contrast, dietary intake of fucoxanthin in mice accumulated in the heart and liver as fucoxanthinol and in adipose tissue as amarouciaxanthin A (Hashimoto *et al.*, 2009). However, fucoxanthinol further converted into amarouciaxanthin A by short-chain dehydrogenase or reductase in the mice liver within 24 hours and rapidly transported to the other tissues. No adverse side effects from fucoxanthin were reported in the mice study. In an animal study, Sugawara *et al.* (2009), fucoxanthin also appeared to stimulate liver to produce docosahexaenoic acid (DHA), a type of omega-3 fatty acid, at levels comparable to fish oil supplementation. Hence, the animal experiments with fucoxanthin stimulated researchers to recommend human clinical trials. In placebo-controlled trials, a supplement containing a 5% fucoxanthin (daily dosage 10 mg) did not reveal any harmful effects (Holt, 2008).

Another natural pigment found in seafood is phycobiliproteins, which are water-soluble fluorescent proteins. Phycobiliproteins are used as accessory or antenna pigments for photosynthetic light collection in which energy is absorbed from some of the visible spectrum (450–650 nm) (Sousa *et al.*, 2006). Phycobiliproteins are the principal photoreceptor for photosynthesis in cyanobacteria, red algae and cryptomonads (Glazer, 1994). In many algae, phycobiliproteins are arranged in subcellular structures called phycobilisomes, which allow the pigments to be arranged geometrically in a manner which helps to optimize the capture of light and transfer of energy. The colours of the phycobiliproteins arise from the presence of covalently attached prosthetic groups, bilins, which are linear tetrapyrroles derived biosynthetically from heme via biliverdin. There are three major categories of phycobiliproteins: phycocyanins, allophycocyanins and phycoeryththins, with phycoerythrins as the most abundant phycobiliproteins found in many red algae species (Bogorad, 1975; Glazer, 1994).

6.2.5 Polyunsaturated fatty acids

Marine oils serve as rich source of PUFAs which originated primarily from the body of fatty fish such as mackerel, the liver of white lean fish and the blubber of marine mammals such as seals and whales. PUFAs are also present in certain algal and fungal oils. In addition, by-products from gutting, filleting and other processing operations are also good raw materials for fish meal and oil production.

Fish oil extraction methods and conditions are vital factors affecting the the quality of fish oil. Presently, several methods such high-speed centrifugation, low temperature solvent extraction and supercritical fluid extraction are used to extract fish oil. In addition, wet and steam rendering methods are also used to extract fish oil from fish processing by-products. Separation of omega-3 fatty acids is one of the main concerns in current research. However, due to the presence of complex mixture of triacylglycerols, separation of omega-3 fatty acids becomes complicated. Many separation methods have been developed to isolate them at higher purity including crystallization, distillation, supercritical fluid extraction and chromatography. Column liquid chromatography is frequently used to analyse and separate fatty acids. In addition, the combination of a chromatographic method with urea crystallization enables successful separation of fatty acids. Proper separation techniques and advanced processing methods could promote the production of higher quality fish oil which may play an even more important role in the pharmaceutical and food industry in the near future.

There are two major families of dietary PUFA, the omega-6 and omega-3 families. The omega-6 PUFAs are derived from the parent compound linoleic acid (LA; 18:2(ω6)). They are fatty acids containing at least two double bonds where the first double bond is six carbons from the methyl end of the molecule (Whelan and McEntee, 2004). Meanwhile, the omega-3 PUFAs have the first double bond located in the third carbon from the methyl terminus and contain up to six double bonds. Seafood is particularly rich in ω3 PUFA (Ortiz *et al.*, 2006). Eicosapentanoic acid (EPA; 20:5) and DHA (22:6) are the two important omega-3 PUFAs of seafood, along with the precursor α-linolenic acid (ALA; 18:3). Both EPA and DHA are basically derived from ALA through elongation and desaturation (Ortiz *et al.*, 2006; Ratana-arporn and Chirapart, 2006; Alamsjah *et al.*, 2008). The omega-3 fatty acids play a significant role in the human body where their beneficial effects can be classified into two main areas. First, these fatty acids sustain normal healthy life through the reduction of blood pressure, plasma triglycerides and cholesterol, together with increased blood coagulation time. Both EPA and DHA are important for maintenance of normal blood flow as they lower fibrinogen levels and also prevent platelets from sticking to each other. Second, they alleviate certain diseases such as blood vessel disorders and inflammatory conditions. Deficiency of omega-3 fatty acids causes several disorders such as restrictive growth, abnormality of the skin and hair, damage of the reproductive system and abnormal composition of serum and tissue fatty acids. The human body cannot synthesize omega-3 fatty acids *de novo*; hence, to obtain their potential health-promoting effects, omega-3 fatty acids should be introduced in the diet. Intake of fish oil, which is an excellent source of omega-3 fatty acids, has linked the promotion of human health to the fight against numerous diseases. Researchers are convinced that EPA and DHA are the main protective components of fish oil that act against certain types of diseases, as presented in Table 6.1.

Table 6.1 Heath benefit effects of omega-3 fatty acids

Health benefit effects	References
Prevention of cardiovascular diseases	Kris-Etherton *et al.*, 2002
Chemopreventive agents	Rose and Connolly, 1999
Protection against arrhythmias	Leaf *et al.*, 2003
Prevent relapses in patients with Crohn's disease	Belluzzi *et al.*, 1996
Prevention from atherosclerosis	Angerer *et al.*, 2002
Beneficial for diabetic patients	Montori *et al.*, 2000
Fight against manic-depressive illness	Su *et al.*, 2003
Reduce symptoms in asthma patients	Wong, 2005
Alleviate symptoms of cystic fibrosis	Coste *et al.*, 2007

6.2.6 Vitamins and minerals

Vitamins and minerals are essential for life since their deficiencies lead to various health disorders. Seafood is rich in vitamins and minerals. Marine fish oils are rich sources of vitamins A and D. Marine fish provide a moderate amount of thiamin (B_1). Furthermore, marine fish also contains modest amounts of biotin (B_7), folic acid (B_9), niacin (B_3) and pantothenic acid (B_5). The best sources of pyrodixine (B_5) are salmon and tuna. Fish is particularly rich in vitamin cobalamin (B_{12}), and 100 g of fish normally provides more than 100% of the recommended daily intake. Vitamin B_{12} plays a role in the formation of red blood cells, and insufficient B_{12} levels can lead to a form of anaemia. Most fish species also contain little vitamin C. Surprisingly, water-soluble vitamins such as vitamin C are present in large amounts in sea lettuces. The levels of vitamin C in sea lettuces average from 500 to 3000 mg/kg of dry matter. These levels of vitamin C are comparable with that of parsley, blackcurrant and peppers. In sea lettuces, the highest levels of vitamin C were found in *Ulva fasciata* (22 mg/100 g) (McDermid and Stuercke, 2003). Vitamin C is of interest for many reasons. First, it strengthens the immune defence system, activates the intestinal absorption of iron and acts as a reversible reductant and antioxidant in the aqueous fluid and tissue compartments. Furthermore, this vitamin is specifically required for the activity of eight human enzymes involved in collagen, hormone, amino acid and carnitine synthesis or metabolism (Jacob and Sotoudeh, 2002).

Minerals are inorganic elements that retain their chemical identity in foods. They can be classified into two groups: macro (calcium, phosphorous, potassium, sulfur, sodium, chloride, and magnesium) and trace minerals. Seafood contains a wealth of mineral elements drawn from the sea. The total minerals in raw fish muscles and invertebrates are roughly in the range 0.6–1.5% wet weight (Venugopal, 2008). Calcium is an important nutrient for humans and substantial quantities are especially required for fetal growth, milk production and growth in young children. However, low calcium intakes are reported in many low-income countries, where milk and milk products make up only a small part of the diet. Calcium is accumulated in seafood, its content varying from 6 to 120 mg/100 g depending on the species. Whole small fish with bones are an extremely calcium-rich food (Larsen *et al.*, 2000). The calcium content may be as low as 15 mg in mackerel and 15–50 mg in catfish, haddock and oysters. Surprisingly, calcium content in sea lettuces is higher than in milk, brown rice, spinach, peanuts and lentils (MacArtain *et al.*, 2007). Calcium content in green algae *Ulva lactuca, Ulva reticulate* and *Ulva fasciata* were 32.5, 147 and 0.47 mg/100 g edible portion, respectively. Potassium and sodium are known as electrolytes because of their ability to dissociate into positively and negatively charged ions when dissolved in water. Potassium is the major cation of intracellular fluid. Together with sodium, it maintains normal water balance. In addition, potassium also promotes cellular growth and maintains normal blood pressure. Potential sources of potassium are *Ulva reticulata*, which contains 1540 mg potassium/100 g edible portion (Ratanaarporn and Chirapart, 2006). Most fresh fish contain low sodium levels. However, the sodium content of most processed fish and seafood products is substantially higher due to the conventional onboard handling and processing treatments (Venugopal, 2008). Iodine is an important mineral in metabolic regulation and growth patterns. The recommended daily intake of iodine for adults is 150 μg/day. During pregnancy and lactation, an additional dose of 25 and 50 μg/day, respectively, is recommended.

Notably, iodine deficiency is prevalent worldwide, which corresponds to the worldwide phenomena of brain damage and mental retardation. During pregnancy, infancy and childhood, deficiency may lead to endemic and irreversible cretinism in infants or children. Seafood is naturally rich in iodine. Cod, sea bass, haddock and perch are good sources. Kelp and sea lettuces are the most common vegetable seafood rich in iodine. Dairy products also contain iodine. Other good sources are plants grown in iodine-rich soil. Molluscs and crustaceans are good sources of zinc and copper. An average serving of fish or marine invertebrate can meet the total requirement of essential trace minerals. Oyster and clams provide 45–60% of the daily requirement of minerals.

6.2.7 Fish skin

Fish skin as potential source of collagen Fish skin waste could be used as a potential source of collagen and gelatine, which are currently used in various fields such as the food, cosmetics and biomedical industries. Collagen is structurally formed as a triple helix by three extended protein chains that wrap around one another. The three peptide chains, each of which has a helical structure, together form a triple-stranded helix of three almost identical polypeptide chains consisting of repeating triplets (Glycine-X-Y)$_n$ called tropocollagen, where X and Y are often proline (Pro) or hydroxyproline (Hyp) (Shoulders and Raines, 2009). Collagen is the major structural protein found in the skin and bones of all animals. Most commercial collagens are derived from bovine skin, pig skin and chicken waste. The emergence of bovine spongiform encephalopathy, foot and mouth diseases and religious views has resulted in apprehensions in the use of collagen derived from land-based animal skin. Since the 1980s, gelatin replacement has gained increased attention, especially in Europe, with the emergence of bovine spongiform encephalopathy. The use of collagen and gelatin from fish skin is expected to attract the interest of the industry as an alternative source. Fish collagen and gelatin have a relatively a low risk of possessing unknown pathogens such as of bovine spongiform encephalopathy. Collagen is generally extracted with acid treatment and solubilized without altering its triple helix (Yoshimura *et al.*, 2000).

Collagen is commonly used in medical and pharmaceutical industries as a carrier molecule for drugs, proteins and genes. Long-term maintenance of drug concentration and controlled release at target sites promote the utilization of collagen as effcient drug carriers (Kim and Mendis, 2006). In addition, collagen film/matrix has recently been used as a gene delivery agent promoting bone and cartilage formation. Further, collagen has been reported to play a role in the formation of tissues and organs and the functional expression of cells. Clinical investigations suggest that ingestion of collagen/gelatin hydrolysates reduces pain in patients suffering from osteoarthritis and hydrolysed collagen has been involved in cartilage matrix synthesis (Moskowitz, 2000). The main clinical and experimental applications of collagen include treatment and prophylaxis of bone and soft tissue infections, wound healing, as well as ophthalmic and periodontal treatment (Ruszczak and Friess, 2003).

Fish skin as potential source of gelatin Collagen and gelatin are different forms of the same macromolecule; gelatin is the partially hydrolysed form of collagen. Gelatin is an important industrial biopolymer because of its utility, particularly as a food ingredient. Heat denaturation easily converts collagen into gelatin. Gelatin is derived from the fibrous protein collagen, which is the principal constituent of animal skin, bone and connective tissue. Gelatin is produced via the partial hydrolysis of native collagen.

Gelatin possesses a characteristic melt-in-the-mouth property that makes it useful in a wide range of applications in the food and pharmaceutical industries. It has many applications including thickening, water holding, colloid stabilization, crystallization control, film formation, whipping and emulsification. Fish gelatin releases a kind of aroma and shows higher digestibility than that of animal gelatin (Gómez-Guillén *et al.*, 2002). Some studies on the food properties of fish gelatin have been conducted. Fish gelatin is heterogeneous in molecular composition and contains α- and β-chains, similar to animal gelatins. Similarly with animal gelatin, gelation of fish gelatin involves electrostatic interactions which are important in the stabilization of gelation gel network. However, fish gelatin gels generally have considerably lower storage modulus, gelling (4–5 °C), and melting temperature (12–13 °C) (Venugopal, 2008). The physicochemical and functional properties of fish gelatin have been evaluated, especially with respect to its rheological properties (Badii and Howell, 2006) as well as its emulsifying, foaming, film-forming and sensory properties (Karim and Bhat, 2009).

6.2.8 Fish bone

Calcium sources Fish bone, the non-edible part separated after removal of muscle proteins from the skeletal frame, is a valuable storehouse of various health-promoting components. The organic component of fish bone, which accounts for 30% of the material, is made up of collagen. Fish bone is also considered an excellent source for the isolation of collagen and gelatin. In addition, fish bone is 60–70% inorganic substances, mainly calcium phosphate and hydroxyapatite. Hence, fish bone is a potential source of calcium.

Up to now, only a few studies have been carried out to identify the bioavailability of fish bone calcium and its potential applications. Fish bone material derived from processing large fish provides a useful quantity of calcium. In order to incorporate fish bone into calcium-fortified food it should be converted into an edible form by softening its structure. This can be achieved using different methods including hot water treatment, hot acetic acid solutions and superheated steam to reduce the loss of soluble components from fish tissue and to enable better recovery of bone within a shorter period (Kim and Mendis, 2006; Techochatchawal *et al.*, 2009).

Calcium-fortified supplements Calcium is generally obtained from the diet and it is severely deficient in most regular diets. Therefore, it is essential to take in calcium as a food supplement. Several calcium-fortified products are available in the market and demands for these products are growing fast; however, most of these products are expensive. Alaska pollack (*Theragra chalcogramma*) and hoki backbones discarded from industrial processing have been demonstrated as a source of soluble calcium and a potential calcium-fortified supplement as an alternative to calcium from dairy products (Jung *et al.*, 2006b, 2006c).

Fish bone minerals in medicinal science Hydroxyapatite (HA; $Ca_{10}(PO_4)_6(OH)_2$), has achieved significant applications as a bone graft material in a range of medical and dental applications (Porter *et al.*, 2003). It is the major mineral component of bone and teeth. It can promote rapid bone regeneration and direct bonding to regenerated bone without intermediate connective tissue and its synthetic form is one of the most widely used biomaterials for reconstruction of the skeleton as it has no local or systemic toxicity and possesses osteoconductive properties.

Fish bone material is an important source for biomedical applications due to the presence of hydroxyapatite as the major inorganic constituent. Unlike other calcium phosphates, hydroxyapatite does not break under physiological conditions. In fact, it is thermodynamically stable at physiological pH and actively takes part in bone bonding. This property has been exploited for rapid bone repair after major trauma or surgery. Attempts have been taken to isolate fish-bone-derived hydroxyapatite and use it as an alternate for synthetic hydroxyapatite. Fish-bone ceramics resulting from the heat treatment of fish bone at 600–1300 °C have a major hydroxyapatite phase and contain macropores with a sintered wall (Ozawa and Suzuki, 2002). Such ceramics could be useful as inexpensive ceramic media for biologically and environmentally compatible materials. Fish-originated hydroxyapatite is a potential new ceramics resource worldwide, which also suggests the possibility of materials recycling technology for future waste management and ecology (Huang *et al.*, 2011; Kongsri *et al.*, 2013).

6.2.9 Fish viscera

Fish viscera represent rich sources of enzymes, and many of them exhibit high catalytic activity at relatively low concentrations (Byun *et al.*, 2002). Marine organisms have adapted excellently to diverse extreme environmental conditions, such as high salt concentration, low or high temperature, high pressure and low nutrient availability. Therefore, fish proteinases are reported to possess better properties such as higher catalytic efficiency at low temperatures, lower sensitivity to substrate concentrations and greater stability at broader pH ranges (Kim and Mendis, 2006). These characteristics of fish enzymes have made them suitable for different applications in many food processing operations. Because of the specific characteristics of these enzymes, fish processing by-products are currently used for enzyme extraction.

A range of proteolytic enzymes including pepsin, trypsin, chymotrypsin and collagenases are commercially extracted from marine fish viscera on a large scale. Carnivorous fishes such as Atlantic cod contain high levels of stomach pepsin. In addition, a concentrate of trypsin-like enzymes can be obtained by ultrafiltration of fish sauce produced by salt fermentation of cod intestines; 7 l of enzyme concentrate and 50 l of fish sauce can be produced from 100 kg of cod intestines within 16 days of fermentation at 27 °C (Gildberg, 1992). Chitinases as well as chitosanases can also be isolated from the digestive tract and other organs of some marine fish species (Matsumiya *et al.*, 2006; Ikeda *et al.*, 2009). These enzymes promote the recovery from marine by-products of chitin and chitosan, which are necessary for a wide array of biomedical applications. Use of these enzymes could provide an economical method for isolating bioactive compounds from marine shell wastes. Even though marine fish-derived enzymes do not have direct applications in the field of functional foods or nutraceuticals, they can be used to produce bioactive components on a large scale.

6.2.10 Crustacean shells and shellfish wastes

Chitin One important category of seafood processing by-products is crustacean shells and shellfish wastes. Efficient utilization of these marine by-products has become an environmental priority due to the increased quantities accumulating from processing plants as well as the slow natural degradation of these materials. Chitin is one major structural component of these shell wastes and has been identified as a bioactive polysaccharide and is thus valuable for many applications. These shell wastes are potential sources for the isolation of chitin and are currently utilized for commercial-scale chitin production as well as production of chitosan and their oligomers. Chitin is a high-molecular weight linear polymer of *N*-acetyl-D-glucosamine (*N*-acetyl-2-amino-2-deoxy-D-glucopyranose) units and can be easily processed into many other bioactive derivatives.

Chitosan and chito-oligosaccharides Among them, the most common form is chitosan, which results from the removal of a considerable amount of acetyl groups from chitin. According to the chemical structure, chitosan is a positively charged heteropolymer of D-glucosamine (GlcN) and *N*-acetylglucosamine (GlcNAc) units. Generally, chitin and chitosan oligomers are produced either by chemical or microbiological treatments; however, current commercial preparations of chitin and chitosan utilize thermochemical treatments. The molecular weight as well as the degree of deacetylation of chitosan is largely dependent on the conditions utilized during the production process. However, chitin and chitosan have poor solubility, making them difficult to use in food and biomedical applications (Jeon *et al.*, 2001). Considering this property limitation, some researchers are interested in converting them into oligosaccharides (Jeon *et al.*, 2000). Chito-oligosaccharides (COS), oligosaccharide forms of chitosan, are readily soluble in water due to their shorter chain lengths and free amino groups in D-glucosamine units (Turan and Nagata, 2006; Prabaharan, 2008). Similarly to chitosan, COS have positive charges resulting from the removal of acetyl units from D-glucosamine residues. These properties enable it to interact with negatively charged polymers, macromolecules and polyanions in an aqueous environment (Jeon and Kim, 2000; Jeon *et al.*, 2001). Both chitosan and COS are known to possess many biological activities such as antibacterial (Suzuki *et al.*, 1986), immunoenhancing (Je *et al.*, 2004), antioxidant (Kim and Kim, 2006; Rajapakse *et al.*, 2006; Van Ta *et al.*, 2006), MMP inhibition (Liu *et al.*, 2007a), antidiabetic (Artan *et al.*, 2008), anti-HIV (Yang *et al.*, 2010), anti-inflammatory (Liu *et al.*, 2007b), neuroprotective activities (Pangestuti and Kim, 2010; Pangestuti *et al.*, 2011) and drug delivery (Kim and Rajapakse, 2005). Chemical modification will enhance and open up ways to various uses of chitin, chitosan and COS that are not restricted only to these activities (Khodagholi *et al.*, 2010).

Glucosamine Glucosamine (GlcN) is produced from chitin that is isolated from shells of marine crustaceans, and the vast majority of industrial processes are based on the chemical processing of shellfish. Recent advances have provided insights into several health benefits of GlcN, including protective effects against infections and controlling arthritis (Rajapakse *et al.*, 2008). Specially, multiple clinical trials on GlcN have been carried out as a medical therapy for osteoarthritis because it is a precursor for glycosaminoglycans, and glycosaminoglycans are a major component of joint cartilage. Hence, currently a great deal of attention has been focused on improving the functional properties and biological effects of GlcN for different therapeutic applications.

6.3 Conclusion

In conclusion, seafood is highly nutritious. Therefore, consumption of adequate quantities of seafood can help humans derive significant health benefits. Furthermore, seafood processing by-products are used in many industries and their commercial applications are expanded every year. Identification of the nutraceutical potential of natural bioactive materials is a growing field and use of seafood processing by-products makes it a novel approach for developing more commercial applications. So far, a limited number of bioactivities have been identified from isolated materials and further studies are needed to develop methods to apply them for human health promotion.

Acknowledgments

This study was supported by a grant from the Marine Bioprocess Research Center of the Marine Bio 21 Project funded by the Ministry of Land, Transport and Maritime, Republic of Korea.

References

Alamsjah, M.A., Hirao, S., Ishibashi, F., Oda, T. and Fujita, Y. (2008). Algicidal activity of polyunsaturated fatty acids derived from *Ulva fasciata* and *U. pertusa* (Ulvaceae, Chlorophyta) on phytoplankton. *Journal of Applied Phycology*, 20, 713–720.

Aneiros, A. and Garateix, A. (2004). Bioactive peptides from marine sources: Pharmacological properties and isolation procedures. *Journal of Chromatography B*, 803, 41–53.

Angerer, P., Kothny, W., Störk, S. and Von Schacky, C. (2002). Effect of dietary supplementation with ω-3 fatty acids on progression of atherosclerosis in carotid arteries. *Cardiovascular Research*, 54, 183–190.

Artan, M., Karadeniz, F., Karagozlu, M.Z., Kim, M.M. and Kim, S.K. (2010). Anti-HIV-1 activity of low molecular weight sulfated chitooligosaccharides. *Carbohydrate Research*, 345, 656–662.

Artan, M., Li, Y., Karadeniz, F. *et al.* (2008). Anti-HIV-1 activity of phloroglucinol derivative, 6,6′-bieckol, from *Ecklonia cava*. *Bioorganic and Medicinal Chemistry*, 16, 7921–7926.

Asai, A., Sugawara, T., Ono, H. and Nagao, A. (2004). Biotransformation of fucoxanthinol into amarouxanthin a in mice and hepG2 cells: Formation and cytotoxicity of fucoxanthin metabolites I. *Drug Metabolism and Disposition*, 32, 205–211.

Badii, F. and Howell, N.K. (2006). Fish gelatin: structure, gelling properties and interaction with egg albumen proteins. *Food Hydrocolloids*, 20, 630–640.

Belluzzi, A., Brignola, C., Campieri, M. *et al.* (1996). Effect of an enteric-coated fish-oil preparation on relapses in Crohn's disease. *New England Journal of Medicine*, 334, 1557–1560.

Bogorad, L. (1975). Phycobiliproteins and complementary chromatic adaptation. *Annual Review of Plant Physiology*, 26, 369–401.

Bohn, T. (2008). Bioavailability of non-provitamin a carotenoids. *Current Protein and Food Sciences*, 4, 240–258.

Byun, H.G., Park, P.J., Sung, N.I. and Kim, S.K. (2002). Purification and characterization of a serine proteinase from the tuna pyloric caeca. *Journal of Food Biochemistry*, 26, 479–494.

Costa, L., Fidelis, G., Cordeiro, S. *et al.* (2010). Biological activities of sulfated polysaccharides from tropical seaweeds. *Biomedicine and Pharmacotherapy*, 64, 21–28.

Coste, T.C., Armand, M., Lebacq, J. *et al.* (2007). An overview of monitoring and supplementation of omega 3 fatty acids in cystic fibrosis. *Clinical Biochemistry*, 40, 511–520.

Cui, Y., Zhang, L., Zhang, T. *et al.* (2010). Inhibitory effect of fucoidan on nitric oxide production in lipopolysaccharide activated primary microglia. *Clinical and Experimental Pharmacology and Physiology*, 37, 422–428.

Delgado-Vargas, F., Jiménez, A. and Paredes-López, O. (2000). Natural pigments: carotenoids, anthocyanins, and betalains – characteristics, biosynthesis, processing, and stability. *Critical Reviews in Food Science and Nutrition*, 40, 173–289.

Fallarero, A., Loikkanen, J.J., Männistö, P.T., Castañeda, O. and Vidal, A. (2003). Effects of aqueous extracts of *Halimeda incrassata* (Ellis) Lamouroux and *Bryothamnion triquetrum* (S.G.Gmelim) Howe on hydrogen peroxide and methyl mercury-induced oxidative stress in GT1–7 mouse hypothalamic immortalized cells. *Phytomedicine*, 10, 39–47.

Ferruzzi, M.G. and Blakeslee, J. (2007). Digestion, absorption, and cancer preventative activity of dietary chlorophyll derivatives. *Nutrition Research*, 27, 1–12.

Gildberg, A. (1992). Recovery of proteinases and protein hydrolysates from fish viscera. *Bioresource Technology*, 39, 271–276.

Glazer, A.N. (1994). Phycobiliproteins – a family of valuable, widely used fluorophores. *Journal of Applied Phycology*, 6, 105–112.

Gómez-Guillén, M., Turnay, J., Fernández-Dıaz, M. *et al.* (2002). Structural and physical properties of gelatin extracted from different marine species: a comparative study. *Food Hydrocolloids*, 16, 25–34.

Gross, J. (1991). *Pigments in Vegetables: Chlorophylls and Carotenoids*. Van Nostrand Reinhold.

Hashimoto, T., Ozaki, Y., Taminato, M. *et al.* (2009). The distribution and accumulation of fucoxanthin and its metabolites after oral administration in mice. *British Journal of Nutrition*, 102, 242–248.

Holdt, S.L. and Kraan, S. (2011). Bioactive compounds in seaweed: functional food applications and legislation. *Journal of Applied Phycology*, 23, 543–597.

Holt, S. (2008). Fucose complexes, fucoxanthin, fucoid and fat storage. *Townsend Letter*, 87–92.

Huang, Y.C., Hsiao, P.C. and Chai, H.J. (2011). Hydroxyapatite extracted from fish scale: Effects on MG63 osteoblast-like cells. *Ceramics International*, 37, 1825–1831.

Ikeda, M., Miyauchi, K., Mochizuki, A. and Matsumiya, M. (2009). Purification and characterization of chitinase from the stomach of silver croaker *Pennahia argentatus*. *Protein Expression and Purification*, 65, 214–222.

Ioannou, E. and Roussis, V. (2009). Natural products from seaweeds, in *Plant-derived Natural Products: Synthesis, Function, and Application* (eds A.E. Osbourn and V. Lanzotti). Springer, pp. 51–81.

Iwai, K. (2008). Antidiabetic and antioxidant effects of polyphenols in brown alga *Ecklonia stolonifera* in genetically diabetic KK-A y mice. *Plant Foods for Human Nutrition (Formerly Qualitas Plantarum)*, 63, 163–169.

Jacob, R.A. and Sotoudeh, G. (2002). Vitamin C function and status in chronic disease. *Nutrition in Clinical Care*, 5, 66–74.

Je, J.Y., Park, P.J. and Kim, S.K. (2004). Free radical scavenging properties of heterochitooligosaccharides using an ESR spectroscopy. *Food and Chemical Toxicology*, 42, 381–387.

Jeffrey, S.W., Mantoura, R.F.C. and Wright, S.W. (1997). *Phytoplankton Pigments in Oceanography*. UNESCO-Paris.

Pangestuti, R. and Kim, S.K. (2011a). Biological activities and health benefit effects of natural pigments derived from marine algae. *Journal of Functional Foods*, 3, 255–266.

Pangestuti, R. and Kim, S.K. (2011b). Neuroprotective effects of marine algae. *Marine Drugs*, 9, 803–818.

Panlasigui, L., Baello, O., Dimatangal, J. and Dumelod, B. (2003). Blood cholesterol and lipid-lowering effects of carrageenan on human volunteers. *Asia Pacific Journal of Clinical Nutrition*, 12, 209–214.

Pisani, P., Bray, F. and Parkin, D. (2002). Estimates of the world-wide prevalence of cancer for 25 sites in the adult population. *International Journal of Cancer*, 97, 72–81.

Porter, A., Patel, N., Skepper, J., Best, S. and Bonfield, W. (2003). Comparison of *in vivo* dissolution processes in hydroxyapatite and silicon-substituted hydroxyapatite bioceramics. *Biomaterials*, 24, 4609–4620.

Prabaharan, M. (2008). Review paper: chitosan derivatives as promising materials for controlled drug delivery. *Journal of Biomaterials Applications*, 23, 5–36.

Rajapakse, N., Kim, M.M., Mendis, E., Huang, R. and Kim, S.K. (2006). Carboxylated chitooligosaccharides (CCOS) inhibit MMP-9 expression in human fibrosarcoma cells via down-regulation of AP-1. *Biochimica et Biophysica Acta (BBA) – General Subjects*, 1760, 1780–1788.

Rajapakse, N., Kim, M.M., Mendis, E. and Kim, S.K. (2008). Inhibition of inducible nitric oxide synthase and cyclooxygenase-2 in lipopolysaccharide-stimulated RAW264.7 cells by carboxybutyrylated glucosamine takes place via down-regulation of mitogen-activated protein kinase-mediated nuclear factor-κB signaling. *Immunology*, 123, 348–357.

Ratana-arporn, P. and Chirapart, A. (2006). Nutritional evaluation of tropical green seaweeds *Caulerpa lentillifera* and *Ulva reticulata*. *Kasetsart Journal: Natural Sciences*, 40, 75–83.

Rha, C.K. (2007). Antioxidant activity of sulfated polysaccharides isolated from *Sargassum fulvellum*. *Journal of Food Science and Nutrition*, 12, 65–73.

Rose, D.P. and Connolly, J.M. (1999). Omega-3 fatty acids as cancer chemopreventive agents. *Pharmacology & Therapeutics*, 83, 217–244.

Ruszczak, Z. and Friess, W. (2003). Collagen as a carrier for on-site delivery of antibacterial drugs. *Advanced Drug Delivery Reviews*, 55, 1679–1698.

Ryu, B.M., Qian, Z.J. and Kim, S.K. (2010). Purification of a peptide from seahorse, that inhibits TPA-induced MMP, iNOS and COX-2 expression through MAPK and NF-[kappa] B activation, and induces human osteoblastic and chondrocytic differentiation. *Chemico-Biological Interactions*, 184, 413–422.

Sachindra, N.M., Sato, E., Maeda, H. *et al.* (2007). Radical scavenging and singlet oxygen quenching activity of marine carotenoid fucoxanthin and its metabolites. *Journal of Agricultural and Food Chemistry*, 55, 8516–8522.

Sailasree, R., Abhilash, A., Sathyan, K.M. *et al.* (2008). Differential roles of p16INK4A and p14ARF genes in prognosis of oral carcinoma. *Cancer Epidemiology Biomarkers and Prevention*, 17, 414–420.

Sangeetha, R., Bhaskar, N., Divakar, S. and Baskaran, V. (2010). Bioavailability and metabolism of fucoxanthin in rats: structural characterization of metabolites by LC-MS (APCI). *Molecular and Cellular Biochemistry*, 333, 299–310.

Shahidi, F. (2008). Bioactives from Marine Resources. *ACS Publications*, 987, 24–34.

Shahidi, F. and Alasalvar, C. (2011). Marine oils and other marine nutraceuticals, in *Handbook of Seafood Quality, Safety and Health Applications.* Wiley Online Library, Chapter 36.

Shahidi, F. and Brown, J.A. (1998). Carotenoid pigments in seafoods and aquaculture. *Critical Reveiws in Food Science*, 38, 1–67.

Shahidi, F. and Janak Kamil, Y. (2001). Enzymes from fish and aquatic invertebrates and their application in the food industry. *Trends in Food Science and Technology*, 12, 435–464.

Shahidi, F. and Zhong, Y. (2008). Bioactive peptides. *Journal of AOAC International*, 91, 914–931.

Shoulders, M.D. and Raines, R.T. (2009). Collagen structure and stability. *Annual Review of Biochemistry*, 78, 929–958.

Sousa, I., Batista, A.P., Raymundo, A. and Empis, J. (2006). Rheological characterization of coloured oil-in-water food emulsions with lutein and phycocyanin added to the oil and aqueous phases. *Food Hydrocolloids*, 20, 44–52.

Strand, A., Herstad, O. and Liaaen-Jensen, S. (1998). Fucoxanthin metabolites in egg yolks of laying hens. *Comparative Biochemistry and Physiology – Part A: Molecular and Integrative Physiology*, 119, 963–974.

Su, K.P., Huang, S.Y., Chiu, C.C. and Shen, W.W. (2003). Omega-3 fatty acids in major depressive disorder: a preliminary double-blind, placebo-controlled trial. *European Neuropsychopharmacology*, 13, 267–271.

Sugawara, T., Baskaran, V., Tsuzuki, W. and Nagao, A. (2002). Brown algae fucoxanthin is hydrolyzed to fucoxanthinol during absorption by caco-2 human intestinal cells and mice. *The Journal of Nutrition*, 132, 946–951.

Sugawara, T., Yamashita, K., Asai, A. *et al.* (2009). Esterification of xanthophylls by human intestinal caco-2 cells. *Archives of Biochemistry and Biophysics*, 483, 205–212.

Suzuki, K., Mikami, T., Okawa, Y. *et al.* (1986). Antitumor effect of hexa-*N*-acetylchitohexaose and chitohexaose. *Carbohydrate Research*, 151, 403–408.

Swing, J. (2003). What future for the oceans? *Foreign Affairs*, 82, 139–152.

Techochatchawal, K., Therdthai, N. and Khotavivattana, S. (2009). Development of calcium supplement from the bone of nile tilapia (*Tilapia nilotica*). *Food Innovation Asia Conference Bangkok-Thailand*, 2, 539–546.

Terasaki, M., Hirose, A., Narayan, B. *et al.* (2009). Evaluation of recoverable functional lipid components of several brown seaweeds (Phaeophyta) from Japan with special reference to fucoxanthin and fucosterol contents. *Journal of Phycology*, 45, 974–980.

Turan, K. and Nagata, K. (2006). Chitosan-DNA nanoparticles: the effect of cell type and hydrolysis of chitosan on *in vitro* DNA transfection. *Pharmaceutical Development and Technology*, 11, 503–12.

Van Ta, Q., Kim, M.M. and Kim, S.K. (2006). Inhibitory effect of chitooligosaccharides on matrix metalloproteinase-9 in human fibrosarcoma cells (HT1080). *Marine Biotechnology*, 8, 593–599.

Venugopal, V. (2008). *Marine Products for Healthcare: Functional and Bioactive Nutraceutical Compounds from the Ocean*. CRC-Taylor and Francis.

Vidal Novoa, A., Motidome, M., Mancini Filho, J. *et al.* (2001). Antioxidant activity related to phenolic acids in the aqueous extract of the marine seaweed *Bryothamnin triquetrum* (SG Gmelim) Howe. *Revista Brasileira de Ciencias Farmaceuticas (Impr.)*, 37, 373–382.

Whelan, J. and McEntee, M.F. (2004). Dietary (*n*-6) PUFA and intestinal tumorigenesis. *The Journal of Nutrition*, 134, 3421S.

Wijesekara, I., Yoon, N. and Kim, S. (2010). Phlorotannins from *Ecklonia cava* (Phaeophyceae): Biological activities and potential health benefits. *BioFactors*, 36, 408–414.

Wijesinghe, W.A.J. P. and Jeon, Y.J. (2011). Enzyme-assistant extraction (EAE) of bioactive components: A useful approach for recovery of industrially important metabolites from seaweeds: A review. *Fitoterapia*, 83, 6–12.

Wong, K.W. (2005). Clinical efficacy of *n*-3 fatty acid supplementation in patients with asthma. *Journal of the American Dietetic Association*, 105, 98–105.

Yan, X., Chuda, Y., Suzuki, M. and Nagata, T. (1999). Fucoxanthin as the major antioxidant in *Hijikia fusiformis*, a common edible seaweed. *Bioscience, Biotechnology, and Biochemistry*, 63, 605–607.

Yang, E.J., Kim, J.G., Kim, J.Y. *et al.* (2010). Anti-inflammatory effect of chitosan oligosaccharides in RAW 264.7 cells. *Central European Journal of Biology*, 5, 95–102.

Yoshimura, K., Terashima, M., Hozan, D. and Shirai, K. (2000). Preparation and dynamic viscoelasticity characterization of alkali-solubilized collagen from shark skin. *Journal of Agricultural and Food Chemistry*, 48, 685–690.

Yuan, Y. and Walsh, N. (2006). Antioxidant and antiproliferative activities of extracts from a variety of edible seaweeds. *Food and Chemical Toxicology*, 44, 1144–1150.

Zhang, R., Kang, K.A., Piao, M.J. *et al.* (2008). Eckol protects V79-4 lung fibroblast cells against γ-ray radiation-induced apoptosis via the scavenging of reactive oxygen species and inhibiting of the c-Jun NH2-terminal kinase pathway. *European Journal of Pharmacology*, 591, 114–123.

Zhu, W., Chiu, L.C.M., Ooi, V.E.C., Chan, P.K.S. and Ang Jr, P.O. (2006). Antiviral property and mechanisms of a sulphated polysaccharide from the brown alga *Sargassum patens* against *Herpes simplex* virus type 1. *Phytomedicine*, 13, 695–701.

7

Food Processing By-products as Sources of Functional Foods and Nutraceuticals

Nina Karla M. Alparce and Anil Kumar Anal
Asian Institute of Technology, Pathum Thani, Thailand

7.1 Introduction

The process of transforming raw ingredients into food that is more convenient and safer for human as well as livestock consumption and has a longer shelf life dates back to prehistoric times. Early methods of food processing include fermenting, drying, salting and various types of cooking (e.g. roasting and smoking). These processes evolved and gave rise to more sophisticated and efficient processes enabling production of a wide variety of processed food. Commonly used methods nowadays include canning, freezing, dehydration and aseptic processing.

The world's food requirement is directly related to population and population growth. However, the crop-pattern, demand for semiprocessed and processed foods and food consumption keep changing. Hence, food processing is, perhaps, one of the most dynamic and fastest growing industries. And as the world population continues to rise, the volume of food processed every day also needs to increase and keep up with demand.

The very nature of raw agricultural ingredients (e.g. fruits, vegetables, cereals), that is, they are seasonal, highly perishable and some are not even edible in their unprocessed form, makes processing indispensible. Rough rice, for instance, is grown only twice a year, so the harvest is available for only a few months if it is kept unprocessed. To make this commodity available all year round, it has to be dehulled and whitened. While brown rice can be cooked and consumed and is healthier, it is susceptible to oxidation and thus it has a shorter shelf life, requires longer cooking time and is

Functional Foods and Dietary Supplements: Processing Effects and Health Benefits, First Edition.
Edited by Athapol Noomhorm, Imran Ahmad and Anil Kumar Anal.

preferred by few. Hence, the bran layer is removed leaving mostly endosperm for consumption.

Whilst cereals may be considered durables, fruits and vegetables are especially perishable and must be consumed a few days or weeks after harvest. These commodities are also prone to mechanical and insect damage that renders a significant proportion of the total production unmarketable. Hence, some sound yet unappetizing pieces may be processed into juices or purees and other products to reduce the losses, utilize the nutrients and maximize profits. Marine and meat products also cannot be stored for a long time, hence they are processed into canned goods, frozen slabs or fillets, etc.

Most foods are necessary for the basic nutrition of human beings, but some may also contain bioactive compounds that provide health benefits beyond nourishment. Studies have shown that some of these bioactive compounds are also present or, in some cases, concentrated in by-products that are often discarded after food processing. Albeit most of these by-products are not suitable for human or animal consumption, they can be utilized in many other ways instead of being disposed off in the environment where they contribute to pollution. This review outlines information based on recent studies about by-products of food processing that are potential sources of functional foods and nutraceuticals.

7.2 By-products of plant food processing

Plants have been used for food throughout history but some plants have been extensively utilized for medicinal purposes since ancient times. For a long time, natural products obtained mainly from plants have been prominent sources of prophylactic agents for the prevention and treatment of diseases in both humans and animals (Bernal *et al.*, 2011). But in the twentieth century, synthetic chemicals dominated the pharmaceutical industry replacing natural extracts (Raskin *et al.*, 2002).

However, prevalence of chronic diseases, for which truly effective drugs without adverse side effects have not been developed, may have led to the increasing emphasis on the health benefits of plant products. Such diseases include cardiovascular diseases (CVD) and cancer, which are the leading causes of death in both developed and developing countries. Regular consumption of fruits and vegetables or any plant-based foods has been strongly associated with a reduced risk from major chronic diseases and with slowing age-related functional decline (Martin *et al.*, 2011).

The rediscovery of the connection between plants and health has launched a new generation of botanical therapeutics that include plant-derived pharmaceuticals, multicomponent botanical drugs, dietary supplements, functional foods and plant-produced recombinant proteins (Raskin *et al.*, 2002). But the health-promoting constituents in plants have proved difficult to identify with certainty, confounding the precision of dietary recommendations so many researchers have investigated which particular components are responsible for the beneficial properties of plant-based foods or products. By-products of plant food processing represent a major disposal problem for the industry but are of interest as potential sources of compounds with favourable technological and nutritional properties.

Such studies have identified various bioactive compounds in plants such as flavonoids, phenolics, liminoids, carotenoids, phytosterols and even proteins and peptides. Bioactive peptides are of particular interest today as they have antimicrobial, antioxidative, antithrombic, antihypertensive and immunostimulatory activities.

Bioactive peptides have been defined as specific protein fragments that positively affect body functions or conditions and, ultimately, health. Their effects depend on their amino acid content. Furthermore, recent findings in animals and humans have suggested that, in gastrointestinal digestion, peptides may mediate many of the actions of parent proteins by acting as regulatory compounds with hormone-like activities (Hettiarchchy, 2011).

7.2.1 Cereal grains

Some cereal grains are staple foods in many countries. Rice, in particular, is part of almost every meal in some parts of Asia. Wheat, on the other hand, is a main ingredient in bread making. To make these raw materials edible or consumable, rice and wheat must be milled, which involves removal of the hull and the germ layers. Cereal grains are known to possess high-quality protein, which is broken down by gastrointestinal proteolytic enzymes to release bioactive peptides when it is consumed (Hettiarchchy, 2011; Kitts and Weiler, 2003).

Depending on their amino acid content and sequence, bioactive peptides administered orally may affect major body systems such as the cardiovascular, digestive, immune and nervous system. Bioactive peptides already identified from cereal grains include exorphins, or opioid peptides derived from wheat gluten following digestion with pepsin. Such peptides have a similar structure to endogenous opioid peptides with a tyrosine residue located at the amino terminal or bioactive site (Kitts and Weiler, 2003).

7.2.2 Rice

Generally, the aleuronic layer of the grains is removed during processing, particularly in rice milling. The aleuronic layer, often called bran, is therefore a by-product of rice milling but it contains protein and other health-promoting components. Hence, this processing waste is a potent source of bioactive peptides. In fact, enzymatic hydrolysates prepared from rice bran showed growth inhibitory effects to certain types of cancer cells *in vitro*. Kannan *et al.* (2010) separated and purified single peptides from rice bran that show significant anticancer effects.

Their experiments using MTS dye assay showed nearly 75% inhibition on colon and liver cancer cells, 68% on breast cancer cells and 60% on lung cancer cells. However, the pure peptides exhibited increased inhibition, i.e. 80 and 85% inhibition of breast and liver cancer cells, respectively and 69% inhibition of lung cancer cells. Moreover, there was an increase in inhibition pattern as the dosage of pure peptide increased but it seemed to level off beyond 600 μg/ml.

It was found that arginine (Arg), proline (Pro) and glutamic acid (Glu) are predominant in the purified peptides. The amino acid sequence, Arg-Pro-Arg was found in the C-terminus, Glu-Gln at the N-terminus, and Glu-Gln-Arg-Pro-Arg was found to be the *de novo* sequence. The activity of biofunctional peptides is based on their inherent amino acid composition and sequence. The shorter the peptide chains, the higher the solvent accessibility, exposing the functional groups to impart functional properties. The presence of Pro signifies more accessibility to solvent owing to its predominance in turns of a polypeptide chain and it is thought to significantly contribute to the bioactivity of the peptide. The presence of charged (Glu) and heterocyclic amino acid (Pro) in the sequence could have attributed anticancer properties to the peptide.

Hettiarchchy (2011) has published a patent entitled 'Bioactive Pentapeptides from Rice Bran and Use Thereof.' In general, the invention relates to the novel bioactive pentapeptides from heat stabilized defatted rice bran having anticancer, antiobesity, anti-Alzheimer and other health-promoting activities of proteins. Defatted rice bran has approximately 20% protein, with the proteins and their peptide fragments complexed within carbohydrates and lipids providing difficulties in protein extraction.

Bioactive pentapeptide isolated from heat-stabilized defatted rice bran has a sequence Glu-Gln-Arg-Pro-Arg as in the study described previously (Kannan *et al.*, 2010). It may have an inhibitory activity on proliferation of human colon, liver, breast and/or lung cancer cell lines. It is therefore desirable to provide purified bioactive pentapeptides from defatted rice bran that have anticancer, antiobesity, anti-Alzheimer and other health-promoting activities and which can be incorporated as an active ingredient into pharmaceutical, nutraceutical and food compositions.

7.2.3 Corn

Other researchers also found bioactive peptides in an equally common cereal grain – corn. Suh, Whang and Lee (1999) and Yang *et al.* (2007) isolated a hexapeptide (Pro-Ser-Gly-Gln-Tyr-Tyr) and a dipeptide (Ala-Tyr) from corn gluten meal (CGM) hydrolysate. CGM, a by-product of the starch industry with abundant protein, is mainly composed of zein ($\approx$40%) and glutelin ($\approx$40%). Several peptides were also separated from α-zein hydrolysate including a tripeptide with the sequence Leu-Arg-Pro.

These bioactive peptides isolated from CGM were found to have angiotensin-I-converting enzyme (ACE)-inhibitory activity and thus have a blood-pressure lowering effect. Synthetic ACE inhibitors (e.g. captopril, enalapril and lisinopril) are effective in lowering blood pressure but are reported to have side effects such as dizziness, coughing, headache, abnormal taste (metallic or salty taste) and kidney and liver problems. Hence, in terms of toxicological safety and side effects, natural ACE inhibitors have an advantage over synthetic ones.

Huang *et al.* (2011) investigated the use of ultrafiltration membrane reactors for production of corn protein hydrolysate with ACE-inhibitory activity, evaluated the operation stability and hydrolysate product quality, and evaluated the *in vivo* antihypertension effects of purified peptides on spontaneously hypertensive rats. Membrane separation techniques have been widely used for enrichment of peptides with a specific molecular weight range. Ultrafiltration is routinely employed to enrich bioactive hydrolysates.

The researchers pointed out that the molecular size of the ACE-inhibitory peptide plays an important role in its inhibitory activity. In fact, ACE inhibitors have been categorized by mechanisms in which size has an effect. They may be competitive or non-competitive. Competitive inhibitors compete with available ACE substrate to interact with ACE and are usually composed of more than four amino acids. Non-competitive ACE inhibitors that combine with the ACE bioactive region to inhibit its enzymatic activity are usually made of two to three amino acids.

Furthermore, molecular size and structural properties, such as hydrophobicity, affect the major transport route of peptides. Research findings indicated that peptides with two to six amino acids were most easily absorbed in comparison with protein and free amino acids. Roberts *et al.* (1999) reported that small (di- and tripeptides) and large (10–51 amino acids) peptides could cross the intestinal barrier intact and exhibit their biological functions at the tissue level. In the current study, the Mw<3 kDa fraction not only exhibited the highest ACE-inhibitory activity, but also the highest OH scavenging activity.

ACE exists in the vascular endothelium of various organs. In order to exert an antihypertensive effect after oral ingestion, bioactive peptides must be absorbed from the intestine intact and be resistant to degradation by plasma peptidases so they reach the target sites. The mixture of peptides in this current study not only showed potent ACE-inhibitory activity *in vitro*, but also decreased blood pressure significantly in 1 h and the effect lasted for 5 h. Findings demonstrated that corn peptides (CP) not only had a good long-term antihypertensive effects but also had no side effects on small rats. CP derived from CGM demonstrated more potent antihypertensive effects through synergist action.

7.2.4 Wheat

Wheat germ, a by-product from the milling industry, is also one of the most potent sources of plant or vegetable proteins with a protein content of about 27.8–30 g/100 g. Defatted wheat germ hydrolysates or proteins (DWGP) were also found to have ACE-inhibitory activities. Jia *et al.* (2010) investigated the use of ultrasonic pretreatment in the extraction of bioactive peptides and found that it affects the release of peptides from DWGP during enzymatic hydrolysis.

The findings also indicated that ultrasonic pretreatment could result in an increase in surface hydrophobicity of DWGP and loosening of the protein tissue, facilitating the release of hydrophobic amino acids during enzymatic hydrolysis. The amino acid composition further showed that the hydrolysate of ultrasound-pretreated DWGP had more hydrophobic amino acids and Pro, which play important roles in the activities of ACE-inhibitory peptides, than that without ultrasonic pretreatment.

7.2.5 Other cereal grains

A number of bioactive peptides from other cereal grains were also identified. One of which, lunasin, was originally isolated from soybean but was also found in barley and wheat. According to Hernandez-Ledesma *et al.* (2008), lunasin contains eight Asp residues in its carboxyl end which are responsible for its antimitotic effect after they bind to regions of hypoacetylated chromatin, such as those found in centromeres. As a result, the kinetechore complex does not form properly and the microtubules fail to attach to the centromeres, leading to mitotic arrest and eventually to cell death.

Lunasin also contains the cell adhesion motif Arg-Gly-Asp, known to allow attachment to the extracellular matrix, and a predicted helix with structural homology to a conserved region of chromatin binding proteins. Chemical carcinogenesis and viral oncogenesis have been found to share common mechanism(s) involving changes in chromatin status that lunasin disrupts to suppress cancer formation.

This 43-amino-acid-long peptide also has antioxidant and anti-inflammatory properties and can enter target tissues. They were found to be biostable, bioactive and thermostable after oral administration in animals. Its potential as a nutraceutical and functional food is considerable, hence, other researchers have tried to find other sources. Nakurte *et al.* (2012) tested the presence of lunasin in triticale, a cross-breed of wheat (*Triticum*) and rye (*Secale*). This crop has the functionality and high yield of wheat and durability of rye but is produced mainly as animal food. It is also not suitable for leavened products due to the production of weak and sticky gluten.

The researchers investigated various genotypes of triticale grown in Latvia and determined whether winter rye and wheat grown in the Latvian climate produce the peptide in comparable amounts with that in genotypes grown in Korea. Other published data on the occurrence of lunasin in cereals were obtained in barley, rye and wheat genotypes grown in Korea and also *S. nigrum* L., a plant indigenous to Northeast Asia (Hernandez-Ledesma *et al.*, 2008; Nakurte *et al.*, 2012).

7.2.6 Other bioactive compounds in cereal grains

Cereal grains also contain many other bioactive components such as phenolic compounds. These are any compound containing a benzene ring with one or more hydroxyl groups. They have antioxidant properties and can protect against degenerative diseases such as cancer and heart diseases in which reactive oxygen species are involved (Dykes and Rooney, 2007). They can potentially inhibit platelet aggregation and prevent oxidative damage of lipid and low-density lipoproteins (Butsat and Siriamornpun, 2009). In cereal grains, these compounds are located mainly in the pericarp and they can be concentrated by decorticating the grain to produce bran, which can be incorporated into a food product with increased dietary fibre levels and nutraceutical properties (Dykes and Rooney, 2007).

According to Adom and Liu (2002, as cited by Butsat and Siriamornpun, 2009), cereal grains, especially rice, contain special phenolic acids (e.g. ferulic acid, *p*-coumaric and diferulate) that are not present in significant quantities in fruit and vegetables. These compounds are found in distinct fractions from milling the grains. Rice bran was reported as a rich source of steryl ferulate esters, commonly referred to as oryzanols. It is also a potential source of tocopherols, tocotrienols and phenolic compounds, which show antioxidant activity (Butsat and Siriamornpun, 2009).

Rice husk, on the other hand, is also a low-value by-product of commercial milling. The husks are inedible and hence used mostly in non-food applications. However, they offer the valuable nutritional advantage that they contain an antioxidant defence system to protect the rice seed from oxidative stress. Jeon *et al.* (2006, cited by Butsat and Siriamornpun, 2009) have reported that phenolic compounds from methanolic extracts of rice husk exhibit high antioxidant activity against scavengers of singlet oxygen and inhibit high hydrogen peroxide-induced damage to cellular DNA in human lymphocytes. While Lee *et al.* (2003, cited by Butsat and Siriamornpun, 2009) demonstrated that the antioxidant activity of rice husks was increased by far-infrared radiation, when using them for cooking turkey breast (Butsat and Siriamornpun, 2009).

In a study conducted by Butsat and Siriamornpun (2009), it was found that the concentrations of bioactive components (i.e. phenolic acids, γ-oryzanols and tocopherols), were found in greater amounts in the external layers. The ability to scavenge DPPH radical by rice fractions was in the order of bran > husk > brown rice > milled rice for all samples. Moreover, the bran fraction had the greatest ferric reducing ability followed by husk, brown rice and then milled rice.

Furthermore, it was found that the bran fractions contained the highest level of ferulic acid, while vanillic acid and *p*-coumaric acid were the most dominant phenolic acids in husk fractions. In addition, ferulic, *p*-hydroxybenzoic, protocatechuic and chlorogenic acids were minor constituents in the husk. These results indicate that the concentrations of phenolic acids increase from endosperm to the aleurone layer. Moreover, they support the concept that *p*-coumaric acid is primarily cross-linked with the lignin of the husk cell walls. Therefore rice husk, as a valuable source of phenolic acids, is also a good source of natural antioxidants.

Similarly, Moheb *et al.* (2013) reported that wheat hulls can be considered a rich and cheap source of tricin, particularly from winter wheat varieties. Reportedly, this 'waste by-product' of wheat can be exploited as a source of this rare chemopreventive flavonoid. Tricin is a naturally occurring flavone with a relatively rare and sporadic distribution. It was mainly found in cereal grains, for example wheat, rice, barley, oat and corn.

Tricin was described as the most potent anticlonogenic (anti-colony forming) agent of human-derived tumour breast cell lines and human-derived colon carcinoma cell lines. This property was attributed to its ability to inhibit cyclooxygenase activity and its interference with intestinal carcinogenesis in mice. Jeong *et al.* (2007) reported that tricin inhibited P-glycoprotein activity in adriamycin-resistant human breast cancer cells, thus delaying spontaneous mammary tumorigenesis and suppressing oxidative stress-induced apoptosis.

Moheb *et al.* (2012) reported that the yellow hull powder of winter wheat can be incorporated into bread and other bakery products in order to obtain a high quality food that provides the combined benefits of richness in dietary fibre and tricin. The hull powder can also be integrated into a suitable pharmaceutical dosage form as a food supplement. Using tricin in such a manner can stop the progression of cirrhosis in a fibrotic liver of targeted liver patients (Seki *et al.*, 2012 as cited by Moheb *et al.*, 2012). More generally, the consumption of winter wheat hull rich in both tricin and dietary fiber can prevent colon cancer (Moheb *et al.*, 2012).

While the outer bran layers of wheat kernels may be rich in antioxidant compounds, several contaminants such as mycotoxins, principally deoxynivalenol, or synthetic contaminants such as heavy metals (cadmium and lead) and pesticides are also concentrated in the outer layers. However, dietary fibre, free phenolic acids and total antioxidant activity decreased progressively from the external to the internal layers (Sovrani *et al.*, 2011). A previous study demonstrated that the phenolic content, which is highly correlated to the total antioxidant activity (TAA), progressively decreases as the pearling (bran removal or debranning) progresses through the aleurone layer into the inner parts of the kernel (Liyana-Pathirana *et al.*, 2006).

The protective effects of cereal fibres depend on their solubility. Soluble fibre, particularly β-glucans, can reduce blood cholesterol, while insoluble fibres shorten the transit time through the intestinal tract, decreasing the contact between carcinogens and the epithelial cells in the colon (Fardet, Rock and Rémésy, 2008 as cited by Sovrani *et al.*, 2011). Nonetheless, whole grain foods are not so attractive to consumers, because the higher bran content in whole grain flour reduces the sensory value of the end-use products. The high fibre content, on the other hand, is the main cause of the negative technological properties of whole grain bread, with a reduction in loaf volume, an increase in crumb firmness and a dark colour.

food-borne pathogens when added into beef patties (Sagdic *et al.*, 2011 as cited by Tseng and Zhao, 2013). Furthermore, research has indicated that WGP seed extracts show better antioxidant activities than the synthetic antioxidants BHA and BHT (Baydar, Ozkan, and Yasar, 2007 as cited by Tseng and Zhao, 2013).

ADF may be incorporated with flour for making high dietary fibre bakery goods, while the polyphenols in ADF could act as antioxidants for improving colour, aroma and taste of the product. Tseng and Zhao (2013) also outlined the following examples of ADF application:

(1) mango peel powders used for preparing macaroni to enhance the antioxidant properties (Ajila *et al.*, 2010);
(2) apple pomace incorporated into wheat flour as a fibre source to improve the rheological characteristics of cake (Sudha *et al.*, 2007 as cited by Tseng and Zhao, 2013).
(3) grape pomace mixed with sourdough for rye bread (Mildner-Szkudlarz *et al.*, 2011 as cited by Tseng and Zhao, 2013); and
(4) grape seed flour used for cereal bars, pancakes and noodles (Rosales Soto *et al.*, 2012 as cited by Tseng and Zhao, 2013)

The functional compounds in three legume by-products – pea pod (*Pisum sativum* L.), broad bean pod (*Vicia faba* L.) and okara from soybean (*Glycine max* L.) – were also investigated. Mateos-Aparicio *et al.* (2010) reported that these by-products can be considered as sources of dietary fibre because it is their major constituent, i.e. more than 50% for pea pod and okara and 40% for broad bean pod. Moreover, the high quantity of vegetable protein in okara (more than 30%) and the considerable amount of fat rich in linoleic and oleic acids found make this by-product a candidate for food fortification. Both pod by-products present an important amount of vegetable protein and also a remarkable concentration of potassium; moreover, iron is higher than potassium in pea pod. In addition, α-galactosides were found in broad bean pod and okara. Inulin was also found in okara. The presence of this large amount of dietary fibre and the other nutritive compounds provides an important added value. It may be possible to balance nutritional food requirements using these by-products, which could have an advantage over using isolated functional ingredients.

Most studies on the functional components of fruits and vegetables indicate that they are rich sources of antioxidant compounds such as those mentioned in the studies presented earlier in this review. However, some fruits were also found to contain peptides that may have functional activities. Kissper, a 39-residue peptide, was isolated from kiwi fruit (*Actinidia deliciosa*) by Ciardiello *et al.* (2008). Its primary structure, elucidated by direct protein sequencing, is identical to the *N*-terminal region of kiwellin, a recently reported kiwi fruit allergenic protein, suggesting that kissper derives from the *in vivo* processing of kiwellin. The peptide does not show high sequence identity with any other polypeptide of known function. However, it displays a pattern of cysteines similar, but not identical, to those observed in some plant and animal proteins, including toxins involved in defence mechanisms. A number of these proteins also act on mammalian cells (Ciardiello *et al.*, 2008).

Pihlanto *et al.* (2008) isolated proteins from potato tubers at different physiological states and by-products from the potato industry and evaluated their ACE-inhibitory and radical scavenging potencies. The enzymes alcalase, neutrase and esperase were used to hydrolyse and autolyse the protein isolates and by-products.

It was found that hydrolysis increased the inhibition of ACE and radical-scavenging activity. Moreover, the ACE-inhibitory potencies of the hydrolysates were reportedly high. The by-product fractions also showed ACE inhibition before hydrolysis. However, all samples exhibited low radical-scavenging activity and prolonged hydrolysis with proteases was needed to produce an increase in the activity. Ultrafiltration through 3–10 kDa membranes efficiently separated the ACE-inhibitory compounds into permeate fractions. The results of this study suggest that potato is a promising source for the production of bioactive compounds to be used as ingredients for developing functional foods beneficial to cardiovascular health (Pihlanto *et al.*, 2008).

7.4 By-products of oil extraction from plant materials

Over the century, cases of cancer, a leading cause of death, has continuously risen. Cancer treatment is expensive and involves drugs that have adverse side effects and toxicity complications. Hence, cheaper alternative methods using bioactive peptides could improve the economics of cancer prevention and therapy. Bioactive peptides derived from food ingredients are highly acceptable due to their non-toxic nature. In a study conducted by Rayaprolu *et al.* (2013), peptide hydrolysates were prepared from high oleic acid soy protein isolates (SPIs), tested for gastrointestinal resistance, fractionated based on molecular size and tested for multiple site cancer inhibiting activities.

Soybean meal, a co-product after oil extraction from seeds, is rich in protein. Protein isolates were prepared at alkaline pH and hydrolysed using alcalase enzyme to generate peptide hydrolysates. After determining the gastrointestinal resistance of the peptide hydrolysates, they were fractionated into definite molecular sizes and tested against human colon, liver and lung cancer cell lines. Results led to the conclusion that peptide fractions derived from meals of high oleic acid soybean lines have the property of inhibiting cancer cell growth in human cell lines and could have potential nutraceutical use against colon, liver and lung cancers (Rayaprolu *et al.*, 2012).

Defatted sunflower meal, generated as a by-product of sunflower oil extraction, is usually used as animal feed. However, its high protein content (about 30%) makes it a desirable source of protein isolates that can be subjected to hydrolytic treatments to produce hydrolysates with increased nutritional and functional properties. Megias *et al.* (2009), obtained sunflower protein hydrolysates by treatment with the endoprotease alcalase followed by treatment with the endo/exoprotease flavourzyme. The sequential use of the two enzymatic preparations was adopted to increase the degree of hydrolysis.

The researchers reported a dramatic increase in the generation of ACE-inhibitory peptides at the beginning of the hydrolysis with alcalase, the maximum ACE inhibition observed after 5 minutes of hydrolysis. After this, ACE-inhibitory activity rapidly decreased, probably reflecting hydrolysis of many of the ACE-inhibiting peptides that were generated during the initial minutes of hydrolysis. The ACE-inhibitory peptides were purified by affinity purification using pig lung ACE immobilized on 4% BCL glyoxyl-agarose. Covalent binding to agarose resulted in immobilization not only of ACE, but also of other proteins and molecules carrying a reactive amino group that are present in pig lung extracts.

Therefore, a specific eluting solvent is needed to recover ACE binding properties without releasing peptides binding to other immobilized molecules. This was accomplished by employing an affinity purification method with captopril, which is a specific ACE competitive inhibitor. In the preparative reverse-phase chromatography, hydrolysates containing peptides that eluted last had the highest ACE-inhibitory activity. It was proposed that this is due to the fact that ACE-inhibitory peptides are rich in hydrophobic amino acids, resulting in higher retention times in reverse-phase chromatography.

The fractions prepared by analytical reverse-phase chromatography were found to be rich in Asp, Ser, Gly, Thr and Val residues compared to the original protein hydrolysate. Some fractions also showed a higher content of Ala, Met, Ile, Leu or Phe residues confirming that ACE-inhibitory peptides are rich in hydrophobic amino acids. It was concluded that purification of ACE-inhibitory peptides by affinity chromatography followed by high-performance liquid chromatography (HPLC) results in a more effective purification of bioactive peptides from food sources than procedures using a combination of gel filtration chromatography and HPLC.

Similarly, ACE-inhibitory peptides and antioxidative hydrolysates were extracted from defatted rapeseed meal. Rapeseed is one of the most important oil-seed crops worldwide and also represents the world's second leading source of protein meal. Makinen *et al.* (2012) used various proteolytic enzymes to extract hydrolysates from the defatted rapeseed meal.

The hydrolysate generated by alcalase displayed the highest ACE-inhibitory activity (IC_{50} 0.02 mg/ml) as well as high inhibitory capacity against lipid oxidation in a liposomal model. This hydrolysate was fractionated using step-wise solid-phase extraction into three fractions of which the hydrophobic fractions possessed the highest ACE-inhibitory activity. Moreover, the ACE-inhibitory peptides in alcalase hydrolysate exhibited good stability in an *in vitro* digestion model using human gastric and duodenal fluids. They were also found to have an uncompetitive mechanism against ACE. Overall, the results suggested that defatted rapeseed meal is a potential source of ACE-inhibitory compounds for use in functional foods.

7.5 By-products of processing fish and marine products

Fisheries and aquaculture play a vital role in the global, national and rural economy. They contribute significantly to food security and nutrition as they are important sources of protein for about 17% of the world's population and nearly 25% for low-income food deficit countries (FAO, 2012a). FAO has reported that in 2010, capture fisheries and aquaculture supplied the world with about 148 million tons of fish, of which about 128 million tons was for human use. On the other hand, the preliminary data for 2011 indicated an increase in production to154 million tons, of which 131 million tons was utilized as food (FAO, 2012b).

Like any other biological materials, fish and marine organisms have a wide range of species and product forms. Once harvested or caught, fish quickly perish and so require timely procurement, efficient transportation, and advanced storage, processing and packaging facilities for marketing. Specific requirements and preservation techniques must be employed to prolong their shelf life, minimize the activity of spoilage as well pathogenic microorganisms, prevent losses and preserve their quality and nutritional content (FAO, 2012a).

Fish and other marine organisms can be processed into a variety of products with increased economic value. Fish, for instance, may be distributed live, fresh, chilled, frozen, heat-treated, fermented, dried, smoked, salted, pickled, boiled, fried, freeze-dried, minced, powdered or canned, or as a combination of two or more of these forms (FAO, 2012a). The processes used to add value to fish and marine products results in increasing amounts of by-products or residues. According to Kim (2013), approximately 25% of the fish and shellfish caught annually are discarded as waste. It was also estimated that only 43% of crustacean and mollusc catches are utilized as products for human consumption.

7.5.1 Fish by-products

Processing by marine capture fisheries produces left-overs such as trimmings, fins, frames, heads, skins and viscera while marine bioprocessing left-overs include shells of crustaceans and shellfish. These by-products or left-overs are not normally saleable but can be recycled after appropriate treatments. Presently, most of these by-products are utilized in the production of fish oil, fishmeal, fertilizer, pet food and silage. However, these products are of low economic value (Kim and Mendis, 2005).

In recent studies, a number of bioactive compounds have been identified in remaining fish muscle proteins, collagen and gelatin, fish oil, fish bone, internal organs and shells of crustaceans and shellfish. Fish frames and cutoffs resulting from mechanically deboned fish contain considerable amounts of muscle proteins which are nutritionally valuable, are easily digestible and have a well-balanced amino acid composition. (Kim and Mendis, 2005)

Tuna frame proteins, for instance, are usually discarded as processing waste or used as animal feed because of their poor functional properties. However, frame proteins can be converted to value-added products by enzymatic hydrolysis and can be widely used to improve the functional and nutritional properties of proteins. Lee *et al.* (2010) extracted ACE inhibitory peptides from tuna frame protein. The enzymatic hydrolysis was performed using various commercial enzymes, for example alcalase, a-chymotrypsin, papain, pepsin, Neutrase and trypsin, at their corresponding optimal condition.

In this study, the isolated ACE inhibitory peptide from the purified tuna frame hydrolysate (PTFP) was composed of Gly-Asp-Leu-Gly-Lys-Thr-Thr-Thr-Val-Ser-Asn-Trp-Ser-Pro-Pro-Lys-Try-Lys-Asp-Thr-Pro with a MW of 2482 Da. It exhibited a higher or similar activity (IC_{50} = 11.28 μM) compared to similar peptides in other studies. The identified ACE inhibitory peptides from other food processing by-products include Ile-Val-Tyr (IC_{50} = 0.48 μM) from wheat germ hydrolysate; Leu-Gln-Pro (IC_{50} = 9.6 μM) from zein; Glu-Val-Met-Ala-Gly-Asn-Leu-Try-Pro-Gly (IC_{50} = 2.98 μM) from sauce of fermented blue mussel; Leu-Gly-Phe-Pro-Thr-Thr-Lys-Thr-Tyr-Phe-Pro-His-Phe (IC_{50} = 4.92 μM) and Val-Val-Tyr-Pro-Trp (IC_{50} = 6.02 μM) from porcine haemoglobin; Trp-Pro-Glu-Ala-Ala-Glu-Leu-Met-Met-Glu-Val-Asp-Pro from bigeye tuna dark muscle (IC_{50} = 21.6 μM). Furthermore, a single oral administration (10 mg/kg) of PTFP showed a strong suppressive effect on the systolic blood pressure of spontaneously hypertensive rats and this antihypertensive activity was similar to that shown by captopril but without observed side effects.

Generally, ACE inhibitors contain one or more molecular functionalities such as zinc binding ligands (usually either a phosphate or carboxylate oxygen, or thiol sulphur), a hydrogen-bond donor and carboxyl-terminal group (Andrews *et al.*, 1985 as cited by Sang-Hoon Lee *et al.*, 2010). In the case of ACE inhibitory peptides, the most potent and specific peptide inhibitors have similar structures and ACE activity is strongly influenced by the C-terminal tripeptide sequence (Kim, 2013). The tripeptides with Trp, Tyr, Phe, Pro and a hydrophobic amino acid at the C-terminal were effective for ACE inhibitory activity because of the interaction between three subsites at the active site of ACE (Pihlanto, 2000 as cited by Sang-Hoon Lee *et al.*, 2010).

Aside from being recognized as low-value resources with negligible market value, fish processing by-products present other problems, particularly environmental pollution due to improper disposal. However, fish protein hydrolysates have been shown to have potential for nutritional or pharmaceutical applications. *Sphyrna lewini,* which belongs to the family Triakidae, for instance, is a valuable fishery resource containing plenty of bioactive proteins, glycosaminoglycans, squalenes and lipids. However, large quantities of *S. lewini* muscle protein from cut-off fins are discarded as waste due to its lower economic value.

In a study conducted by Hong-Yu Luo *et al.* (2012), antioxidative peptides were prepared, separated and purified from *S. lewini* muscle proteins. The peptide with the highest antioxidative activity (SAP) from the samples was reported to be composed of the hydrophobic amino acid residue of Leu, which might have contributed in inhibiting lipid peroxidation by increasing peptide solubility in the lipid, thereby facilitating better interaction with radical species. And it was reported that antioxidant hydrophobicity is important for accessing hydrophobic targets. Moreover, it was assumed that Leu can increase interaction between peptides and fatty acids. Additionally, the presence of Asp seems to play an important role, regardless of its position, as observed in several antioxidative peptide sequences.

Lipid and fatty acid oxidation generates free radicals which lead to the development of undesirable off-flavours, odours and potentially toxic reaction products. Furthermore, cancer, coronary heart disease and Alzheimer's diseases are also reported to be partly caused by oxidation or free radical reactions in the body. According to Rajapakse *et al.* (2005), lipid peroxidation is thought to proceed via radical-mediated abstraction of hydrogen atoms from methylene carbons in polyunsaturated fatty acids (Hong-Yu Luo *et al.*, 2012). It was then presumed that the smaller size of SAP may have contributed to its higher antioxidative activity in the lipid peroxidation model system. This was expected due to the higher possibility of effective interaction between smaller antioxidant molecules and free radicals and therefore of inhibiting the propagation cycles of lipid peroxidation.

Two antioxidative peptides with sequences Leu-Pro-Thr-Ser-Glu-Ala-Ala-Lys-Tyr (978 Da) and Pro-Met-Asp-Tyr-Met-Val-Thr (756 Da) were also extracted from tuna dark muscle by-product in a study conducted by Hsu (2010). This protein-rich by-product has limited uses due to its dark colour, susceptibility to oxidation and off-flavour. They are usually discarded from canned tuna processing and are mainly utilized to produce low-market value products such as fish waste meal and fertilizer.

Another group of researchers has reported that antihypertensive and antioxidative peptides were obtained by hydrolysing tuna dark muscle with pepsin, an aspartic protease, which mainly acted on the N-terminal aromatic amino acids. In Kuo-Chiang's (2009) study, two commercial proteases (orientase and protease XXIII) were used. Orientase (OR), an endopeptidase prepared from *Bacillus subtilis,* is classified as both serine protease and metalloprotease. Protease XXIII (PR), on the other hand, is an endopeptidase prepared from *Aspergillus melleus* and is classified as the mixture of aspartic protease, metalloprotease, serine protease and carboxypeptidase. OR has broad specificity and acts mainly on Leu-, Phe-NH2 and Tyr-COOH; while, PR has very broad specificity.

The study has demonstrated that the OR and PR protein hydrolysates of tuna dark muscle by-product and their fractions, separated via a column chromatographic and two-step HPLC procedure, possessed strong DPPH radical-scavenging capacity and antioxidative activity. It was reported that the purified peptides contained Pro, Leu, Ala, Val, Met and Tyr in the sequence, which may have contributed to the antioxidative activity. More importantly, results from this study indicate that it is feasible to produce natural antioxidants from tuna dark muscle by-product by enzymatic hydrolysis. These natural antioxidants may then be used as food ingredients and in nutraceutical applications.

Another by-product of canned tuna processing is the tuna liver which is also used to produce fish meal and animal feed or is directly discarded as processing waste. Je *et al.* (2009) produced hydrolysates from this by-product using commercially available proteases such as Flavourzyme, Alcalase, Protamex and Neutrase. The bioactive peptides from the hydrolysates were reported to have antioxidative and antihypertensive properties.

All hydrolysates significantly exhibited antioxidant activities against DPPH, hydroxyl radical and hydrogen peroxide scavenging; ferrous chelating capacity and reducing power; and protected hydroxyl radical-induced oxidative DNA damage. Furthermore, the hydrolysates also showed potential antihypertensive activity measured by ACE inhibition assay.

After filleting, the fish backbone still holds a considerable amount of muscle that can be used as a raw material for further processing in products like surimi, burgers and fish cakes. But even after mechanically scraping the remaining muscles from the backbone, there is still protein-rich material left on the bones, in the tail region and near the fins which can be made soluble by hydrolysis. Fish protein hydrolysates were obtained from cod backbones (Slizyte *et al.*, 2009). The product was in the form of light yellow powder with a fishy odour and good functional, antioxidative and bioactive properties. It could potentially enhance product stability by preventing oxidative deterioration. The DPPH scavenging activity showed that antioxidative activity of hydrolysates could be due to the ability to scavenge lipid radicals. An increased degree of hydrolysis (DH) resulted in slightly increased DPPH radical scavenging activity.

The researchers proved that it is also possible to obtain bioactive molecules from cod backbones by protein hydrolysis. The obtained molecules (gastrin/CCK- and CGRP-like peptides) could make the cod hydrolysates useful for incorporation in functional foods. Similarly, Naqash and Nazeer (2010) evaluated the antioxidant, antiproliferative and antimicrobial properties of flying fish (*Exocoetus volitans*) backbone hydrolysed by three different enzymes, namely papain, pepsin and trypsin. The peptic protein hydrolysate showed maximum free radical scavenging potential and lipid peroxidation inhibition. Moreover, the amino acid composition of the potent purified fraction was determined by HPLC and was found to contain essential and nonessential amino acids with glutamic acid (24.10%), lysine (23.62%), glycine (12.05%) and threonine (10.41%) as the dominant amino acids. Though the potent purified fraction did not show any cytotoxic effect for Vero cell lines, it exerted a significant antiproliferative effect on Hep G_2 cell lines (Naqash and Nazeer, 2010).

Fish scales also contribute significantly to the amount of by-products in fish processing. They are dermally derived, specifically in the mesoderm, and composed of highly ordered type I collagen fibres and hydroxyapatite $Ca_{10}(OH)_2(PO_4)_6$. Fish scales are stiff, and most of them are discarded during processing. However, they can be hydrolysed to release biologically active peptides. With the continuous increase in fish production or capture, the amount of fish scales will also increase and add to waste disposal problems. It is therefore desirable to efficiently utilize them for nutraceutical and functional food applications.

Zhang *et al.* (2009) purified grass carp fish scale peptides (FSP) with ACE inhibitory activities using macroporous resins (MARs). Generally, enzyme hydrolysates are purified first by fractionation based on their molecular weight using ultrafiltration, size exclusion chromatography, or both. However, purification processes are limited by low capacity and film blocking and more importantly, they don't take into consideration the hydrophobic amino acid content, which is the important characteristic of ACE inhibitory peptides. However, MARs have good recovery due to their unique adsorption properties and other advantages, including ideal pore structure and availability of various surface functional groups, low operational cost and easy regeneration. Furthermore, the main interactions between the absorbent and absorbate are known to be hydrophobic, electrostatic and hydrogen-bonding forces.

The researchers used specific MARs to desalt grass carp fish scale peptides (FSPs) and enrich the peptides with *in vitro* ACE inhibitory ability from the hydrolysates in order to provide purification information that may be useful for the industry. It was found that crude hydrolysates of the grass carp fish scales without desalting had negative inhibitory activity at lower concentrations, which indicates that the salt in the hydrolysates increases the activity of the ACE. Moreover, *in vitro* results showed that ACE inhibition increased with FSP concentrations.

As suggested, most naturally occurring ACE inhibitory peptides contain Pro, Lys or aromatic amino acid residues that are mostly hydrophobic. It was found that the content of hydrophobic amino acids (Ile, Tyr, Phe, Pro, Leu, Val and Lys) in FSP was greater in the fraction eluted with the higher ethanol concentration, and the hydrophobicity of each eluted fraction also increased. Thus, it was deduced that the separation of FSPs with non-polar residues via ethanol gradient elution was based on hydrophobicity and that the *in vitro* ACE inhibitory ability of the FSPs was closely related to amino acid hydrophobic properties.

Marine collagen peptides, which are found in some of the fish by-products discussed earlier, for example bones and scales, are also found in fish skin and fins which are very often discarded as processing by-products. Collagen and gelatin are unique proteins compared to fish muscle proteins and their uniqueness lies in their amino acid content. They are particularly rich in non-polar amino acids (>80%) such as Gly, Ala, Val and Pro (Kim, 2013). Type I collagen is the main component of extracellular matrices and gives strength and resistance to biological materials. Moreover, it also plays an important role in physiological regulation of the cell environment (Ikoma *et al.*, 2003).

The industrial use of collagen has expanded and now includes health foods, cosmetics and biomedical materials. It is also commonly used in medical and pharmaceutical industries as a carrier molecule for drugs, proteins and genes. Long-term maintenance of drug concentration and controlled release at target sites promote the utilization of collagen as efficient drug carriers (Kim, 2013).

Collagen used in the industry is mainly from bovine and pig skins (Nagai *et al.*, 2000). However, these two sources are disadvantaged by some religious restraints and risks posed by, bovine spongiform encephalopathy, commonly referred to as mad cow disease. However, fish collagen and gelatin have a relatively low risk of possessing unknown pathogens (Kim, 2013). Many studies about collagen in marine vertebrates as well as invertebrates have already been conducted. Type I collagens have been extracted from the skin of aquatic species, such as jellyfish, starfish, octopus, paper nautilus, cuttlefish, purple sea urchin and others (Ikoma *et al.*, 2003).

Even before 1956, collagen was already of interest for several researchers. Eastoe (1957) reported the amino acid composition of collagens from sturgeon, cod, shark and the Australian lung fish. The fish collagens showed amino acid distribution that is similar to that of mammalian collagen, with lower amounts of proline and hydroxyproline and higher amounts of serine, threonine and, in some cases, methionine and hydroxylysine. Although, collagen as a whole is used in various applications, its peptides, when released, exhibit beneficial properties such as antihypertensive and antioxidative activities, among many others.

In one recent study, marine collagen peptides (MCP) derived from chum salmon (*Oncorhynchus keta*) skin were found to dose-dependently inhibit the age-related decrease in antioxidant activities and the age-related increase in the levels of lipid peroxidation in both male and female Sprague-Dawley rats. This antoxidative property was reported to be responsible for the increase in life span and decreased spontaneous tumour incidence in the subjects fed with MCP-supplemented diets (Liang *et al.*, 2010).

Many other studies reported that MCPs have biological functions including antihypertension, anti-ulcer, anti-skin ageing and extending the life span. Hepatoprotective agents are known to have antioxidative properties; hence, the effects of MCP on early alcoholic liver injury in rats were investigated. Early liver injury was induced in rats by administering alcohol at a dose of 6 g/kg body weight intragastrically per day. Lin *et al.* (2012a) reported that treatment with MCP could reverse the increased level of serum transferase and reduce hepatic histological damage. Moreover, MCP attenuated the alteration in serum superoxide dismutase and malondialdehyde levels and counteracted the increased levels of total cholesterol. The results suggested that MCPs have a protective effect on early alcoholic liver injury in rats brought about by their antioxidative properties and thus their ability to improve lipid metabolism (Lin *et al.*, 2012a).

Peptides with antioxidant properties were also purified from skin protein hydrolysates of horse mackerel and croaker (Sampath Kumar *et al.*, 2012). The sequence of the peptide from the skin protein hydrolysate of horse mackerel was Asn-His-Arg-Tyr-Asp-Arg (856 Da) and that of croaker was Gly-Asn-Arg-Gly-Phe-Ala-Cys-Arg-His-Ala (1101.5 Da). Both peptides exhibited higher activity against peroxidation of polyunsaturated fatty acid than the natural oxidant α-tocopherol. Thus, these antioxidative peptides may be utilized as food additives and pharmaceutical agents.

Supplementation of MCPs, also derived from chum salmon, was also reported to increase the size, mineral density, dry weight, ash weight, amount of most minerals and both stiffness and toughness of femurs in male growing rats. The effects were also observed in female rats but at milder degrees. According to Xu *et al.* (2010), the increase in mineral density was likely to be related to increased osteoblast activity rather than to a decreased rate of bone resorption, as an increase in serum osteocalcin and bone-specific alkaline phosphatase content was observed. Therefore, MCP supplementation could promote the development of long bones in growing male rats. This study suggests that MCP could potentially improve skeletal development during growth as absorption rates of many bone-related minerals are relatively low from traditional diets, especially Asian and African diets (Xu *et al.*, 2010).

Pei *et al.* (2010) also reported that MCP from chum salmon can facilitate learning and memory in aged mice through reduction of the oxidative damage in the brain and increasing the expression level of brain-derived neurotrophic factor and of postsynaptic density protein 95. Cognitive deficits such as learning impairment and delayed amnesia may be brought about by age-related degeneration in brain function. While most dietary interventions are aimed at the more common chronic diseases including diabetes and CVDs, the number of aged people with neurodegenerative diseases, for example Alzheimer's disease and Parkinson's disease, is rapidly growing and deserves some public concern. Mounting evidence suggests that lifestyle factors, especially diet, may have a considerable influence on the development of neurodegenerative diseases. Hence, the need for functional food and drugs that are proven effective in improving memory retrieval, reinforce, the importance and practical value of the neuroprotective effect of MCP.

Gelatin peptides, on the other hand, have a repeated unique Gly-Pro-Ala sequence in their structure which is presumably associated with their observed antioxidative and antihypertensive properties. These peptides have also been shown to accelerate absorption of dietary calcium in animal models increasing calcium bioavailability (Kim, 2013). Thus, they can also be developed for applications that will address problems in skeletal development during growth.

7.5.2 Other seafood and aquaculture processing by-products

Whilst fish form the largest group of animals used as a source of animal-based foods, with more than 700 species commercially fished and utilized for food production, several species of crustaceans, molluscs, seaweeds and microalgae are also used as food for humans (Alasalvar *et al.*, 2011). Generally, marine organisms comprise approximately half of the total global diversity; hence the sea offers a wide variety of novel compounds. The natural habitat of these organisms is characterized by a highly competitive and aggressive surrounding giving rise to situations that demand the production of quite specific and potent active molecules. This is perhaps the main reason why marine organisms are a rich source of structurally diverse bioactive compounds with various biological activities. Among the many functional materials that can be obtained from marine organisms, polyunsaturated fatty acids, polysaccharides, minerals and vitamins, antioxidants, enzymes and bioactive peptides are generally of interest (Kim and Wijesekara, 2010).

Seafood is one of the most popular sources of protein worldwide. The demand is overwhelming such that more than half, by volume, of the seafood for human consumption is farmed while the other half is still caught wild. Aquaculture's contribution is expected to rise while the wild caught supply is expected to diminish or remain stable, as fisheries have reached their maximum production limits (Shrimp Aquaculture Dialogue, 2011).

Fish by-products have been extensively studied and numerous bioactive peptides isolated from fish sources have been reported. Other marine organisms such as mollusc and crustacean are not as widely investigated. Some recent studies, mostly about bioactive peptides from processing by-products of other marine organisms, are briefly described in the following section.

7.5.3 Molluscs

Molluscs are one of the largest and most successful groups of animals and they are characterized by their soft bodies usually covered by a shell made of calcium carbonate. Familiar representatives of this group include chitons, snails, clams, octopods and squid. Other marine organisms that belong to this group such as oysters, scallops and conchs are common food animals for humans (Karleskint *et al.*, 2010).

Scallop is an economically important edible shellfish widely cultured in East Asia. The adductor muscle is the main edible part of a scallop body. It is considered a delicacy and has high nutritive value. During processing, approximately 60% of the scallop body which includes shell, mid-gut gland, mantle lobe and gonad (ovary and testis) is discarded as waste. These processing by-products contain many bioactive materials including proteins and, therefore, peptides. To reduce the contribution of these by-products to waste disposal and ultimately to environmental problems, efforts have been made to add value to and effectively utilize these materials (Jin *et al.*, 2012).

Gelation-like protein hydrolysates from scallop male gonads were obtained by enzymatic hydrolysis using nutrease (Jin *et al.*, 2012). The scallop male gonads and their hydrolysates were found to be rich in glycine, lysine, alanine, glutamic acid and aspartic acid, containing all the essential amino acids. The hydrolysates, with their desirable characteristics, i.e. water holding capacity, oil holding capacity, gelation property, solubility and surface hydrophobicity, make them a potential multifunctional and nutritive ingredient in the food industry. Scallop skirt peptide extracts were also reported to have dose-dependent effects of lipid adjustment and anti-hyperoxidation and can potentially offer liver protection (Bai *et al.*, 2008).

After harvest of scallops and abalones, low-quality ones that are typically smaller or broken are often discarded or sold at a lower price. However, these rejected products can be effectively utilized or subjected to value addition. Hydrolysis of abalone foot muscle and scallop adductor muscle with papain and neutral protease, respectively, yielded hydrolysates that act as radical quenchers, hydrogen donors and transitional metal ion sequesters (Zhou *et al.*, 2012a). The antioxidant activities of the resulting hydrolysates were evaluated based on DPPH and hydroxyl radicals scavenging abilities, reducing power and ferrous ion chelating capacity. Moreover, it was reported that limited hydrolysis of proteins can increase their antioxidant activity, whereas extensive hydrolysis can decrease it.

Pacific Abalone is also economically important and widely cultured in East Asia. Its viscera, which are normally discarded as industrial waste, account for 15–25% of the abalone's total body weight. In China alone, approximately 4500 tonnes of viscera are produced as waste from 30 000 tonnes of abalone. In an effort to alleviate disposal problems, Zhou *et al.* (2012b) hydrolysed abalone viscera using commercially available proteases, i.e. alkali protease, papain, neutral protease, pepsin and trypsin, and evaluated the antioxidant activity of the resulting hydrolysates. The hydrolysate fractions were reportedly effective antioxidants. Hence, abalone viscera are a potential source of antioxidant peptides.

Although the freshwater environment is not as exigent as the wide, exceedingly diverse oceans, organisms thriving there also produce compounds, though not as exotic as in the marine environment, that are beneficial to humans. This has been demonstrated in the studies presented in the previous section as some of the processed fishes from which the useful by-products have been derived are from fresh water. Solid wastes from freshwater clam, for instance, including mainly mantle, were hydrolysed yielding peptides that have strong ACE-inhibitory activity (Sun *et al.*, 2011).

Squid processing is also a major part of the seafood industry. Squid processing by-products include heads, viscera, skin and fins, with abundant endogenous proteases (Xu *et al.*, 2008). Squid skin is usually used as animal feed. However, about 70–80% of the squid skin dry matter is collagen. Hence, it can be used in other more valuable applications. Collagen was boiled to convert it to gelatin, which in turn was hydrolysed with pepsin. The ACE-inhibitory activity of the gelatin peptides was measured by spectrophotometric assay. The gelatin peptides that are less than 2 kDa showed the most potent ACE-inhibitory activity *in vitro* (with IC_{50} of 0.33 mg/ml). After oral administration of the gelatin peptides, the systolic and diastolic blood pressure of the renovascular hypertensive rats decreased, indicating an intense effect in the reduction of blood pressure *in vivo* (Lin *et al.*, 2012b).

Meanwhile, β-chitin was isolated from squid (*Illex argentines*) pens (Cortizo *et al.*, 2008) and from jumbo squid (*Dosidicus gigas*) pens (Jung and Zhao, 2011). The major components (dry weight basis) of squid pen are protein (61%), chitin (38%) and minerals (1%) (Wang *et al.*, 2010). Chitin is the main supporting structure in a wide variety of organisms, for example in the exoskeleton or cuticle of different invertebrates and the cellular wall of algae and fungi. It is a homopolymer of *N*-acetyl-D-glucosamine residues and is the most abundant renewable natural polymer after cellulose. Chitin and its derivative are now widely recognized and hold great economic value due to their versatile biological activities and agrochemical applications (Wang, 2012). β-chitin has a parallel arrangement, held by weak, intra-sheet hydrogen bonds.

Chitin has been extensively studied and used in non-food applications such as moisture-retaining agents in cosmetics and collection of metals from industrial wastewater. But chitin, along with chito-oligosaccharides (from the hydrolysis of squid pen by proteases and chitinases) and peptides from squid pen waste, reportedly have antioxidant (Wang *et al.*, 2010) and anticarcinogenic properties and thus can be utilized in the production of functional foods. Wang *et al.* (2010) found antioxidant activities and a high total phenolic content in the culture supernatant of *Serratia ureilytica* TKU013 with squid pen. These bacteria utilized squid pen as the sole carbon/nitrogen source. It was demonstrated that the ethyl acetate-soluble extract of the fermented supernatant is a fairly active fraction for *in vitro* DPPH free radical scavenging activity.

7.5.4 Crustaceans

Marine crustaceans are a group of free-living and sessile invertebrates living in salt or brackish water best known for their hard outer shell, for example lobsters, crabs and shrimp. There is a high demand for these crustaceans, especially shrimp, which it is now being farmed extensively in many developing countries such as China, Thailand, India, Vietnam, Brazil, Ecuador and Bangladesh. Shrimp is the most valuable traded marine product in the world today. In 2005, farmed shrimp was a US$10.6-billion industry. Today, production is growing at a rate of approximately 10% per annum, which is one of the highest growth rates in aquaculture (WWF, 2013).

Shrimp by-products have been identified as proteinaceous materials that are also good sources of chitin and astaxanthin. Only 65% of the shrimp body is edible and the rest discarded as inedible waste. Therefore, the overwhelming demand for shrimp produces an enormous volume of wastes or by-products of head and body carapace that must be discarded. Utilization of such large quantities of shrimp processing discards for recovery of bioactive molecule would not only reduce the disposal problems associated with these wastes, but also enhance the economy of shrimp processing (Sowmya and Sachindra, 2011).

Many studies have reported that bioactive peptides were isolated from shrimp by-products. In one such study by Bueno-Solano *et al.* (2009), protein hydrolysates were prepared through lactic acid fermentation of the cephalothorax and exoskeleton of shrimp. The protein-rich hydrolysate was further processed into concentrated paste through vacuum evaporation or was processed into a dry powder using a spray drying method.

The liquid hydrolysate, concentrated paste and dry powder containing a high content of essential amino acids and ash, suggest that the protein hydrolysates, derived from the lactic fermentation of shrimp by-products, have a high nutritional content, as well as a low metal and microorganism content. It was reported that products obtained from processing shrimp by-products can be incorporated as high-value supplements in human and animal diets.

Although the common antioxidative, ACE-inhibitory and anticancer, biological activities of peptides have been well studied, other properties that are also greatly beneficial to humans have not yet been investigated as extensively. One such activity, iron-binding, has been observed in a particular peptide from shrimp processing waste. Iron is an essential trace nutrient in plants, animals and humans alike. It is structurally important in cytochromes and some enzymes and is also a component of haeme groups in haemoglobin and myoglobin. One of its major roles is to transport oxygen and electrons inside the human body (Lee and Song, 2009).

It has been reported that nearly one-fifth of the world population has nutritional problems due to iron deficiency, particularly among women, children and the aged. Iron deficiency generates several adverse conditions such as iron deficiency anaemia and reduced physical and intellectual working capacity. Generally, iron deficiency is caused by insufficient intake (mainly a plant-based diet) and the low bioavailability of iron. Iron can be supplied in salts, elemental iron, metal chelates and iron-binding proteins or peptides. The most popular means is through intake of iron salts, yet they have low bioavailability in the body because of their reactivity with other food components. Meanwhile, recent studies indicate that iron-chelated peptides are more stable and result in increased absorption and bioavailability of iron (Lee and Song, 2009).

Huang *et al.* (2012) isolated such iron-binding peptides by hydrolysing shrimp processing by-products with flavourzyme. The researchers suggested that the amino acids Ser, Lys and Pro in the sequence Leu-Pro-Thr-Gly-Pro-Lys-Ser might contribute to iron-binding capacity. Results indicated that iron binding peptides obtained from shrimp processing by-products could be used for high-value bioproducts in health care such as a supplement for improved iron absorption in the human body.

As well as bioactive peptides, there are significant amounts of carotenoids present in crustaceans, especially in their exoskeleton. Carotenoids have the ability to protect cells and tissues from the damaging effects of free radicals and singlet oxygen, thus acting as antioxidants (Sowmya and Sachindra, 2012). They have been known to provide protection against diseases and age-related phenomena. They exhibit biological activities including anticancer, anti-inflammatory and even anti-obesity effects. Furthermore, the main carotenoid found in crustaceans, astaxanthin, has been shown to have important applications in the functional food, cosmetic and food industries.

Crude carotenoid extracts have been obtained by solvent extraction from shrimp processing discards and their fractions were evaluated for antioxidant activity by *in vitro* assays and in a membrane model system. Sowmya and Sachindra (2012) reported strong antioxidant activity in the crude extract and the astaxanthin-rich fractions. The antioxidant activity of shrimp carotenoid extract demonstrates its potential for use as a natural antioxidant in food and biomedical applications.

Carotenoids present in shrimp and other crustaceans may be in the form of carotenoproteins, which are stable complexes of carotenoids bound to high-density lipoproteins (Sowmya *et al.*, 2011). These carotenoproteins could be utilizable as pharmacological agents due to their astaxanthin content. Carotenoprotein isolation was attempted using various methods such as hydrolysis with proteases and through fermentation. Efforts have also been made to disrupt the protein–carotenoid bond using proteolytic enzymes to increase carotenoid recovery.

Cahú *et al.* (2012) reported a process developed for recovering bioactive molecules from shrimp heads through autolysis. Protein hydrolysates were recovered and lyophilized from shrimp heads. Carotenoids were also recovered as ethanolic extracts. In addition, chitin and chitosan were recovered, the latter was characterized and found to exhibit a variable degree of deacetylation. Sulfated glycosaminoglycans that exhibited electrophoretic migration similar to mammalian standards were also recovered and their degradation products suggested the presence of C6-sulfated heparan sulfate. The results suggested the feasibility of an integrated process for isolating highly bioactive molecules, such as sulfated- and amino-polysaccharides, with a broad spectrum of applications from shrimp processing waste (Cahú *et al.*, 2012).

Similarly, in a study conducted by Sowmya *et al.* (2011), protein hydrolysates from shrimp head were prepared using autolysis. Head waste, comprising digestive organs, accounts for approximately 35–45% of the whole shrimp weight. Hydrolytic enzymes such as proteases found in biological materials become active upon cell death and rapidly hydrolyse the tissue in the process of autolysis since the cell's own enzymes are involved in the hydrolysis. The viscera in the shrimp heads contain most of the endogenous enzymes, hence, shrimp heads undergo autolysis by the action of *in situ* proteases. The researchers reported that the optimum autolysis condition for obtaining antioxidant activity rich carotenoprotein from shrimp heads was found to be a waste to buffer (pH 8.0) ratio of 1 : 5 and an autolysis time of 2 h at 50 °C. The isolated carotenoprotein was found to have antioxidant activity with respect to singlet oxygen quenching, reducing power and metal chelating activity.

Isolation of carotenoproteins can also be achieved through a relatively new method called pH shift, which has been used for isolating protein. The process isolates protein from other components based on charge characteristics. It creates repulsive forces which drive the molecules of the protein to unfold. Proteins are extracted in either acidic or alkaline pH and are subsequently precipitated at an isoelectric point. Most sarcoplasmic and myofibrillar proteins are recovered. This allows for higher protein recoveries than the conventional method (Tadpitchayangkoon, 2008).

Khumallambam *et al.* (2011) compared the antioxidant activity of the protein isolate obtained by the pH shift method from unhydrolysed waste with that obtained from the waste hydrolysed with Alcalase®. The DPPH scavenging activity of protein isolate after enzyme hydrolysis was significantly higher than that of protein isolate from unhydrolysed waste. With respect to recovery of total antioxidant activity, protein isolated from unhydrolysed waste was superior to hydrolysed waste due to a higher yield (Khumallambam *et al.*, 2011).

Seafoods, especially marine fishes, are quite well known for their omega-3 polyunsaturated fatty acids (PUFAs). Research on long chain PUFAs, found primarily in fish oils, has increased substantially in recent years and considerable evidence suggests a wide range of beneficial effects in a number of health conditions ranging from cardiovascular disease and cancer to autoimmune diseases and mental health disorders. Omega-3 PUFAs have anti-inflammatory, antithrombotic, antiarrhythmic, hypolipidemic and vasodilatory properties (Shahidi and Miraliakbari, 2004, 2005 as cited by Amiguet *et al.*, 2012). Moreover, there is now considerable demand for eicosapentoic acid (EPA) and docosahexaenoic acid (DHA) because of their preventive and curative therapies. Clinical studies have reported that EPA and DHA from fish oil help support cognitive health, brain function, cardiovascular health, help reduce serum triglycerides and, in conjuction with conventional therapy, help reduce the pain of rheumatoid arthritis (Amiguet *et al.*, 2012).

Conventionally, PUFA is extracted by solvent extraction, enzymatic extraction, urea complexation or molecular distillation. The high temperatures and toxic solvents used in these methods has spurred efforts to develop alternative extraction technologies. Extraction and fractionation of PUFAs from fish oil with supercritical fluid extraction (SFE) using carbon dioxide has been of great interest for generating cleaner (residue-free), higher quality PUFA extracts (Sahena *et al.*, 2009 as cited by Amiguet *et al.*, 2012). SFE using non-polar CO_2 is especially well suited to this application as the mild conditions, critical temperature (C_T) = 31 °C, critical pressure (C_P) = 7.38 MPa and low oxygen setting provides an environment favourable for heat-sensitive and easily oxidized substances such omega-3 PUFAs. In addition, SFE using CO_2 does not produce any distinct taste, is odourless, non-toxic and non-flammable and, generally regarded as safe (GRAS status).

Amiguet *et al.* (2012) investigated the potential use of northern shrimp by-products including heads, shell and tail as a source of omega-3 PUFA. Supercritical CO_2 extraction of the said by-products at 35 MPa and 40 °C generated a deep red oil, rich in omega-3 PUFAs, specifically 7.8 $\pm$ 0.06% EPA and 8.0 $\pm$ 0.07% DHA.

Snow crabs are harvested and processed throughout the Atlantic Provinces. They are sold fully precooked and frozen, as cocktail claws or sections while some are processed such that leg meat, salad meat, or leg and shoulder meat are sold in packs. Recently, a snow crab by-product hydrolysate has demonstrated antibacterial properties due to a peptide with a molecular weight of about 800 Da, but only at high concentration on several gram-negative and gram-positive bacteria (Beaulieu *et al.*, 2010). Among the bacterial strains tested, peptide fractions demonstrated inhibitory activity against gram-negative bacteria such as *Aeromonas caviae, Aeromonas hydrophila, Campylobacter jejuni, Listonella anguillarum, Morganella morganii, Shewanella putrefasciens, Vibrio parahaemolyticus and Vibrio vulnificus* and against a few gram-positive bacteria such as *Listeria monocytogenes, Staphylococcus epidermidis* and *Streptococcus agalactiae.*

The antibacterial peptide fractions were generated via proteolytic processing and the amino acid content revealed that arginine (4.6%), glutamic acid (5.3%) and tyrosine (4.8%) residues were represented in the highest composition in the antibacterial peptide fraction. The optimal inhibitory activity was observed at alkaline pH. The active peptide fraction was reportedly a complex of molecules consisting of several amino acids and other organic compounds. In addition, copper was the main metal found in the active peptide fraction. It was reported that the production of antibacterial molecules from crustacean by-products supports further applications for high-value bioproducts in several areas such as food and health (Beaulieu *et al.*, 2010).

Doyen *et al.* (2012) also recovered antibacterial peptides from snow crab by-products by electrodialysis with ultrafiltration membranes (EDUF). This method allows separation of molecules according to their charges (electrodialysis) and molecular weight (membrane filtration cut-off), which that is not only used to recover but also to concentrate the active fraction. Doyen *et al.* (2011) also separated a mixture of polypeptides from snow crab by-products with anticancer properties using the same method. EDUF has recently been patented and was developed as an alternative to inefficient separation processes such as ultrafiltration, nanofiltration and microfiltration that are currently used. These processes present different drawbacks, they are expensive and applicable only to a small volume, i.e. chromatography. In pressure-driven processes, on the other hand, accumulation of particles on membranes leads to the formation of fouling and to a modification in membrane transport selectivity.

EDUF is reportedly an effective alternative to conventional food processing for peptide separation in snow crab by-products. Results showed that peptides could migrate in selective ways through ultrafiltration membranes under the effect of an electrical field applied between the electrodes. There was no fouling in EDUF and the process also allowed a selective and a simultaneous separation of anionic and cationic peptides present in an uncharacterized concentrated polypeptide mixture of snow crab by-products hydrolysate. The peptide fractions recovered exhibited anticancer activities on three cancerous cell lines. The researchers hypothesized that the anticancer activity is due to the peptide sequence containing His residues (Doyen *et al.*, 2011).

References

Ajila, C.M., Naidu, K.A., Bhat, S.G. and Prasada Rao, U.J.S. (2007). Bioactive compounds and antioxidant potential of mango peel extract. *Food Chemistry*, 105 (3), 982–988.

Alasalvar, C., Miyashita, K., Shahidi, F. and Wanasundara, U. (eds) (2011). *Handbook of Seafood Quality, Safety and Health Applications*. Blackwell Publishing Ltd.

Amiguet, V.T., Kramp, K.L., Mao, J.Q. *et al.* (2012). Supercritical carbon dioxide extraction of polyunsaturated fatty acids from Northern shrimp (*Pandalus borealis Kreyer*) processing by-products. *Food Chemistry*, 130, 853–858.

Bai, L.-F., Lui, J.-S. and Zhou, P.-G. (2008). Effects of the scallop skirt peptide extract in regulating blood lipid and anti-oxidation of rats with hyperlipidemia. *Journal of Anhui Agricultural University*, 35 (4), 615–618.

Beaulieu, L., Thibodeau, J., Desbiens, M. *et al.* (2010). Evidence of antibacterial activities in peptide fractions originating from snow crab (*Chionoecetes opilio*) by-products. *Probiotics and Antimicrobial Proteins*, 2, 1–13.

Bernal, J., Mendiola, J.A., Ibáñez, E. and Cifuentes, A. (2011). Advanced analysis of nutraceuticals. *Journal of Pharmaceutical and Biomedical Analysis*, 55, 758–774.

Bueno-Solano, C., López-Cervantes, J., Campas-Baypoli, O.N. *et al.* (2009). Chemical and biological characteristics of protein hydrolysates from fermented shrimp by-products. *Food Chemistry*, 112, 671–675.

Butsat, S. and Siriamornpun, S. (2009). Antioxidant capacities and phenolic compounds of the husk, bran and endosperm of Thai rice. *Food Chemistry*, 119, 606–613.

Cahú, T.B., Santos, S.D., Mendes, A. *et al.* (2012). Recovery of protein, chitin, carotenoids and glycosaminoglycans from Pacific white shrimp (*Litopenaeus vannamei*) processing waste. *Process Biochemistry*, 47 (4), 570–577.

Ciardiello, M.A., Meleleo, D., Saviano, G. *et al.* (2008). Kissper, a kiwi fruit peptide with channel-like activity: Structural and functional features. *Journal of Peptide Science*, 14, 742–754.

Cortizo, M.S., Berghoff, C.F. and Alessandrini, J.L. (2008). Characterization of chitin from *Illex argentinus* squid pen. *Carbohydrate Polymers*, 74 (1), 10–15.

Doyen, A., Saucier, L., Beaulieu, L., Pouliut, Y. and Bazinet, L. (2011). Demonstration of in vitro anticancer properties of peptide fractions from a snow crab by-products hydrolysate after separation by electrodialysis with ultrafiltration membranes. *Separation and Purification Technology*, 78, 321–329.

Doyen, A., Saucier, L., Beaulieu, L., Pouliut, Y. and Bazinet, L. (2012). Electroseparation of an antibacterial peptide fraction from snow crab by-products hydrolysate by electrodialysis with ultrafiltration membranes. *Food Chemistry*, 132, 1177–1184.

Dykes, L. and Rooney, L.W. (2007). Phenolic compounds in cereal grains and their health benefits. *Cereal Foods World*, 52 (3), 105–111.

Eastoe, J.E. (1957). The amino acid composition of fish collagen and gelatin. *Biochemistry Journal*, 65 (2), 363–368.

FAO (2012a). Fisheries and Aquaculture – enabling a vital sector to contribute more. Food and Agriculture Organization, Rome. http://www.fao.org/news/story/en/item/150839/icode/ [accessed 8July 2013].

FAO (2012b). *The State of World Fisheries and Aquaculture 2012*. Food and Agriculture Organization, Rome. 209 pp.

Hernandez-Ledesma, B. Hsieh, C., de Lumen, B.O. 2008. Lunasin, a novel seed peptide for cancer prevention. *Peptides*. Vol 30 (2009), pp. 426–430.

Hettiarachchy, N.S. (2011). Bioactive pentapeptides from rice bran and use thereof. US Patent 2011/0152180, filed November 24, 2011, and published June 23, 2012.

Hsu, K.C. (2010). Purification of antioxidative peptides prepared from enzymatic hydrolysates of tuna dark muscle by-product. *Food Chemistry*, 122 (1), 42–48.

Huang, G.-R., Ren, Z.-Y., Jiang, J.-X. and Chen, W.-W. (2012). Purification of a hepta-peptide with iron binding activity from shrimp processing by-products hydrolysates. *Advance Journal of Food Science and Technology*, 4 (4), 207–212.

Huang, W.-H., Sun, J., He, H., Dong, H.-W. and Li, J.-T. (2011). Antihypertensive effect of corn peptides produced by a continuous production in enzymatic membrane reactor, in spontaneously hypertensive rats. *Food Chemistry*, 128, 968–973.

Ikoma, T., Kobayashi, H., Tanaka, J., Walsh, D. and Mann, S. (2003). Physical properties of type I collagen extracted from fish scales of *Pagrus major* and *Oreochromis niloticas*. *International Journal of Biological Macromolecules*, 32(3–5), 199–204.

Je, J.-Y., Lee, K.-H., Lee, M.H. and Ahn, C.-B. (2009). Antioxidant and antihypertensive protein hydrolysates produced from tuna liver by enzymatic hydrolysis. *Food Research International*, 42, 1266–1272.

Jeong, Y.H., Chung, S.Y., Han, A.-R. *et al.* (2007). P-Glycoprotein inhibitory activity of two phenolic compounds, (−)-syringaresinol and tricin from *Sasa borealis*. *Chemistry & Biodiversity*, 4, 12–16.

Jia, J., Ma, H., Zhao, W., Wang, Z., Tian, W., Luo, L., He, R. 2010. The use of ultrasound for enzymatic preparation of ACE-inhibitory peptides from wheat germ protein. *Food Chemistry*, 119, 336–342.

Jin, W.-G., Wu, H.-T., Zhu, B.-W. and Ran, X.-Q. (2012). Functional properties of gelation-like protein hydrolysates from scallop (*Patinopecten yessoensis*) male gonad. *European Food Research and Technology*, 234 (5), 863–872.

Jung, J. and Zhao, Y. (2011). Characteristics of deacetylation and depolymerization of β-chitin from jumbo squid (*Dosidicus gigas*) pens. *Carbohydrate Research*, 346, 1876–1884.

Kannan, A., Hettiarchchy, N.S., Lay, J.O. and Liyanage, R. (2010). Human cancer cell proliferation inhibition by a pentapeptide isolated and characterized from rice bran. *Peptides*, 31, 1629–1634.

Karleskint, G., Jr., Turner, R. and Small, J.W., Jr. (2010). *Introduction to Marine Biology*. Brooks/Cole, Cengage Learning, USA.

Khumallambam, M., Rama, S., Karuppannan, R.R., Manjabhat, S.N. (2011). Antioxidant activity of carotenoprotein isolate from shrimp processing discards. *Journal of Aquatic Food Product Technology*, 20, 209–221.

Kim, S.-K. (ed.) (2013). *Marine Proteins and Peptides: Biological Activities and Applications*. John Wiley & Sons, Ltd, Chichester.

Kim, S.-K. and Mendis, E. (2005). Bioactive compounds from marine processing by-products – a review. *Food Research International*, 39, 383–393.

Kim, S.-K. and Wijesekara, I. (2010). Development and biological activities of marine-derived bioactive peptides: a review. *Journal of Functional Foods*, 2, 1–9.

Kitts, D.D. and Weiler, K. (2003). Bioactive proteins and peptides from food sources. applications of bioprocesses and in isolation and recovery. *Current Pharmaceutical Design*, 9 (16), 1309–1323.

Lata, B. and Tomala, K. (2007). Apple peel as a contributor to whole fruit quantity of potentially healthful bioactive compounds: cultivar and year implication. *Journal of Agricultural and Food Chemistry*, 55 (26), 10795–10802.

Lee, S.-H., Qian, Z.-J. and Kim, S.-K. (2010). A novel angiotensin I converting enzyme inhibitory peptide from tuna frame protein hydrolysate and its antihypertensive effect in spontaneously hypertensive rats. *Food Chemistry*, 118, 96–102.

Lee, S.-H. and Song, K.B. (2009). Purification of an iron-binding nona-peptide from hydrolysates of porcine blood plasma protein. *Process Biochemistry*, 44, 378–381.

Liang, J., Pei, X.R., Wang, N. *et al.* (2010). Marine collagen peptides prepared from chum salmon (*Oncorhynchus keta*) skin extend the life span and inhibit spontaneous tumor incidence in Sprague-Dawley Rats. *Journal of Medicinal Food*, 13(4), 757–770.

Lin, B., Zhang, F., Yu, Y. *et al.* (2012a) Marine collagen peptides protect against early alcoholic liver injury in rats. *The British Journal of Nutrition*, 107 (8), 1160–1166.

Lin, L., Lv, S. and Li, B. (2012b). Angiotensin-I-converting enzyme (ACE)-inhibitory and antihypertensive properties of squid skin gelatin hydrolysates. *Food Chemistry*, 131(1), 225–230.

Liyana-Pathirana, C., Dexter, J. and Shahidi, F. (2006). Antioxidant properties of wheat as affected by pearling. *Journal of Agricultural and Food Chemistry*, 54(17), 6177–6184.

Luo, H.-Y., Wang, B., Li, Z.-R. *et al.* (2013). Preparation and evaluation of antioxidant peptide from papain hydrolysate of *Sphyrna lewini* muscle protein. *LWT – Food Science and Technology*, 51, 281–288.

Makinen, S., Johannson, T., Gerd, E.V., Pihlava, J.M. and Pihlanto, A. (2012). Angiotensin I-converting enzyme inhibitory and antioxidant properties of rapeseed hydrolysates. *Journal of Functional Foods*, 4, 575–583.

Martin, C., Butelli, E., Petroni, K. and Tonelli, C. (2011). How can research on plants contribute to promoting human health? *The Plant Cell*, 23, 1685–1699.

Mateos-Aparicio, I., Redondo-Cuenca, A., Villanueva-Suárez, M.J., Zapata-Revilla, M.A. and Tenorio-Sanz, M.D. (2010). Pea pod, broad bean pod and okara, potential sources of functional compounds. *LWT—Food Science and Technology*, 43 (9), 1467–1470.

Megias, C., Pedroche, J., del Mar Yust, M. *et al.* (2009). Stability of sunflower protein hydrolysates in simulated gastric and intestinal fluids and Caco-2 cell extracts. *LWT – Food Science and Technology*, 42 (9), 1496–1500.

Moheb, A., Grondin, M., Ibrahim, R.K., Roy, R. and Sarhan, F. (2013). Winter wheat hull (husk) is a valuable source for tricin, a potential selective cytotoxic agent. *Food Chemistry*, 138 (2–3), 931–937.

Nagai, T., Worawattanamateekul, W., Suzuki, N. *et al.* (2000). Isolation and characterization of collagen from rhizostomous jellyfish (*Rhopilema asamushi*). *Food Chemistry*, 70 (2), 205–208.

Naqash, S.Y. and Nazeer, R.A. (2010). Evaluation of bioactive properties of peptide isolated from *Exocoetus volitans* backbone. *International Journal of Food Science and Technology*, 46 (1), 37–43.

Nakurte, I., Klavins, K., Kirhnere, I. *et al.* (2012). Discovery of lunasin peptide in triticale (X Triticosecale Wittmack). *Journal of Cereal Science*, 56, 510–514.

Pei, X., Yang, R., Zhang, Z. *et al.* (2010). Marine collagen peptide isolated from chum salmon (*Oncorhynchus keta*) skin facilitates learning and memory in aged C57BL/6J mice. *Food Chemistry*,118 (2), 333–340.

Pihlanto, A., Akkanen, S. and Korhonen, H.J. (2008). ACE-inhibitory and antioxidant properties of potato (Solanum tuberosum). *Food Chemistry*, 109 (1), 104–112.

Rajapakse, N., Mendis, E., Jung, W.J., Je, J.Y. and Kim, S.K. (2005). Purification of a radical scavenging peptide from fermented mussel sauce and its antioxidant properties. *Food Research International*, 38, 175–182.

Raskin, I., Ribnicky, D.M., Komarnytsky, S. *et al.* (2002). Plants and human health in the twenty-first century. *Trends in Biotechnology*, 20 (12), 522–531.

Rayaprolu, S.J., Hettiarchchy, N.S., Chen, P., Kannan, A. and Mauromostakos, A. (2013). Peptides derived from high oleic acid soybean meals inhibit colon, liver and lung cancer cell growth. *Food Research International*, 50 (1), 282–288.

Roberts, P.R., Burney, J.D., Black, K.W. and Zaloga, G.P. (1999). Effect of chain length on absorption of biologically active peptides from the gastrointestinal tract. *Digestion*, 60, 332–338.

Rupasinghe, H.P.V., Erkan, N. and Yasmin, A. (2010). Antioxidant protection of eicosapentaenoic acid and fish oil oxidation by polyphenolic-enriched apple skin extract. *Journal of Agricultural and Food Chemistry*, 58 (2), 1233–1239.

Sairam, S., Krishna, A.G.G., Urooj, A. (2011). Physico-chemical characteristics of defatted rice bran and its utilization in a bakery product. *Journal of Food Science and Technology*, 48 (4), 478–483.

Sampath Kumar, N.S., Nazeer, R.A. and Jaiganesh, R. (2012). Purification and identification of antioxidant peptides from the skin protein hydrolysate of two marine fishes, horse mackerel (*Magalaspis cordyla*) and croaker (*Otolithes ruber*). *Amino Acids*, 42 (5), 1641–1649.

Shrimp Aquaculture Dialogue (2011). Draft Standards for Responsible Shrimp Aquaculture. http://assets.worldwildlife.org/publications/429/files/original/ShAD_Standard_Final_Draft. pdf?1346186260 [accessed 7 July 2013].

Slizyte, R., Mozuraityte, R., Martinez-Alvarez, O. *et al.* (2009). Functional, bioactive and antioxidative properties of hydrolysates obtained from cod (*Gadus morhua*) backbones. *Process Chemistry*, 44, 668–677.

Sovrani, V., Blandino, M., Scarpino, V. *et al.* (2012). Bioactive compound content, antioxidant activity, deoxynivalenol and heavy metal contamination of pearled wheat fractions. *Food Chemistry*, 135 (1), 39–45.

Sowmya, R. and Sachindra, N.M. (2012). Evaluation of antioxidant activity of carotenoid extract from shrimp processing by-products by *in vitro* assays and in membrane model system. *Food Chemistry*, 134, 308–314.

Sowmya, R., Rathinaraj, K. and Sachindra, N.M. (2011). An autolytic process for recovery of antioxidant activity rich carotenoprotein from shrimp heads. *Marine Biotechnology*, 13 (5), 918–927.

Suh, H.J., Whang, J.H. and Lee, H. 1999. A peptide from corn gluten hydrolysate that is inhibitory toward angiotensin enzyme. *Biotechnology Letters*. 21, 1055–1058.

Sun, Y., Hayakawa, S., Ogawa, M. *et al.* (2011). Evaluation of angiotensin I-converting enzyme (ACE) inhibitory activities of hydrolysates generated from by-products of freshwater clam. *Food Science and Biotechnology*, 20 (2), 303–310.

Tadpitchayangkoon, P. (2008). Effect of pH and pH Shift process on conformational changes and gelation of sarcoplasmic proteins from striped catfish (*Pangasius hypophthalmus*). Doctoral dissertation. Suranaree University of Technology. http://sutir.sut.ac.th:8080/sutir/bitstream/123456789/3136/2/fulltext.pdf [accessed 7 July 2013].

Tseng, A. and Zhao, Y. (2013). Wine grape pomace as antioxidant dietary fibre for enhancing nutritional value and improving storability of yogurt and salad dressing. *Food Chemistry*, 138, 356–365.

Wang, S.-L. (2012). Microbial reclamation of squid pen. *Biocatalysis and Agricultural Biotechnology*, 1 (2), 177–180.

Wang, S.-L., Liu, K.-C., Liang, T.-W., Kuo, Y.-H. and Wang, C.-Y. (2010). *In vitro* antioxidant activity of liquor and semi-purified fractions from fermented squid pen biowaste by *Serratia ureilytica* TKU013. *Food Chemistry*, 119 (4), 1380–1385.

Wolfe, K.L. and Liu, R.H. (2003). Apple peels as a value-added food ingredient. *Journal of Agricultural and Food Chemistry*, 51 (6), 1676–1683.

WWF (2013). Farmed Shrimp Overview. World Wide Fund. http://worldwildlife.org/industries/farmed-shrimp [accessed 7 July 2013].

Xu, Y., Han, X. and Li, Y. (2010). Effect of marine collagen peptides on long bone development in growing rats. *Journal of the Science of Food and Agriculture*, 90, 1485–1491.

Xu, W., Lv, Y.-T., Xue, C.-H. *et al.* (2008). Optimization of autohydrolysing conditions of endogenous proteases from squid byproducts. *CNKI Journal*, http://en.cnki.com.cn/Article_cn/CJFDTOTAL-SPKJ200808050.htm [accessed 26 July 2013].

Yang, Y.J., Tao, G.J., Liu, P.J. and Liu, J. (2007). Peptide with angiotensin I-converting enzyme inhibitory activity from hydrolysed corn gluten meal. *Agricultural and Food Chemistry*, 55, 7891–7895.

Zhang, F., Wang, Z. and Xu, S. (2009). Macroporous resin purification of grass carp fish (*Ctenopharyngodon idella*) scale peptides with *in vitro* angiotensin-I converting enzyme (ACE) inhibitory ability. *Food Chemistry*, 117 (3), 387–392.

Zhou, D.-Y., Tang, Y., Zhu, B.-W. *et al.* (2012a). Antioxidant activity of hydrolysates obtained from scallop (*Patinopecten yessoensis*) and abalone (*Haliotis discus hannai Ino*) muscle. *Food Chemistry*, 132, 815–822.

Zhou, D.-Y., Zhu, B.-W., Qiao, L. *et al.* (2012b). *In vitro* antioxidant activity of enzymatic hydrolysates prepared from abalone (*Haliotis discus hannai* Ino) viscera. *Food and Bioproducts Processing*, 90 (2), 148–154.

8 Functionality of Non-starch Polysaccharides (NSPs)

Kelvin K. T. Goh[1], Ramesh Kumar[2] and Shen-Siung Wong[2]
[1]*Institute of Food, Nutrition and Human Health, Massey University, Palmerston North, New Zealand*
[2]*Massey University, Singapore Campus*

8.1 Introduction

Polysaccharides, which are classified as carbohydrates, are long-chain molecules that are made up of simple sugar molecules connected by glycosidic linkages. In nature, there is a wide range of polysaccharide molecular structures with different functional properties as these macromolecules differ in the type of glycosidic linkages, their monosaccharide composition, their degree of polymerization and the presence of side groups. Because of the diverse molecular structures and sugar compositions, polysaccharides are commonly categorized as starches and non-starch polysaccharides (NSPs). Starch, which is the most common carbohydrate in the human diet, is derived from plants. Its molecular structure consists of glucose units linked by alpha linkages. NSP is used to describe the remaining carbohydrate polymers other than starches. NSPs include cellulose, hemicellulose, gums and mucilages.

In monogastric animals, NSP cannot be digested in the small intestine so it is also a major component of dietary fibre (as well as lignin and resistant starch). NSPs can be further categorized as soluble fibre and insoluble fibre. Soluble NSP can be fermented by microorganisms in the large intestine of monogastric animals to produce short-chain fatty acids, which are beneficial to the host animal. Some of these soluble NSPs are considered to be prebiotics because they are capable of promoting the growth of intestinal microflora. Insoluble fibre generally provides bulking and facilitates stool movement through the large intestine.

Apart from their important function in human nutrition, many soluble NSPs play a major role as additives in the food industry, because they possess important

Functional Foods and Dietary Supplements: Processing Effects and Health Benefits, First Edition.
Edited by Athapol Noomhorm, Imran Ahmad and Anil Kumar Anal.

physicochemical properties that can be used thicken, stabilize, gel and emulsify food products (Hemar *et al.*, 2001a,b; Dickinson, 2003; Dickinson *et al.*, 2003). The physicochemical properties of these polysaccharides have been studied extensively over the past several decades. It is well established that the factors that influence the physicochemical properties of these macromolecules in solution include molar mass, molecular conformation, polydispersity, charge density, concentration, pH, ionic strength, temperature, solvent quality and the nature of molecular (intra-/inter-) interactions (Tolstoguzov, 1997; Doublier *et al.*, 2000; de Kruif and Tuinier, 2001).

The physical properties of food systems are complex because components such as polysaccharides, proteins, fats, minerals, pigments and flavouring compounds are present (either naturally or as added ingredients). These components are either entrapped or involved in physical and/or chemical interactions. The assembly of these components, which form unique microstructures and macrostructures, can influence the sensorial perception of foods and can influence consumers' food choices. When eaten, these complex macrostructures are broken down in the mouth to meet consumers' sensorial expectations in terms of flavour release characteristics and textural attributes. In addition, the rates at which these macrostructures are broken down and the efficiency with which the nutrients are released and absorbed in the gastrointestinal tract will depend on the extent to which these nutrients are held or trapped within the microstructures.

NSP plays a crucial role in the food systems in which it is present because it has the ability to control the mobility of free water or to form a three-dimensional network structure in foods. In addition, NSP is capable of interacting with different components in a food system, which can further influence the type of microstructures and macrostructures formed. All these ultimately influence the physical functionality, sensory attributes and nutritional value of the foods.

This chapter provides a brief review of some of the recent advances in the field of NSP research. It begins with an overview of the different commercial NSPs that are commonly used in the food industry. Key functional properties and the molecular parameters for each NSP type are summarized in a table. This is meant to be a quick reference for undergraduates, food scientists and food product developers because it is important to relate molecular characteristics to functional properties in applications.

The second section provides a brief overview of a number of novel NSPs from non-commercial sources, mainly of Middle Eastern, Asian and Asia–Pacific origin. Uncovering polysaccharides from new sources is important not only for their unique functionalities (e.g. gelling, thickening, water-holding capacity, etc.) but also to allow sustainable use of resources through diversification.

The third section gives an overview of the recent work carried out on modifying NSPs. Different modification approaches, broadly categorized as chemical, enzymatic and physical techniques, are briefly discussed, with a greater emphasis on the more environmentally friendly physical techniques. Polysaccharide modification is an important field as it provides avenues for enhancing or modifying the functional properties of known NSPs.

The fourth section briefly presents the biological importance of NSPs in relation to human health. The discussion is based on recent studies on how NSPs influence human health. The section focuses on the function of NSPs as prebiotics and immunostimulants and their influence on starch digestibility.

The final section of this chapter broadly discusses the interactions of NSPs with other food ingredients (e.g. starch, colourants, flavour compounds, salt and sugar). We have deliberately omitted NSP–protein interactions as this information is widely available in recent reviews. Knowledge in the area of NSP interactions is particularly important for food scientists and food product developers because these components are present in many food systems. Understanding these interactions is necessary for determining optimum processing methods and conditions, selecting appropriate ingredients in formulating food products and designing food products for optimum nutrition.

8.1.1 Functionality of commercial hydrocolloids

Many NSPs are available commercially as food additives to provide thickening, gelling or emulsifying properties. These NSPs are often called 'hydrocolloids' because of their ability as polymers to bind a large amount of water compared with their own mass. The sources of commercial hydrocolloids are largely seaweeds, seeds, woods, fruits, plant exudates and microorganisms. Table 8.1 provides a list of commercially available NSPs and includes a compilation of key functionalities, including their sugar compositions, rheological behaviours and molecular parameters, and serves mainly as a quick reference. It is useful and important to be able to relate the molecular characteristics of these biopolymers in different applications. It is essential to note that some of the published values could vary among the sources of NSPs and the methods used to characterize them.

8.2 Novel NSPs of Asian and Oceania origins

Various plant materials (i.e. leaves, roots, stems, seeds, etc.) have been used as culinary ingredients and traditional medicines for centuries. In recent years, these plants have been reported to contain functional NSPs that can be used as potential food hydrocolloids. The following provides an overview of the various sources of NSPs and their functional properties that have been reported in the past decade. These new sources of NSPs may potentially become commercial ingredients because new physical functionality is continually required by food product developers to meet the demands of consumers.

8.2.1 Arugula (*Eruca sativa*) seed mucilage

Arugula or salad rocket (*Eruca sativa*) is a common weed that is found in India and southern Europe. The seeds are capable of forming a layer of mucilage, which surrounds each seed when soaked in water (Koocheki *et al.*, 2012). In a recent study, an attempt was made to optimize the extraction of the mucilage layer. The mucilage was reported to be composed of 68.0% carbohydrates, 12.3% moisture, 10.0% ash, 9.7% protein and 0% fat (Koocheki *et al.*, 2012). In the study, the optimum extraction was a procedure that was carried out at 65.5 °C, at pH 4, using a water to seed ratio of 60 : 1 (Koocheki *et al.*, 2012). Under these optimum conditions, the maximum

Table 8.1 Key commercial NSPs and their physicochemical properties

NSP	Major Sugar Composition	Molecular Weight (Da)	Main Rheological Behaviour	Cold Water Solubility (25°C)	Main Functional Properties	Gel Properties	Charge at Neutral pH	Intrinsic Viscosity (mL/g)	Radius of Gyration (nm)	Molecular Conformation	References
Exudates											
Gum Arabic	Galactose, Arabinose, Rhamnose and Glucuronic Acid	$2.0–7.9 \times 10^5$ (Idris *et al.*, 1998) 2.5×10^5 (Hoefler, 2004)	Newtonian	Yes	Emulsifying	N/A	Negative	10.4–19.8 (Idris *et al.*, 1998)	7.1–16.4 (Idris *et al.*, 1998)	Branched	Idris *et al.*, 1998; Williams and Phillips, 2001; Ramsden, 2003; Hoefler, 2004
Gum Ghatti	Arabinose, Galactose, Mannose, Xylose, Rhamnose and Glucuronic Acid	8.9×10^7 (Kaur *et al.*, 2009)	Pseudoplastic	Yes	Emulsifying	N/A	Negative	92.0 (Kaur *et al.*, 2009)	140 (Kaur *et al.*, 2009)	Branched	Kaur *et al.*, 2009; Sakai *et al.*, 2013
Gum Karaya	Galactose, Rhamnose, Arabinose, Galacturonic Acid and Glucuronic Acid	Water-soluble fraction: $2.0–5.0 \times 10^6$ (Le Cerf *et al.*, 1990) $0.3–1.0 \times 10^6$ (Hoefler, 2004)	Pseudoplastic	No	Thickening	N/A	Negative	700–1100 (Le Cerf *et al.*, 1990)	210–320 (Le Cerf *et al.*, 1990)	Branched	Le Cerf *et al.*, 1990; Ramsden, 2003; Hoefler, 2004; Williams *et al.*, 2006
Gum Tragacanth	Fucose, Arabinose, Glucose, Galacturonic Acid, Mannose, Xylose and Galactose	8.4×10^5 (Gralén and Kärrholm, 1950) 5.02×10^5 (Hoagland *et al.*, 1993)	Pseudoplastic	No	Thickening, Emulsifying	N/A	Negative	720 (Hoagland *et al.*, 1993)	26.5–96 (Mohammadi-far *et al.*, 2006)	Branched	Gralén and Kärrholm, 1950; Hoefler, 2004; Chenlo *et al.*, 2009

Algal polysaccharides										
Agarose	D-Galactose and 3,6-Anhydro-L-Galactose	$3.6-14.4 \times 10^4$ (Rochas and Lahaye, 1989)	N/A	No	Gelling	Thermo-reversible	Neutral	127–363 (Rochas and Lahaye, 1989)	N/A	Random Coil	Rochas and Lahaye, 1989; Ramsden, 2003; Hoefler, 2004
Sodium Alginate	Guluronic Acid and Mannuronic Acid	1.9×10^5 (Strand *et al.*, 1982)	Pseudoplastic	Yes	Gelling (presence of Ca^{2+})	Thermo-reversible	Negative	145C (Villay *et al.*, 2012)	50 (Strand *et al.*, 1982)	Random Coil	Strand *et al.*, 1982; Ramsden, 2003; Hoefler, 2004
κ-Carrageenan (sodium salt)	3,6-Anhydro-D-Galactose (non-sulfated)	3.00×10^5 (Harding *et al.*, 1997; Nickerson *et al.*, 2004) $3.3-3.5 \times 10^5$ (Slootmaekers *et al.*, 1988; Slootmaekers *et al.*, 1991)	N/A	No	Gelling (presence of K^+) Rigid and Brittle Gel	Thermo-reversible	Negative	570–690 (Harding *et al.*, 1997; Nickerson *et al.*, 2004) 650–690 (Slootmaekers *et al.*, 1991)	64.8–86.8 (Vanneste *et al.*, 1996)	Random Coil	Slootmaekers *et al.*, 1988, 1991; Vanneste *et al.*, 1996; Harding *et al.*, 1997; Ramsden, 2003; Hoefler, 2004; Nickerson *et al.*, 2004
λ-Carrageenan (sodium salt)	2-Sulfated Galactose	$6.00-6.14 \times 10^5$ (Slootmaekers *et al.*, 1991)	Pseudoplastic	No	Thickening	N/A	Negative	930–970 (Slootmaekers *et al.*, 1991)	87.7–115.9 (Vanneste *et al.*, 1996)	Random Coil	Slootmaekers *et al.*, 1991; Vanneste *et al.*, 1996; Ramsden, 2003; Hoefler, 2004
ι-Carrageenan (sodium salt)	3,6-Anhydro-Galactose (sulfated at C-2)	2.0×10^5 (Bongaerts *et al*, 2000)	N/A	No	Gelling (presence of Ca^{2+}) Elastic and Cohesive Gel	Thermo-reversible	Negative	500 (Norton *et al.*, 1933)	46 ± 5 (Norton *et al.*, 1983)	Random Coil	Bongaerts *et al.*, 2000; Ramsden, 2003; Hoefler, 2004

(*continued*)

Table 8.1 (*Continued*)

NSP	Major Sugar Composition	Molecular Weight (Da)	Main Rheological Behaviour	Cold Water Solubility (25°C)	Main Functional Properties	Gel Properties	Charge at Neutral pH	Intrinsic Viscosity (mL/g)	Radius of Gyration (nm)	Molecular Conformation	References
Crustacean polysaccharide											
Chitosan	Glucosamine	DA (7%): 1.47×10^5 (Berth *et al.*, 1998) DA (25%): 6.38×10^4 (Berth *et al.*, 1998)	Pseduoplastic	No	Thickening Gelling (presence of multivalent anions)	Thermo-irreversible	Positive	650 (Berth *et al.*, 1998) 333 (Berth *et al.*, 1998)	47.1 (Berth *et al.*, 1998) 27.9 (Berth *et al.*, 1998)	Random Coil	Berth *et al.*, 1998; Izydorczyk *et al.*, 2005; Várum and Smidsr d, 2006
Microbial polysaccharides											
Curdlans	Glucose	$5.3 \times 10^4 - 2.0 \times 10^6$ (Nakata *et al.*, 1998)	–	No	Gelling	Thermo-irreversible (high-set gel)	Neutral	38–665 (Nakata *et al.*, 1998)	96.6 (0.1 N NaOH) 377.4 (0.01 N NaOH) (Norton *et al.*, 1983)	Random Coil	Nakata *et al.*, 1998; Yotsuzuka, 2001; Sutherland, 2005
Gellan Gum	Glucose, Glucuronic Acid and Rhamnose	5.0×10^5 (Sutherland, 2005) $1.0 - 2.0 \times 10^6$ (Hoefler, 2004) High Acyl: 5.2×10^5 (Goh *et al.*, 2006)	–	No (~95°C)	Gelling (in the presence of Na^+ or Ca^{2+})	Thermo-reversible	Negative	High Acyl: 3950 (Goh *et al.*, 2006)	~82 (Goh *et al.*, 2006)	Semi-flexible	Hoefler, 2004; Takahashi *et al.*, 2004; Izydorczyk *et al.*, 2005; Sutherland, 2005; Goh *et al.*, 2006
Xanthan Gum	Glucose, Mannose and Gucuronic Acid	4.05×10^6 (Viturawong *et al.*, 2008) 2.94×10^6 (Coviello *et al.*, 1986) $0.3–8 \times 10^6$ (Izydorczyk *et al.*, 2005) 3.0×10^6 (Hoefler, 2004)	Thixotropic	Yes	'Weak' Gel/ Thickening	N/A	Negative	11 230 (Achayuthakan *et al.*, 2006) 11 034 (Viturawong *et al.*, 2008)	289 (Coviello *et al.*, 1986)	Stiff	Coviello *et al.*, 1986; Hoefler, 2004; Izydorczyk *et al.*, 2005; Sutherland, 2005; Achayuthakan *et al.*, 2006; Viturawong *et al.*, 2008

Legume Seed galactomannans										
Fenugreek Gum	Galactose: Mannose ratio of 1:~1	2.28×10^6 (Youssef *et al.*, 2009)	Pseudoplastic	Yes	Thickening (low viscosity) Emulsifying	N/A	Neutral	1070 (Youssef *et al.*, 2009) 1510 (Wu *et al.*, 2009)	90 (Youssef *et al.*, 2009) 42.13 (Wu *et al.*, 2012)	Random Coil	Brummer *et al.*, 2003; Ramsden, 2003; Jiang *et al.*, 2007; Wu *et al.*, 2009; Youssef *et al.*, 2009; Wu *et al.*, 2012b
Guar Gum	Galactose: Mannose ratio of 1:~2	1.87×10^6 (Picout *et al.*, 2001) $2.0–3.0 \times 10^6$ (Ellis *et al.*, 2001) $0.15–1.5 \times 10^6$ (Hoefler, 2004) $0.5–8.0 \times 10^6$ (Mahungu and Meyland, 2008)	Pseudoplastic	Yes	Thickening	N/A	Neutral	1210 (Gaisford *et al.*, 1986) 1270 (Launay *et al.*, 1998; Picout *et al.*, 2001) 1580 (Wu *et al.*, 2009)	31.05 (Wu *et al.*, 2012) 133 (Picout *et al.*, 2001)	Random Coil	Gaisford *et al.*, 1986; Launay *et al.*, 1998; Ellis *et al.*, 2001; Picout *et al.*, 2001; Ramsden, 2003; Hoefler, 2004; Wu *et al.*, 2009; Wu *et al.*, 2012b
Tara Gum	Galactose: Mannose ratio of 1:~3	2.25×10^6 (Picout *et al.*, 2002) $0.3–1.0 \times 10^6$ (Hoefler, 2004)	Pseudoplastic	No (~80°C)	Thickening	N/A	Neutral	1455 (Wu *et al.*, 2009) 1420 (Picout *et al.*, 2002)	29.61 (Wu *et al.*, 2012) 141 (Picout *et al.*, 2002)	Random Coil	Picout *et al.*, 2002; Ramsden, 2003; Wu *et al.*, 2009; Wu *et al.*, 2012b
Locust Bean Gum	Galactose: Mannose ratio of 1:~4	$2.3–3.9 \times 10^6$ (Lazaridou *et al.*, 2001) 1.05×10^6 (Picout *et al.*, 2002) $0.4–1.0 \times 10^6$ (Hoefler, 2004) $0.5–3.0 \times 10^6$ (Mahungu and Meyland, 2008)	Pseudoplastic	No (~60°C)	Thickening	N/A	Neutral	1420 (Wu *et al.*, 2009) 1103 (Sittikijyothin *et al.*, 2005) 815–1302 (Lazaridou *et al.*, 2001) 1260 (Picout *et al.*, 2002)	59.18 (Wu *et al.*, 2012) 127 (Picout *et al.*, 2002)	Random Coil	Lazaridou *et al.*, 2001; Picout *et al.*, 2002; Ramsden, 2003; Hoefler, 2004; Sittikijyothin *et al.*, 2005; Wu *et al.*, 2009; Mathur, 2011b; Wu *et al.*, 2012b

(*continued*)

Table 8.1 (*Continued*)

NSP	Major Sugar Composition	Molecular Weight (Da)	Main Rheological Behaviour	Cold Water Solubility (25°C)	Main Functional Properties	Gel Properties	Charge at Neutral pH	Intrinsic Viscosity (mL/g)	Radius of Gyration (nm)	Molecular Conformation	References
Root polysaccharides											
Konjac Mannan	Glucose: Mannose ratio of 1:~1.6	$7.7–9.6 \times 10^5$ (Ratcliffe *et al.*, 2005) $0.2–2.0 \times 10^6$ (Hoefler, 2004)	Pseudoplastic	No (~90°C)	Thickening (with acetyl groups) Gelling (without acetyl groups)	Not Thermo-reversible	Neutral	1600–2000 (Ratcliffe *et al.*, 2005)	80–95 (Ratcliffe *et al.*, 2005)	Random Coil	Jacon *et al.*, 1993; BeMiller, 2001; Hoefler, 2004; Ratcliffe *et al.*, 2005
Plant Wall polysaccharides											
β-Glucan	Glucose	Wheat: 3.29×10^5 (Li *et al.*, 2006) Barley: $2.31–2.53 \times 10^5$ (Gómez *et al.*, 1997) Oat: 2.78×10^5 (Gómez *et al.*, 1997)	Pseudoplastic	Yes	Thickening Gelling (6%; low temperature)	Thermo reversible	Neutral	Wheat: 455 (Li *et al.*, 2006) Barley: 270–280 (Gómez *et al.*, 1997) Oat: 280 (Gómez *et al.*, 1997)	Wheat: 45.6 (Li *et al.*, 2006) Barley: 27–28.2 (Gómez *et al.*, 1997) Oat: 35.0 (Gómez *et al.*, 1997)	Random Coil	Gómez *et al.*, 1997; Ramsden, 2003; Cui and Wang, 2005; Li *et al.*, 2006
Low Ester Pectin	Galacturonic Acid, Rhamnose, Arabinose and Galactose	$0.96–2.05 \times 10^5$ (Corredig *et al.*, 2000) $1.8–1.9 \times 10^5$ (Plashchina *et al.*, 1985) 2.26×10^5 (Yoo *et al.*, 2006) $1.13–2.90 \times 10^5$ (Li *et al.*, 2013)	N/A	No (~60°C)	Gelling	Not Thermo-reversible	Negative	2940 (Yoo *et al.*, 2006) 2900–4900 (Li *et al.*, 2013) 2450 (Sato *et al.*, 2008)	53–57 (Corredig *et al.*, 2000) 43–54 (Plashchina *et al.*, 1985)	Random Coil	Plashchina *et al.*, 1985; Corredig *et al.*, 2000; MacDougall and Ring, 2003; Hoefler, 2004; Yoo *et al.*, 2006; Sato *et al.*, 2008; Li *et al.*, 2013

High Ester Pectin	Galacturonic Acid, Rhamnose, Arabinose and Galactose	$1.81-2.00 \times 10^5$ (Corredig *et al.*, 2000) $1.9-2.0 \times 10^5$ (Plashchina *et al.*, 1985) 1.38×10^5 (Yoo *et al.*, 2006)	N/A	No (~60°C)	Gelling	Not Thermo-reversible	Negative	2150 (Yoo *et al.*, 2006)	52–56 (Corredig *et al.*, 2000) 45–60 (Plashchina *et al.*, 1985)	Random Coil	Plashchina *et al.*, 1985; Corredig *et al.*, 2000; MacDougall and Ring, 2003; Hoefler, 2004; Yoo *et al.*, 2006
Carboxymethyl cellulose	Glucose	2.6×10^4 (Villay *et al.*, 2012)	Pseudoplastic	Yes	Thickening/ Gelling (with Al^{3+})		Negative	546 (Villay *et al.*, 2012)	39 (Villay *et al.*, 2012)	Random Coil	Hoefler, 2004; Izydorczyk *et al.*, 2005
Methylcellulose	Glucose	3.5×10^4 (El Ghzaoui *et al.*, 2001)	Pseudoplastic	Yes	Gelling (at 40–70°C) Thickening (at 25°C)	Thermo-reversible	Neutral	456 (El Ghzaoui *et al.*, 2001)	77 (El Ghzaoui *et al.*, 2001)	Random Coil	Hoefler, 2004; Izydorczyk *et al.*, 2005
Hydroxypropyl-methylcellulose	Glucose	$4.0-5.5 \times 10^4$ (El Ghzaoui *et al.*, 2001)	Pseudoplastic	Yes	Gelling, Thickening	Thermo-reversible	Neutral	382–753 (El Ghzaoui *et al.*, 2001)	75–82 (El Ghzaoui *et al.*, 2001)	Random Coil	Hoefler, 2004; Izydorczyk *et al.*, 2005
Microcrystalline cellulose	Glucose		Thixotropic and Pseudo-plastic	Yes	'Weak' Gel		Neutral			Stiff	Hoefler, 2004; Izydorczyk *et al.*, 2005

N/A: not applicable; DA: degree of acetylation.

extraction yield, viscosity, emulsion stability, foam stability, solubility and water absorption capacity were reported to be 10.3%, 357 mPa s, 87.0%, 87.5%, 28.5% and 9.3 g/g respectively (Koocheki *et al.*, 2012). Currently, no further information is available on the sugar composition of the NSP, its solution properties or the rheological behaviour of this novel mucilage.

8.2.2 Chubak (*Acanthophyllum bracteatum*) gum

The chubak plant (*Acanthophyllum bracteatum*) is endemic to Iran. Its roots have been used as a detergent because they contain large amounts of saponin (Jahanbin *et al.*, 2012). The native gum extracted from the roots consists of 84.3% total sugar, 13.2% moisture, 1.5% ash and 0.9% protein (Jahanbin *et al.*, 2012). The NSP was identified as a gluco-arabinogalactan-type polysaccharide that comprises galactose, glucose, arabinose, rhamnose and uronic acid in the ratio of about 16.0 : 7.2 : 3.0 : 1.0 : 3.1, respectively (Jahanbin *et al.*, 2012). The soluble NSP fraction has a weight-average molecular weight of $\sim 2.6 \times 10^4$ Da (Jahanbin *et al.*, 2011). Newtonian behaviour was observed for solutions with gum concentrations of $\leq 5\%$ over the shear rate range 1–300/s. However, shear-thinning behaviour was observed for solutions with gum concentrations of $> 5\%$ (Jahanbin *et al.*, 2012). The study also reported that, when the temperature was increased from 10 to 70 °C, the viscosity dropped by ~49%, from 73.5 to 37.5 mPa s. The native pH of a 1% gum solution was 6.85. The viscosity was at its highest at a neutral pH of 6–7 (Jahanbin *et al.*, 2012). The gum was noted to possess poorer emulsification properties than gum arabic, which was attributed to the lower protein content and/or the poor quality of the proteins in the gum structure (Jahanbin *et al.*, 2012). However, the authors suggested that chubak gum has the potential to be used in food systems to improve foaming properties; it has moderate foaming capacity and relatively high foaming stability because of the viscosity contributed by the gum (Jahanbin *et al.*, 2012). More studies are required to understand the foaming application of this novel gum.

8.2.3 Cincau Hijau (*Cyclea barbata*) gum

Cyclea barbata belongs to the *Menispermaceae* family. In some parts of South East Asia and India, *Cyclea barbata* is considered to be a medicinal plant. The water extract from the leaves is capable of forming a firm and brittle gel, called 'Cincau Hijau' (in Bahasa Indonesia; see Figure 8.1). The gel is consumed as a dessert or a traditional remedy for stomach ailments (Lemmens and Horsten, 1999). The ability of the polysaccharide extract to gel at room temperature is possibly due to the presence of cations naturally present in the leaves and/or the water used to extract the polysaccharide (Figure 8.1). One study reported that the gel was thermo-reversible and had a natural pH of 3.4 (Arkarapanthu *et al.*, 2005). The purified gum is composed of 79.9% carbohydrates, 8.5% moisture, 9.5% ash, 2.0% protein and 0.1% fat (Arkarapanthu *et al.*, 2005). The main polymer in the gum was identified as polygalacturonic acid with 66.3% methylation and a molecular weight of 7.41×10^5 Da (Arkarapanthu *et al.*, 2005). The phenolic compounds in the extract have also been reported to influence the gelling ability and the gel strength (Arkarapanthu *et al.*, 2005). The gel formation

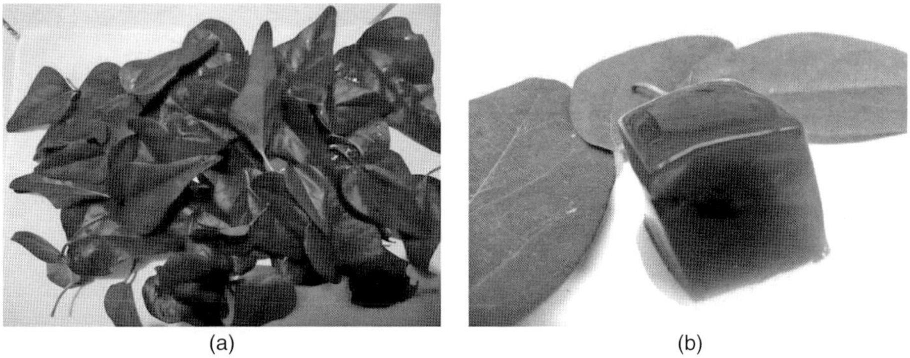

Figure 8.1 (a) Fresh leaves of *Cyclea barbata*. (b) Firm gel formed by the extract from the leaves, using 10 leaves in 100 g of water. For colour details, see the colour plates section

has been proposed to be due to: (i) hydrogen bonds formed between polygalacturonic acid chains; (ii) linkages between the polygalacturonic acid chains via phenolic compounds; (iii) electrostatic interactions between the polygalacturonic acid chains via divalent cations; (iv) intermolecular hydrophobic bonds between methylated groups on the polygalacturonic acid chains (Arkarapanthu *et al.*, 2005).

8.2.4 Cress (*Lepidium sativum*) seed gum

Garden cress (*Lepidium sativum*) is a herb that is grown in West Asia, Europe and the United States (Karazhiyan *et al.*, 2011). The mucilage extracted from the seeds is composed of 77.0% carbohydrates, 11.5% ash, 7.2% moisture, 2.5% protein and 1.8% fat (Karazhiyan *et al.*, 2009). The monosaccharide composition of the gum consists of mannose (38.9%), arabinose (19.4%), galacturonic acid (8.0%), fructose (6.8%), glucuronic acid (6.7%), galactose (4.7%), rhamnose (1.9%) and glucose (1.0%) (Karazhiyan *et al.*, 2009). The hydrocolloid was identified as a glycoprotein with a weight-average molecular weight of 5.4×10^4 Da, an intrinsic viscosity of 550–1330 ml/g and a radius of gyration of 75 nm (Karazhiyan *et al.*, 2009). The mucilage solution exhibited Newtonian behaviour at $< 0.1\%$ concentration, pseudoplastic characteristics at $< 6\%$ concentration and thixotropy at $> 6\%$ concentration (Karazhiyan *et al.*, 2009). In another study, (Naji *et al.*, 2012) reported that the mucilage was stable to heat treatment (even at 121 °C for 15 min) as the textural attributes of samples formed from the mucilage remained similar. They suggested that the hydrocolloid can be used in foods that require high temperature processing.

8.2.5 Basil (*Ocimum basilicum*) seed gum

Basil seeds are commonly used in beverages and as a medicine throughout Asia. When the seeds are soaked in water, a thick gel layer is observed to surround each seed (see Figure 8.2). The gel from the seeds is composed of 79.6% carbohydrates, 9.1% moisture, 6.5% ash, 4.4% fat and 1.3% protein (Hosseini-Parvar *et al.*, 2010). The NSP was reported to be a heteropolysaccharide that contained glucomannan,

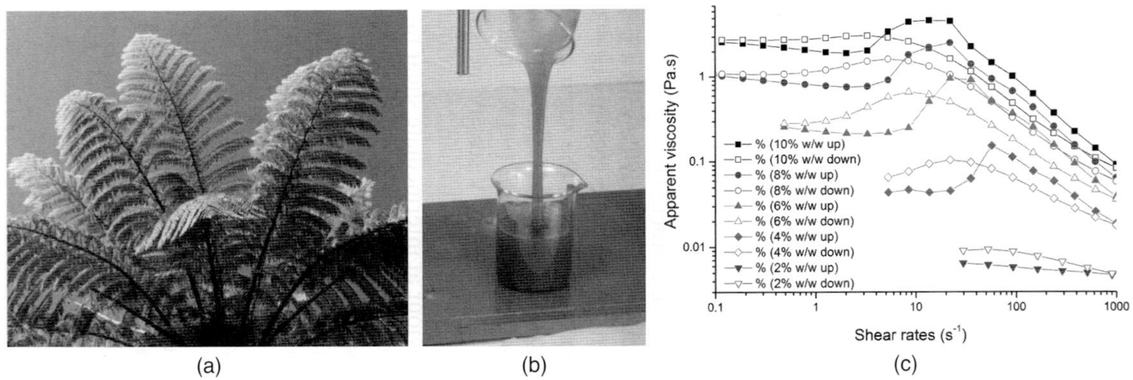

Figure 8.3 (a) Mamaku, the black tree fern (*Cyathea medullaris*). (b) Viscoelastic properties of 7% w/w solution of mamaku extract, illustrated by decanting from one beaker to another. (c) Viscosity curves of solutions of mamaku extract (2, 4, 6, 8 and 10% w/w) as a function of shear rate at 20 °C. The viscosity measurements were carried out using a double-gap attachment to obtain 'up-curves' (filled symbols) and 'down-curves' (open symbols). *Source:* Goh *et al.*, 2007. Reproduced with permission from the American Chemical Society. For colour details, see the colour plates section

The mucilage layer exhibited pseudoplastic behaviour (Koocheki *et al.*, 2009b) and was found to have good emulsifying properties (Koocheki *et al.*, 2009a; Koocheki and Kadkhodaee, 2011). Further work is required to characterize the molecular and rheological properties of this gum.

8.2.11 Malva (*Sterculiae lychnophorae*) nut gum

The seeds of the malva (*Sterculiae lychnophorae*) tree are used in traditional medicine in China, Taiwan and South East Asia. They are commonly added as an ingredient in a dessert known as 'Cheng Tng' (in Hokkien, a Chinese dialect). When submerged in water, the seed swells into a reddish-brown, seaweed-like, gelatinous mass. Three NSP fractions were isolated: water-soluble, alkali-soluble and insoluble fractions (Ai *et al.*, 2012). The water-soluble extract consisted of both neutral and acidic fractions. The neutral NSP fraction consisted of mainly glucose (85.86%), with small amounts of galactose, arabinose and xylose. The acidic NSP fraction was composed mainly of galacturonic acid (40.13%) along with rhamnose, arabinose, galactose and small amounts of xylose and glucose (Wu *et al.*, 2007). The acidic fraction was identified as a pectic polysaccharide with 68% degree of esterification. This NSP fraction required a co-solute under acidic conditions to form a gel (Wu *et al.*, 2012a). Recent studies also reported that the NSP from the seeds possessed anti-inflammatory properties in murine models (Wu *et al.*, 2007; Ai *et al.*, 2012).

8.2.12 Wild sage (*Salvia macrosiphon*) seed gum

Wild sage, which is native to West Asia, is traditionally used as a medicine. When the seeds are soaked in water, a mucilage layer forms around each seed (Razavi *et al.*, 2010). The molar mass of the mucilage fraction has recently been reported to be $\sim 1.5 \times 10^6$ Da (Razavi *et al.*, 2012). The rheological properties of the gum dispersion showed a high zero-shear-rate viscosity accompanied by a strong shear-thinning characteristic over a wide range of concentration, when compared with xanthan gum (Razavi *et al.*, 2011). The gum can potentially be used as an effective stabilizer and thickener in food systems (Razavi *et al.*, 2011).

8.2.13 Cashew (*Anacardium occidentale*) gum

The cashew tree (*Anacardium occidentale*) is widely grown in some tropical countries for the seeds found in the fruits. These seeds are commonly known as 'cashew nuts'. The bark of the cashew tree secretes a polysaccharide exudate (Zakaria and Rahman, 1996; de Paula *et al.*, 1998). The polysaccharide fraction of the exudate has a molar mass of 1.13×10^5 Da (de Paula *et al.*, 1998) and is composed of 70% galactose, 5% arabinose, 11% glucose, 4% rhamnose, 1% mannose and 6% glucuronic acid (de Paula and Rodrigues, 1995). Cashew gum solutions exhibited a unique lower viscosity characteristic compared with the other common exudate gums such as arabic and tragacanth. However, their viscosity exhibited non-Newtonian behaviour even at concentrations less than 1%. In addition, the gum has good emulsifying properties and can be utilized as a substitute for gum arabic to stabilize emulsions (de Paula *et al.*, 1998).

as determined by gel filtration. It was identified as a hetero-polysaccharide consisting of β-D-xylose, α-D-glucose and 4-*O*-methyl-α-D-glucuronic acid in the ratio 2:1:1 (Lin *et al.*, 1994). Muñoz *et al.* (2012) recently found that hydration of chia seed gum reached a maximum when the solution temperature was 80 °C and that hydration of the gel layer was maximum at pH 9 and at low salt concentration. The gel layer obtained from chia seed has not been well characterized to date. Further work is required to characterize the physicochemical properties of the gel to determine potential areas of application.

8.3 Modification of physical and functional properties of NSPs

A number of studies on the modification of polysaccharide molecular structures have been reported over the past decade. The aim is to improve or alter the physicochemical properties of NSPs. Knowledge of the NSP structure–function relationship is important as it can help to determine suitable regimes for modifying polysaccharides to achieve the desired properties. Generally, the options available are enzymatic, chemical and physical methods alone or in combination. In chemical and enzymatic modifications, solvents and enzymes respectively are required. However, in physical modification, no additives are usually needed. This last option is preferred from a 'green' perspective. However, it must be noted that applying a physical technique does not imply the absence of chemical changes taking place even though no chemical reagents are added.

8.3.1 Chemical modification

Commercially, chemical modification of polysaccharides has been applied widely to starches but not substantially to NSPs. The most common chemical derivation is the conversion of insoluble non-ionic cellulose to water-soluble anionic carboxymethylcellulose, which is achieved by introducing carboxymethyl ether at regular intervals on the polymer backbone (Mathur, 2011a). Other functional groups that are substituted along NSP chains (e.g. guar gum and locust bean gum) include methyl, ethyl, hydroxypropyl, phosphate esters, sulfate esters and quaternary ammonium (Lindblad and Albertsson, 2004). All these require different chemical reagents such as methyl chloride, ethylene oxide, propylene oxide and trimethyl ammonium chloride (Mathur, 2011a). Chemical modification has great potential, especially in the non-food industry, where the specific functional properties of NSPs can be enhanced chemically, consequently reducing the cost of manufacture through improved functionality. However, when these modified NSPs are proposed as food additives, considerable cost and time will be required to obtain approval by government agencies and legislators to ensure that the modified NSPs do not cause harm to humans.

8.3.2 Enzymatic modification

Enzymatic modification to alter the functional properties of NSPs has also been applied. Several early studies successfully used enzymes to improve the gelling properties of pectins from sugar beet by cleaving the acetyl groups (Williamson *et al.*, 1990; Oosterveld *et al.*, 2000, 2002). Recent studies reported the use of enzymes to depolymerize guar gum to achieve an improved printing quality of the ink used in the textile industry (Baldaro *et al.*, 2012). Food scientists have also reported the use of enzymes to partially depolymerize NSPs to be used as a source of dietary fibre without significantly increasing the viscosity of food products (Mudgil *et al.*, 2012). In addition, the enzyme α-galactosidase has been added to guar gum to remove some of the galactose residues. The modified guar gum has been shown to synergistically form stronger gels with xanthan gum (Pai and Khan, 2002; Mao *et al.*, 2012). In another study related to guar gum, Mahammad *et al.* (2007) reported the sequential addition of three enzymes, i.e. β-mannosidase (specifically cleaves a single mannose unit from the non-reducing end of the guar molecule), β-mannanase (cleaves the interior glycosidic bonds between adjacent mannose units) and α-galactosidase (cleaves the galactose side branches), which acted synergistically in the hydrolysis of guar molecules. Li *et al.* (2009) reported an enzyme-modified konjac glucomannan that interacted synergistically with xanthan gum. The enzymatic degradation of the konjac gum resulted in strong intermolecular interaction caused by hydrogen bonds between xanthan gum and the hydrolysed konjac gum. The gel strength was found to increase with lower molar mass of the konjac gum although the thermal stability of the gel was poorer.

Because of their specificity, the use of enzymes to alter the chemical structure of NSPs is an effective way to produce NSPs with customized functional properties. Thus, knowing the specific cleavage sites of enzymes along the NSP molecular structure can be an effective tool for researchers to understand the structure–function relationship of NSPs. Persin *et al.* (2011) aptly wrote in a recent review that 'enzymes with hydrolytic, oxidative/reductive and transferase activity as well as the development of selective enzymatic cleavage and attachments of chains, side groups and branches' are important future pathways for the modification of NSPs with specific functionality.

8.3.3 Physical modification

The most favourable method of modifying polysaccharide functionality from the perspective that it is environmentally friendlier and does not require the use of the volatile organic solvents that are commonly employed in chemical methods, is by physical means. Physical methods include mechanical, thermal, thermomechanical, electromagnetic and electrochemical methods. This section focuses mainly on three physical techniques: ultrasonication, high pressure treatment and pulsed electric field.

Ultra-high pressure The use of ultra-high pressure treatment has received significant attention in recent years (Rastogi *et al.*, 2007). High pressure treatment can be categorized into two main groups: dynamic high pressure treatment and hydrostatic high pressure treatment. The former involves a homogenizer, which can achieve a pressure of only 50 MPa in conventional models. However, in more recent designs such as a microfluidizer, the pressure can go up to 250 MPa. In a hydrostatic high pressure machine, samples are typically subjected to pressures of between 100 and 800 MPa (Bigikocin *et al.*, 2011). It is important to note that dynamic high pressure homogenization differs markedly from hydrostatic high pressure treatment as the former involves high shear elongation, turbulence and cavitation when a liquid is forced through a minute gap between a seat and a valve at very short residence times (Stang and Schubert, 2001; Villay *et al.*, 2012). The effect of ultra-high pressure on proteins (Fernandes and Raemy, 1996; Galazka *et al.*, 2001; Michel and Autio, 2002; Rastogi *et al.*, 2007) and polysaccharides (Lagoueyte and Paquin, 1998; Floury *et al.*, 2002; Kasaai *et al.*, 2008; Kivelä *et al.*, 2010; Souza *et al.*, 2013) has been studied extensively over the past decade. High pressure treatment causes depolymerization of polysaccharides. In a recent study, dynamic high pressure was applied to a number of NSPs including sodium alginate, guar gum, gum arabic, hydroxyethylcellulose and sodium carboxymethylcellulose. The effect of high pressure was found to be dependent on the structure and conformation of the polysaccharides. Gum arabic was found not to be affected by the high pressure treatment, probably because of its branched and globular structures. In contrast, a linear stiff polymer underwent depolymerization with a reduction in polydispersity while retaining its native conformation (Villay *et al.*, 2012). High pressure homogenization resulted in thickening and gelation of inulin, which was attributed to a reduction in particle size and the formation of an agglomerated network in solution (Ronkart *et al.*, 2010).

Hydrostatic high pressure treatment applied to NSPs alone has not been widely studied to date, probably because of the less drastic effect of high pressure on polysaccharides than on proteins or protein–polysaccharide systems. Ahmed and Ramaswamy (2004) applied hydrostatic high pressure ranging from 80 to 400 MPa for 30 min at ~20 °C to xanthan gum. In contrast to heat treatment, the apparent viscosity was maximum at a pressure of 550 MPa and a gum concentration of 1.8% w/w but no significant effects ($p < 0.05$) on the flow behaviour index and the yield stress were observed. Teramoto and Fuchigami (2000) reported that konjac gum that was subjected to high pressure freezing–thawing (freezing under high pressure and subsequently thawing at atmospheric pressure) at 200–400 MPa differed markedly from the original gel or gels frozen at from −20 to 180 °C (Fuchigami *et al.*, 2006). They observed an increase in the rupture stress but a decrease in the gel rupture strain (Teramoto and Fuchigami, 2000). They also reported that an agar gel subjected to pressure-shift freezing at 200–400 MPa, holding for 63 min and subsequently thawing at atmospheric pressure was less coarse and had less syneresis than gels treated at between 0.1 and 100 MPa and from 500 to 686 MPa. This was attributed to the size and number of ice crystals formed during the freezing process at different pressures (Fuchigami and Teramoto, 2003; Fuchigami *et al.*, 2006).

Panteloglou *et al.* (2010) recently applied hydrostatic high pressure to a gum arabic dispersion (40% w/w) at 800 MPa for 10 min at below 30 °C and showed considerable changes in the rheological behaviour of the gum arabic under different pH conditions. In an acidic environment (pH 2.8), a weaker gel structure than in the unpressurized native sample was observed. However, at a higher pH of 4.2, the viscoelasticity of the pressure-treated samples increased. The high pressure treatment did not alter the overall sugar or protein composition of the gums. Panteloglou *et al.* (2010) attributed the change in the rheological behaviour to the conformation and the extent of denaturation of the protein fraction in gum arabic.

Pulsed electric field Pulsed electric field (PEF) has recently been reported to have an effect on the structural and functional properties of pectin (Ma and Wang, 2013). The study showed that PEF pectin reacted with arachidic anhydride in the absence of any solvent resulted in a significant increase in the degree of esterification (from DE 61 to DE 76) and improved thermal stability. The structural modification was attributed to redox electrochemical reactions (Sato and Ohshima, 2006; Seo *et al.*, 2010). The electric field intensity varied from 8 to 30 kV/cm and the total specific energy input ranged from 124 to 345 J/ml. The use of PEF has also been reported to cause degradation of chitosan polymer molecules, resulting in smaller molar mass fractions (Luo *et al.*, 2010). In another study, PEF was reported to cause changes in the crystalline region of starch granules to an amorphous structure. The pulsed field applied was between 30 and 50 kV/cm (Han *et al.*, 2012). The use of this technique to modify NSPs is relatively new and to date appears to be promising. Further studies involving different field intensities, pulse widths, numbers of pulses, durations of treatment etc. are required to evaluate the potential of using this technique as a tool to improve the functionality of NSPs.

Ultrasonication Ultrasonication using high-intensity ultrasound treatment to extract, mix, homogenize, emulsify, modify viscosity and inactivate microorganisms has been increasingly applied in food processing (Rastogi, 2011). It uses low frequency ultrasound (16–100 kHz) with energies above 10 W/cm^2, which generates alternating high pressure (i.e. compression) and low pressure (i.e. rarefaction) cycles. During rarefaction, high-intensity sonic waves create small vacuum bubbles or voids in the liquid, which then collapse violently when they reach a critical size (i.e. cavitation) during compression, creating very high local temperatures and shear (Mason and Lorimer, 2002). Generally, ultrasonication is an economical, eco-friendly technique for the controlled fragmentation of polymer chains.

The effect of ultrasound on gelling polysaccharides was first investigated using agarose, κ-carrageenan and ι-carrageenan (Min-Feng *et al.*, 1996). Aqueous polysaccharide solutions were treated with ultrasound waves of 35 kHz at 50 °C. The authors reported that ultrasound treatment could affect the storage moduli and the rate of gelation of the three polysaccharides. The ultrasonicated agarose gel retained higher thermal stability than the heated gel but no significant change was observed for the carrageenan gels. The application of ultrasonic irradiation at a frequency of 20 kHz to chitosan showed that the rate of fragmentation increased with an increase in the ultrasound power and the solution temperature and at lower chitosan concentration. Ultrasonication of chitosan caused partial depolymerization of the polymer molecules. However, there was no noticeable effect on the chemical structure and polydispersity (Kasaai *et al.*, 2008). In a recent study, Souza *et al.* (2013) reported a decrease in the moisture permeability of a chitosan film after a solution of chitosan (30 ml) was ultrasonicated (sonic model 750 W with 0.5 inch tip, 50% amplitude) up to 60 min. This was due to the reduction in the molar mass of the chitosan polymers.

Another study (Wong *et al.*, (2010) revealed the ability of ultrasound to modify NSPs beyond the conventional depolymerization. It was found that ultrasonication is capable of promoting sulfation of curdlan in the presence of sulfuric acid. By sonicating curdlan in 50% sulfuric acid, the degree of sulfation was almost four times higher than that of the non-sonicated sample. This is more environmentally friendly than the conventional chemical synthesis (which usually requires the utilization of toxic chemicals and solvents) for producing sulfated polysaccharides.

8.4 Polysaccharides and human health

8.4.1 Source of dietary fibre

Generally, NSPs cannot be digested in the small intestine but are fermented into short-chain fatty acids by the microflora in the colon and caecum. These short-chain fatty acids lower the pH of the colon, inhibit the growth of pathogens, increase mineral absorption, maintain normal bowel function, stimulate repair in damaged colon and colonic blood flow and promote fluid and electrolyte uptake (Kumar *et al.*, 2012c). The current suggested dietary NSP intake for a healthy individual is 12.8–17.8 g/day (Green, 2000). NSPs incorporated into daily meals have been suggested to reduce the risk of constipation, diabetes mellitus, cardiovascular diseases, colo-rectal cancer, tumour formation and breast cancer (Yoshida, 2004; Chiu *et al.*, 2011; Kumar *et al.*, 2012c). Kumar *et al.* (2012c) present a comprehensive review on the health benefits of NSPs.

8.4.2 Effect of NSPs on starch digestibility

Starch is a major component of any staple diet. Based on the rate of digestion, starch can be classified as rapidly digestible starch, slowly digestible starch and resistant starch (Englyst and Hudson, 1996). The rate at which these starches are digested can affect the blood glucose level, which has a major implication on human health. Diets that mostly include slowly digestible starches have been associated with a reduced risk of coronary heart disease and type 2 diabetes (Chiu *et al.*, 2011). Currently, there is a growing trend in the use of NSPs in starch-rich foods, aimed at reducing the glucose level in the bloodstream, especially from the rapidly digestible starches.

The effect of NSPs on starch digestibility requires further elucidation. The mechanism involved in the interactions between NSP and starch, which ultimately affect the post-prandial rise in blood glucose, requires further validation. Several mechanisms have been proposed.

(1) The increased viscosity of the digesta contributed by NSPs can retard mixing effects generated by peristalsis, which therefore slows down interactions between enzymes and starch (Singh *et al.*, 2010).
(2) Possible interactions between NSP and starch provide a physical barrier that reduces α-amylase hydrolysis activity (Brennan *et al.*, 1996). This is further discussed in section 8.5.
(3) The expansion of NSP in the upper gastrointestinal tract because of hydration can lead to an increase in the viscosity of the digesta. The viscosity increment could reduce the rate of glucose absorption, reduce insulin secretion and inhibit gastric polypeptide secretion (Ellis *et al.*, 1995; Singh *et al.*, 2010).

Further information on the effect of NSPs (xanthan gum, guar gum, konjac glucomannan and pectin) on the *in vitro* digestibility of starch can be found in recent publications (Kumar *et al.*, 2012c; Sasaki and Kohyama, 2012).

8.4.3 Antitumour and immuno-stimulating functions of NSPs

Some NSPs have been reported to possess biological activities that influence immunological function. Polysaccharides from various sources have been studied over the past few decades for their bioactivities. Most notable of NSPs that possess immuno-stimulating functions are β-glucan from oats (Daou and Zhang, 2012), polysaccharide–protein complexes from *Coriolus versicolor* (known as 'Yun Zhi' in Mandarin Chinese) (Sun *et al.*, 2012; Sekhon *et al.*, 2013) and NSPs from *Lentinus edodes* ('Shitake' mushroom), *Ganoderma lucidum* ('Lingzhi' in Mandarin Chinese), *Cordyceps senensis* ('Dong Chong Xia Cao' in Mandarin Chinese) (Song *et al.*, 2013) and *Grifola frondosa* ('Maitake' in Japanese) (Wu *et al.*, 2013). It has now become a common trend, particularly in Asia, to use bioactive compounds from medicinal mushrooms as supportive treatments in conventional cancer therapies (De Silva *et al.*, 2012).

The immuno-stimulating and immuno-modulating functions of NSPs have been reviewed recently (Wasser, 2011; De Silva *et al.*, 2012; Ren *et al.*, 2012). These bioactive NSPs have been reported to stimulate the immune system against cancer cells by increasing immunoglobulin, NK cells, killer T-cells, B-cells, neutrophils and macrophage. Stimulation of host immune defence systems by bioactive polymers from medicinal mushrooms has significant effects on the maturation, differentiation and proliferation of different immune cells in the host (Wasser, 2011). The immuno-stimulating and immuno-modulating abilities of these NSPs are influenced by the molecular structure, molecular mass, degree of branching and conformation. These attributes are important to explain the correlation between the structural features and the biological functions (Ren *et al.*, 2012). Extensive research is necessary to carry out all three phases of clinical trials to understand the exact mechanism involved so that the appropriate concentration and characteristics of NSPs can be used more effectively in alternative cancer therapy than is current practice.

8.5 Interactions of NSPs with other food components

This section reviews the interactions of NSPs with other components commonly found in foods. The interactions between NSPs and proteins are omitted because the topic has already been comprehensively reviewed (Tolstoguzov, 2002; Dickinson, 2006; Goh *et al.*, 2009; Schmitt *et al.*, 2009; Corredig *et al.*, 2011; Jones and McClements, 2011; Rodriguez Patino and Pilosof, 2011; Schmitt and Turgeon, 2011). The following subsections focus on the interactions of NSPs with starch, colourants and food ingredients that affect taste sensations.

8.5.1 NSP–starch interaction

The addition of NSP has become increasingly common in starch-based food products. For example, NSP–starch mixtures are used in the formation of edible coatings for fruits. The addition of NSP in starch-based foods can also increase the water-holding capacity and reduce syneresis and retrogradation. In addition, NSP has been shown

sweetener molecules to the taste receptors because of an increase in viscosity (Baines and Morris, 1987). In another study, Mälkki *et al.* (1993) investigated the effects of oat gum and guar gum on the extent of the perceived sweetness of fructose, sucrose and aspartame. The thickener solutions (containing 10% sucrose) were prepared to give equivalent viscosity (500 MPa s) at a shear rate of 50/s. The results indicated that the type of NSP could influence the perception of sweetness. In addition, different sweeteners were affected differently by the type of NSP. The sweetness intensity of 10% sucrose was highest in oat gum solution, followed by carboxymethylcellulose, and was lowest in guar gum solution. The exact mechanisms affecting sweetness perception seemed to be dependent on some interactions between sweetener molecules and NSP molecules, depending on the reactive groups available. In addition, the physical characteristics of some NSPs, such as the stickiness observed in oat gum, could imply a longer residence time of oat gum on the taste buds than of guar gum and carboxymethylcellulose (Mälkki *et al.*, 1993).

Saltiness Both the ionic nature of the NSPs and the viscosity increment play a crucial role in the perception of saltiness. Cook *et al.* (2002) reported that the perception of the saltiness of sodium chloride (0.35% w/w) was significantly reduced in a non-ionic HPMC solution above the c* of 0.57% w/w. Interestingly, when the sodium chloride concentration in the sample above the c* was increased to 0.45% w/w, the sensory panellists indicated that there was no significant difference in saltiness (Cook *et al.*, 2002). In another study, it was reported that both non-ionic HPMC and ionic λ-carrageenan reduced the perceived saltiness at high NSP concentration (Cook *et al.*, 2003). The sodium ions from sodium chloride could have bound with the ionic λ-carrageenan, resulting in fewer ions available to induce the salty perception. However, in the case of HPMC, which is a non-ionic NSP, the reduction in salty perception was attributed to the viscosity effect. Studies using nuclear magnetic resonance (NMR) spectroscopy have shown that sodium ions are less mobile in ionic systems (xanthan gum and κ-carrageenan) than in non-ionic systems (locust bean gum and guar gum) (Rosett *et al.*, 1994). In another study, at equivalent molar concentrations of added ions, ^{23}Na NMR transverse relaxation rates showed an increase in average sodium ion mobility with the addition of potassium or calcium ions to ionic NSP systems. It was determined that divalent cations such as Ca^{2+} have greater affinity for the anionic groups on the ionic NSP, followed by K^+ and then Na^+ (Rosett *et al.*, 1995). Therefore, combining Na^+ with Ca^{2+} or K^+ would competitively free the Na^+ and reduce the suppression of saltiness (Rosett *et al.*, 1995). These findings strongly suggest that to achieve maximum saltiness in a thickened food system, a non-ionic NSP or a competitive ion such as potassium or calcium can possibly be incorporated into the formulation (Rosett *et al.*, 1994, 1995).

Sourness and bitterness Cook *et al.* (2002) reported that neither the acidity of citric acid nor the bitterness of quinine hydrochloride was affected by the c* transition in HPMC solution. Interestingly, even though bitter and sweet taste transduction mechanisms share common features, sweetness, but not bitterness, was suppressed at the c* transition in HPMC. It has been suggested that the brain probably relates viscous consistency to the perception of sweetness, but not to sour or bitter tastes, which usually have a thinner mouthfeel (Christensen, 1980). Therefore, when a viscous solution is consumed, the sensory input for viscosity arouses the expectation of sweetness. This psychological element may possibly explain the perceived suppression of sourness and bitterness (Cook *et al.*, 2002).

Savouriness Cook *et al.* (2003) reported that mushroom and garlic flavours (with added sodium chloride) were perceived to be significantly more intense when the concentrations of both λ-carrageenan and HPMC solutions decreased. However, when the sodium chloride concentration in the more viscous sample was increased to 3 g, the garlic flavour intensities of the low and high viscous systems were not significantly different, suggesting a 'perceptual interaction' between salt taste and garlic flavour. *In vivo* aroma release measurements using atmospheric pressure ionization mass spectrometry showed that the NSP concentration did not significantly alter the amount of mushroom or garlic aroma released when the solutions were consumed (Cook *et al.*, 2003). Therefore, the addition of NSP had limited effects on the aroma whereas perceived saltiness drove the reduction in savoury flavour perception (Cook *et al.*, 2003).

Astringency Condensed tannins (polyphenolic compounds) are found naturally in fruits, grains, tea, red wine and beer. These polyphenolic compounds can interact with human salivary protein (proline-rich) in the mouth, involving hydrophobic and hydrogen bonds to form insoluble aggregates/precipitates. These aggregates are believed to be the cause of the sensation of astringency (Bennick, 2002; de Freitas *et al.*, 2003; Soares *et al.*, 2012). The presence of NSPs such as pectin, gum arabic and polygalacturonic acid was reported to inhibit the formation of aggregates but to different degrees. Pectin and polygalacturonic acid are similar in structure and thus are capable of forming a ternary complex of salivary protein–polyphenol–NSP. This complex has enhanced solubility in an aqueous medium and therefore reduces the extent of perceived astringency (McRae and Kennedy, 2011; Soares *et al.*, 2012). Compared with polygalacturonic acid, pectin had a greater effect in reducing astringency as it is more esterified, thus favouring hydrophobic interactions with the hydrophobic polyphenols (Soares *et al.*, 2012). In the case of gum arabic, because of structural differences, the interaction mechanism is different as it competes with the salivary protein for tannin binding instead (Soares *et al.*, 2012). Gum arabic has protein moieties that allow hydrophobic interactions, whereas the charged polysaccharide allows electrostatic and hydrogen bond formation with the polyphenols as well (McRae and Kennedy, 2011; Soares *et al.*, 2012). This NSP–polyphenol interaction can be observed during the fruit ripening process, whereby the astringency of fruits decreases because of the increase in polysaccharide concentration (McRae and Kennedy, 2011). In addition, wine also contains neutral arabinogalactan and pectins, which help to reduce the astringency (Carvalho *et al.*, 2006; McRae and Kennedy, 2011).

8.6 Conclusions

It is evident that much research is still needed to optimize current uses and to explore new applications of NSPs in foods. Current research trends have shown that NSPs do not merely provide thickening, gelling and stabilizing functions. These biomacromolecules from nature have a lot more to offer, as new insights and understanding in the structure–function relation continue to unfold. Improved isolation techniques and new tools to characterize these polymers and their interactions will help to accelerate the process of advancing our knowledge of the functionality of

NSPs. The following are a few areas that are likely to continue to dominate future research in NSPs.

(1) NSPs will continue to play an important role in the assembly and disassembly of food structures at both the nanoscale and the macroscale to facilitate optimum nutrient release and absorption in both humans and animals. Understanding the interactions of NSPs with other food components (e.g. starches) and at interfaces is important in developing foods with improved or customized functionality.
(2) Improved isolation, purification and characterization techniques will continue to provide avenues to obtain better yields of NSPs with the desired functionality.
(3) Modification of existing NSPs using new processing techniques will provide significant opportunities to obtain NSPs with different physicochemical properties.
(4) The biological activities of NSPs from existing, modified or new sources in relation to immunological functions in the human body require further work. This will require a cross-functional approach involving medical professionals, physicists, chemists and other scientists from various fields.

Acknowledgements

The authors thank Dr Claire Woodhall for proofreading this article. The authors also thank Dr Oni Yiliarti and Miss Wenying Lim for the permission to use the pictures in Figure 8.1 and Figure 8.4, respectively.

References

Achayuthakan, P. and Suphantharika, M. (2008). Pasting and rheological properties of waxy corn starch as affected by guar gum and xanthan gum. *Carbohydrate Polymers*, 71 (1), 9–17.

Achayuthakan, P., Suphantharika, M. and Rao, M.A. (2006). Yield stress components of waxy corn starch–xanthan mixtures: effect of xanthan concentration and different starches. *Carbohydrate Polymers*, 65 (4), 469–478.

Ahmed, J. and Ramaswamy, H.S. (2004). Effect of high-hydrostatic pressure and concentration on rheological characteristics of xanthan gum. *Food Hydrocolloids*, 18 (3), 367–373.

Ai, L., Wu, J., Che, N., Wu, Y. and Cui, S.W. (2012). Extraction, partial characterization and bioactivity of polysaccharides from boat-fruited sterculia seeds. *International Journal of Biological Macromolecules*, 51 (5), 815–818.

Amid, B.T. and Mirhosseini, H. (2012). Optimisation of aqueous extraction of gum from durian (*Durio zibethinus*) seed: a potential, low cost source of hydrocolloid. *Food Chemistry*, 132 (3), 1258–1268.

Amid, B.T. and Mirhosseini, H. (2013). Shear flow behaviour and emulsion-stabilizing effect of natural polysaccharide-protein gum in aqueous system and oil/water (O/W) emulsion. *Colloids and Surfaces B: Biointerfaces*, 103, 430–440.

Amid, B.T., Mirhosseini, H. and Kostadinovi, S. (2012). Chemical composition and molecular structure of polysaccharide-protein biopolymer from Durio zibethinus seed: extraction and purification process. *Chemistry Central Journal*, 6 (3), 117–130.

Amin, A.M. and Arshad, R. (2009). Proximate composition and pasting properties of durian (Durio zibethinus) seed flour. *International Journal of Postharvest Technology and Innovation*, 1 (4), 367–375.

Amin, A.M., Ahmad, A.S., Yin, Y.Y., Yahya, N. and Ibrahim, N. (2007). Extraction, purification and characterization of durian (*Durio zibethinus*) seed gum. *Food Hydrocolloids*, 21 (2), 273–279.

Amiza, M.A., Aziz, Y., Ong, B.C., Wong, V.L. and Pang, A.M. (2004). *CHIEF: cheap high fibre flour from local fruit seed.* Paper presented at Expo Science, Technology and Innovation, 2004. PWTC. Kuala Lumpur, 27–29 August 2004.

Appelqvist, I.A.M. and Debet, M.R.M. (1997). Starch-biopolymer interactions – a review. *Food Reviews International*, 13 (2), 163–224.

Arkarapanthu, A., Chavasit, V., Sungpuag, P. and Phuphathanaphong, L. (2005). Gel extracted from Khruea-ma-noi (Cyclea barbata Miers) leaves: chemical composition and gelation properties. *Journal of the Science of Food and Agriculture*, 85 (10), 1741–1749.

Bahramparvar, M., Haddad Khodaparast, M.H. and Razavi, S.M. (2009). The effect of Lallemantia royleana (Balangu) seed, palmate-tuber salep and carboxymethylcellulose gums on the physicochemical and sensory properties of typical soft ice cream. *International Journal of Dairy Technology*, 62 (4), 571–576.

Bahramparvar, M., Razavi, S.M. and Mazaheri Tehrani, M. (2012). Optimising the ice cream formulation using basil seed gum (Ocimum basilicum L.) as a novel stabiliser to deliver improved processing quality. *International Journal of Food Science and Technology*, 47 (12), 2655–2661.

Baines, Z.V. and Morris, E.R. (1987). Flavour/taste perception in thickened systems: the effect of guar gum above and below c*. *Food Hydrocolloids*, 1 (3), 197–205.

Baldaro, E., Gallucci, M., Formantici, C. *et al.* (2012). Enzymatic improvement of guar-based thickener for better-quality silk screen printing. *Coloration Technology*, 128 (4), 315–322.

BeMiller, J. (2001). Classification, structure, and chemistry of polysaccharides of foods, in: *Handbook of Dietary Fiber* (eds S.S. Cho and M. Dreher), Chapter 31. Marcel Dekker, New York, NY, pp. 604–611.

BeMiller, J.N. (2011). Pasting, paste, and gel properties of starch-hydrocolloid combinations. *Carbohydrate Polymers*, 86 (2), 386–423.

Bennick, A. (2002). Interaction of plant polyphenols with salivary proteins. *Critical Reviews in Oral Biology and Medicine*, 13 (2), 184–196.

Berth, G., Dautzenberg, H. and Peter, M.G. (1998). Physico-chemical characterization of chitosans varying in degree of acetylation. *Carbohydrate Polymers*, 36 (2–3), 205–216.

Bigikocin, E., Mert, B. and Alpas, H. (2011). Effect of high hydrostatic pressure and high dynamic pressure on stability and rheological properties of model oil-in-water emulsions. *High Pressure Research*, 31 (3), 462–474.

Bongaerts, K., Paoletti, S., Denef, B. *et al.* (2000). Light scattering investigation of ι-carrageenan aqueous solutions. Concentration dependence of association. *Macromolecules*, 33 (23), 8709–8719.

Brennan, C.S., Blake, D.E., Ellis, P.R. and Schofield, J.D. (1996). Effects of guar galactomannan on wheat bread microstructure and on the in vitro and in vivo digestibility of starch in bread. *Journal of Cereal Science*, 24 (2), 151–160.

Brooker, S.G., Cambie, R.C. and Cooper, R.C. (1987). *New Zealand Medicinal Plants.* Reed Publishing (NZ) Ltd, Auckland.

Brummer, Y., Cui, W. and Wang, Q. (2003). Extraction, purification and physicochemical characterization of fenugreek gum. *Food Hydrocolloids*, 17 (3), 229–236.

Carvalho, E., Mateus, N., Plet, B. *et al.* (2006). Influence of wine pectic polysaccharides on the interactions between condensed tannins and salivary proteins. *Journal of Agricultural and Food Chemistry*, 54 (23), 8936–8944.

Chao, S.J. and Lai, L.S. (1999). Effects of salt on the gelling behavior of hsian-tsao (*Mesona procumbens* Hemsl) leaf gum as studied using rapid-visco analyzer. *Food Science (Taiwan)*, 26 (2), 228–239.

Chen, C.H., Kuo, W.S. and Lai, L.S. (2009). Rheological and physical characterization of film-forming solutions and edible films from tapioca starch/decolorized hsian-tsao leaf gum. *Food Hydrocolloids*, 23 (8), 2132–2140.

Chenlo, F., Moreira, R., Pereira, G. and Silva, C. (2009). Rheological modelling of binary and ternary systems of tragacanth, guar gum and methylcellulose in dilute range of concentration at different temperatures. *LWT – Food Science and Technology*, 42 (2), 519–524.

Chiu, C.J., Liu, S., Willett, W.C. *et al.* (2011). Informing food choices and health outcomes by use of the dietary glycemic index. *Nutrition Reviews*, 69 (4), 231–242.

Christensen, C.M. (1980). Effects of taste quality and intensity on oral perception of viscosity. *Perception and Psychophysics*, 28 (4), 315–320.

Cook, D.J., Hollowood, T.A., Linforth, R.S.T. and Taylor, A.J. (2002). Perception of taste intensity in solutions of random-coil polysaccharides above and below c*. *Food Quality and Preference*, 13 (7–8), 473–480.

Cook, D.J., Linforth, R.S.T. and Taylor, A.J. (2003). Effects of hydrocolloid thickeners on the perception of savory flavors. *Journal of Agricultural and Food Chemistry*, 51 (10), 3067–3072.

Corredig, M., Kerr, W. and Wicker, L. (2000). Molecular characterization of commercial pectins by separation with linear mix gel permeation columns in-line with multi-angle light scattering detection. *Food Hydrocolloids*, 14 (1), 41–47.

Corredig, M., Sharafbafi, N. and Kristo, E. (2011). Polysaccharide-protein interactions in dairy matrices, control and design of structures. *Food Hydrocolloids*, 25 (8), 1833–1841.

Coviello, T., Kajiwara, K., Burchard, W., Dentini, M. and Crescenzi, V. (1986). Solution properties of xanthan. 1. Dynamic and static light scattering from native and modified xanthans in dilute solutions. *Macromolecules*, 19 (11), 2826–2831.

Cui, S. and Wang, Q. (2005). Understanding the physical properties of food polysaccharides. In: *Food Carbohydrates: Chemistry, Physical Properties, and Applications* (Cui, S.W. ed.), Chapter 4. CRC Press, Boca Raton, FL, pp. 161–218.

Daou, C. and Zhang, H. (2012). Oat beta-glucan: its role in health promotion and prevention of diseases. *Comprehensive Reviews in Food Science and Food Safety*, 11 (4), 355–365.

De Silva, D.D., Rapior, S., Fons, F., Bahkali, A.H. and Hyde, K.D. (2012). Medicinal mushrooms in supportive cancer therapies: an approach to anti-cancer effects and putative mechanisms of action. *Fungal Diversity*, 55 (1), 1–35.

Delgado-Vargas, F., Jiménez, A.R., Paredes-López, O. and Francis, F.J. (2000). Natural pigments: carotenoids, anthocyanins, and betalains—characteristics, biosynthesis, processing, and stability. *Critical Reviews in Food Science and Nutrition*, 40 (3), 173–289.

Dickinson, E. (2003). Hydrocolloids at interfaces and the influence on the properties of dispersed systems. *Food Hydrocolloids*, 17 (1), 25–39.

Dickinson, E. (2006). Colloid science of mixed ingredients. *Soft Matter*, 2 (8), 642–652.

Dickinson, E., Radford, S.J. and Golding, M. (2003). Stability and rheology of emulsions containing sodium caseinate: combined effects of ionic calcium and non-ionic surfactant. *Food Hydrocolloids*, 17 (2), 211–220.

Doublier, J.L., Garnier, C., Renard, D. and Sanchez, C. (2000). Protein–polysaccharide interactions. *Current Opinion in Colloid & Interface Science*, 5 (3–4), 202–214.

Eidam, D., Kulicke, W.-M., Kuhn, K. and Stute, R. (1995). Formation of maize starch gels selectively regulated by the addition of hydrocolloids. *Starch – Stärke*, 47 (10), 378–384.

El Ghzaoui, A., Trompette, J.L., Cassanas, G., Bardet, L. and Fabregue, E. (2001). Comparative rheological behavior of some cellulosic ether derivatives. *Langmuir*, 17 (5), 1453–1456.

Ellis, P.R., Roberts, F.G., Low, A.G. and Morgan, L.M. (1995). The effect of high-molecular-weight guar gum on net apparent glucose absorption and net apparent insulin and gastric inhibitory polypeptide production in the growing pig: relationship to rheological changes in jejunal digesta. *British Journal of Nutrition*, 74 (4), 539–556.

Ellis, P.R., Wang, Q., Rayment, P., Ren, Y. and Ross-Murphy, S.B. (2001). Guar gum, in *Handbook of Dietary Fiber* (eds S.S. Cho and M. Dreher), Chapter 32. Marcel Dekker, New York, NY, pp. 612–657.

Englyst, H.N. and Hudson, G.J. (1996). The classification and measurement of dietary carbohydrates. *Food Chemistry*, 57 (1), 15–21.

Feng, T., Gu, Z., Jin, Z. and Zhuang, H. (2010). Rheological properties of rice starch–Mesona blumes gum mixtures. *Journal of Texture Studies*, 41 (5), 685–702.

Fernandes, P.B. and Raemy, A. (1996). High pressure treatment of whey protein/ polysaccharide systems. In:Progress in Biotechnology, Volume 13, *High Pressure Bioscience and Biotechnology* (Hayashi, R. and Balny, C. eds), pp. 337–342. Elsevier Science, Amsterdam.

Floury, J., Desrumaux, A., Axelos, M.A.V. and Legrand, J. (2002). Degradation of methylcellulose during ultra-high pressure homogenisation. *Food Hydrocolloids*, 16 (1), 47–53.

Freitas, R.A., Martin, S., Santos, G.L. *et al.* (2005). Physicochemical properties of seed xyloglucans from different sources. *Carbohydrate Polymers*, 60 (4), 507–514.

de Freitas, V., Carvalho, E. and Mateus, N. (2003). Study of carbohydrate influence on protein-tannin aggregation by nephelometry. *Food Chemistry*, 81 (4), 503–509.

Fuchigami, M. and Teramoto, A. (2003). Changes in temperature and structure of agar gel as affected by sucrose during high-pressure freezing. *Journal of Food Science*, 68 (2), 528–533.

Fuchigami, M., Teramoto, A. and Jibu, Y. (2006). Texture and structure of pressure-shift-frozen agar gel with high visco-elasticity. *Food Hydrocolloids*, 20 (2–3), 160–169.

Funami, T., Kataoka, Y., Omoto, T. *et al.* (2005a). Effects of non-ionic polysaccharides on the gelatinization and retrogradation behavior of wheat starch. *Food Hydrocolloids*, 19 (1), 1–13.

Funami, T., Kataoka, Y., Omoto, T. *et al.* (2005b). Food hydrocolloids control the gelatinization and retrogradation behavior of starch. 2a. Functions of guar gums with different molecular weights on the gelatinization behavior of corn starch. *Food Hydrocolloids*, 19 (1), 15–24.

Gaisford, S.E., Harding, S.E., Mitchell, J.R. and Bradley, T.D. (1986). A comparison between the hot and cold water soluble fractions of two locust bean gum samples. *Carbohydrate Polymers*, 6 (6), 423–442.

Galazka, V.B., Dickinson, E. and Ledward, D.A. (2001). Influence of high pressure processing on protein-polysaccharide interactions in emulsions, in *Food Colloids: Fundamentals of Formulation* (eds E. Dickinson and R. Miller). Royal Society of Chemistry, Cambridge, pp. 315–322.

Gidley, M.J., Lillford, P.J., Rowlands, D.W. *et al.* (1991). Structure and solution properties of tamarind-seed polysaccharide. *Carbohydrate Research*, 214 (2), 299–314.

Goh, K.K.T., Haisman, D.R. and Singh, H. (2006). Characterisation of a high acyl gellan polysaccharide using light scattering and rheological techniques. *Food Hydrocolloids*, 20 (2–3 Special Issue), 176–183.

Goh, K.K.T., Matia-Merino, L., Hall, C.E., Moughan, P.J. and Singh, H. (2007). Complex rheological properties of a water-soluble extract from the fronds of the black tree fern, *Cyathea medullaris*. *Biomacromolecules*, 8 (11), 3414–3421.

Goh, K.K.T., Sarkar, A. and Singh, H. (2009). Milk protein-polysaccharide interactions, in *Milk Proteins: from Expression to Food* (eds A. Thompson, M. Boland and H. Singh). Elsevier, New York, NY, pp. 347–376.

Goh, K.K.T., Matia-Merino, L., Pinder, D.N., Saavedra, C. and Singh, H. (2011). Molecular characteristics of a novel water-soluble polysaccharide from the New Zealand black tree fern (*Cyathea medullaris*). *Food Hydrocolloids*, 25 (3), 286–292.

Gómez, C., Navarro, A., Manzanares, P., Horta, A. and Carbonell, J.V. (1997). Physical and structural properties of barley (1→3), (1→4)-β-D-glucan. Part I. Determination of molecular weight and macromolecular radius by light scattering. *Carbohydrate Polymers*, 32 (1), 7–15.

Gralén, N. and Kärrholm, M. (1950). The physicochemical properties of solutions of gum tragacanth. *Journal of Colloid Science*, 5 (1), 21--36.

Green, C.J. (2000). Fiber in enteral nutrition. *South African Journal of Clinical Nutrition*, 13 (4), 150–160.

Han, Z., Zeng, X.A., Fu, N., Yu, S.J., Chen, X.D. and Kennedy, J.F. (2012). Effects of pulsed electric field treatments on some properties of tapioca starch. *Carbohydrate Polymers*, 89 (4), 1012–1017.

Harding, S.E., Day, K., Dhami, R. and Lowe, P.M. (1997). Further observations on the size, shape and hydration of kappa-carrageenan in dilute solution. *Carbohydrate Polymers*, 32 (2), 81–87.

Hemar, Y., Tamehana, M., Munro, P.A. and Singh, H. (2001a). Influence of xanthan gum on the formation and stability of sodium caseinate oil-in-water emulsions. *Food Hydrocolloids*, 15 (4–6), 513–519.

Hemar, Y., Tamehana, M., Munro, P.A. and Singh, H. (2001b). Viscosity, microstructure and phase behavior of aqueous mixtures of commercial milk protein products and xanthan gum. *Food Hydrocolloids*, 15 (4–6), 565–574.

Hoagland, P.D., Fishman, M.L., Konja, G. and Clauss, E. (1993). Size exclusion chromatography with viscosity detection of complex polysaccharides: component analysis. *Journal of Agricultural and Food Chemistry*, 41 (8), 1274–1281.

Hoefler, A.C. (2004). *Hydrocolloids: Practical Guides for the Food Industry*. American Association of Cereal Chemists, St. Paul, MN.

Hollowood, T.A., Linforth, R.S.T. and Taylor, A.J. (2002). The effect of viscosity on the perception of flavour. *Chemical Senses*, 27 (7), 583–591.

Hosseini-Parvar, S.H., Matia-Merino, L., Goh, K.K.T., Razavi, S.M.A. and Mortazavi, S.A. (2010). Steady shear flow behavior of gum extracted from *Ocimum basilicum* L. seed: effect of concentration and temperature. *Journal of Food Engineering*, 101 (3), 236–243.

Hubbermann, E.M., Heins, A., Stöckmann, H. and Schwarz, K. (2006). Influence of acids, salt, sugars and hydrocolloids on the colour stability of anthocyanin rich black currant and elderberry concentrates. *European Food Research and Technology*, 223 (1), 83–90.

Idris, O.H.M., Williams, P.A. and Phillips, G.O. (1998). Characterisation of gum from *Acacia senegal* trees of different age and location using multidetection gel permeation chromatography. *Food Hydrocolloids*, 12 (4), 379–388.

Izydorczyk, M., Cui, S. and Wang, Q. (2005). Polysaccharide gums: structures, functional properties, and applications, in *Food Carbohydrates* (ed. S.W., Cui). CRC Press, Boca Raton, FL, pp. 263–307.

Jacon, S.A., Rao, M.A., Cooley, H.J. and Walter, R.H. (1993). The isolation and characterization of a water extract of konjac flour gum. *Carbohydrate Polymers*, 20 (1), 35–41.

Jahanbin, K., Gohari, A.R., Moini, S., Emam-Djomeh, Z. and Masi, P. (2011). Isolation, structural characterization and antioxidant activity of a new water-soluble polysaccharide from *Acanthophyllum bracteatum* roots. *International Journal of Biological Macromolecules*, 49 (4), 567–572.

Jahanbin, K., Moini, S., Gohari, A.R., Emam-Djomeh, Z. and Masi, P. (2012). Isolation, purification and characterization of a new gum from *Acanthophyllum bracteatum* roots. *Food Hydrocolloids*, 27 (1), 14–21.

Jiang, J.X., Zhu, L.W., Zhang, W.M. and Sun, R.C. (2007). Characterization of galactomannan gum from fenugreek (*Trigonella foenum-graecum*) seeds and its rheological properties. *International Journal of Polymeric Materials*, 56 (12), 1145–1154.

Jones, O.G. and McClements, D.J. (2011). Recent progress in biopolymer nanoparticle and microparticle formation by heat-treating electrostatic protein-polysaccharide complexes. *Advances in Colloid and Interface Science*, 167 (1–2), 49–62.

Karazhiyan, H., Razavi, S.M.A., Phillips, G.O. *et al.* (2009). Rheological properties of *Lepidium sativum* seed extract as a function of concentration, temperature and time. *Food Hydrocolloids*, 23 (8), 2062–2068.

Karazhiyan, H., Razavi, S.M.A. and Phillips, G.O. (2011). Extraction optimization of a hydrocolloid extract from cress seed (*Lepidium sativum*) using response surface methodology. *Food Hydrocolloids*, 25 (5), 915–920.

Kasaai, M.R., Arul, J. and Charlet, G. (2008). Fragmentation of chitosan by ultrasonic irradiation. *Ultrasonics Sonochemistry*, 15 (6), 1001–1008.

Kaur, L., Singh, J. and Singh, H. (2009). Characterization of gum ghatti (Anogeissus latifolia): a structural and rheological approach. *Journal of Food Science*, 74 (6), E328–E332.

Khounvilay, K. and Sittikijyothin, W. (2012). Rheological behaviour of tamarind seed gum in aqueous solutions. *Food Hydrocolloids*, 26 (2), 334–338.

Kivelä, R., Pitkänen, L., Laine, P., Aseyev, V. and Sontag-Strohm, T. (2010). Influence of homogenisation on the solution properties of oat β-glucan. *Food Hydrocolloids*, 24 (6–7), 611–618.

Koocheki, A. and Kadkhodaee, R. (2011). Effect of *Alyssum homolocarpum* seed gum, Tween 80 and NaCl on droplets characteristics, flow properties and physical stability of ultrasonically prepared corn oil-in-water emulsions. *Food Hydrocolloids*, 25 (5), 1149–1157.

Koocheki, A., Kadkhodaee, R., Mortazavi, S.A., Shahidi, F. and Taherian, A.R. (2009a). Influence of *Alyssum homolocarpum* seed gum on the stability and flow properties of O/W emulsion prepared by high intensity ultrasound. *Food Hydrocolloids*, 23 (8), 2416–2424.

Koocheki, A., Mortazavi, S.A., Shahidi, F., Razavi, S.M.A. and Taherian, A.R. (2009b). Rheological properties of mucilage extracted from *Alyssum homolocarpum* seed as a new source of thickening agent. *Journal of Food Engineering*, 91 (3), 490–496.

Koocheki, A., Razavi, S.M.A. and Hesarinejad, M.A. (2012). Effect of extraction procedures on functional properties of *Eruca sativa* seed mucilage. *Food Biophysics*, 7 (1), 84–92.

de Kruif, C.G. and Tuinier, R. (2001). Polysaccharide protein interactions. *Food Hydrocolloids*, 15 (4–6), 555–563.

Kumar, C.S. and Bhattacharya, S. (2008). Tamarind seed: properties, processing and utilization. *Critical Reviews in Food Science and Nutrition*, 48 (1), 1–20.

Kumar, R., Rajarajeshwari, N. and Narayana Swamy, V.B. (2012a). *Borassus flabellifer* fruit mucilage: potential biodegradable carrier for colon specific drug delivery. *International Journal of Pharmacy and Pharmaceutical Sciences*, 4 (4), 522–531.

Kumar, R., Rajarajeshwari, N. and Narayana Swamy, V.B. (2012b). Exploitation of *Borassus flabellifer* fruit mucilage as novel natural gelling agent. *Der Pharmacia Lettre*, 4 (4), 1202–1213.

Kumar, V., Sinha, A.K., Makkar, H.P.S., de Boeck, G. and Becker, K. (2012c). Dietary roles of non-starch polysaccharides in human nutrition: a review. *Critical Reviews in Food Science and Nutrition*, 52 (10), 899–935.

Lagoueyte, N. and Paquin, P. (1998). Effects of microfluidization on the functional properties of xanthan gum. *Food Hydrocolloids*, 12 (3), 365–371.

Lai, L.S. and Chiang, H.F. (2002). Rheology of decolorized hsian-tsao leaf gum in the dilute domain. *Food Hydrocolloids*, 16 (5), 427–440.

Lai, L.S. and Liao, C.L. (2002). Steady and dynamic shear rheological properties of starch and decolorized hsian-tsao leaf gum composite systems. *Cereal Chemistry*, 79 (1), 58–63.

Lai, L.S., Tung, J. and Lin, P S. (2000). Solution properties of hsian-tsao (*Mesona procumbens* Hemsl) leaf gum. *Food Hydrocolloids*, 14 (4), 287–294.

Launay, B., Cuvelier, G. and Martinez-Reyes, S. (1998). Viscosity of locust bean, guar and xanthan gum solutions in the Newtonian domain: a critical examination of the log (ηsp)o-log C[η]o master curves. *Carbohydrate Polymers*, 34 (4), 385–395.

Lazaridou, A., Biliaderis, C.G. and Izydorczyk, M.S. (2001). Structural characteristics and rheological properties of locust bean galactomannans: a comparison of samples from different carob tree populations. *Journal of the Science of Food and Agriculture*, 81 (1), 68–75.

Le Cerf, D., Irinei, F. and Muller, G. (1990). Solution properties of gum exudates from *Sterculia urens* (Karaya gum). *Carbohydrate Polymers*, 13 (4), 375–386.

Lemmens, R.H.M.J. and Horsten, S.F.A.J. (1999). *Cyclea barbata* MiersIn, in *Plant Resources of South-East Asia*, No. 12 (1), *Medicinal and Poisonous Plants* (eds L.S. de Padua, N. Bunyapraphatsara and R.H.M. J. Lemmens). Backhuys Publishers, Leiden, pp. 221–222.

Li, W., Cui, S.W. and Wang, Q. (2006). Solution and conformational properties of wheat β-D-glucans studied by light scattering and viscometry. *Biomacromolecules*, 7 (2), 446–452.

Li, Q., Qi, W., Su, R. and He, Z. (2009). Preparation and characterization of enzyme-modified konjac glucomannan/xanthan blend films. *Journal of Biomaterials Science, Polymer Edition*, 20 (3), 299–310.

Li, X., Al-Assaf, S., Fang, Y. and Phillips, G.O. (2013). Characterisation of commercial LM-pectin in aqueous solution. *Carbohydrate Polymers*, 92 (2), 1133–1142.

Lim, W.Y. (2010). Screening and partial characterisation of novel stabilisers from plant sources in Asia. Bachelor of Food Technology Honours Year Thesis. Massey University, Palmerston North.

Lin, K.Y., Daniel, J.R. and Whistler, R.L. (1994). Structure of chia seed polysaccharide exudate. *Carbohydrate Polymers*, 23 (1), 13–18.

Lindblad, M.S. and Albertsson, A.-C. (2004). Chemical modification of hemicelluloses and gums, in *Polysaccharides: Structural Diversity and Functional Versatility*, 2nd edn (ed S. Dumitriu). CRC Press, Boca Raton, FL, pp. 491–508.

Liu, H., Eskin, N.A.M. and Cui, S.W. (2003). Interaction of wheat and rice starches with yellow mustard mucilage. *Food Hydrocolloids*, 17 (6), 863–869.

Luo, W.B., Han, Z., Zeng, X.A., Yu, S.J. and Kennedy, J.F. (2010). Study on the degradation of chitosan by pulsed electric fields treatment. *Innovative Food Science & Emerging Technologies*, 11 (4), 587–591.

Ma, S. and Wang, Z.-H. (2013). Pulsed electric field-assisted modification of pectin from sugar beet pulp. *Carbohydrate Polymers*, 92 (2), 1700–1704.

MacDougall, A.J. and Ring, S.G. (2003). Pectic polysaccharides, in *Chemical and Functional Properties of Food Saccharides* (ed. P. Tomasik), Chapter 12. CRC Press, Boca Raton, FL, pp. 181–195.

Mahammad, S., Comfort, D.A., Kelly, R.M. and Khan, S.A. (2007). Rheological properties of guar galactomannan solutions during hydrolysis with galactomannanase and alpha-galactosidase enzyme mixtures. *Biomacromolecules*, 8 (3), 949–956.

Mahungu, S.M. and Meyland, I. (2008). Cassia gum, chemical and technical assessment (CTA). http://www.fao.org/fileadmin/templates/agns/pdf/jecfa/cta/71/cassia-gum.pdf [accessed 15 July 2013].

Maiani, G., Castón, M.J.P., Catasta, G. *et al.* (2009). Carotenoids: actual knowledge on food sources, intakes, stability and bioavailability and their protective role in humans. *Molecular Nutrition and Food Research*, 53 (Suppl. 2), 194–218.

Maier, T., Fromm, M., Schieber, A., Kammerer, D.R. and Carle, R. (2009). Process and storage stability of anthocyanins and non-anthocyanin phenolics in pectin and gelatin gels enriched with grape pomace extracts. *European Food Research and Technology*, 229 (6), 949–960.

Mälkki, Y., Heiniö, R.L. and Autio, K. (1993). Influence of oat gum, guar gum and carboxymethyl cellulose on the perception of sweetness and flavour. *Food Hydrocolloids*, 6 (6), 525–532.

Mao, C.F., Zeng, Y.C. and Chen, C.H. (2012). Enzyme-modified guar gum/xanthan gelation: an analysis based on cascade model. *Food Hydrocolloids*, 27 (1), 50–59.

Mason, T.J. and Lorimer, J.P. (2002). *Applied Sonochemistry: The Uses of Power Ultrasound in Chemistry and Processing*. Wiley-VCH, Weinheim.

Mathur, N.K. (2011a). Derivatization of polysaccharides, in *Industrial Galactomannan Polysaccharides*. CRC Press, Boca Raton, FL, pp. 49–60.

Mathur, N.K. (2011b). Locust bean gum, or carob gum, in *Industrial Galactomannan Polysaccharides*. CRC Press, Boca Raton, FL, pp. 93–114.

Matia-Merino, L., Goh, K.K.T. and Singh, H. (2012). A natural shear-thickening water-soluble polymer from the fronds of the black tree fern, *Cyathea medullaris*: influence of salt, pH and temperature. *Carbohydrate Polymers*, 87 (1), 131–138.

McRae, J.M. and Kennedy, J.A. (2011). Wine and grape tannin interactions with salivary proteins and their impact on astringency: a review of current research. *Molecules*, 16 (3), 2348–2364.

Michel, M. and Autio, K. (2002). Effects of high pressure on protein- and polysaccharide-based structures. In: *Ultra High Pressure Treatments of Foods* (Hendrickx, M.E.G. and Knorr, D., eds), pp. 189–214. Kluwer Academic/Plenum Publishers, New York, NY.

Min-Feng, L., Meng, I.K., Chin-Fung, L. and Cheng-Yi, L. (1996). Ultrasonication and heat effects on the chemical and gelling properties of red algal polysaccharides. *Food Science, Taiwan*, 23 (5), 717–729.

Miyazaki, Y., Yakou, S. and Takayama, K. (2004). Study on jelly fig extract as a potential hydrophilic matrix for controlled drug delivery. *International Journal of Pharmaceutics*, 287 (1–2), 39–46.

Moghaddam, T.M., Razavi, S.M.A. and Emadzadeh, B. (2011). Rheological interactions between *Lallemantia royleana* seed extract and selected food hydrocolloids. *Journal of the Science of Food and Agriculture*, 91 (6), 1083–1088.

Mohammad Amini, A. and Razavi, S.M.A. (2012). Dilute solution properties of Balangu (*Lallemantia royleana*) seed gum: effect of temperature, salt, and sugar. *International Journal of Biological Macromolecules*, 51 (3), 235–243.

Mohammadifar, M.A., Musavi, S.M., Kiumarsi, A. and Williams, P.A. (2006). Solution properties of targacanthin (water-soluble part of gum tragacanth exudate from *Astragalus gossypinus*). *International Journal of Biological Macromolecules*, 38 (1), 31–39.

Mudgil, D., Barak, S. and Khatkar, B.S. (2012). Effect of enzymatic depolymerization on physicochemical and rheological properties of guar gum. *Carbohydrate Polymers*, 90 (1), 224–228.

Muñoz, L.A., Cobos, A., Diaz, O. and Aguilera, J.M. (2012). Chia seeds: microstructure, mucilage extraction and hydration. *Journal of Food Engineering*, 108 (1), 216–224.

Naji, S., Razavi, S.M.A., Karazhiyan, H. and Koocheki, A. (2012). Influence of thermal treatments on textural characteristics of cress seed (*Lepidium sativum*) gum gel. *Electronic Journal of Environmental, Agricultural and Food Chemistry*, 11 (3), 222–237.

Nakata, M., Kawaguchi, T., Kodama, Y. and Konno, A. (1998). Characterization of curdlan in aqueous sodium hydroxide. *Polymer*, 39 (6–7), 1475–1481.

Nickerson, M.T., Paulson, A.T. and Hallett, F.R. (2004). Dilute solution properties of κ-carrageenan polysaccharides: effect of potassium and calcium ions on chain conformation. *Carbohydrate Polymers*, 58 (1), 25–33.

Norton, I.T., Goodall, D.M., Morris, E.R. and Rees, D.A. (1983). Role of cations in the conformation of iota and kappa carrageenan. *Journal of the Chemical Society, Faraday Transactions 1: Physical Chemistry in Condensed Phases*, 79 (10), 2475–2488.

Oosterveld, A., Beldman, G., Searle-van Leeuwen, M.J.F. and Voragen, A.G.J. (2000). Effect of enzymatic deacetylation on gelation of sugar beet pectin in the presence of calcium. *Carbohydrate Polymers*, 43 (3), 249–256.

Oosterveld, A., Beldman, G. and Voragen, A.G.J. (2002). Enzymatic modification of pectic polysaccharides obtained from sugar beet pulp. *Carbohydrate Polymers*, 48 (1), 73–81.

Pai, V.B. and Khan, S.A. (2002). Gelation and rheology of xanthan/enzyme-modified guar blends. *Carbohydrate Polymers*, 49 (2), 207–216.

Panteloglou, A.G., Bell, A.E. and Ma, F. (2010). Effect of high-hydrostatic pressure and pH on the rheological properties of gum arabic. *Food Chemistry*, 122 (4), 972–979.

Patel, T.R., Morris, G.A., Ebringerová, A. *et al.* (2008). Global conformation analysis of irradiated xyloglucans. *Carbohydrate Polymers*, 74 (4), 845–851.

de Paula, R.C.M., Heatley, F. and Budd, P.M. (1998). Characterization of *Anacardiumo ccidentale* exudate polysaccharide. *Polymer International*, 45 (1), 27–35.

de Paula, R.C.M. and Rodrigues, J.F. (1995). Composition and rheological properties of cashew tree gum, the exudate polysaccharide from *Anacardium occidentale* L. *Carbohydrate Polymers*, 26 (3), 177–181.

Persin, Z., Stana-Kleinschek, K., Foster, T.J. *et al.* (2011). Challenges and opportunities in polysaccharides research and technology: the EPNOE views for the next decade in the areas of materials, food and health care. *Carbohydrate Polymers*, 84 (1), 22–32.

Picout, D.R., Ross-Murphy, S.B., Errington, N. and Harding, S.E. (2001). Pressure cell assisted solution characterization of polysaccharides. 1. Guar gum. *Biomacromolecules*, 2 (4), 1301–1309.

Picout, D.R., Ross-Murphy, S.B., Jumel, K. and Harding, S.E. (2002). Pressure cell assisted solution characterization of polysaccharides. 2. Locust bean gum and tara gum. *Biomacromolecules*, 3 (4), 761–767.

Plashchina, I.G., Semenova, M.G., Braudo, E.E. and Tolstoguzov, V.B. (1985). Structural studies of the solutions of anionic polysaccharides. IV. Study of pectin solutions by light-scattering. *Carbohydrate Polymers*, 5 (3), 159–179.

Ramsden, L. (2003). Plant and algal gums and mucilages, in *Chemical and Functional Properties of Food Saccharides* (ed. P. Tomasik), Chapter 15. CRC Press, Boca Raton, FL, pp. 231–254.

Ramu, G., Mohan, G.K. and Jayaveera, K. (2011). Preliminary investigation of patchaippasali mucilage (*Basella alba*) as tablet binder. *International Journal of Green Pharmacy*, 5 (1), 24–27.

Rastogi, N.K. (2011). Opportunities and challenges in application of ultrasound in food processing. *Critical Reviews in Food Science and Nutrition*, 51 (8), 705–722.

Rastogi, N.K., Raghavarao, K.S.M.S., Balasubramaniam, V.M., Niranjan, K. and Knorr, D. (2007). Opportunities and challenges in high pressure processing of foods. *Critical Reviews in Food Science and Nutrition*, 47 (1), 69–112.

Ratcliffe, I., Williams, P.A., Viebke, C. and Meadows, J. (2005). Physicochemical characterization of konjac glucomannan. *Biomacromolecules*, 6 (4), 1977–1986.

Razavi, S.M.A., Bostan, A. and Rahbari, R. (2010). Computer image analysis and physico-mechanical properties of wild sage seed (*Salvia macrosiphon*). *International Journal of Food Properties*, 13 (2), 308–316.

Razavi, S.M.A., Taheri, H. and Quinchia, L.A. (2011). Steady shear flow properties of wild sage (*Salvia macrosiphon*) seed gum as a function of concentration and temperature. *Food Hydrocolloids*, 25 (3), 451–458.

Razavi, S.M.A., Moghaddam, T.M., Emadzadeh, B. and Salehi, F. (2012). Dilute solution properties of wild sage (*Salvia macrosiphon*) seed gum. *Food Hydrocolloids*, 29 (1), 205–210.

Ren, L., Perera, C. and Hemar, Y. (2012). Antitumor activity of mushroom polysaccharides: a review. *Food & Function*, 3 (11), 1118–1130.

Rochas, C. and Lahaye, M. (1989). Average molecular weight and molecular weight distribution of agarose and agarose-type polysaccharides. *Carbohydrate Polymers*, 10 (4), 289–298.

Rodriguez Patino, J.M. and Pilosof, A.M.R. (2011). Protein-polysaccharide interactions at fluid interfaces. *Food Hydrocolloids*, 25 (8), 1925–1937.

Ronkart, S.N., Paquot, M., Deroanne, C. *et al.* (2010). Development of gelling properties of inulin by microfluidization. *Food Hydrocolloids*, 24 (4), 318–324.

Rosett, T.R., Shirley, L., Schmidt, S.J. and Klein, B.P. (1994). Na^+ binding as measured by ^{23}Na nuclear magnetic resonance spectroscopy influences the perception of saltiness in gum solutions. *Journal of Food Science*, 59 (1), 206–210.

Rosett, T.R., Wu, Z., Schmidt, S.J., Ennis, D.M. and Klein, B.P. (1995). KCI, $CaCI_2$, Na^+ binding, and salt taste of gum systems. *Journal of Food Science*, 60 (4), 849–853.

Sakai, E., Katayama, T., Ogasawara, T. and Mizuno, M. (2013). Identification of *Anogeissus latifolia* Wallich and analysis of refined gum ghatti. *Journal of Natural Medicines*, 67 (2), 276–280.

Sasaki, T. and Kohyama, K. (2012). Influence of non-starch polysaccharides on the *in vitro* digestibility and viscosity of starch suspensions. *Food Chemistry*, 133 (4), 1420–1426.

Sato, M. and Ohshima, T. (2006). Applications of high-voltage pulsed electric field in bioprocesses. Paper presented at Asia-Pacific International Symposium on Air and Water Treatment by Green Oxidation/Reduction Technologies, Dalian, China.

Sato, A.C.K., Oliveira, P.R. and Cunha, R.L. (2008). Rheology of mixed pectin solutions. *Food Biophysics*, 3 (1), 100–109.

Schmitt, C. and Turgeon, S.L. (2011). Protein/polysaccharide complexes and coacervates in food systems. *Advances in Colloid and Interface Science*, 167 (1–2), 63–70.

Schmitt, C., Aberkane, L. and Sanchez, C. (2009). Protein-polysaccharide complexes and coacervates, in *Handbook of Hydrocolloids*, 2nd edn (eds G.O. Phillipsand P.A. Williams), Chapter 16. Woodhead Publishing, Cambridge, pp. 420–476.

Sekhon, B.K., Sze, D.M.-Y., Chan, W.K. *et al.* (2013). PSP activates monocytes in resting human peripheral blood mononuclear cells: immunomodulatory implications for cancer treatment. *Food Chemistry*, 138 (4), 2201–2209.

Seo, H.N., Jeon, B.Y., Tran, H.T., Ahn, D.H. and Park, D.H. (2010). Influence of pulsed electric field on growths of soil bacteria and pepper plant. *Korean Journal of Chemical Engineering*, 27 (2), 560–566.

Singh, J., Dartois, A. and Kaur, L. (2010). Starch digestibility in food matrix: a review. *Trends in Food Science and Technology*, 21 (4), 168–180.

Sittikijyothin, W., Torres, D. and Gonçalves, M.P. (2005). Modelling the rheological behaviour of galactomannan aqueous solutions. *Carbohydrate Polymers*, 59 (3), 339–350.

Slootmaekers, D., De Jonghe, C., Reynaers, H., Varkevisser, F.A. and Bloys van Treslong, C.J. (1988). Static light scattering from κ-carrageenan solutions. *International Journal of Biological Macromolecules*, 10 (3), 160–168.

Slootmaekers, D., van Dijk, J.A.P.P., Varkevisser, F.A., van Treslong, C.J.B. and Reynaers, H. (1991). Molecular characterisation of κ- and λ-carrageenan by gel permeation chromatography, light scattering, sedimentation analysis and osmometry. *Biophysical Chemistry*, 41 (1), 51–59.

Soares, S., Mateus, N. and de Freitas, V. (2012). Carbohydrates inhibit salivary proteins precipitation by condensed tannins. *Journal of Agricultural and Food Chemistry*, 60 (15), 3966–3972.

Song, D., He, Z., Wang, C. *et al.* (2013). Regulation of the exopolysaccharide from an anamorph of *Cordyceps sinensis* on dendritic cell sarcoma (DCS) cell line. *European Journal of Nutrition*, 52 (2), 687–694.

Souza, H.K.S., Campiña, J.M., Sousa, A.M.M., Silva, F. and Gonçalves, M.P. (2013). Ultrasound-assisted preparation of size-controlled chitosan nanoparticles: characterization and fabrication of transparent biofilms. *Food Hydrocolloids*, 31 (2), 227–236.

Stang, M. and Schubert, H. (2001). Emulsification in high-pressure homogenizers. *Chemical Engineering and Technology*, 24 (10), 151–157.

Strand, K.A., Bøe, A., Dalberg, P.S., Sikkeland, T. and Smidsrød, O. (1982). Dynamic and static light scattering on aqueous solutions of sodium alginate. *Macromolecules*, 15 (2), 570–579.

Sun, C., Rosendahl, A.H., Wang, X.D., Wu, D.Q. and Andersson, R. (2012). Polysaccharide-K (PSK) in cancer – old story, new possibilities? *Current Medicinal Chemistry*, 19 (5), 757–762.

particularly in the liver, muscle and adipose tissue – and influence weight management as well.

Applications of RS in food are of interest especially to food formulators and nutritionists for two reasons: first, the potential physiological benefits and second, the high quality of the final products, which is not attainable with traditional insoluble fibres. Physicochemical properties, particularly the low water-holding capacity, make RS a functional ingredient that provides good handling, stability at high processing temperatures (type RS III) and improves texture in the final products. Worldwide, people are now very much concerned about foods for a healthier life, which pressurizes the food industry to produce foods with nutritionally functional ingredients, beneficial physiological effects as well as high organoleptic acceptability. The diversity and the enormous variety of food products require starches that can tolerate a wide range of processing techniques and preparation conditions. Native starches are modified using chemical, physical and enzymatic methods (Betancur and Chel, 1997) for the formation of RS, indigestible residues. To make the utmost use of RS, it is essential to know about its properties, factors influencing its formation, the consequences of such formation, methods of preparation and methods of estimation.

9.2 Starch, composition and its structure

Starch is the most consumed carbohydrate in the human diet and is present in many food plants. Traditional staple foods such as cereals, roots and tubers are the main source of dietary starch. The green leaves of plants produce starch from excess glucose by photosynthesis and store it for further use. Physically, starch is a soft, white, granular, tasteless organic chemical that is insoluble in cold water, alcohol or other solvents. Starch is a polysaccharide comprising glucose monomers joined in α-1,4 and α-1,6 linkages with the chemical formula $(C_6H_{10}O_5)_n$. The simplest form of starch is the linear polymer called amylose; amylopectin is the branched form of the glucose polymer. Amylose and amylopectin associate through hydrogen bonding and arrange themselves radially in layers to form granules. Starch primarily consists of amylose and amylopectin. Moreover it also contains some minor components such as proteins, lipids, inorganic substances and non-starch polysaccharides. Some starches also contain a group of intermediate materials between amylose and amylopectin.

9.2.1 Amylose

Amylose is made up of a linear chain of α(1→4) bound glucose molecules. The carbon atoms on glucose are numbered, starting at the aldehyde (C=O) carbon, so, in amylose, the 1-carbon on one glucose molecule is linked to the 4-carbon on the next glucose molecule (α(1→4) bonds). Many amylose molecules have a very few α(1→6) bound glucose molecules that may occur once in every 180–320 units, or 0.3–0.5% of the linkages. The number of repeated glucose subunits (n) is usually in the range of 300–3000, but can be many thousands. The chains can easily form single or double helices. The amylose chain gives the molecules a right-handed spiral or helical shape. The inside of the helix contains predominantly hydrogen atoms and is lipophilic, while the hydrophilic hydroxyl groups are positioned on the outside of coil (Whistler and BeMiller, 1997).

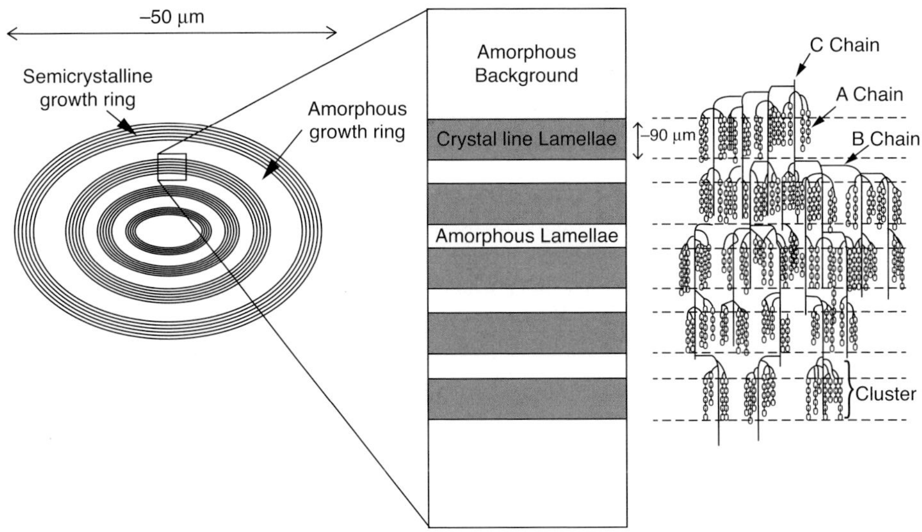

Figure 9.1 Semicrystalline growth ring consisting of amorphous and crystalline lamellae and also consisting of A, B and C chain of amylopectin. *Source:* Adapted from Donald *et al.*, 1997 with permission from the author

9.2.2 Amylopectin

Amylopectin is a soluble polysaccharide and highly branched polymer of glucose with an average molecular weight range from 10^7 to 5×10^8 g/mol and degree of polymerization (DP) of 2×10^6. This makes it one of the largest polymers in nature found in plants. Glucose units are linked in a linear way with $\alpha(1\rightarrow4)$ glycosidic bonds. Branching takes place with $\alpha(1\rightarrow6)$ bonds occurring every 24–30 glucose units, resulting in a soluble molecule that can be quickly degraded as it has many end-points for enzymes to attach. An amylopectin molecule consists of a main chain – the C chain – which carries the one reducing end-group and numerous branches, termed A chains and B chains (Figure 9.1).

Short chains (A chains) of DP 12–16 that can form double helices are arranged in clusters. The clusters consist of 80–90% of the chain and are linked by longer chains (B chains) that form the other 10–20% of the chain. Most B chains extend into two (DP about 40) or three clusters (DP about 70), but some extend into more clusters (DP about 110) (Thompson, 2000). From X-ray diffraction experiments, starch granules are seen to have a semicrystalline character, which indicates a high degree of orientation of the glucan molecules. About 70% of the mass of starch granules is regarded as amorphous and about 30% as crystalline. The amorphous regions contain the main amount of amylose but also a considerable part of the amylopectin. The crystalline region consists primarily of amylopectin.

9.2.3 Intermediate materials

A group of components may present between amylose and amylopectin in some starches called intermediate material, which contains the same types of glucosidic linkages as amylose and amylopectin but their functional properties and molecular weight are different. Amylose with up to 20 or more branch points on average may be considered as intermediate material (Hizukuri, 1996). The amount and structural features of these intermediate materials vary with starch sources.

9.2.4 Minor components

Starches from different sources vary in their content of minor components. Cereal starches in general contain lipids that seem to be associated with the amylose fraction, whereas tuber starches have very low lipid contents. Three categories of materials are allied with starches as minor components, namely: (i) particulate material; (ii) surface components, removable by extraction procedures; and (iii) internal components (Buléon *et al.*, 1998).

Particulate material is usually made up of cell-wall fragments. Lipids are the most important fraction associated with the starch granules of cereals. For example, 0.8–1.2% lipids are associated in wheat starch. The main constituents of surface components are proteins, enzymes, amino acids and nucleic acids that are usually removable by extraction methods. Some components can be extracted without granule disruption: approximately 10% of proteins and 10–15% of lipids. Minor components have great impact on the physicochemical properties of the starch granule though they present at very low levels. Non-starch polysaccharides in starch are susceptible to binding water and developing viscosity. The presence of proteins in starch can participate in Maillard reactions between free amino acid groups and reducing sugars producing unwanted flavours or colours. In addition, surface charge and interactions between starch granules and hydrolytic enzymes may also be affected by protein.

Lipids can form an amylose–lipid complex that enhances the resistance of starch to enzyme hydrolysis. Lipid may be present on the surface or inside the starch granule, depending on the plant source. The basic composition of starch ash is phosphorus, calcium (CaO), potassium (K_2O), sodium (Na_2O), and silicon (SiO_2) (Leszczynski, 1989).

9.3 Classification of starch

9.3.1 Based on the action of enzymes

As a result of the activity of amylolytic enzymes of the gastrointestinal tract (also *in vitro*) starch undergoes hydrolysis as shown in Table 9.1.

9.3.2 Based on X-ray diffraction

On the basis of their X-ray diffraction patterns, starch can be classified into four main categories.

Type A: This type of structure has chain lengths of 23–29 glucose units in amylopectin. A type has densely packed double helices and contains 4 water molecules per 12 glucose residues (Lebail *et al.*, 2000). A-starch is found chiefly in cereals.

Type B: This type of structure has chain lengths of 30–44 glucose units in amylopectin. B type has loosely packed double helices and contains 36 water molecules per 12

Table 9.1 Starch classification

Starch fraction	Rapidly digestible starch (RDS)	Slowly digestible starch (SDS)	Resistant starch (RS) Types 1–4
Digestion timeline (in vitro)/place	Within 20 min; mouth and small intestine	20–120 min; Small intestine	>120 min; colon
Examples	Freshly cooked or baked food such as bread, potato	Native waxy maize starch, gelatinized starch	Raw potato and plantain starch
Maize starch (Tate & Lyle)	22.4%	53%	22.6%
Main physiological property	Rapid source of energy	Slow and sustained source of energy and sustained blood glucose	Fermented by gut bacteria in the large intestine acting as prebiotics
Structure	Mainly amorphous	Amorphous/ crystalline	Depending on the type, mainly crystalline

Source: Adapted from Englyst *et al.*, 1992.

glucose residues (Lebail, *et al.*, 2000). This is the usual pattern of starches in tuber and banana.

Type C: The type C structure is made up of amylopectin of chain lengths of 26–29 glucose molecules. This type is found in peas and beans.

Type V: An additional type which is a single helical structure initiated in amylose complexed with lipids or other agents (Zobel, 1988; Lebail *et al.*, 2000). It is found in swollen granules.

9.4 Types and structure of RS

RS is the part of consumed starch that is digested incompletely and in the intact form or as products of its partial hydrolysis, escapes the small intestine and enters the large bowel. It is measured from the difference between the amount of starch subjected to the activity of amylolytic enzymes and the amount of glucose (as starch equivalent) produced as a result of hydrolysis with those enzymes. According to the definition and the physical characteristics of RS which exist, it can be divided into four subtypes (Englyst *et al.*, 1992; Nugent, 2005; Sajilata *et al.*, 2006) as described here. Figure 9.2 represents the structural view of different types of resistant starch.

RS I RS II RS III RS IV

Figure 9.2 Structural view of four type of resistant starch. *Source:*Asp, 1992 and Englyst *et al.*, 1992. Both reproduced with permission from Nature

9.4.1 Resistant starch type 1 (RS I)

RS I is found in the plant cells of undamaged cell walls such as unground cereal grain. Amylolytic enzymes cannot degrade RS I because the gastrointestinal tract enzymes are not capable of degrading cellulose, hemicelluloses, lignins and other constituents of plant cell walls (Leszczynski, 2004) which pass to the small intestine in the intact form. RS I is heat stable in most normal cooking operations, which enables its use as an ingredient in a wide variety of conventional foods.

9.4.2 Resistant starch type 2 (RS II)

RS II includes granules of raw starch of some plant species, for example potato or banana. In raw starch granules, starch is tightly packed in a radial pattern and is relatively dehydrated. This compact structure limits the accessibility of digestive enzymes, various amylases, and accounts for the resistant nature of RS II, such as ungelatinized starch.

These starches contain relatively high amounts of amylopectin and demonstrate a relatively high degree of crystallization. The amylolytic enzymes first degrade the amorphous regions; hence, crystallinity of starch granules could have been the reason for their resistance to the activity of those enzymes. However, the degree of starch crystallinity is not always linked with its resistance to the activity of amylases.

The resistance of starch granules may be improved by annealing starch, a process of keeping the starch for longer in water with a temperature lower than that for gelatinization. At annealing temperatures, the granules are not damaged but change their properties. The resultant changes depend on the botanical origin of the starch, the temperature and time of annealing, as well as on the concentration of the starch suspension in water. The annealing of starches result in an increased and strengthened degree of crystallinity by 'stiffening' and ordering of starch chains both in the crystalline and amorphous layer. The changes in the starch granule structure increase the starch gelatinization temperature and the enthalpy of that process (Leszczyñski, 2004).

9.4.3 Resistant starch type 3 (RS III)

RS III is produced by precipitation from starch paste or gel in the retrogradation process. At first, starch granules are disrupted by heating in excess water, commonly known as gelatinization. The molecular order of the granule is gradually and irreversibly destroyed during gelatinization. Amylose mostly leaches out from the granule when it is further heated, and then partial solubilization occurs. Upon cooling, starch undergoes a relatively slow re-association process commonly termed retrogradation. During retrogradation, starch molecules re-associate as double helices and can form a tightly packed structure stabilized by hydrogen bonding (Eerlingen and Delcour, 1995). The association process can be driven further by dehydration and these structures (B-type crystalline structures) are thermally very stable, and can only be rehydrated at 80–150 °C. Apart from this structure, starch paste also contains an amorphous phase made of loose amylose chains with a DP of 6–30 (Leloup *et al.*, 1992). This amorphous fraction experiences hydrolysis and further ordering of amylose chains during gel treatment with amylolytic enzymes, in contrast to the crystalline fraction built of those chains, leftovers are resistant to the enzymatic activity (Colquhoun *et al.*, 1995).

The formation of RS III is hampered if native starch contains lipid substances, which form inclusive complexes with amylose, penetrating into its chains. This type of amylose cannot bind into double helices to produce crystalline structures upon aggregation. Therefore, less RS is formed as a fewer insoluble crystallites of amylose are precipitated in the retrogradation process (Eerlingen *et al.*, 1994). Amylopectin gels are also partly crystalline. A net is formed within short outer branch-points of amylopectin with a DP of 14–20 into crystalline structures. This crystallization of amylopectin happens very slowly and is less stable than that of amylose. Unlike amylose, their dissolution temperature is also low, ranging from 55 to 70 °C (Eerlingen and Delcour, 1995).

The formation of RS has a great impact on the storage temperature of starch paste. When paste is stored for several hours at a low temperature, more RS is formed than upon paste storage at high temperatures. On the other hand, long storage of paste at about 100 °C results in the formation of higher amounts of RS than is formed within the same time but at lower temperatures (Eerlingen *et al.*, 1993). But RS formed at low temperatures demonstrates the B-type of crystallinity, whereas that produced during starch paste storage at boiling temperature is the A-pattern of crystallinity (Shamai *et al.*, 2003). At low temperatures, a major part of the amylose is subject to retrogradation and precipitation from the solution; at higher temperatures, those processes proceed only in a small fraction of the amylose with a low degree of polymerization (Lu *et al.*, 1997).

9.4.4 Resistant starch type 4 (RS IV)

RS IV or cross-linked starch is an example of chemically modified starch. Chemical modification is anticipated to smooth the progress of intramolecular and intermolecular bonds at random locations in the starch granules for their stabilization (Singh *et al.*, 2007; Carmona-Garcia *et al.*, 2009) that is more resistant to shear and acidic conditions. Cross-linked starch is generally produced by treating granular starch with multifunctional reagents capable of forming either ether or ester intermolecular linkages between the hydroxyl groups of the starch molecules. The main cross-linking reagents are sodium trimetaphosphate, monosodium phosphate, sodium tripolyphosphate, phosphoryl chloride ($POCl_3$), a mixture of adipic acid, acetic anhydride and vinyl chloride (Singh *et al.*, 2007; Ratnayake and Jackson, 2009). The functional properties of treated starch depend on the type of cross-linking agent because different cross-linking agents produce cross-linked starch with different molecular structures (Seker and Hanna, 2006; Ratnayake and Jackson, 2009). Therefore, based on the reagent used for cross-linking, the final product is generally divided into three types: (i) mono-starch phosphate produced by esterification of starch with orthophosphoric acid, sodium or potassium orthophosphate, or sodium tripolyphosphate; (ii) di-starch phosphate produced with sodium trimetaphosphate or phosphorous oxychloride; (iii) phosphated di-starch phosphate produced by combined treatments of mono-starch phosphate and di-starch phosphate (Seker and Hanna, 2006; Jyothi *et al.*, 2006). The chemical modification of starch for food application is precisely restricted not only by the type of chemical reactions used but also by the extent of changes in starch macromolecules (FAO, 1997). The restrictions mentioned are recommended by Joint FAO/WHO Expert Committee on Food Additives (JECFA) with the aim of protecting consumers against the intake of objectionable food. However, changes in the molecular and supermolecular structure of starch, caused by chemical modification and the changing rate of digestion could be advantageous, for example in manufacturing functional food designed for people with diabetes.

9.5 Factors affecting RS content and its digestibility by enzymes

The resistance of starches and their formation is influenced by several parameters and factors.

9.5.1 Intrinsic properties of starch granules

Source of starch Starch granules come in a wide variety of sources and structures. Different types of raw starch granules influence the formation of RS. Potato, plantain and high amylose maize starch are very resistant *in vitro* and incompletely absorbed *in vivo*, while most cereal starches are almost entirely digested and absorbed *in vivo* though this happens slowly (Holm *et al.*, 1987).

Starch granule configuration Granular shape, size, surface characteristics and surface volume ratio greatly affects the action of the enzyme (Ring *et al.*, 1988). The rate of enzyme hydrolysis is augmented by reducing the granule size (in the order of wheat starch > maize starch > pea starch > potato starch). (Lehmann and Robin, 2007). Smaller granules have a larger specific surface area that may amplify the scope of enzyme binding (Tester *et al.*, 2006). The shape of starch granules influences the specific surface area extensively as it may be circular, spherical, oval or polyhedral (Singh *et al.*, 2010). The individual characteristics of the granule surface such as pin holes, equatorial grooves and small nodules are important factors for enzymatic hydrolysis (Singh *et al.*, 2010). For example, potato, plantain and high amylose starches have an even surface and less holes that help to resist digestion by amylases (Tester *et al.*, 2006; Lehmann and Robin, 2007).

Polymorphism of starch A, B and C type polymorphism or crystallinity of starch depends on the length of the chains making up the amylopectin lattice, the density of packing within the granules and the presence of water (Wu and Sarko, 1978). The crystallites or polymorph structures of A and B are the same type of double helical conformation but differ in packing arrangement and crystalline water content. The crystallinity of native type B starch granules present in potato and amylomaize starch are more resistant to that of type A. Different treatments such as gelatinization, break down of the integrity of the plant cell or tissue structure (e.g. milling) increase enzyme availability and reduce the content of RS, whereas recrystallization and chemical modification tend to increase the RS.

Proportion of amylose and amylopectin A higher content of amylose increases the formation of RS, which lowers the digestibility of starch (Berry, 1986; Sievert and Pomeranz 1989). According to Åkerberg *et al.* (1998), amylose/amylopectin ratio greatly influences the retrogradation process and, accordingly, RS3 formation in bread samples. The greater the content of amylose, the more difficult it is to gelatinize the starch and the more susceptible it is to retrogradation (Topping *et al.*, 2003).

Retrogradation of amylase If starch is heated with water to about 50 °C, the amylose in the granule swells, the crystalline structure of the amylopectin disintegrates and the granule ruptures rendering the starch easily digestible. On cooling/drying, recrystallization (retrogradation) that takes place very fast for the amylose portion occurs as the linear structure facilitates cross-linkages by means of hydrogen bonds. On the other hand, the branched nature of amylopectin inhibits its recrystallization to some extent and it takes place over several days. The level of RS formation is strongly related to the amylose content, and the retrogradation of amylose was identified as the main mechanism for the formation of RS. Higher amounts of RS can be produced by repeated autoclaving (Berry 1986; Bjorck *et al.,* 1990). During storage, the dispersed polymers of gelatinized starch are said to undergo retrogradation to semicrystalline forms that resist digestion by pancreatic α-amylase.

9.5.2 Presence of other components with starch

The existence of some non-starchy substances such lipid, proteins and dietary fibre over the granule surface may also influence the rate of enzymatic hydrolysis.

Lipid Asp (1994) and Crowe *et al.* (2000) found that amylose–lipid complexes had a reduced digestibility compared to free amylose as they are usually found on the surface of the granule thus reducing contact between enzyme and substrate. The level of this decline depends mainly on the type of lipid (monoglycerides form complexes highly resistant to amylolysis) (Sajilata *et al.,* 2006) and the amylose–amylopectin ratio, degree of amylose polymerization, lipid chain length and complexation temperature (Singh *et al.,* 2010).

Protein Surface proteins present at 3 g/kg of starch or lower may also reduce the rate of enzymatic hydrolysis by covering the adsorption sites of starch granules (Tester *et al.,* 2006; Singh *et al.,* 2010). Escarpa *et al.* (1997) found that during autoclaving and cooling of potato starch mixed with albumin, starch–protein interaction reduces RS content. The physical barrier created by the protein network in cereal-based products limits the accessibility of starch to amylase and delays *in vitro* starch hydrolysis, resulting in increased resistance (Hoebler *et al.,* 1999).

Ions Potassium and calcium ions have a great impact on RS production since these ions may prevent the formation of hydrogen bonds between amylose and amylopectin chains. In the presence of calcium and potassium ions, the production of RS in potato starch gels was reduced compared with those with no added constituent (Escarpa *et al.,* 1997).

Sugars The level of crystallization and the yields of RS formation are reduced in the presence of soluble sugars such as glucose, maltose, sucrose and ribose (Buch and Walker, 1988; I'Anson *et al.,* 1990; Kohyama and Nishinari, 1991). Eerlingen *et al.,* (1994) showed that sugars influenced the retrogradation process only at high concentrations (starch–water–sugar ratio of 1:10:5 w/w). The mechanism of retrogradation inhibition was the interaction between sugar molecules and the starch molecular chains, which change the matrix of gelatinized starch (the sugars act as anti-plasticizers and increase the glass transition temperature).

Dietary fibre Some insoluble dietary fibre such as cellulose and lignin has little impact on RS production (Escarpa *et al.,* 1997). Guar and xanthan gums influence the gelatinization properties of starches and therefore they affect the retrogradation process as well (Achayuthakan and Suphantharika, 2008).

Enzyme inhibitors A wide variety of food crops such as wheat, rye, triticale and sorghum (not rice, barley and maize) contain amylase inhibitors which may inhibit the pancreatic alpha-amylase (Singh *et al.,* 2010). Thompson and Yoon (1984) reported that polyphenols, phytic acid and lectins restrain *in vitro* starch hydrolysis and reduce the glycaemic index. Also, tannic acid significantly inhibits both amylases and intestinal maltase activity (Bjorck and Nyman, 1987).

9.5.3 Food processing techniques

Research on heat load and the changes in the structure of the starch granules are remarkably important as almost all foods, especially foods containing starch, are heat-treated before being eaten. Production of starch-based products often includes a combination of shear and thermal treatment and leads to molecular breakdown, depolymerization, crystal melting and the disappearance of the granular structure (van den Einde *et al.,* 2004; Barron *et al.,* 2001). The de-structuring of starch granules is shown in Figure 9.3 and Figure 9.4.

At first crystalline structures are melted by internal disorganization of starch granules during thermal processing. At higher temperature and shear, phase fragmentation can be seen and the starch crystalline structure totally disappears and an

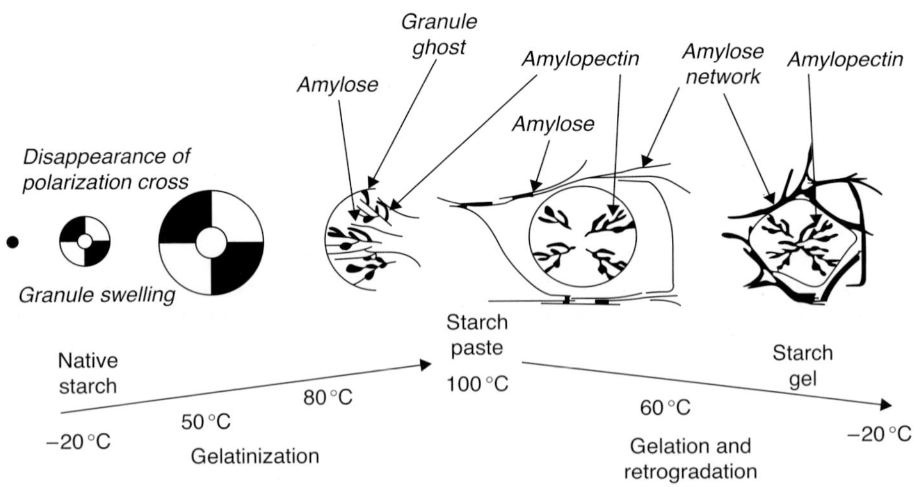

Figure 9.3 De-structuring of starch granules during heat treatment. *Source:* Bornet *et al.*, 1997. Reproduced with permission from Elsevier

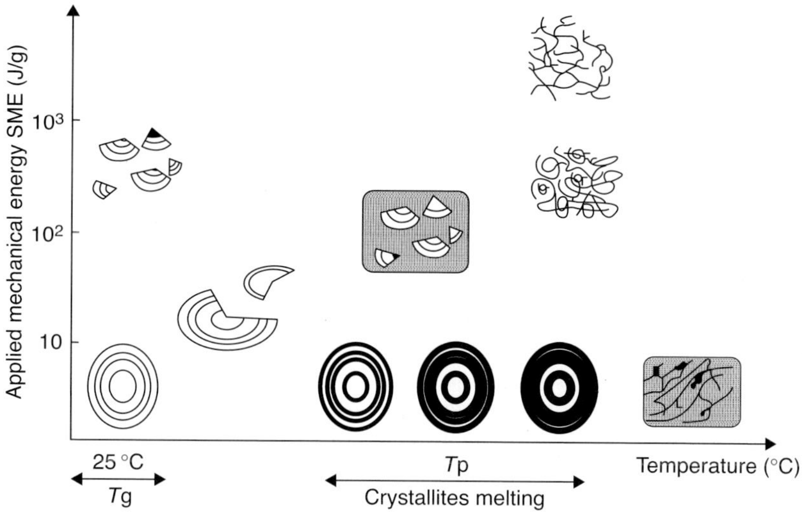

Figure 9.4 Effects of shear and heat on the starch granules. *Source:* Barron *et al.*, 2001. Reproduced with permission from Elsevier

amorphous gel finally forms. According to van den Einde *et al.* (2004), shear stress is the key parameter in the degradation of starch, therefore this parameter has to be taken into account more precisely in the treatment (Figure 9.4).

In different processing treatments such as baking, steaming, microwaving, extrusion cooking, autoclaving and so forth, starch granule structures may be unchanged, partially or wholly gelatinized, or partially retrograded influencing the yield of RS in foods.

Milling, dehulling, polishing and soaking of grain As size reduction increases the surface area, milling results in a higher percentage of hydrolysis. Dehulling, polishing and soaking may enhance the loss of phytic acids, tannins and polyphenols that normally inhibit the activity of alpha-amylase (Singh *et al.*, 2010).

Cooking RS content is notably reduced during cooking with excess water and high temperature by disrupting the crystalline structure (Gelencsér, 2009; Roopa and Premavalli, 2008; Sajilata *et al.*, 2006). RS III shows less sensitivity to heat treatments than others (Gelencsér, 2009; Htoon *et al.*, 2009). Formation of RS is increased by steam cooking. Tovar and Melito (1996) found that several steam-heated legumes were rich in indigestible RS (19–31%, dry matter (DM) basis), which was not observed in raw beans. Similarly, RS measured directly in conventionally and high-pressure steamed beans were three to five times higher than in the raw pulses, suggesting that retrogradation is mainly responsible for the reduction in digestibility.

Autoclaving Autoclaving results in an increase in RS. Siljestrom and Asp (1985) found that autoclaved wheat starch had 9% RS compared with less than 1% in uncooked wheat starch. Autoclaved wheat starch contained 6.2% RS (of DM); this increased to 7.8% after three further reboiling/cooling cycles (Bjorck *et al.*, 1987). The number of cycles exerted the most pronounced effect on RS content; increasing the number of cycles to 20 raised the RS level to >40%.

Baking Like autoclaving, baking amplifies RS content. A product baked at a low temperature for a long-time contained significantly higher amounts of RS than bread baked under ordinary conditions (Liljeberg *et al.*, 1996). In high amylose containing products, more RS may be produced as amylose leached out of starch granules during gelatinization could quickly retrograde in the first hours after baking (Korus *et al.*, 2009). Addition of lactic acid increased RS recovery further, whereas malt had no impact on RS yield.

Extrusion cooking In extrusion cooking, starches are sheared and kneaded vigorously, which leads to the loss of their structural integrity and enhances their enzymatic digestibility (Singh *et al.*, 2010). Faraj *et al.* (2004) found that RS III of the native flours was diminished by extrusion cooking, but not significantly, while storage of extruded flour samples at 4 °C for 24 h before oven drying slightly increased RS III content.

Microwave irradiation Some researchers reported that microwave irradiation enhanced the digestibility of tuber starches, chickpeas and beans, kudzu and maize starches (Sajilata *et al.*, 2006) while Zhang *et al.* (2009) showed that microwave irradiation may increase the development of RS. Actually, amylose content (Lewandowicz *et al.*, 2000) and the structure (Szepes *et al.*, 2005) of the starch are the important parameters for their RS formation.

Storage conditions RS content amplified on storage, especially at low temperatures. Cold storage seems to support an increase in crystalline structure. Niba (2003) reported that whole corn bread and corn bread crumb stored at different temperatures (–20 °C, 4 °C, or 20 °C) for 7 days showed RS contents up to a maximum between 2 and 4 days at all storage temperatures, after which they reduced.

9.6 Production of RS

RS can be prepared by using heat treatment, partial acid hydrolysis with hydrothermal treatment, enzyme treatment, combined heat treatment and enzyme treatment, and chemical treatment.

9.6.1 Heat treatment

Development of RS is greatly affected by the heat treatment of starch. It can be obtained by cooking the starch above the gelatinization temperature and simultaneously drying on heated rolls such as drum driers or even extruders. The optimum amount of RS can be obtained by gelatinizing starch at 120 °C for 20 min, followed by cooling to room temperature (Garcia-Alonso *et al.*, 1999). The starch gels are then frozen overnight at –20 °C and dried at 60 °C before milling. Many researchers treated the starch at different temperatures in their studies. For example, autoclaved temperatures were at 110 °C, 121 °C, 127 °C and 134 °C (Berry, 1986; Bjorck and *et al.*, 1987; Sievert and Pomeranz, 1989), or 148 °C (Sievert and Pomeranz, 1989) for periods ranging from 30 min to 1 h.

9.6.2 Acid modification

Acid modification of starch carried out below the gelatinization temperature (Wang *et al.*, 2003) is widely applied in food, paper, textile and other industries to prepare thin boiling starches. Acid hydrolysis modifies the physicochemical properties of starch, such as increased solubility and gel strength and decreased viscosity (Singh and Ali, 1987; Wang and Wang, 2001; Wang *et al.*, 2003), without destroying its granular structure. By increasing the hydrolysis of acid-thinned starch gels, the retrogradation rate also increased. Zhao and Lin (2009) reported that citric acid hydrolysis of retrograded high-amylose maize starch at room temperature notably amplifies the production of RS. Likewise, acid treatment of gelatinized potato or sweet potato starch was found to increase RS configuration with enhance yield (Shin *et al.*, 2004).

9.6.3 Enzymatic treatment

Two types of enzymes, endo- and exo-acting are brought into play for starch hydrolysis. To change starch into glucose, usually amyloglucosidase (glucoamylase), an exo-enzyme, is applied and gelatinization of starch is needed for complete conversion to glucose (Kitahara *et al.*, 1994; Manelius, 2000). In this conversion, glucoamylase slices consecutive α(1,4) and α(1,6)-D-glucosidic linkages from the non-reducing end to produce glucose (Allen and Spradlin, 1974). Endo-acting amylases could slice haphazardly at α(1,4) linkages, or specifically at α(1,6) linkages. For example, alpha-amylase is an endo-enzyme that cleaves α(1,4)-D-glucosidic linkages in starch hydrolysis and produces glucose, maltose, maltotriose and branched α-limit dextins (pentasaccharides). (Hughes *et al.*, 1963; French *et al.*, 1972) end-products after α-amylase treatment of amylopectin. Pullulanase, another endo-enzyme isolated from *Klebsiella aerogenes*, converts linear pullulan (polymaltotriose) into maltotriose (Marshall and Whelan, 1974; Atwell *et al.*, 1980) by cleaving α(1,6) linkages.

Beta-amylase is an exo-enzyme that acts on α(1,4) glucosidic linkages from the non-reducing end and produces maltose and possibly β-limit dextrins that contain either a branch point of substituents, such as naturally occurring phosphate groups, or added substituent (Manelius, 2000). A debranching enzyme pullulanase was used for digesting starch to produce a RS product that retains the same cooking quality as that found in untreated rice starch or flour, but that has a higher percentage of starch resistant to α-amylase digestion (King and Tan, 2005). In this method, low amylose starches such as rice starch (24%) and rice flour (20%) were used.

9.6.4 Heat and enzyme treatment

Initially, gelatinization of starch is carried out to manufacture RS from high amylose starch and then the starch paste is treated with debranching enzymes like pullulanase and the starch product separated by drying/extrusion. An additional boost of amylase-RS yield can be achieved by the addition of an inorganic salt to the debranched starch before isolation (Chiu *et al.*, 1994). Different research concluded that the optimum amount of RS was obtained at 134 °C, with four heating and cooling cycles and a starch : water ratio of 1 : 3.5. The RS was purified by producing the starch gel and mixing it with an amylase to assimilate non-RS fractions, the remaining RS and then amylase made dormant by heat treatment above 100 °C (Pomeranz and Sievert, 1990).

9.6.5 Chemical treatment

RS is also produced by modifying the starch by cross-linking with chemical agents (Haynes *et al.*, 2000). The reaction of starch with bi- or polyfunctional reagents like sodium trimetaphosphate, phosphorus oxychloride, or mixed anhydrides of acetic acid and dicarboxylic acids such as adipic acid is carried out to get cross-linked starch. Cross-linking occurring between the sulfonate or phosphate group and the hydroxyl group of various starch molecules makes the starch molecules resistant to amylolytic attack.

9.7 Physiological benefit of RS

Physiological effects of RS have been proved to be beneficial for health as follows.

9.7.1 Prevention of cancer

RS helps to retain healthy colon tissue by producing short-chain fatty acids called protective compounds. One of these, butyrate, is particularly important because it is the primary energy source for colonic cells and has anti-inflammatory properties that are important for maintaining healthy colon cells (Scheppach 1994; Andoh *et al.*, 2003). In addition, butyrate acts as an anticarcinogenic substance that may lead to the decreased incidence of colon cancer, atherosclerosis and obesity-related complications in humans (Haralampu, 2000). Research has shown that butyrate restrains the growth and proliferation of tumour cell lines *in vitro* and encourages differentiation of tumour cells, producing a phenotype similar to that of the normal mature cell (Toscani *et al.*, 1988). Moreover, it also provokes apoptosis that leads to the programmed cell death of human colorectal cancer cells (Scharlau *et al.*, 2009). Ferguson *et al.* (2000) reported that faecal pH, bulking agent as well as a greater production of SCFAs in the colon of rats changed dramatically when feeding them with RS preparations. This suggests that RS increases the soluble dietary fibre.

9.7.2 Glycaemic effects

Foods containing RS slow the rate of digestion. The slow digestion of RS helps in controlled glucose release applications. Numerous studies on human health stated that Hi-maize® RS has a positive impact on both postprandial glucose levels as well as insulin response (Noakes *et al.*, 1996; Behall and Hallfrisch, 2002; Granfeldt *et al.*, 1995; Muir *et al.*, 1995). One recent study showed that test beverages with added maize-based RS reduce the relative glycaemic response without any change in palatability (Kendall, 2007). The mechanism may be that a RS ingredient reduces the digestible carbohydrate fraction and improves insulin sensitivity, translating to a lowered glycaemic response (Nugent, 2005).

9.7.3 Prebiotic potential

Food containing RS stimulates healthy bacteria to grow in the bowel and suppresses the growth of potentially harmful bacteria, and, therefore, is called 'prebiotic fibre'. Prebiotics can help to promote bacterial colonization and may well be able to act as enhancers of probiotic bacteria (Topping *et al.*, 2003). RS has prebiotic properties and may provide protection to beneficial *Bifidobacteria in vivo* as it travels through the upper gastrointestinal tract, the 'synbiotic effect' (Wang, 1999). Although there is still much investigation required to develop our understanding in this field, the potential to capture the benefits of prebiotics and probiotics in relation to measurable health outcomes is very exciting.

9.7.4 Inhibition to cholesterol storage

Hypocholesterolaemic effects of RS have been thoroughly proven. In rats, RS diets (25% raw potato) markedly raised the caecal size and the caecal pool of SCFA, as well as SCFA absorption, and lowered plasma cholesterol and triglycerides. Furthermore, there was a lower concentration of cholesterol in all lipoprotein fractions, especially in high-density lipoprotein, (HDL1) and a reduced concentration of triglycerides in the triglyceride-rich lipoprotein fraction (Ranhotra *et al.,* 1997; Kim *et al.,* 2003). The mechanisms are: RS helps to bind the bile acids, leading to increased faecal bile acid excretion, which results in less bile acid being recycled. To compensate for the excreted bile acid, the liver synthesizes new bile acids from cholesterol, thereby reducing the serum cholesterol level.

9.7.5 Weight management

RS can boost fibre content when added to foods such as bread, biscuits, sweet goods, pasta, nutritional bars and cereal without affecting taste or texture. In 2003, the World Health Organization concluded that dietary fibre was the only dietary component that had convincing evidence showing a protective effect against weight gain and obesity (WHO/FAO, 2003). Slavin (2005) reported that the probable mechanisms of reducing weight are its ability to increase satiety and decrease subsequent hunger, along with altering the secretion of hormones related to food digestion. When RS is used to replace flour or other rapidly digested carbohydrates, it lowers the caloric content of foods. Natural RS gives between 2–3 kcal/g (8–12 kJ/g) versus 4 kcal/g (16 kJ/g). (Behall and Howe, 1996; Aust *et al.,* 2001). Consequently, RS is a precious tool to produce low-calorie foods. Multiple recent studies have shown that naturally occurring RS gives satiety and decreases food intake in the short term (within a few hours) and longer-term (for 20–24 h) (Nilsson *et al.,* 2008; Willis *et al.,* 2009; Anderson *et al.,* 2010; Bodinham *et al.,* 2010).

9.7.6 Reducing fat accumulation

RS may promote fat burning and thus help in reducing fat accumulation. Higgins (2004) reported that high-amylose corn RS can amplify fat oxidation after a meal, which has a possible metabolic effect on body weight. Higgins *et al.,* (2004) also reported that trials conducted in the US shows that the consumption of a meal containing 5% RS helped to increase fat oxidation by 23%, and this rise was persistent throughout the day, even when only one meal contained RS. The possible mechanism may be that the insertion of RS altered the order in which the body oxidized the available macronutrients, preferentially oxidizing fat.

9.7.7 Assimilation of minerals

RS could have a positive consequence on intestinal calcium and iron absorption. A study was conducted for intestinal apparent absorption of calcium, phosphorus, iron and zinc in the presence of either RS or digestible starch. The results revealed that the meal that included 16.4% RS had a greater apparent absorption of calcium and iron as compared with a meal that contained completely digestible starch (Morais *et al.*, 1996).

9.8 Functionality of RS in food applications

At present, RS has gained broad worldwide interest for both its potential health benefits and its functional properties. Many findings prove that RS has properties similar to both soluble and non-soluble fibre and shows promising physiological benefits in humans, which may result in disease prevention (Gordon *et al.,* 1997). Such reports have provoked the assessment of RS as a unique ingredient to produce functional foods. For example, application of RS shows improved crispness and expansion in certain products with better mouth feel, colour and flavour over products produced using some traditional insoluble fibres.

Many baked goods and cereals are known to provide a source of fibre, for example high-fibre bread, bran muffins, breakfast cereals, cookies, pastas and brownies are abundant in the marketplace. However, such products can be prepared using RS as a source of fibre. Here are some comparative studies between RS and traditional fibres for physical and sensory characteristics.

9.8.1 RS in bread baking

Bread is a food commonly fortified with dietary fibre. RS has many beneficial properties over conventional fibres as it is tasteless, white and has a fine particle size between 10 and 15 μm. The lower water-holding capacity of RS – the most important property it has over different traditional fibres (Waring, 1998). The rheology of the dough produced with traditional fibres may change because its high water-holding capacity may create difficulties in moulding, baking and slicing and finally may produce bread with dark colour, reduced loaf volume, poor mouth feel and a masked flavour.

Waring (1998) reported that in a study conducted at the American Institute of Baking (AIB), NOVELOSE 240 starch was compared to various traditional fibres in a high-fibre sponge and dough formulation. Breads were supplemented with fibre (10% TDF) or RS (5 g/50 g serving) to obtain a 'high source' of fibre. In the study, fibre or RS was added to the dough portion and water was added to obtain the same consistency. The RS did not increase dough absorption as much as the fibres.

Breads were then subjectively scored one day after baking for symmetry, crust character, crust colour, and break and shred. Scores were also given to describe internal properties of crumb grain, texture, body, colour, taste and aroma, and mouth feel. The maximum scores were obtained by the breads produced with RS for external and internal characteristics and also acquired the highest overall quality score among those breads containing wheat fibre, cellulose, oat fibre and RS. The most remarkable attributes of RS are the white colour and fine particle size giving the prepared bread brighter crumb and better mouth feel, making it different from other traditional fibres.

The internal grain size of the prepared breads was also determined objectively in terms of cell fineness and elongation using Crumb Scan, a computer program developed at the American Institute of Baking. Higher fineness values were scored by RS, the 50/50 blend of RS and oat fibre produced bread than that of other fibres. Among all breads, the maximum loaf volume was also found in the RS bread.

9.8.2 RS as a texture modifier in baked goods

Waring (1998) also reported that RS was tested in a variety of baked goods such as cakes, cake-like muffins or brownies. The overall results confirmed that RS acts as a texture modifier with favourable tenderness to the crumb.

Low-fat loaf cake was prepared with 40% TDF RS (NOVELOSE 240 starch), oat fibre, a blend of oat fibre with NOVELOSE 240 starch in a 50/50 ratio based on TDF contribution, and a 23% TDF RS (HYLON VII starch). In these formulations, RS or fibre replaced both flour and sugar, while the flour-to-sugar ratio and water were maintained as in the control.

The minimum effect on batter rheology, specific gravity and viscosity was found in the 40% TDF RS, similar to the control. The maximum viscosity was found in oat fibre batter, probably due to its higher water-holding capacity. There were no significant differences among the cakes made with RS, oat fibre and the control for moisture loss after baking, height, specific volume and density. The highest sensory overall score was obtained by the cake formulated with 40% TDF RS with best flavour, maximum moisture and most tender of any cake.

A softer texture was also evaluated in a storage study of muffins. Orange-flavoured muffins were prepared containing approximately 4.5% TDF or 2.5 g fibre/55 g serving with NOVELOSE 240 starch as the fibre source. In this formulation, RS replaced an equal weight of flour. The muffins prepared with 40% TDF RS stayed softer than the control during a 2-week storage period although the rate of changes of firmness was approximately the same. But, the panelists reported that the control muffin became noticeably more firm than the RS muffin during the storage period.

The textural difference between traditional fibre and RS was also examined in another study conducted at AIB (Waring, 1998) in cookies. Wire-cut butter cookies were formulated using 23% TDF (HYLON VII starch) and 40% TDF RS (Novelose 240 starch), oat fibre, and a blend of oat fibre with NOVELOSE 240 starch in a 50/50 ratio to get 8% TDF or 2.5 g fibre/30 g serving. Fibre or RS replaced flour, while the level of all other ingredients was maintained as previously.

Among all the different doughs, 23% TDF RS containing dough was very soft and sticky. This may be due to the higher amount of starch material required to obtain 8% TDF and the dilution of gluten in the dough. But, after baking, all of the cookies were similar in height and spread. The cookies containing 40% TDF RS had a tender, shortbread like texture and a richer butter flavour than the control as described by the sensory panel. Their colour was also lighter than others, possibly due to the reduction of flour, which contains reducing sugars and protein that results in colour by browning.

The hardness of the cookies was determined by the Texture Analyser TA.XT2 (Stable Micro Systems, Surrey, UK) 24 hours after baking. The softest texture was found in the cookies with 40% TDF RS as the sole fibre source.

9.8.3 RS as a crisping agent

Another important functional property of RS is that it improves crispness of high temperature heat-processed foods. For example French toast and waffles are this type of surface crispness food. In an AIB study, buttermilk waffle formulations were made to compare the functionality among RS (NOVELOSE 240) and various fibres like wheat fibre, cellulose and oat fibres (Waring, 1998). Traditional fibres or RS replaced with an equal weight of flour to obtain approximately 3% TDF or 2.5 g fibre/85 g serving as previously. Batters were prepared in a mixer and then cooked on a waffle iron until they were firm, but not yet browned. Waffles were then frozen and reconstituted by heating in a toaster. The waffle weights and sizes were similar during cooking. Initial crispness, crispness after 3 minutes, moistness and overall texture of the toasted waffles were scored by a trained sensory panel. The RS waffle obtained the highest score among the samples and was considered to be the crispest with a tender centre. The positive sensory score of the waffles was determined by a puncture test using the Texture Analyser. The maximum force was required to puncture the RS waffle among the samples, indicating highest crispness.

9.8.4 RS as a functional ingredient in extruded materials

In another AIB study, various cereals were formulated using 40% TDF RS (NOVELOSE 240 starch) alone and in combination with oat fibre in ratios of 50/50 and 25/75 based on weight to compare the expansion properties in extruded samples (Waring, 1998). The maximum expansion occurred in cereal containing RS only among the samples.

9.8.5 RS as an encapsulating agent

RS has an important role in the encapsulation of functional food ingredients like probiotics, PUHAs, flavours, etc. Indeed the use of starch in many encapsulation processes has provided solutions to problems such as thermal stabilization, process-induced controlled release and extended shelf life of sensitive compounds (Shimoni, 2008). A symbiotic approach is often accomplished by co-encapsulation of RS as high-amylose maize starch together with the probiotic microorganisms within the microcapsule. Usually, 1–2% insoluble starch grains are added to the probiotic–hydrocolloid precursor directly before the encapsulation process to help maintain the viability of probiotics (Sultana *et al.,* 2000; Iyer and Kailasapathy, 2005). RS has been used to improve encapsulation of viable bacteria in yogurt. Sultana *et al.* (2000) reported that the incorporation of Hi-Maize1 starch (commercial RS) improved encapsulation of viable bacteria (*Lactobacillus acidophilus* and *Bifidobacterium* spp.) in yoghurt, compared with encapsulation without RS.

Lyophilized corn starch (LCS) has been used as capsule-forming material; however, it decomposes after being subjected to pancreatic enzymes (Fanta *et al.,* 2001). RS is not degraded by the pancreatic amylase and enters the intestine in the indigestible form. This specification, apart from giving the microbeads good enteric delivery characteristic (good release of bacterial cells in the large intestine), also gives them prebiotic functionality as they can be used by the probiotic bacteria in the intestine (Kritchevsky, 1995; Muir *et al.,* 1995; Phillips *et al.,* 1995; Silvester *et al.,* 1995; Haralampu, 2000; Thompson, 2000). High-amylose corn starch (HACS) with 20% RS has been recognized as suitable for enteric delivery. By applying hydrothermal and retrogradation processes on the native high-amylose corn starch (NHACS), RS-rich fractions that are suitable for encapsulation can be prepared (Dimantov *et al.,* 2004). It has been reported that fermentation of starch by microorganisms such as bifidobacteria, lactobacilli, streptococci and Entrobacteriaceae reduces the pH of the intestine via formation of SCFAs (Kleessen *et al.,* 1997; Le Blay *et al.,* 1999; Macfarlane and Gummings, 1999). Also, consumption of RS reduces the risk of intestinal cancer because of its dietary fibre functionality (Dimantov *et al.,* 2004).

Culled banana resistant starch (CBRS, made by autoclaving culled banana starch at 135 °C for 30 min followed by cooling and storing at 4 °C for 24 h) has been used in combination with soy protein isolate (SPI) to prepare fish oil emulsions for their sensory quality and oxidative stability (Nasrin and Anal, 2013). Three types of freeze-dried encapsulant materials were mixed with warm (60 °C) water to get three mixtures of 7.5% (w/w) total solid and three mixtures of 10% (w/w) total solids: (i) a mixture of CBRS and SPI; (ii) mixture of Hylon VII and SPI; and (iii) only SPI. Fish oil was added to these six types of mixtures to obtain 15% (w/w) total solid emulsions (2 : 1 : 1 ratio of oil : protein : RS, or 1 : 1 ratio of oil : protein). The final pH of all six emulsions was 7.5 ± 0.2. The oil encapsulant mixture was pre-emulsified using a blender (National, MX-31GN) for 2 min and then a high pressure homogenizer (IKA Labor-pilot, 2000/4) at 1000 bar for two passes. The emulsions were stored in sterilized capped test tubes in the dark at 4 ± 1 °C to investigate their physical and chemical stability.

Emulsions made with the mixture of CBRS and SPI were stable up to the 9th day of storage irrespective of oil load, whereas other emulsions were broken down as shown in Figure 9.5. On the 9th day of storage, the peroxide value (PV) was <5 meq/kg (permissible limit) in the emulsions made by CBRS and SPI but other emulsions produced PV values of ≥10 meq/kg (Figure 9.6). On the other hand, four types of functional muffins were produced using these emulsions as shown in Figure 9.7 (Nasrin, 2013). Control muffins (510) and those made directly with fish oil (301) had the highest and lowest flavour score, respectively. Muffins (709) made with emulsion containing CBRS masked the fishy odour more than those containing Hylon VII (805). Muffins made with emulsion used the same amount of water as the control to produce an emulsion, and wheat flour was replaced with equal amounts of encapsulant materials.

osteoporosis risks (Arjmandi *et al.*, 1996; Zhang *et al.*, 2007), cardiovascular disease (Rimbach *et al.*, 2008), prostate cancer (Nagata *et al.*, 2007), breast cancer (Steiner *et al.*, 2007) and the reduction of postmenopausal syndromes in women (Knight *et al.*, 1996; Adlercreutz and Mazur, 1997; Somekawa *et al.*, 2001; Zhang *et al.*, 2005). Clinical trials and laboratory studies have also suggested that isoflavones exert various pharmacological actions (Hanasaki *et al.*, 1994; Alexandrakis *et al.*, 2003; Zhang *et al.*, 2004a; Liu *et al.*, 2005; Chung *et al.*, 2006, 2008; Chacko *et al.*, 2007; Wang *et al.*, 2009) such as carcinostatic (anticarcinogenic and antiproliferative), antihypertensive, antioxidative, antiallergic (Liu *et al.*, 2005) activities with antiatherosclerotic, antitumourial and antioestrogenic activities (Anderson and Carner, 1997; Scheiber *et al.*, 2001; Messina, 2002; McCue and Kalidas, 2004) gaining increasing interest as functional components of soybeans. Epidemiological data suggest that the low incidence of certain cancers and cardiovascular diseases in Asian populations is partly related to their traditional diet, of which soybean is an important component, with isoflavones often being implicated in such relationships (Adlercreutz *et al.*, 1993). Such health-beneficial properties of soybeans and isoflavones have increased the interest for soybeans and soy-based products in Asia, North America and Europe, and led to their incorporation into a range of commercial functional foods and to the development of numerous non-prescription food supplements (Setchell and Cole, 2003). Nevertheless, there is evidence showing that the type of soy food storage conditions and processing has an effect on the biological activity of isoflavones (Rostagno *et al.*, 2005). This information suggests that incorporating soybeans and isoflavones in the diet is useful for human health.

10.2 Isoflavones: occurrence, biosynthesis, form and structures

10.2.1 Occurrence

In the plant kingdom, isoflavonoids occur primarily in the subfamily Papilionoideae of the Leguminosae. It is still unknown why certain legumes contain isoflavones, whereas some do not. The biological functions of isoflavones in the life cycle of the plant are not well known. There are hundreds of isoflavones in legumes (Dewick, 1993). Kaufman *et al.* (1997) reported the content of genistein and daidzein in the vegetative parts of many legumes, including varieties such as soybean (*Glycine max*), lupin (*Lupinus leteus*), peas (*Pisum sativum*) and mung bean (*Phaseolus aureus*) (Figure 10.1), although isoflavones are also found in various other food legume seeds.

10.2.2 Biosynthesis, form and structures

Isoflavonoids released by soybeans act as signals that attract the rhizobial bacteria (Rolfe, 1988). These are a subclass of the much more common flavonoids, which are members of the large family of polyphenols that are broadly found in plants. Isoflavonoids are formed by the same biosynthetic pathway as flavonoids (Deavours and Dixon, 2005). First, phenylalanine reacts with malonyl CoA to form 4-hydroxycinnamoyl CoA. Chalcone synthase catalyses the reaction of this intermediate with three more molecules of malonyl CoA to form isoliquiritigenin or naringenin chalcone. Chalcone isomerase catalyses the closure of the heterocyclic ring.

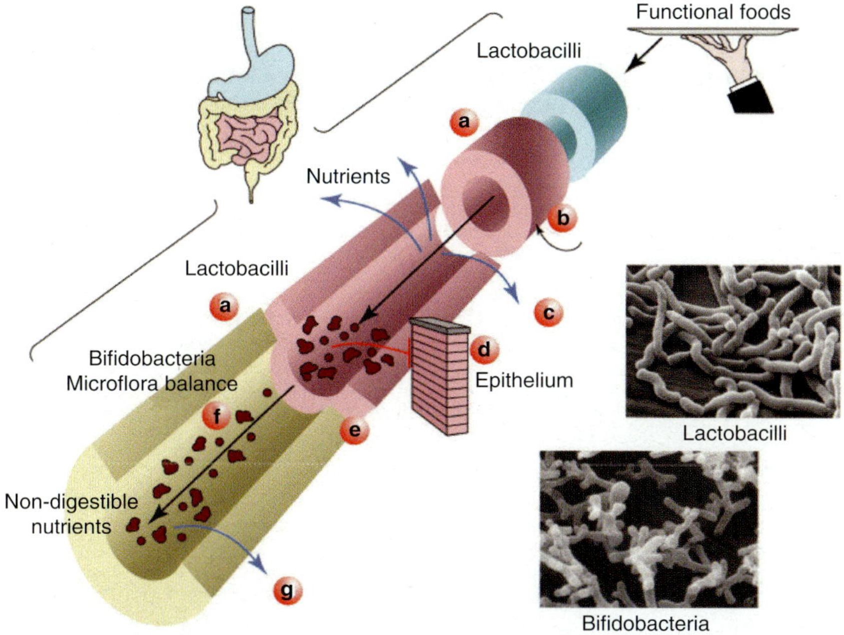

Plate 1.2 Targets throughout the gastrointestinal tract for functional food ingredients. (a) Pre- and probiotics inhibit pathogenic bacteria at various sites, from *Helicobacteria pylori* in the gastric mucosa to *Salmonella* sp. and *Clostridia* sp. in the intestine. (b) Multiple ingredients alter the rate and extent of digestion of nutrients. (c) The absorption of nutrients and anti-nutritional factors throughout the stomach and intestine is affected by the presence, form and activity of functional-food components. (d) Pre- and probiotics modify the barrier functions of the intestinal epithelium. (e) Nutrients, from vitamins and minerals to probiotics, interact with and enhance the functions of gastrointestinal immune cells and, via systemic communication, the entire body's immune system. (f) Pre- and probiotics modulate the overall ecology of the gut microflora. (g) Fermentation products of fibers or non-digestible oligosaccharides and other components from the microflora not only nourish the intestine but also improve the differentiation, maturation and overall health of colonic cells. *Source:* German *et al.*, 1999. Reproduced with permission from Elsevier

Functional Foods and Dietary Supplements: Processing Effects and Health Benefits, First Edition.
Edited by Athapol Noomhorm, Imran Ahmad and Anil Kumar Anal.

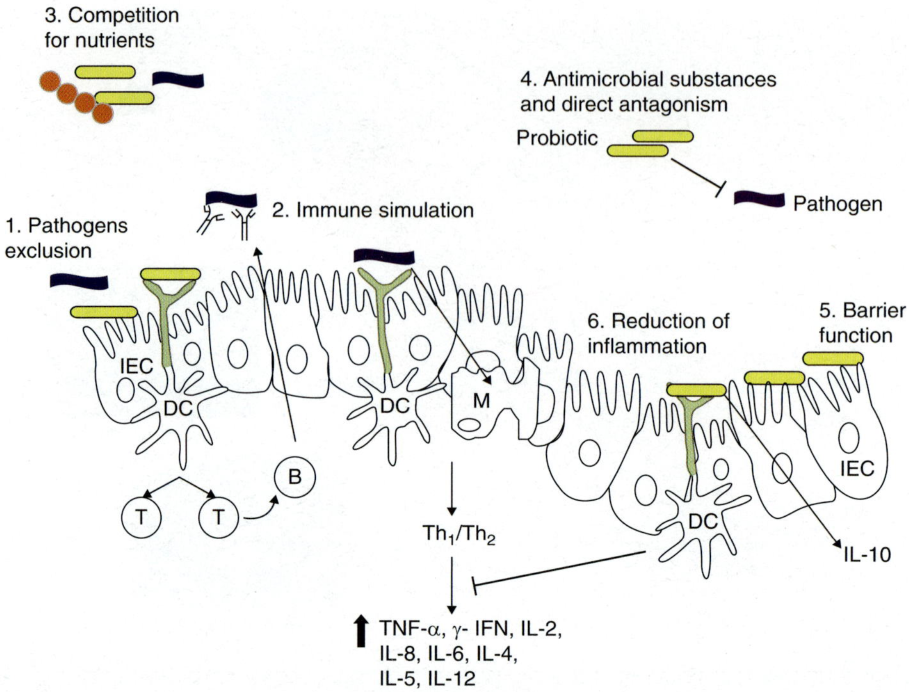

Plate 1.3 Some probiotic mechanisms that induce several beneficial host responses. Most effects consist of (1) Exclusion and competing with pathogen to epithelial cells adhesion, (2) innate immune stimulation, (3) competition for nutrients and prebiotic products, (4) production of antimicrobial substances and thereby pathogen antagonism, (5) protection of intestinal barrier integrity and (6) regulation of anti-inflammatory cytokine and inhibition of pro-inflammatory cytokine production. IEC, intestinal epithelium cells; DC, dendritic cell; IL, interleukin; M, intestinal M cell. *Source:* Saad *et al.*, 2013. Reproduced with permission from Elsevier

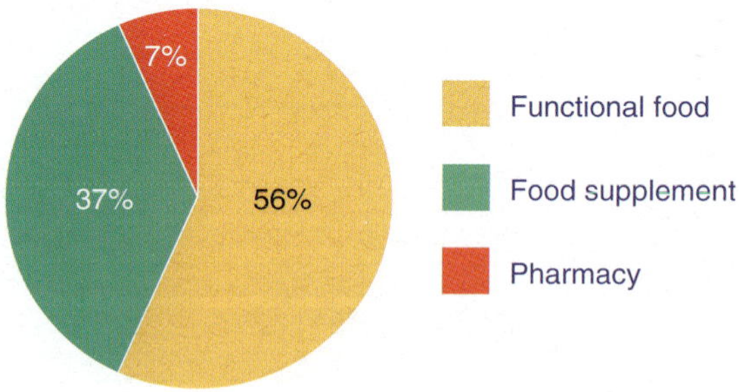

Plate 1.5 The distribution of the probiotics application. *Source:* Ubic Consulting, 2009. Reproduced with permission

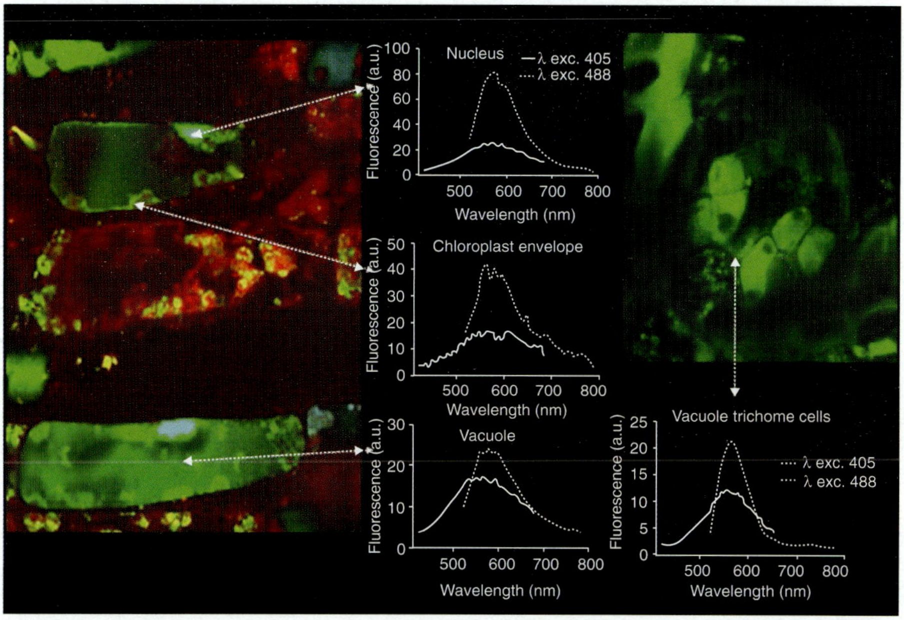

Plate 2.8 Fluorescence micro-imaging of *P. latifolia* leaves showing the subcellular distribution of dihydroxy-substituted phenyl-propanoids. Cross-section, 100 μm-thick, were stained with Naturstoff Reagent and fluorescence recorded with confocal. Views refer to the second layer of palisade parenchyma (at 100 μm depth from the adaxial epidermis) and the glandular trichome cells. The nucleus, the chloroplast envelope and the vacuole of glandular trichome cells are compartments of exclusive accumulation of dihydroxy B-ring-substituted flavonoid glycosides. Indeed, the peak of maximal mission, at approx. 575 nm, did not differ depending on the excitation wavelength. By contrast, in the vacuole of palisade cells which emits at 545 or 575 under 405 or 488 nm excitation, respectively both caffeic acid derivatives (λ_{em} = 525 nm) and di-hydroxy B-ring-substituted flavonoid glycosides are present. Please, note that the light-blue colour associated with the nucleus originates from the dark-blue fluorescence of 4′-6-diamidino-2-phenylindole and the green-fluorescence attributed to flavonoids. *Source:* Agati *et al.*, 2012. Reproduced with permission from Elsevier

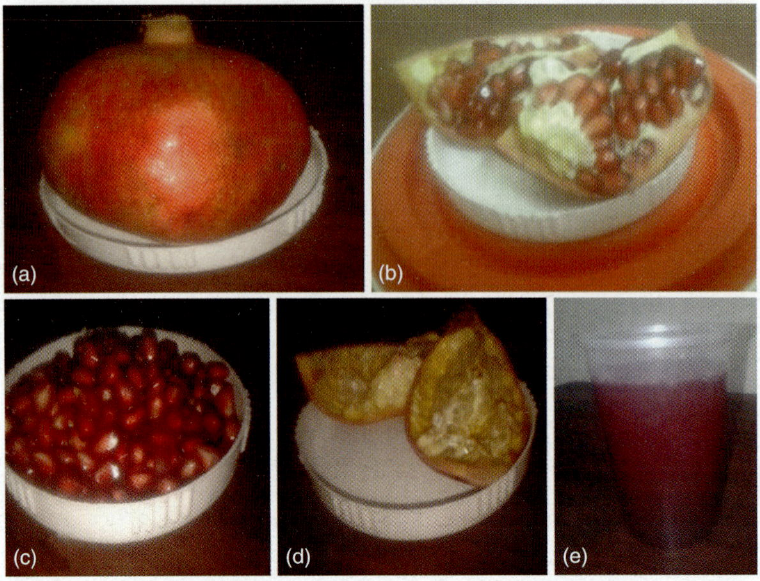

Plate 4.2 (a) Pomegranate fruit; (b) pomegranate internal part; (c) pomegranate arils; (d) pomegranate peel; (e) pomegranate juice (Kaur & Sharma, 2013)

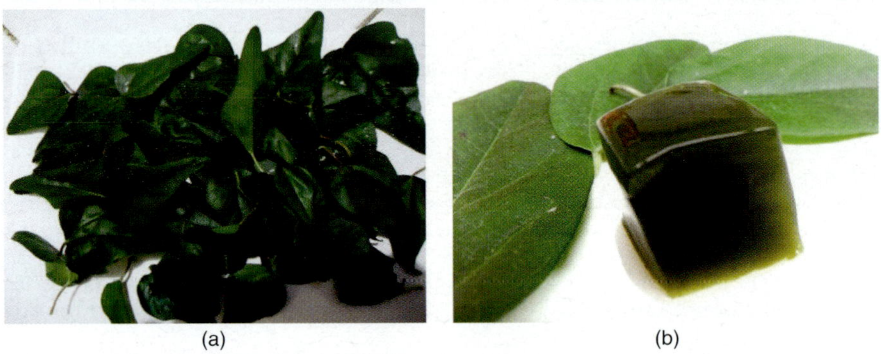

Plate 8.1 (a) Fresh leaves of *Cyclea barbata*. (b) Firm gel formed by the extract from the leaves, using 10 leaves in 100 g of water

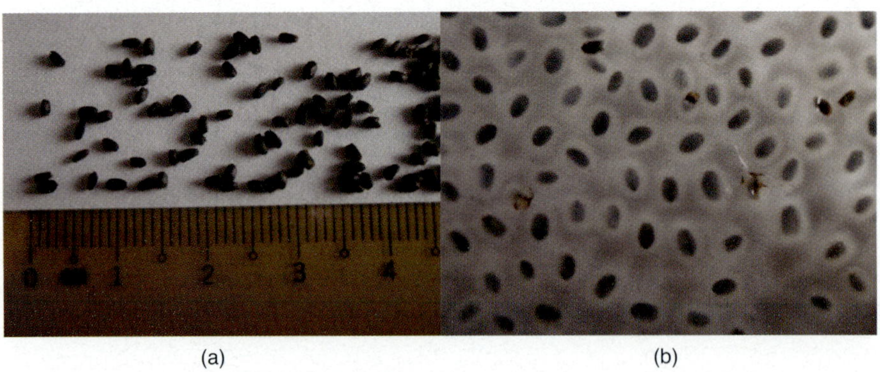

Plate 8.2 (a) Dry basil seeds. (b) Seeds soaked in water with the formation of a thick gel layer surrounding the seeds

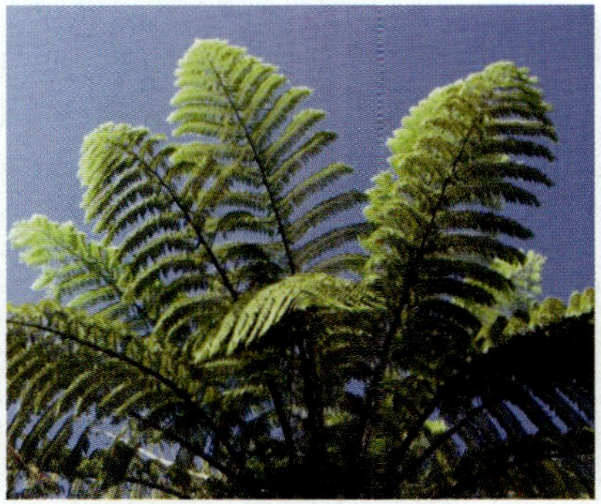

(a)

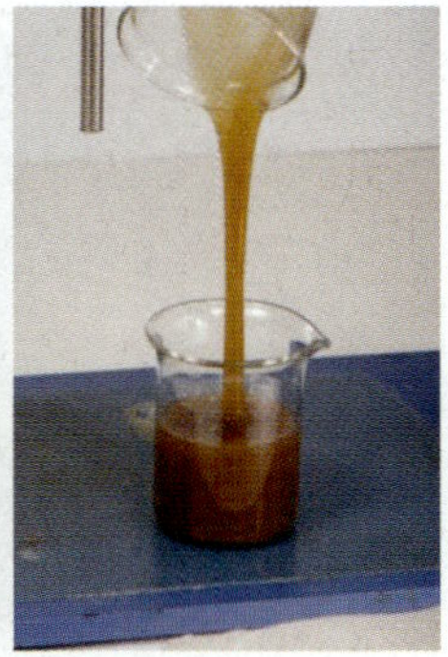

(b)

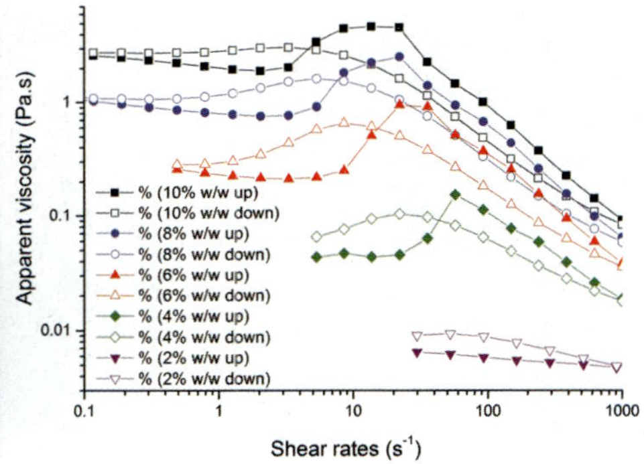

(c)

Plate 8.3 (a) Mamaku, the black tree fern (*Cyathea medullaris*). (b) Viscoelastic properties of 7% w/w solution of mamaku extract, illustrated by decanting from one beaker to another. (c) Viscosity curves of solutions of mamaku extract (2, 4, 6, 8 and 10% w/w) as a function of shear rate at 20 °C. The viscosity measurements were carried out using a double-gap attachment to obtain 'up-curves' (filled symbols) and 'down-curves' (open symbols). *Source:* Goh *et al.*, 2007. Reproduced with permission from the American Chemical Society

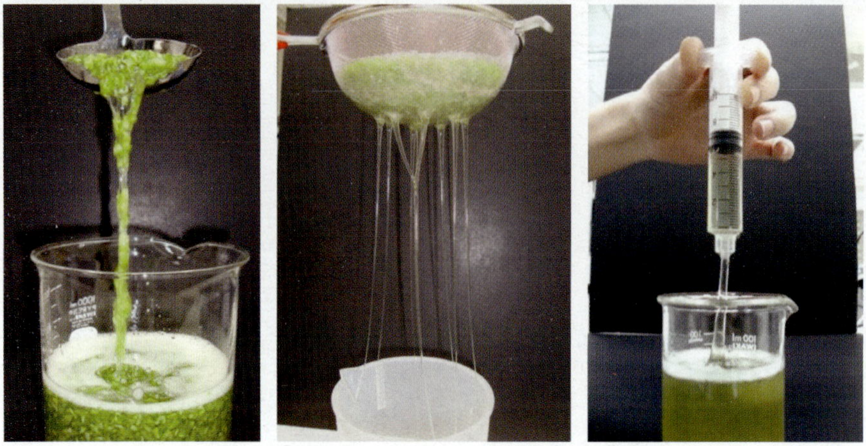

(a) (b) (c)

Plate 8.4 (a) Slimy characteristic of coarsely chopped stems of Malabar spinach dispersed in water (1 : 1 ratio). (b) Clear ropy mucilage obtained by separating the chopped stem using a sieve. (c) Self-siphoning effect observed by withdrawing the mucilage with a syringe. *Source:* Lim, 2010

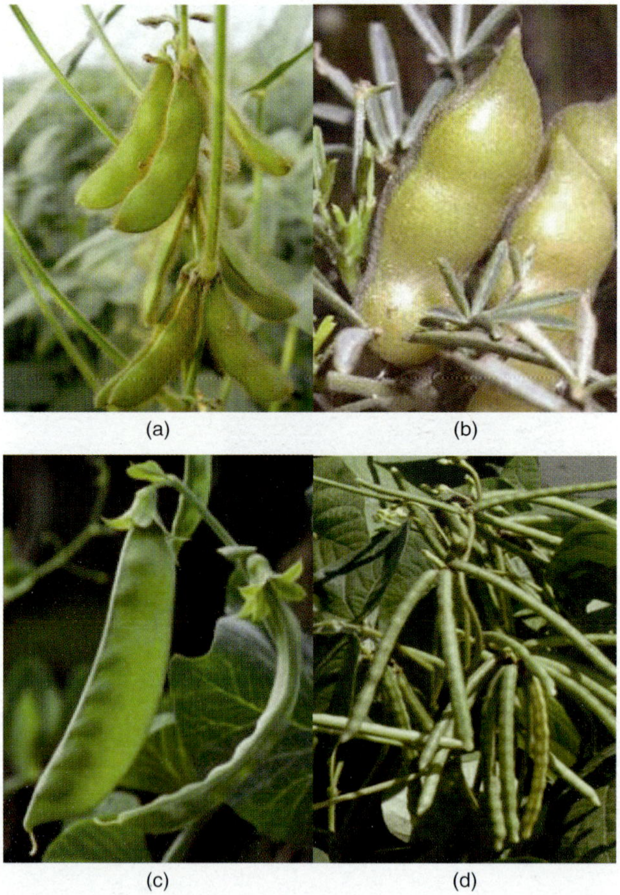

(a) (b)

(c) (d)

Plate 10.1 Different legume varieties: (a) soybean (*Glycine max*), (b) lupin (*Lupinus leteus*), (c) peas (*Pisum sativum*) and (d) mung bean (*Phaseolus aureus*)

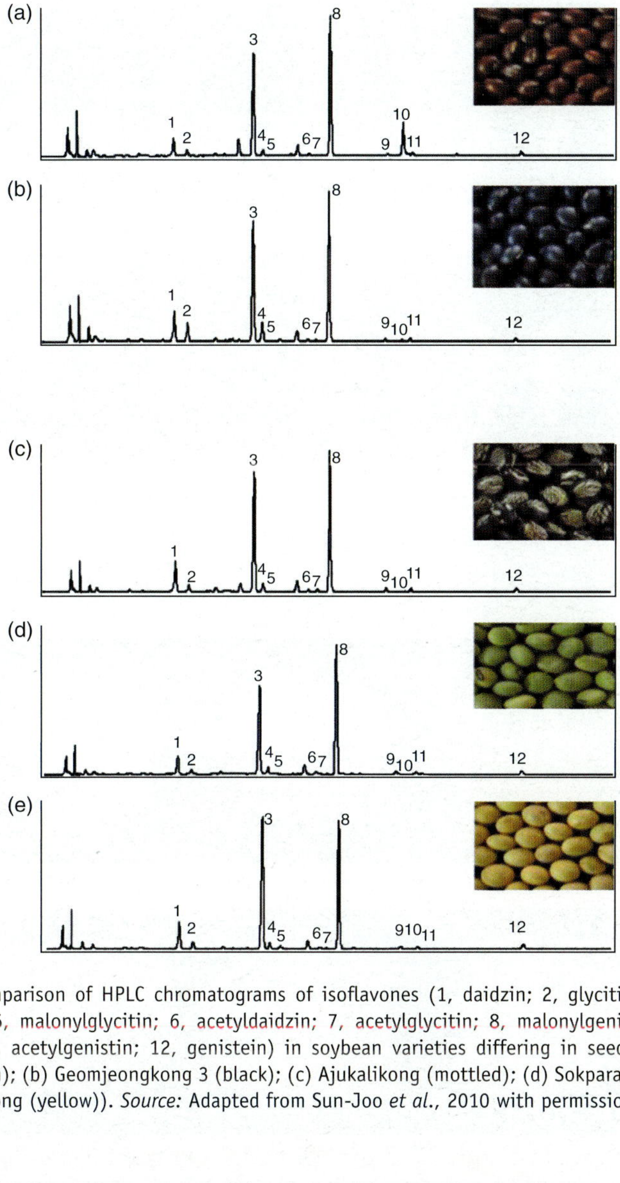

Plate 10.6 Comparison of HPLC chromatograms of isoflavones (1, daidzin; 2, glycitin; 3, genistin; 4, malonyldaidzin; 5, malonylglycitin; 6, acetyldaidzin; 7, acetylglycitin; 8, malonylgenistin; 9, daidzein; 10, glycitein; 11, acetylgenistin; 12, genistein) in soybean varieties differing in seed coat colour: (a) Galmikong (brown); (b) Geomjeongkong 3 (black); (c) Ajukalikong (mottled); (d) Sokparaengikong (green); (e) Hwangkeumkong (yellow)). *Source:* Adapted from Sun-Joo *et al.*, 2010 with permission from Elsevier

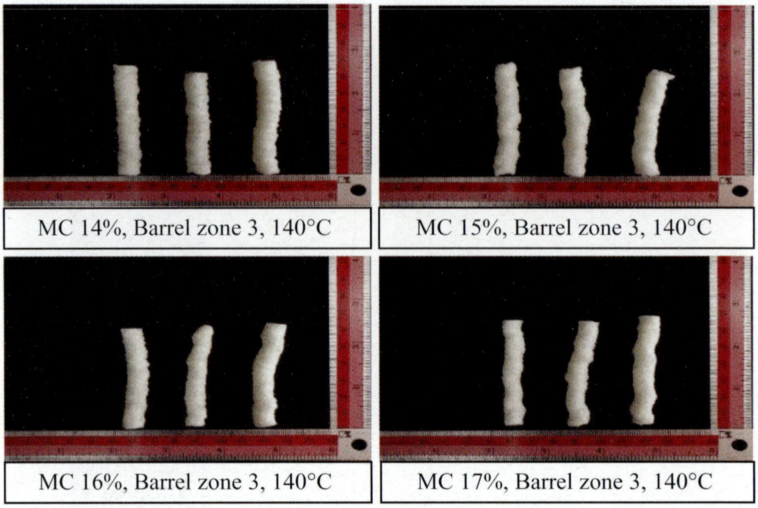

Plate 12.1 Appearance of rice snack extruded from broken rice with different percentage feed moisture content (% MC), feeder speed at 30 rpm, screw speed of 180 rpm and barrel temperature zone 1 : 2 : 3 at 100 : 120 : 140 °C

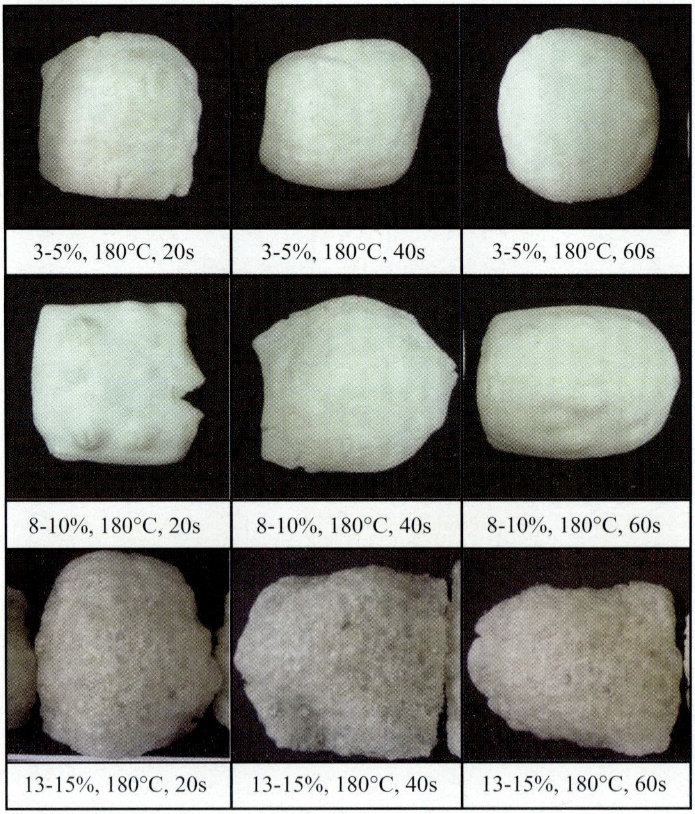

Plate 12.3 Appearance of snack after frying the extruded pellet which were dried to different percentage of moisture content at 180 °C for 20, 40 and 60 s

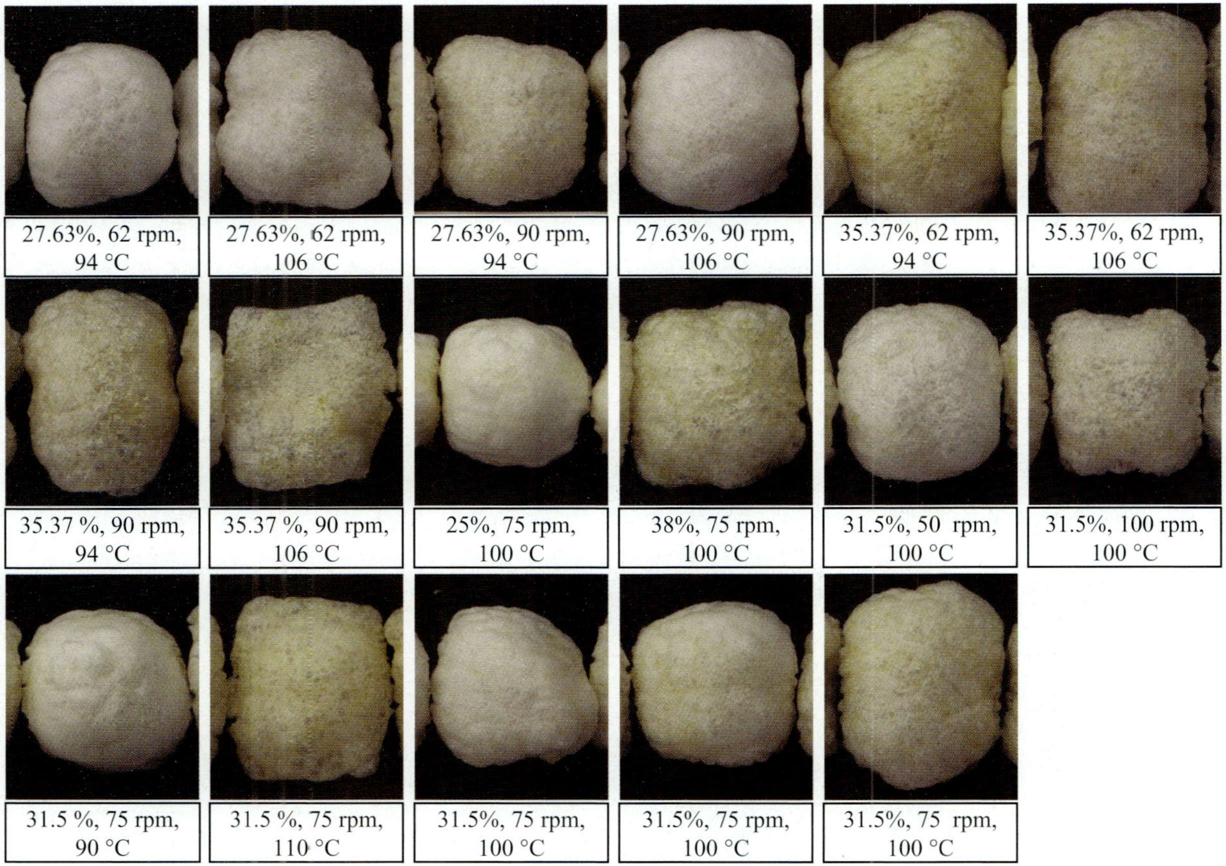

Plate 12.4 Appearance of snack after frying the pellet extruded with different percentage of feed moisture content, screw speed and zone 3 barrel temperature. The pellet from all extrusion conditions were dried to about 8–10% moisture content and fried at 180 °C for 20 s

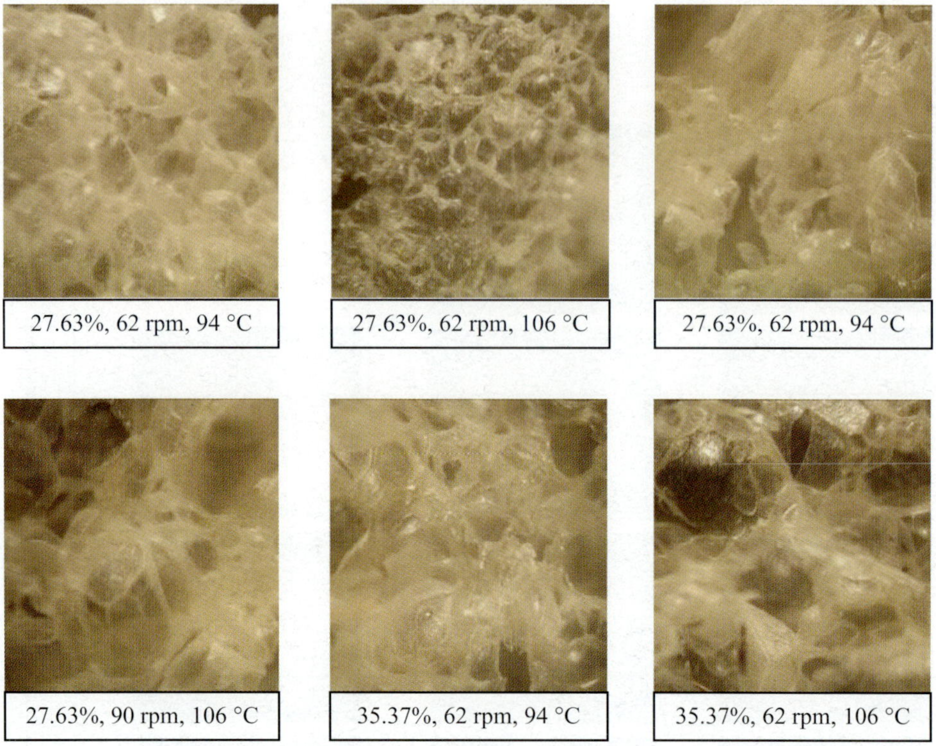

Plate 12.5 Stereomicrograph of air bubbles in the fried snack from the pellet extruded with different percentage of feed moisture content, screw speed and zone 3 barrel temperature ($\times$ 10.5)

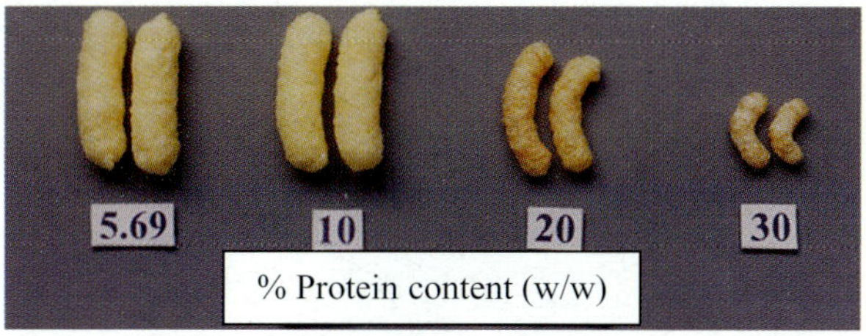

Plate 12.6 Extruded snacks supplemented with dry chicken meat at different percentage of protein content (w/w)

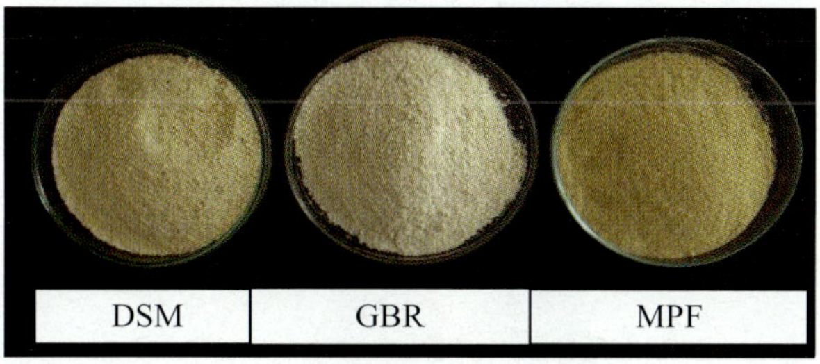

Plate 12.7 Fibre sources from food processing by products: defatted soybean meal (DSM), germinated brown rice meal (GBR) and mango peel fibre (MPF)

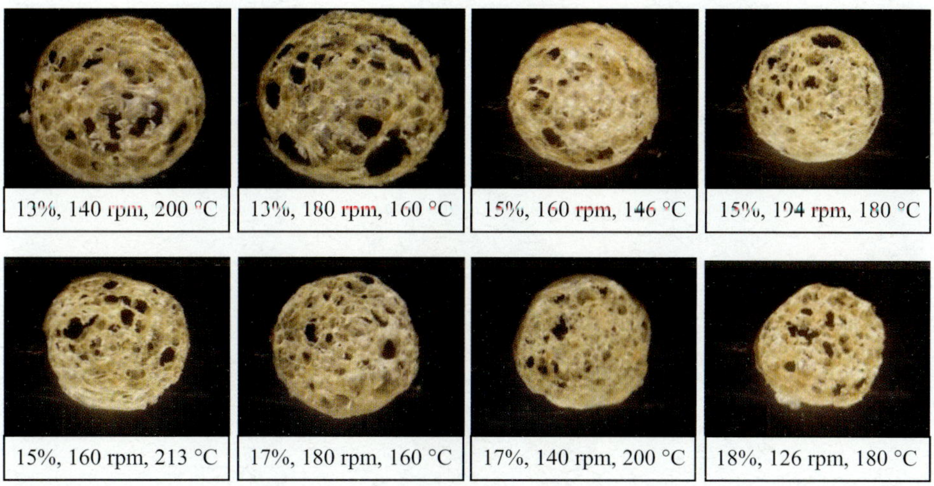

Plate 12.8 Cross-section of fibre contained corn-based snack extruded with different percentage of feed moisture content, screw speed and zone 3 barrel temperature ($\times$ 10.5)

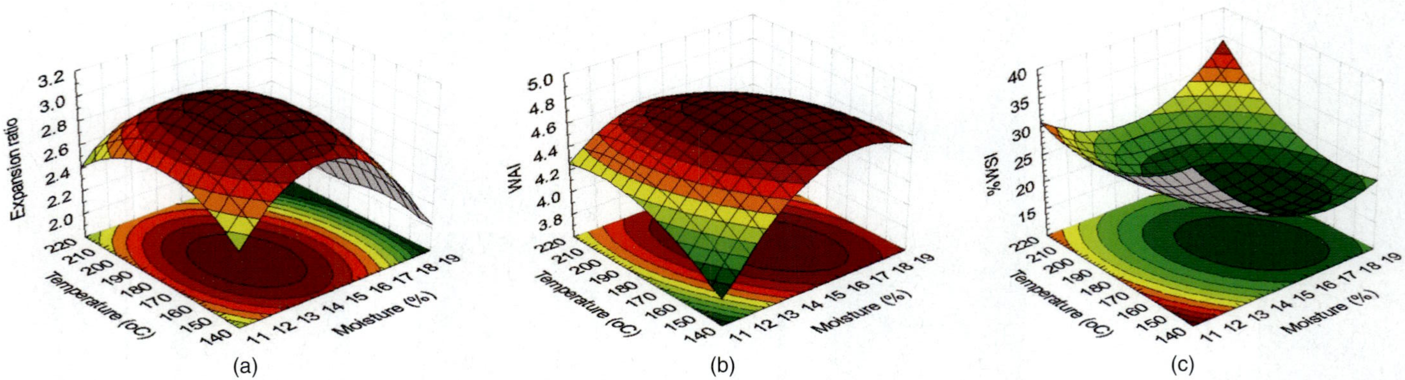

Plate 12.9 RSM on the effects of percentage feed moisture content and barrel temperature of zone 3 on expansion ratio (a), water absorption index (b) and water solubility index (c) of the extruded fiber contained corn based snacks with screw speed 160 rpm

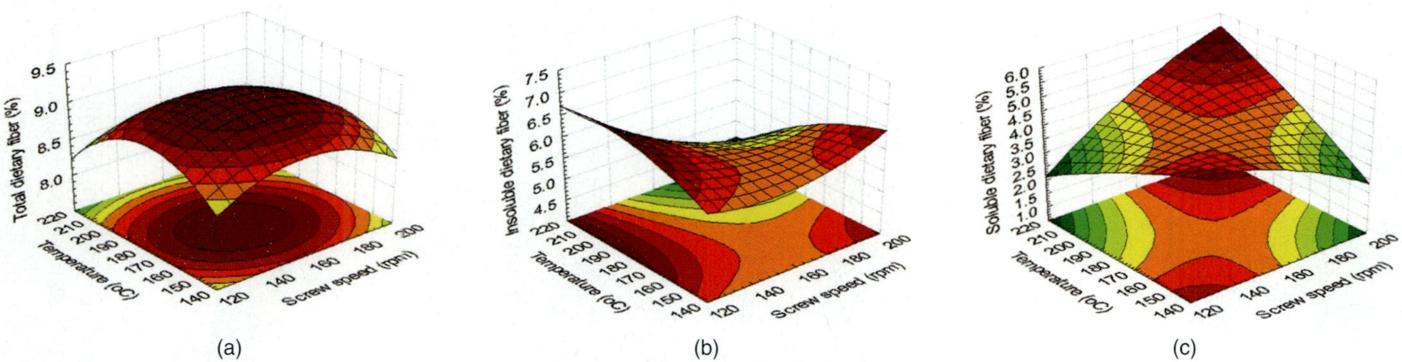

Plate 12.10 RSM on the effects of screw speed and barrel temperature of zone 3 on total dietary fiber (a), insoluble dietary fiber (b) and soluble dietary fiber (c) of the extruded fiber contained corn based snacks with percentage feed moisture content at 13%

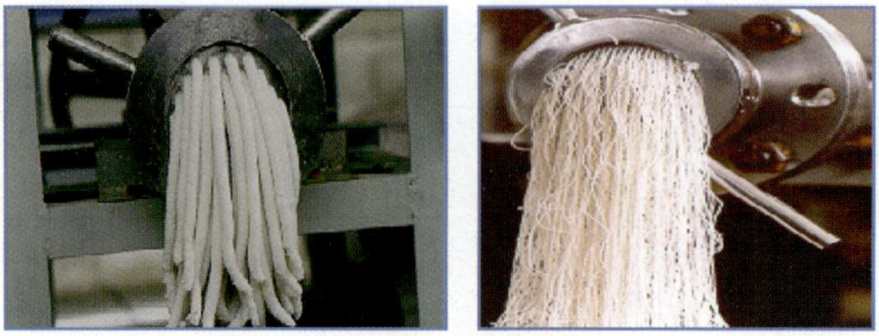

(a) (b)

Plate 12.11 Extrusion of rice cake (a) and after pregelatinized by steaming (b) in most conventional method for rice vermicelli production. *Source:* Yoenyongbuddhagal, S. (2002). The effects of processing condition on ricevermicelli quality, Dissertation No. PH-02-2, Food Engineering and Bioprocess Technology Program, School of Environment, Resources and Development, Asian Institute of Technology, Thailand, 140pp

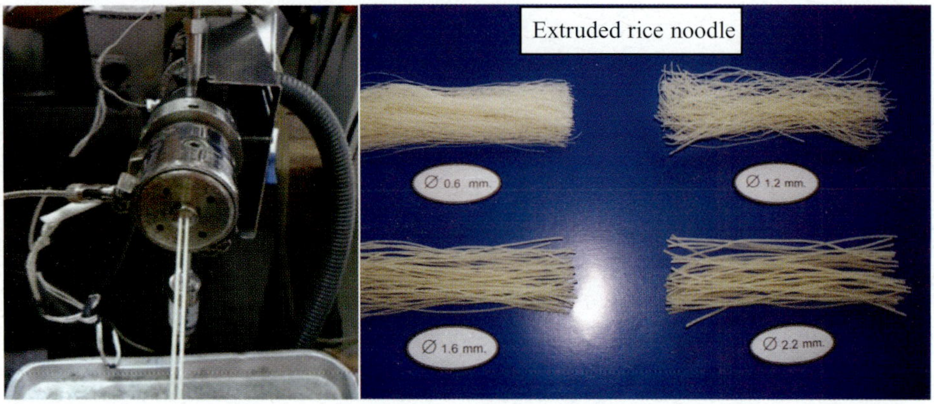

(a) (b)

Plate 12.12 Direct extrusion of rice noodle from rice flour using a Laboratory single screw extruder (a) and the rice noodles extruded through die with different diameter (b)

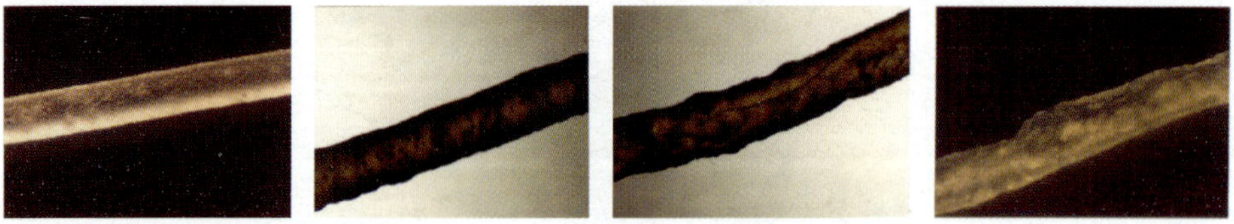

(a) (b) (c) (d)

Plate 12.13 Microscopic observation of rice noodle (diameter 0.6 mm) surface prepared by direct extrusion cooking (a) and commercial products prepared by conventional process (b-d). *Source:* Adapted from Charutigon *et al.*, 2008

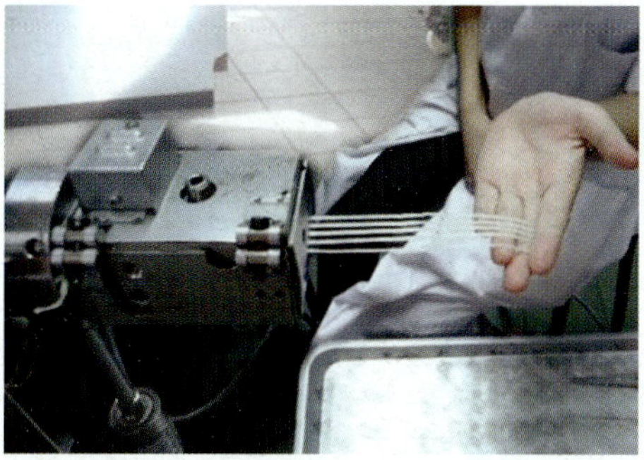

Plate 12.14 Direct extrusion of rice noodle (flat type) from rice flour using a laboratory single screw extruder (Brabender 19/20 DN Model Do-Corder DCE 330, Germany)

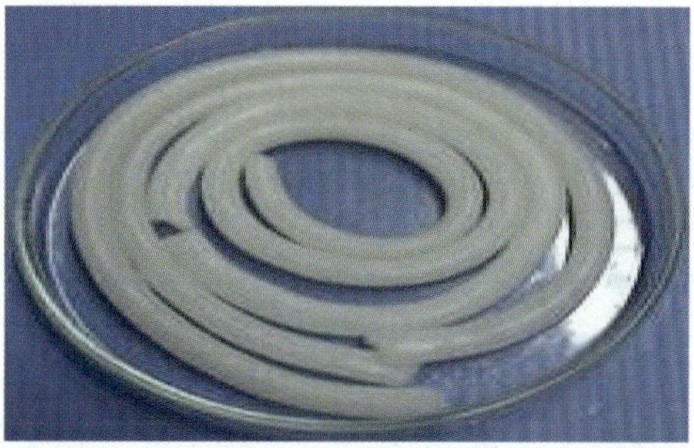

Plate 12.15 Extruded macaroni-like rice noodle after cooking in boiling water for 3.5 min

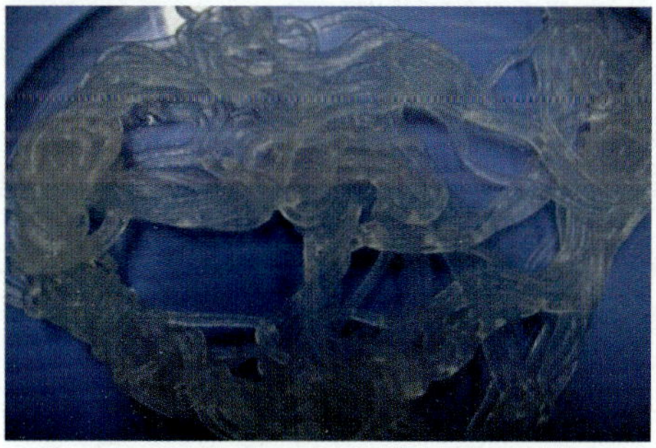

Plate 12.16 Cooked clear glass noodle made from edible canna starch (Japanese Green) using a laboratory single screw with feed moisture content at 30%, barrel temperature of zone 1: 2: 3 at 70: 70: 100 °C, feeder and screw speed at 50 rpm and 30 rpm respectively

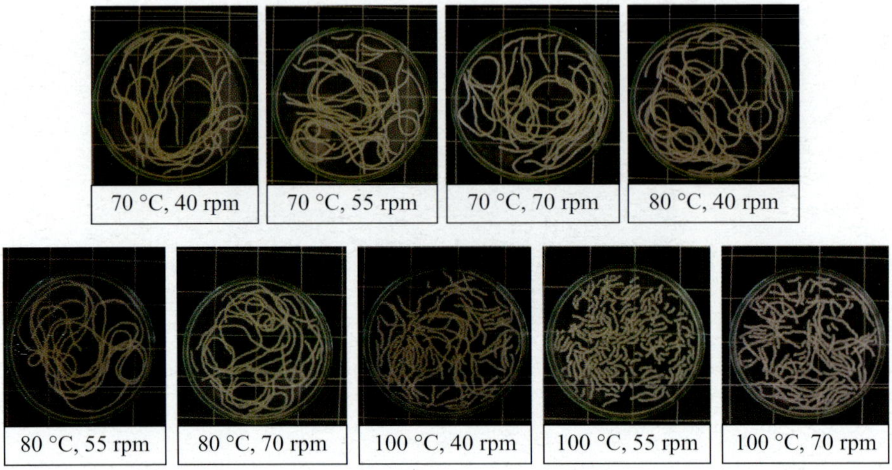

Plate 12.17 Instant wheat noodle, extruded with different barrel temperature of zone 3 and screw speed, after pouring boiling water and kept for 4 minute

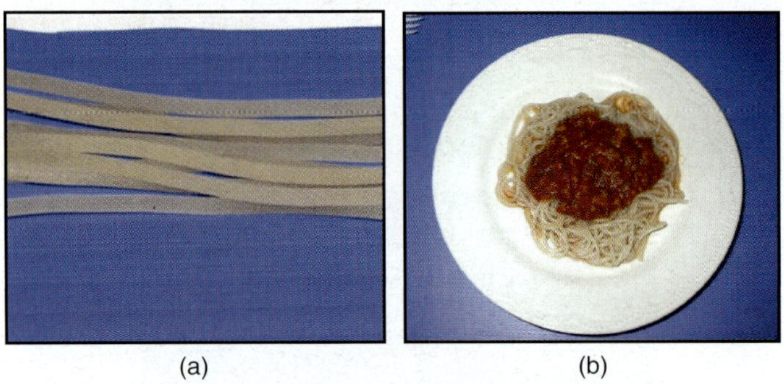

Plate 12.18 Rice spaghetti extruded from rice flour substituted with DSM and Elastitex 3 at 10 and 4 g/100 g flour mix (a) and cooked rice spaghetti with meat sauce on the top (b)

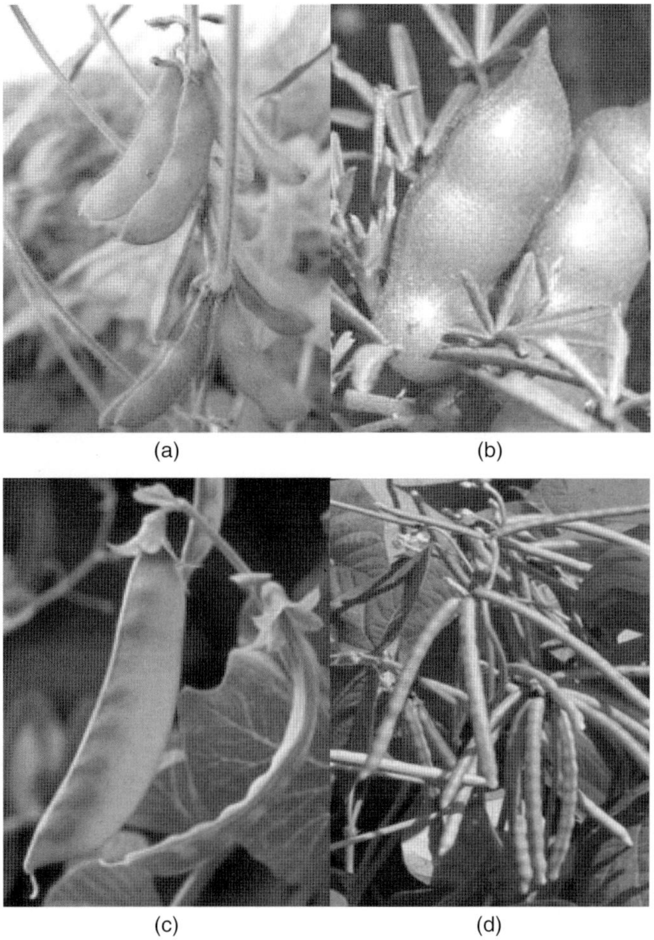

Figure 10.1 Different legume varieties: (a) soybean (*Glycine max*), (b) lupin (*Lupinus leteus*), (c) peas (*Pisum sativum*) and (d) mung bean (*Phaseolus aureus*). For colour details, see the colour plates section

Isoflavone synthase introduces a 2-hydroxyl group, which in turn is removed by an isoflavone dehydratase to yield daidzein (7,4′-dihydroxyisoflavone) and genistein (5,7,4′ trihydroxyisoflavone) (Figure 10.2).

The biosynthesis of glycitein (7,4′-dihydroxy-6-methoxyisoflavone), a major isoflavone in the soy germ (hypocotyls) is not questionable. The numbering scheme for isoflavones is shown in Figure 10.3. Isoflavones in the soybean are converted to 7-*O*-bglucosides by a glucosyltransferase and then to their 6″-omalonates by a malonyl transferase. This form is stored in vacuoles until it is used by the plant and is the major form in harvested soybeans. Although yellow or black soybeans are the most familiar forms, early harvesting before ripening results in a green immature soybean. This is boiled in the pod and is served as edamame; it has similar levels of isoflavones to the yellow and black soybeans (Simonne *et al.*, 2000, Wu *et al.*, 2004b).

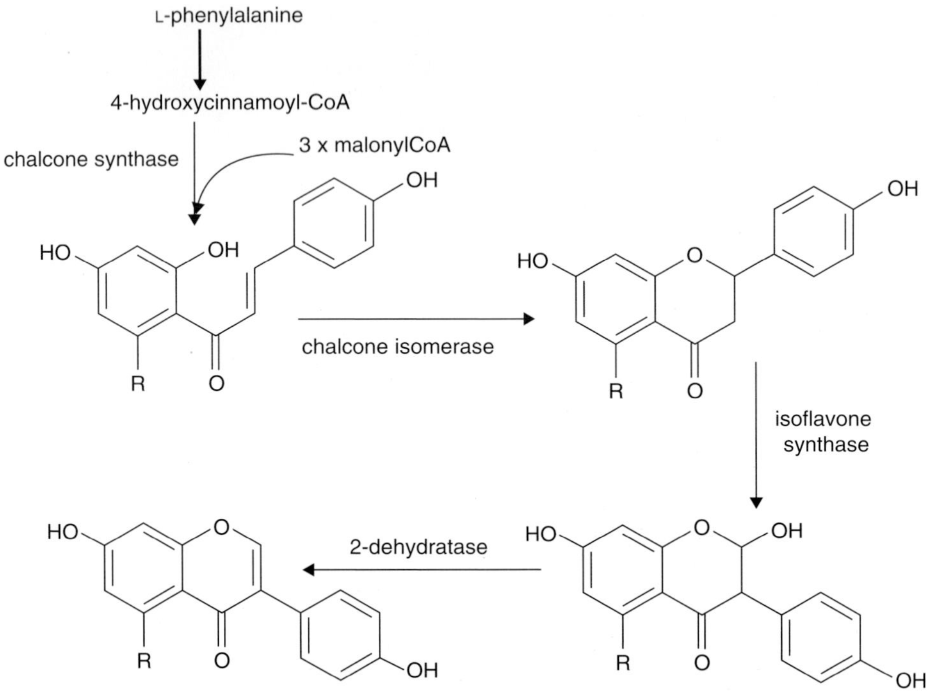

Figure 10.2 The pathway for isoflavone biosynthesis. First phenylalanine reacts with malonyl CoA to produce 4-hydroxycinnamoyl CoA. Under the catalytic control of chalcone synthase 4-hydroxycinnamoyl CoA condenses with three molecules of malonyl CoA to form a chalcone. Chalcone isomerase closes the heterocyclic ring to form naringenin. The B-ring is moved from the 2-position to the 3-position by isoflavone synthase. Isoflavone dehydratase removes water to generate the 2,3 double bond in the heterocyclic ring (see Figure 10.3 for the numbering scheme)

Udgata and Naik (2006) noted 12 isoflavones that have been reported in soybean, including three aglycones – genistein, daidzein and glycitein – and their respective 7-*O*-β-D-glucosides (genistin, daidzin and glycitin), 6″*O*-malonyl-7-*O*-β-D-glucosides (malonylgenistin, malonyldaidzin and malonylglycitin) and 6″*O*-acetyl-7-*O*-β-D-glucosides (acetylgenistin, acetyldaidzin and acetylglycitin) as shown in Figure 10.4.

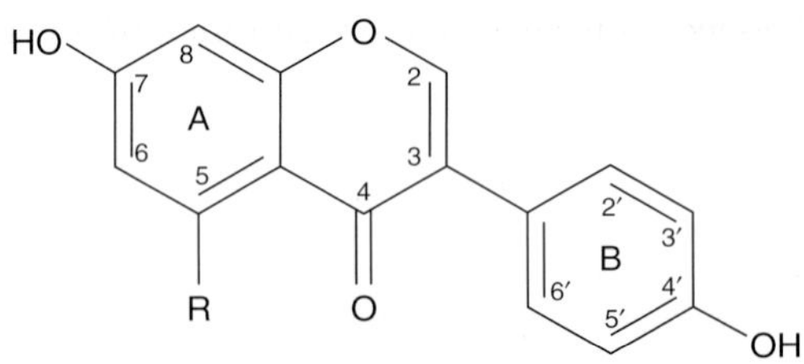

Figure 10.3 The numbering scheme of isoflavones. The scheme starts from the ethereal oxygen in the heterocyclic ring. The B-ring ring has a separate numbering system (1′–6′)

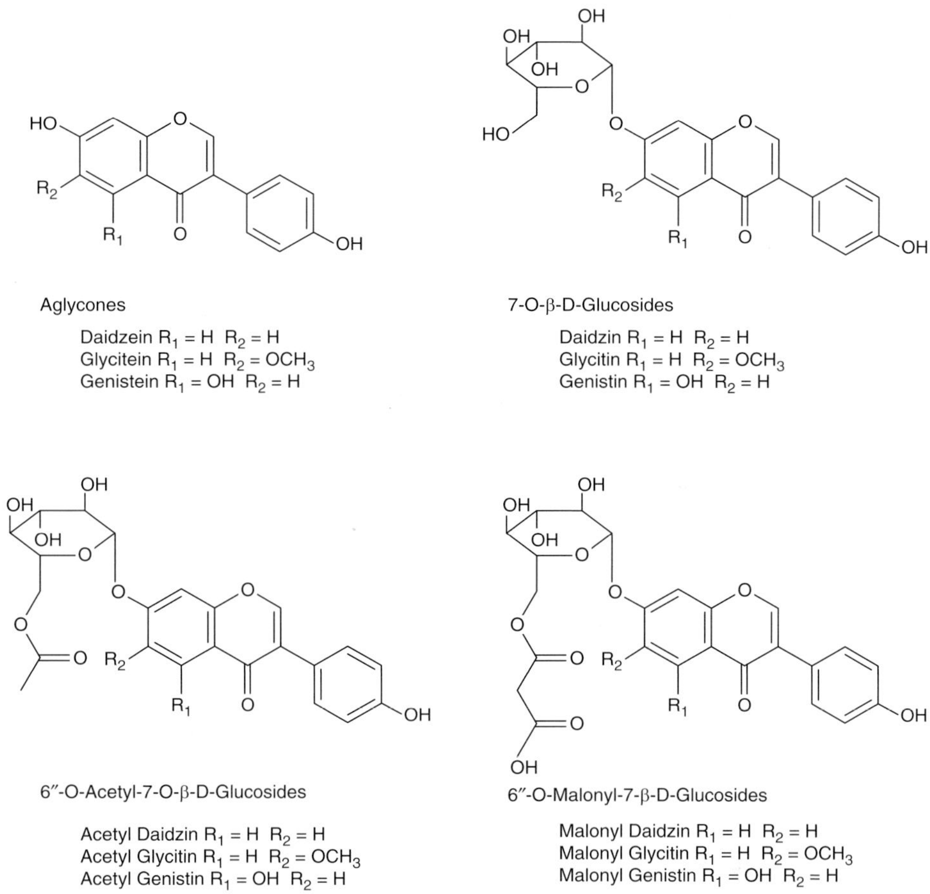

Figure 10.4 Chemical structures of 12 isoflavones isomers

10.2.3 Effect of cultivar and environment on isoflavone content

In soybean, isoflavones exist in the entire plant including the seed coat, cotyledon, hypocotyl and radicle of the seed, and the leaves, stems and roots (Figure 10.5).

In soybean seeds, hypocotyls have a high concentration of isoflavones (Kudou *et al.*, 1991), although the major quantity of isoflavones is in the cotyledons. Similarly, Lee *et al.* (2007) reported that some soybean varieties had isoflavone levels higher in the cotyledons than in roots. In contrast, Kim *et al.* (2004) found that isoflavone content in roots was 2.9-fold higher than in cotyledons. However, Siviengkhek *et al.* (2008) found that isoflavone levels were higher in cotyledons and lowest in the seed coat among the Korean soybean cultivars (Table 10.1).

Numerous researchers have considered isoflavones as the main phenolic soybean compounds and their content in different cultivars may vary from 126.1 to 409.2 mg/100 g of grains (Eldridge and Kwolek, 1983; Coward *et al.*, 1993; Tsukamoto

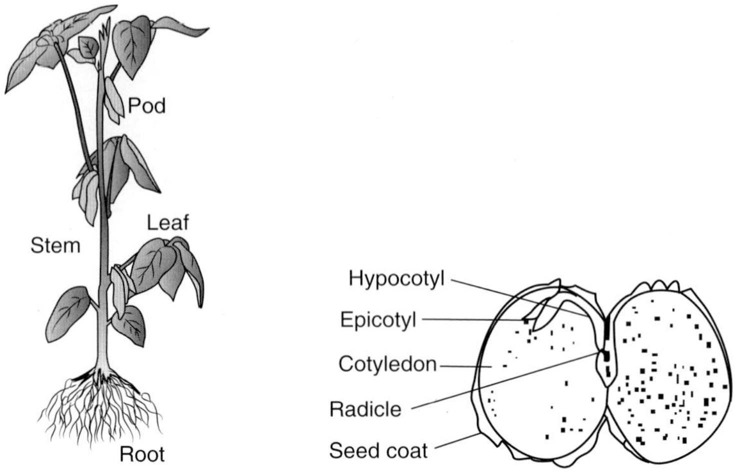

Figure 10.5 Seeds, leaves, stems, seed coat, hypocotyls, radicle and roots of soybean

et al., 1995; Mazur *et al.*, 1998; Wang *et al.*, 2000). The isoflavone content of different soybean cultivars depends on hereditary factors, sowing conditions and geographic location during cultivation (Eldridge and Kwolek, 1983; Tsukamoto *et al.*, 1995; Wang *et al.*, 2000). In addition, environmental factors that can also affect isoflavone content in soybean include air temperature, soil moisture levels, soil fertility (K), CO_2 levels, light quality and pest pressure (Seguin *et al.*, 2007). Despite being highly variable and regulated by multiple environmental and genetic factors, several studies have reported that some varieties may have relatively stable isoflavone content across a variety of environments (Hoeck *et al.*, 2000; Lee *et al.*, 2003; Seguin *et al.*, 2004). Selection and breeding high-isoflavone cultivars is thus underway in several countries (Seguin *et al.*, 2007).

Differences in total isoflavone content between soybeans differing in seed coat colour have been reported; however, results are mostly inconclusive because often a limited number of varieties were compared (Kim *et al.*, 2005, 2007). Further, Wang *et al.* (2000) reported that among 210 North American varieties, while total isoflavone content was not affected by seed coat colour, associations with specific individual isoflavones were observed. Genistin concentration was greater in green soybeans than in black or brown ones, while genistein was lowest in black soybean. In Japan, Sakai *et al.* (2005) reported limited differences in total isoflavone content between 195 varieties grown at one site, with concentrations highest in light-yellow varieties, intermediate in yellow-green, green, grey and black varieties and lowest in yellow varieties. Seed coat colour was associated with differences in flavonoid content and composition in other species (Beninger and Hosfield, 2003). Moreover, results from Sun-Joo *et al.* (2010) have suggested that isoflavone content differences among the Korean soybean cultivars differing in seed coat and cotyledon colour are mainly indicative of environmental and genotype-by-environment effects. Selection and breeding for isoflavones can be carried out irrespective of seed coat and cotyledon colour as shown in Figure 10.6.

Table 10.1 The isoflavone content in different soybean seed components

Variety	Seed component	Isoflavone (μ/g)
Aga3	Radicle	20,304a
	Cotyledon	10,203b
	Seed coat	617c
Aga4	Radicle	14,855a
	Cotyledon	5,524b
	Seed coat	94c
Pungsannanulkong	Radicle	10,154a
	Cotyledon	2,127b
	Seed coat	494c
Taekwangkong	Radicle	14,489a
	Cotyledon	1,502b
	Seed coat	213c
Hwangkeumkong	Radicle	13,131a
	Cotyledon	1,608b
	Seed coat	266c
Cheongjakong	Radicle	11,525a
	Cotyledon	1,035b
	Seed coat	156c
Variety		**
Seed component		**

** Values with different letters (small letter a–c) are significantly different at 5% level by DMRT of seed component within a variety.
Source: Adapted from Phommalth *et al.*, 2008.

According to Kudou *et al.* (1991), accumulation of isoflavone in soybean seeds starts 35 days after flowering and Kitamura *et al.* (1991) reported a lower isoflavone content in early cultivars compared to that from late maturity group cultivars. However, currently no reports are available that relate these isoflavone forms to the number of days required for the seeds to reach maturity (Ribeiro *et al.*, 2007). Tsukamoto *et al.* (1995) reported that the effects of climate temperature contribute significantly to the differences in isoflavone content. Seeds harvested after cultivating in a high-temperature climate had a significantly decreased isoflavone content. Although hypocotyls have a high concentration, most isoflavones are in the cotyledons after the weights of the hypocotyls and the cotyledons are calculated.

10.3 Isoflavones: dietary intakes and supplements

Although soybean-containing foods have become more popular in the United States over the past 50 years, they are in general quite different from the forms of soy consumed in Asia (Synder and Kwon, 1987). In contrast to American soy foods, those in Asia are often fermented. Soybeans are converted using microorganisms to miso (added to soups and stews in Japan), soy paste (in Korea) and tempeh (with a texture like meat in Indonesia). Soy sauce is another familiar soy product and is made either by acid hydrolysis (no isoflavones) or by prolonged fermentation. The proteins

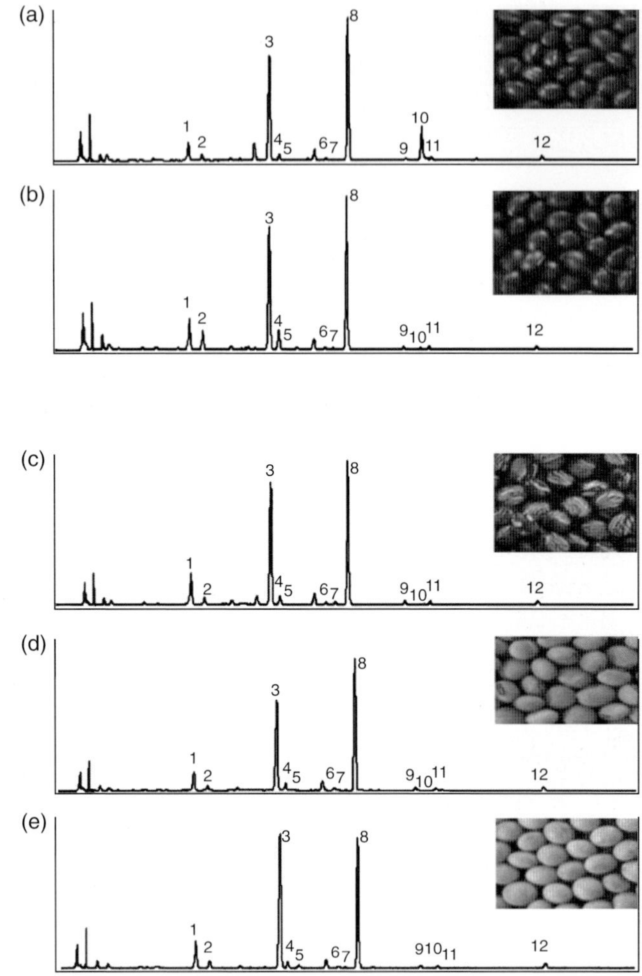

Figure 10.6 Comparison of HPLC chromatograms of isoflavones (1, daidzin; 2, glycitin; 3, genistin; 4, malonyldaidzin; 5, malonylglycitin; 6, acetyldaidzin; 7, acetylglycitin; 8, malonylgenistin; 9, daidzein; 10, glycitein; 11, acetylgenistin; 12, genistein) in soybean varieties differing in seed coat colour: (a) Galmikong (brown); (b) Geomjeongkong 3 (black); (c) Ajukalikong (mottled); (d) Sokparaengikong (green); (e) Hwangkeumkong (yellow)). *Source:* Adapted from Sun-Joo *et al.*, 2010 with permission from Elsevier. For colour details, see the colour plates section

and lipids in soybeans are extracted with boiling water to form soy milk, an important alternative to mother's milk in countries with a high incidence of lactase insufficiency. Soy milk is curdled to prepare tofu, which can be pressed to remove water. Tofu can be fried or added to numerous other dishes.

In order to take in the daily amounts of isoflavones that researchers recommend are desirable for a positive impact on health, it is logical to concentrate on soy-based foods. This may include baking with soy flour (up to 177.89 mg isoflavone/100 g), drinking a soy beverage (109.51 mg/100 g), or eating defatted soybean flakes (125.82 mg/100 g). Good supplementary sources of isoflavones include tofu, such as Mori-Nu silken firm (27.91 mg/100 g) or dried-frozen (67.491 mg/100 g) and tempeh, either cooked (53 mg/100 g) or burgers (29 mg/100 g). Not all beans contain isoflavones. Those that do have low concentrations of isoflavones should be eaten to supplement an isoflavone-rich diet. Navy, pinto, red, fava, garbanza and small white beans contain 0.10–0.74 mg/100 g. Designed for a populace raised on meat and potatoes, significant (often satisfying) changes in cuisine may be required to accomplish the intake reported in clinical studies, including eating miso, tofu and natto. Contrary to popular belief, soya sauce (shoyu), the most important Japanese condiment, is a relatively poor source of isoflavones (1.64 mg/100 g).

Many factors contribute to the variability of isoflavone content in food, including characteristics of the raw material and the procedures used for extraction and analysis. Soybeans are affected by cultivar, location and year of cultivation. Glucoside contents were converted to aglycones by using appropriate molecular weight adjustments. It should be noted that the physiological significance of total content may be different from the individual contents. Although glucosides of isoflavones are readily hydrolysed by the intestinal bacterial enzymes, Setchell (1998) stated that little is known about the biological activity of individual isoflavones. The mean values of the total isoflavone content in selected soy food as reported in the USDA database are summarized in Table 10.2. These mean values are summarized from the results of various labs using different analytical methods.

In general, most isoflavones in soybean are in the form of glucosides or malonyl glucoside conjugates of diadzein and genistein, although total glycitein contributed only 5–10% of the total amount in the soy germ. Aglycones in non-fermented soybean and soy food account for only a very small fraction of the total isoflavone content (Murphy *et al.*, 1999). Aglycones in fermented soy food are the major forms of the isoflavones (Fukutake *et al.*, 1996). Table 10.3 shows the 12 forms of isoflavones in selected soybean and soy food.

10.4 Isoflavones: changing chemistry in soy foods

Depending on processing techniques, soybean products present different forms and concentrations of isoflavones. The fermentation of soybeans is very common making miso, soybean paste and tempeh, as well as soy sauce. Soybeans are used to manufacture full-fat soy milk and tofu. Tofu has several forms depending on how much water is removed. Natto is obtained from the surface layer when generating soy milk. The American products start with a solvent (hexane) extraction procedure to recover the oil from the soybean. The defatted protein-enriched soy flour (50% protein) is the source of soy protein concentrate (70% protein) and soy protein isolate (>90% protein). Soy protein isolate is used to make low-fat soy milk and tofu as well as a fermented isoflavone-protein-enriched product.

Generally, it has been reported that soy isoflavones are stable compounds during cold storage (Morales-de la Peña *et al.*, 2010). No degradation of total isoflavones in soy food has been observed during storage time; nevertheless, they can be subjected to several inter-conversions (Otieno *et al.*, 2007, Uzzan and Labuza, 2004).

Table 10.2 Summary of the mean values of the total isoflavones in soybean and selected foods containing soybean products

Food	Total isoflavones, mg/100 g edible portion
Meatless bacon	12.1
Soy hot dog	15.0
Meatless chicken nuggets, canned, cooked	14.6
Meatless chicken nuggets, canned, raw	12.2
Vegetable protein burger	8.2–9.3
Infant formula of various brands	2.6–26.0
Instant soy beverage, powder	109.5
Miso	69.84
Miso, dry	60.4
Natto, fermented	58.9
Soy cheese of various types	6.4–31.3
Soy fiber	44.4
Soy flour, defatted	131.2
Soy flour, textured	172.55
Soy flour, full-fat	177.9
Soy flour, full-fat, roasted	198.9
Soy meal, defatted	125.8
Soy milk	10.73
Soy film, yuba, Foo-jook, raw	193.9
Soy film, yuba, Foo-jook cooked	50.7
Soy protein concentrate, aqueous wash	102.1
Soy protein concentrate, alcohol wash	12.5
Soy isolate	97.4
Soy sauce, shoyu from soybean and wheat	1.64
Soybean from countries other than the United States	59.8–145.0
Soybean flakes, defatted	125.82
Soybean flakes, full-fat	129.0
Soybean immature, raw	20.4
Soybean mature seeds, raw (U.S. food quality)	128.35
Soybean, mature seeds, raw (U.S. commodity grade)	153.4
Soybean, mature seeds, sprouted, raw	40.7
Tempeh	60.61
Tofu, fresh, soft, film or extra firm of various brands	22.6–31.1
Tofu, frozen-dried, Kori	67.5
Tofu, fried	48.4
Tofu, pressed, semi-dry, Tau kwa	29.5

Source: Data from USDA, 2008. U. S. Department of Agriculture.

Decarboxylation of malonate to acetate, de-esterification of malonate to underivatized glucoside as well as generation of aglycones are some reactions that could take place depending on processing, storage conditions and molecular configuration of the compound (Figure 10.7).

Otherwise, processing soybeans to make foods results in changes in their chemistry. Generally, fermentation causes the removal of the glucosidic group releasing the isoflavone aglucone (Kuo *et al.*, 2006, Chun *et al.*, 2007). Similarly, a study discovered that if fermentation is long-lasting (for miso or some forms of soy sauce this can

Table 10.3 Isoflavone Content of selected Soytean and Commercial Soy Products (mg/g as is Basis)

Soy sample	Daidzin	Genistin	Glycitin	Malonyl Daidzin	Malonyl Genistin	Malonyl Glycitin	Acetyl Daidzin	Acetyl Genistin	Acetyl Glycitin	Daidzein	Genistein	Glycitein
Vinton 81 90H	690	852	56	300	743	50	1	9	nd	26	29	20
Soy flour	147	407	41	261	1023	57	trace	1	32	4	22	19
Soy isolate B	88	301	49	18	88	36	74	215	46	11	36	25
Tofu	25	84	8	159	108	nd[1]	8	1	29	46	52	12
Tempeh	2	65	14	255	104	nd	11	nd	nd	137	193	24
Hozukuri miso	72	123	18	nd	nd	22	1	11	nd	34	93	15
Fermented bean curd	Nd	trace	nd	nd	nd	nd	nd	nd	nd	143	223	23
Soybean hypocotyl	3200	1180	4850	4230	1440	4450	20	1050	1050	1020	35	nd
Soybean cotyledon	450	800	nd	700	1170	nd	20	10	nd	330	480	nd

nd means not detectes.

Source: Data from Kudou *et al.* (1991) and Wang & Murphy (1994a).

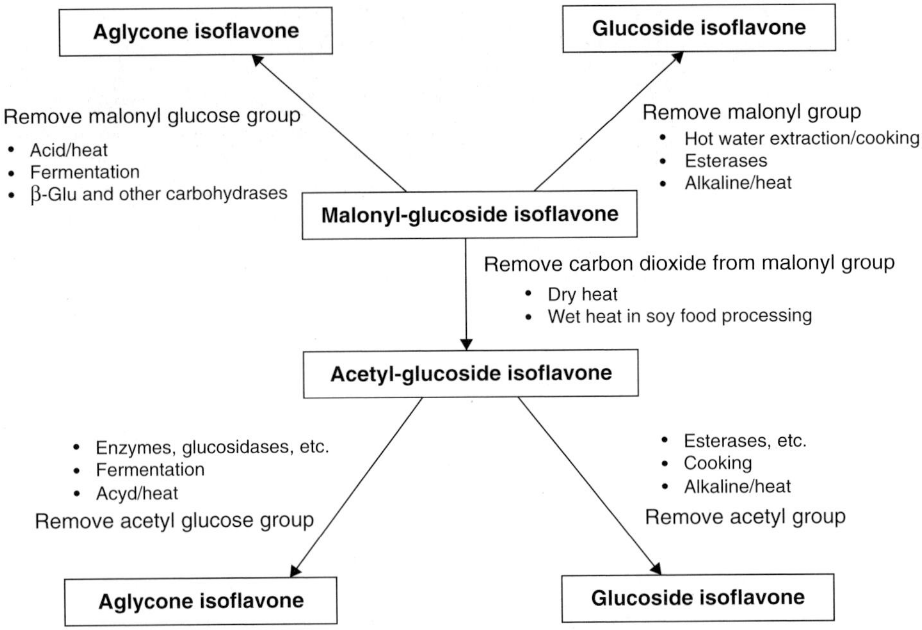

Figure 10.7 Summary of chemical reactions of isoflavones that may occur during food processing and storage as affected by several factors. *Source:* Adapted from Morales-de la Peña *et al.*, 2010 with permission from Elsevier

be up to 9 months), additional oxidative metabolism can occur introducing hydroxyl groups into the 6- and 8-positions on the A-ring (Esaki *et al.*, 1999).

10.4.1 Effect of conventional protein concentration and isolation and traditional food processing

Total isoflavone was found to decrease during processing of defatted flour to protein concentrate and protein isolate. Glucosides daidzein and genistein account for 40–50% of the total isoflavones in the soy flour (Eldridge, 1982a). Alcohol washing during the production of protein concentrate removed most of the isoflavones in the protein products. Aqueous washing had little effect on isoflavones. Approximately 50% of the isoflavones were lost during the manufacture of soy isolate. Moreover, Wang and Murphy (1996) investigated the mass balance of isoflavones and found that soy isolate production lost 47% of the total isoflavone and similarly Wang *et al.* (1998) reported that only 26% of the original soy flour isoflavones were retained in the soy isolate. During three major steps (extraction at an alkaline pH, acid precipitation and aqueous washing) of soy protein isolate production, the losses of the total isoflavones were 19%, 14% and 22%, respectively. The isolate had more aglycones than the soy flour; therefore, alkaline hydrolysis of glycosides may have occurred during processing.

10.4.2 Effect of soaking condition on content of 12 isoflavones in soybean

In a study on the effect of soaking condition on the content of 12 isoflavones in soybean, it was found that the concentration of three aglycones – glycitein, daidzein and genistein – increased (Kao *et al.*, 2004) at a higher soaking temperature and a longer soaking time (Figure 10.8) because acetyl glucosides, glucosides or malonyl glucosides were hydrolysed by the enzyme β-glucosidase in soybean during soaking (Wang & Murphy, 1996).

Interestingly, during soaking genistein changes structure more easily than glycitein and daidzein. In contrast, the other nine forms of isoflavone decreased at the higher temperature and the longer soaking time. A previous study (Murphy *et al.*, 2002) also explained that during soaking of soybean, malonyl glucosides could be changed to acetyl glucosides that could be further converted to aglycones or glucosides depending on soaking time and temperature. Moreover, a higher soaking temperature lead to a quicker conversion of isoflavone glucosides, so the highest aglycone yield was obtained at 45 °C rather than at 25 or 35 °C, possibly because β-glucosidase is able to work more effectively at the higher temperature. In addition, they found that β-glucosidase had its highest activity at 50 °C. In addition, malonyl glucoside decreased and converted to aglycones or glucosides and these were also released into solution because of the large decrease of malonyl glucoside. In conclusion, a higher soaking

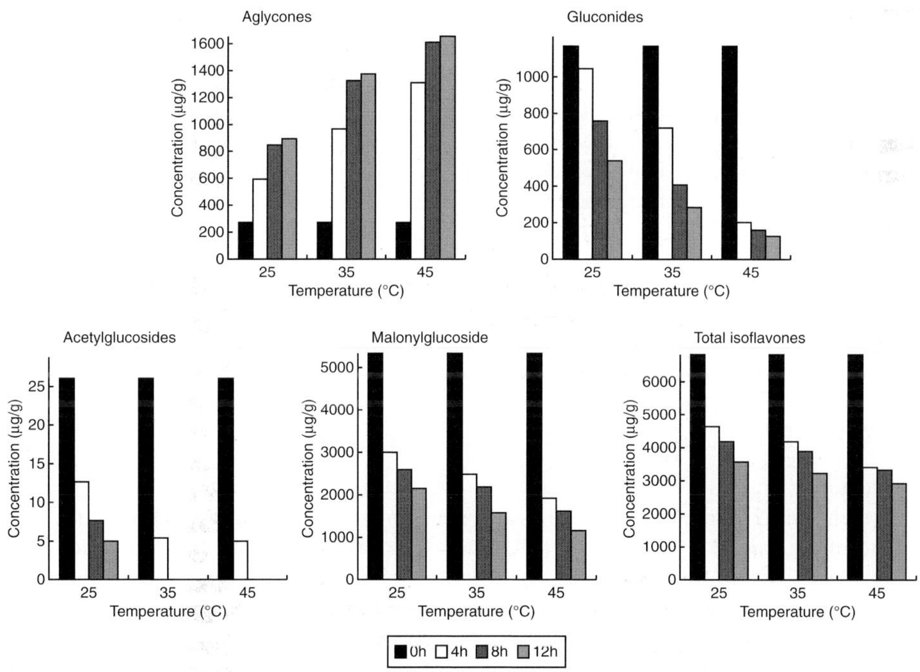

Figure 10.8 Influence of temperature and soaking time on content of varieties of isoflavones and total isoflavones in soybean on a dry weight basis. *Source:* Adapted from Kao *et al.*, 2004 with permission from Elsevier

temperature and a longer soaking time lead to a lower yields of these isoflavones. Similarly, Jackson *et al.* (2002) observed significant losses of isoflavones in the soaking and filtration processes during soy beverage production.

10.4.3 Effect of cooking/heating/toasting/baking on isoflavone structure

Heat treatment involved in the chemical analysis of isoflavones may affect their structure. The soybean was separated into three fractions (seed root, hypocotyls and the cotyledons) and isoflavones extracted using 70% aqueous ethanol at room temperature for 24 h or at 80 °C for 15 h. Total isoflavone concentration in hypocotyls was 5.5–6 times higher than that in the hypocotyls fraction. Most of the malonyl isoflavones were converted to respective glucosides after extraction at 80 °C for 15 h (Kudou *et al.*, 1991). The chemical structure of isoflavones can also be changed during food preparation (Coward *et al.*, 1998). Hot aqueous extraction as well as hot extraction in the making of soy milk and tofu converted some malonyl glucoside to β-glucoside.

Other studies suggested that only one group has examined the changes in distribution of isoflavones during soy bread proofing and baking (Zhang *et al.*, 2003, 2004b, Riedl *et al.*, 2005), and there has been no study evaluating isoflavone retention in all steps of the soy bread production process, particularly starting from soybeans to soy flour and soy protein isolate. Toasting (dry heat) of soybean could convert malonyl forms to acetyl glucosides. Production of low-fat soy milk and low-fat tofu reduced total isoflavones by 57% and 88%, respectively. As food was burnt, total isoflavone decreased with an increase in aglycones. Other studies suggested that the bread making processes did not affect the total isoflavone content, but changed glucosides/acetyl glucosides to aglycones. Malonyl glucosides were stable prior to baking but degraded to acetyl glucosides and further to glucosides during baking. These results provide critical information for the production of functional soy breads that contain varying amounts of soy isoflavones (Suqin *et al.*, 2009).

Currently, it has been found that toasting defatted soy flake at 150 °C for longer periods of time leads to a higher aglycone concentration in the extract; however, 2 h toasting was sufficient prior to high-power ultrasonication (HPU)-assisted extraction (Pananun *et al.*, 2012), as the results in Figure 10.9 show.

10.4.4 Effect of acid and base treatment

Glycosides (simple, malonyl and acetyl forms) of isoflavones can be hydrolysed by acid treatment. Hydrolysis of glucosides was compared under three concentrations, including 1, 2 and 3 N HCl, at 98–100 °C for various times. Conversion of glucosides to aglycone by acid treatment was the best at 1 N HCl for 2 h. A higher concentration of acid than 1 N HCl will decrease the aglycone content beyond 2 h of hydrolysis. Daidzein was found to be more stable than genistein against boiling acid treatment. After boiling for 2 h in 1 N HCl, genistein concentration declined sharply. This may be due to structural degradation of genistein by the acid at a high temperature (Wang *et al.*, 1990). Barbosa *et al.* (2006) showed that different processing parameters, such as ionic strength and pH, resulted in different isoflavone amounts and profile during soy

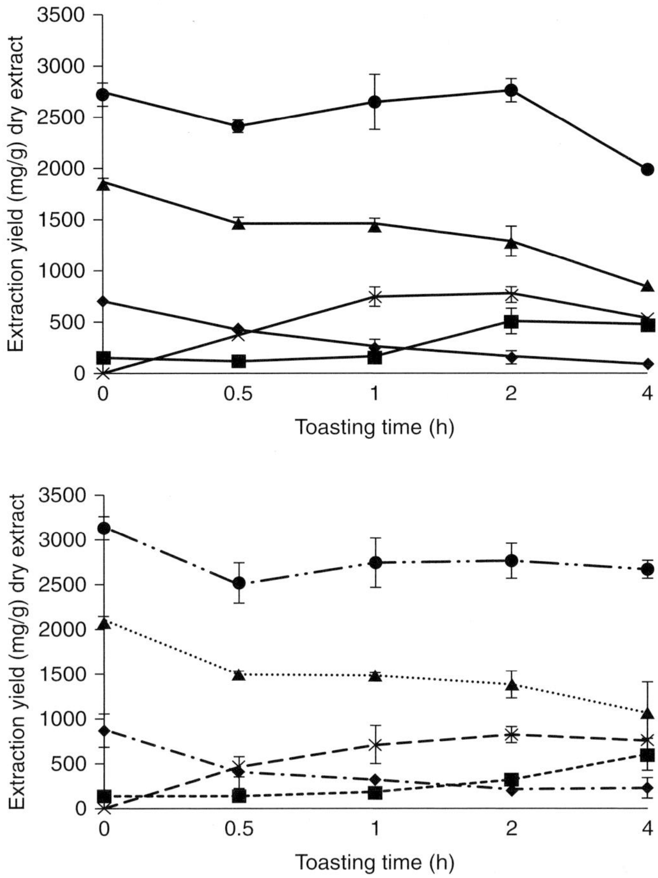

Figure 10.9 Effect of toasting time at 150 °C on isoflavones components and total isoflavones (μg/g dry extract) in defatted soy flakes by conventional mix-stirring extraction (solid lines), and HPU-assisted extraction at 54 μm, 3 min (broken lines). The solid-to-solvent ratio: 0.1 : 1 for both extractions using ACN59 solvent. Symbol key: —●—total isoflavones, —▲—glucosides, —✕—acetyl glucosides, —■—aglycones, and —◆—malonyl glucosides. Aglycone, daidzein + genistein + glycitein; glucosides, daidzin + genistin + glycitin; acetyl glucoside, acetyldaidzin + acetylgenistin + acetylglycitin; malonyl glucoside, malonyldaidzin + malonylgenistin + malonylglycitin; total isoflavones, aglycone + glucosides + acetyl glucoside + malonyl glucoside

protein isolate production and they attributed this to the endogenous ß-glucosidase activity.

10.4.5 Effects of dry heat on soy flour isoflavones

The effects of dry heat on soy flour isoflavones was compared at 80 and 150 °C over a 4-h period. It was shown that for soy flour heated at 80 °C over 4 h, isoflavone concentration did not differ significantly as drying time increased. In soy flour heated at 150 °C, the malonylgenistin group decreased because it was converted to acetylgenistin, but the total mass of genistein remained constant and the glucosides group (genistin) was converted to aglycone group (genistein) by ß-glucoside hydrolysation, leading to an increase in genistein and a reduction in genistin. In addition, the acetylgenistin and genistin form had a similar trend at the longer toasting time (Murphy *et al.*, 2002).

10.4.6 Effects of moist heat of a liquid soy product on isoflavone distribution in soy milk

The effect of moist heat on soy milk isoflavones kept at 80 °C over 3 h was studied. As heating time increased, malonylgenistin decreased because it transformed to acetylgenistin. Also, some genistein was formed because the glucosides group (genistin) was converted to the aglycone group (genistein) by β-glucoside hydrolysation (Murphy *et al.*, 2002). Barnes *et al.* (1994) found hat using hexane extraction to recover the oil fraction did not alter the composition. However, boiling water extraction of soybeans to make soy milk causes hydrolysis of the malonyl group, yielding simple β-glucosides. In contrast, Huang *et al.* (2006) found that the isoflavone content of soy milk significantly decreased during heat treatment.

10.4.7 Effect of enzymes on isoflavone forms and flavour of soybean products

Kudou *et al.* (1991) determined the bitterness taste threshold values for the 12 forms of isoflavones. Generally, the threshold values are in the order of malonyl glucosides $<$ acetyl glucosides $=$ aglycones $<$ glucosides. Therefore, in the production of soy milk, measures need to be taken to reduce the malonyl forms to improve the taste of the product. Additionally, during the production of soy milk, the natural β-glucosidase present in soybean may convert some glucosides to the aglycone forms to contribute to an increase of objectionable flavour (Matsuura *et al.*, 1989). The enzymes should be inactivated as rapidly as possible during or after soy milk extraction to improve the quality of soy milk. Further, the enzyme was also stable from pH 4.0 to 6.0 at 5 °C (Matsuura *et al.*, 1995). However, soaking in water or in 0.25% sodium bicarbonate at 50 °C promoted the production of aglycones due to β-glucosidase hydrolysis and promoted the production of volatiles due to lipoxygenase-catalysed peroxidation. Soaking in boiling water containing sodium bicarbonate inhibited the production of aglycones and the undesirable volatile flavours (Ha *et al.*, 1992).

10.5 Isoflavones: extraction and analytical methods

Due to the enormous endeavours made in the past few years to evaluate isoflavone composition in foods and its relation with nutritional issues and health effects, it is of ultimate importance to develop reliable and accurate methods for the quantification of these compounds in foods. Because of the increasing complexity of the food supply, there are major challenges in collecting reliable food consumption data for phyto-oestrogen intake estimates. Several extraction methods have been used for quantification purposes without sufficient validation of the extraction procedure and

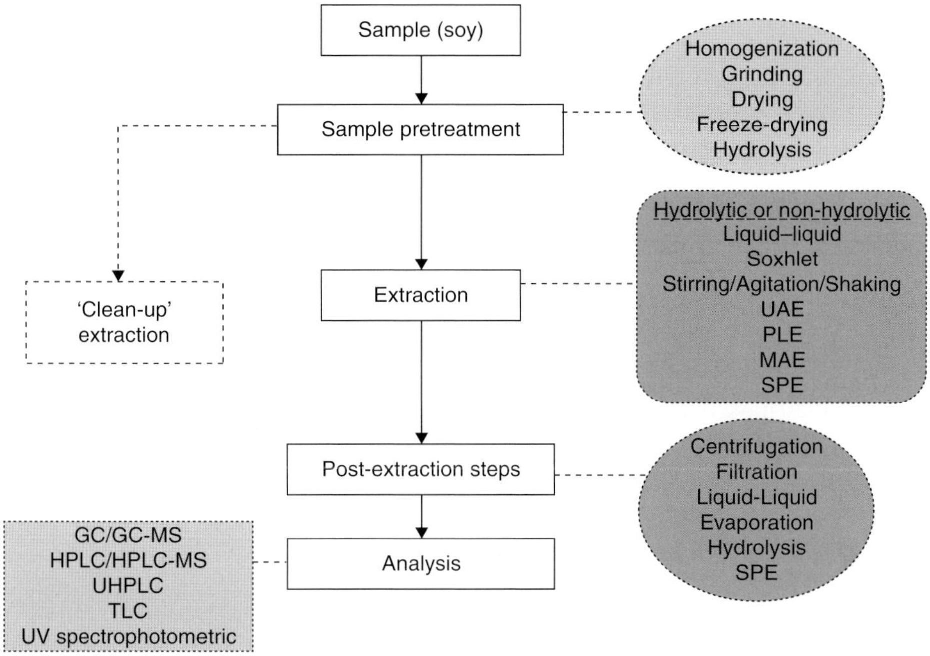

Figure 10.10 Most common steps for sample preparation for the determination of soy isoflavones. *Source:* Adapted from Rostagano *et al.*, 2002 with permission from Elsevier. UAE, ultrasound-assisted extraction; PLE, pressurized liquid extraction; MAE, microwave-assisted extraction; SPE, solid-phase extraction; GC, gas chromatography; GC-MS, gas chromatography mass spectrometry; HPLC, high performance liquid chromatography; HPLC-MS, high performance liquid chromatography mass spectrometry; TLC, thin layer chromatography; UHPLC, ultra high pressure/performance liquid chromatography

far from optimized extraction conditions, which can lead to fallacious measurements and calculations. In addition, optimal extraction conditions can be used to save time, resources and provide reliable information. The four common steps for any analytical method are sampling, sample preservation, sample preparation and analysis. Figure 10.10 presents a general overview of the most common steps for sample preparation for the determination of soy isoflavones.

Sample preparation may consist of multiple steps such as drying, homogenization, sieving, extraction of target compounds, pre-concentration and hydrolysis. Sample preparation can seek several objectives: to increase the efficiency of an assay procedure, to eliminate or reduce potential interferences, to enhance the sensitivity of the analytical procedure by increasing the concentration of the analyte in the assay mixture, and sometimes to transform the analyte of interest to a more suitable form that can be easily separated, detected and/or quantified. Isoflavone determination is complex since its concentration in the sample depends on several variables which may make determination difficult. Overall, the ultimate goal is to obtain a concentrated extract of all isoflavones that is free of interfering compounds from the matrix. The extraction phase is extremely important and the process will depend on analyte liberation from the matrix, which will allow quantitative determinations of the target compounds. Moreover, the extract should resemble the original isoflavone composition and profile as much as possible. For efficient extraction, several parameters such as the solvent, temperature, sample amount and time should be defined.

10.5.1 Extraction techniques and methods

As the 12 different soy isoflavones have different polarities, developing an optimized extraction procedure for all isoflavones has been challenging. Extraction is an extremely important process for production of isoflavone concentrate from rich sources. Different researchers have deployed various solvents and techniques for extraction of isoflavones from soybeans. Among the extraction methods, solid phase extraction (SPE) is one of the most widely used techniques for separating functional materials. Because of their excellent sorption characteristics, Amberlite-XAD-2 and Diaion HP-20 have been used to separate isoflavones (Choi and Kim, 2005; Fedeniuk and Shand, 1998; Hennion, 1999). Liquid–liquid extraction (LLE) also has been used to separate functional materials. In LLE, hydrophobic ingredients in the raw materials are extracted from aqueous samples with a water-immiscible organic phase. A variety of volatile organic solvents are used, including pentane, hexane, ethyl ether, ethyl acetate, chloroform and methylene chloride (Pedersen-Bjergaard *et al.*, 2000). In addition, a wide variation in extraction–solvent composition (methanol, ethanol and acetonitrile with different proportions of acidified and non-acidified water) has been used. The extraction processes are affected by process variables such as solvent, extraction temperature, amount of solvent and extraction time. Furthermore, several researchers have used different extraction equipment or techniques such as multi-wrist shaker, rotary shaker, stirring, sonicator and Soxhlet for extraction of isoflavones from soybeans. Thus wide variations in the usage of different solvent mixtures and techniques have been applied for the extraction of isoflavones from soybeans and other plant matrices. Novel extraction methods including ultrasound-assisted extraction (UAE), microwave-assisted extraction (MAE), supercritical fluid extraction (SFE) and accelerated solvent extraction (ASE) are quick and efficient for extracting chemicals from solid plant matrixes (Wang and Weller, 2006). Different research groups use different methodologies for isoflavone extraction, which are briefly summarized here.

Superheated water extraction (SWE) method Superheated water extraction is a method based on the use of water as an extractant, at temperatures between 100 and 374 °C and at a pressure high enough to retain the liquid state. At the laboratory scale, SWE can be performed using 1–5 g of air-dried solid samples, a 5–20 ml stainless steel extraction cell, 0.5–5.0 ml/min flow rate, temperatures of 100–175 °C, a pressure of 15–60 bar and 15–60 min of extraction time. SWE has numerous advantages over organic solvent extraction, for example, the solvent is environmentally friendly and the procedure is economical and simple. SWE is therefore a technique of interest and is currently receiving increased attention. Penalvo *et al.* (2004) have used SWE to extract five important isoflavones from defatted soybean flakes (DSF) as a viable alternative means of extraction. Suitable conditions for SWE are 110 °C, 641 psi (4520 kPa) over 2.3 h of extraction. Under optimum conditions, 3937 total isoflavones (TIF) μg/g DSF were produced. An efficient way to recover and purify the resulting samples was by using solid-phase Amberlite XAD16-HP resin adsorption.

Pressurized liquid extraction (PLE) method Pressurized liquid extraction is a sample method for the extraction of analytes from solid materials (Wan and Wong, 1996). Recently, Delgado-Zamarreño *et al.* (2012) achieved optimal extraction of formononetin and biochanin-A from chickpeas with PLE using Hydromatrix as a dispersant agent, methanol/water (50 : 50), at 90 °C and three cycles. The contents obtained for daidzin in lentils using the proposed method were not significantly different from those obtained using another official method of analysis. Also, phenolic compounds can be extracted from grape seeds and apple using the PLE method. For isoflavones, it was found that malonyl glucoside forms increased while glucosides decreased because they transformed to malonyl glucosides when the temperature was higher than 100 °C. The optimum protocol for isoflavone extraction from freeze-dried soy matter is: sample 0.1 g, 100 °C, three static extraction cycles, 7 min and 70% ethanol as the extracting solvent.

Solid-phase extraction (SPE) method Solid-phase extraction is an accelerated, cost-efficient method that requires less sample handling than other methods such as UAE and soxhlet methods. The results obtained from this method are more reproducible. As the procedure is performed in a closed system, there is less chance of sample oxidation or solvent evaporation. As a result, extraction can be performed relatively quickly (Rostagno *et al.*, 2005). This method typically eliminates interferences and objectionable matrix components. SPE has mainly replaced classical liquid–liquid extractions which necessitate large quantities of organic solvents and are not environmentally friendly. In SPE, solids are partitioned between a mobile phase and a stationary phase that has a greater affinity for the analytes of interest. SPE cartridges with several different stationary phases are commercially available. Rostagno *et al.* (2005) have developed an automated SPE procedure for concentration and clean-up of soy isoflavones extract achieving very high recoveries (99.37%) and reproducibility (>98%) with a concentration factor of approximately 6 : 1 in less than 10 min.

Supercritical fluid extraction (SFE) method Supercritical fluids can be used to extract analytes from samples. SFE is one method that is economical, extracts the analytes quicker and is more environmentally friendly than organic solvents, so supercritical fluid CO_2 is the reagent broadly used as the supercritical solvent. For extraction of genistein and genistin at 70 °C/200 bar, comparison of conventional extraction methods (soxhlet and ultra-sonification) with supercritical carbon dioxide (SC-CO_2), showed that conventional extraction methods were more effective and cost less. Analytical results additionally showed that temperature significantly affects the amount of genistein and genistin extracted by SC-CO_2. In generally, daidzein extracted at 50 °C/360 bar affected the higher values achieved with traditional methods and also can observe advantages effect of the pressure. The total isoflavone extraction maximum for each technique was: soxhlet 212.86, ultra-sonication 311.55, and SC-CO_2 86.28 μg/g.

Microwave-assisted extraction (MAE) method Another alternative method for the extraction of phytonutrient compounds from plant materials and foods is microwave-assisted extraction. This method is the selective and rapid heating of moisture in the samples because localized heating and pressure builds up within the cell material, resulting in an easier transfer of the cell material to the extraction solvent. Rostagno *et al.* (2007) developed a quick and reliable analytical method for soy isoflavones extraction using MAE, performed on a microwave extractor ETHOS 1600 (Milestrone, Sorisole, Italy) as two different solvent systems (ethanol or methanol, with different water), including different solvent volume, various sample size and varying the extracting temperatures (50–150 °C). Moreover, Terigar *et al.* (2010) designed an optimized continuous MAE by investigating temperature and processing time during and after microwave exposure, in which the parameters for isoflavones extraction were different temperatures (55 and 73 °C) and extraction times (0, 4, 8 and 12 min).

Ultrasound-assisted extraction (UAE) method Recently, ultrasound-assisted extraction has attracted increased attention because it can accelerate the extracting process and improve the extraction yield of bioactive compounds (Wu *et al.*, 2001; Li *et al.*, 2005a, 2005b, 2010; Chen *et al.*, 2007; Bhandari *et al.*, 2008; Boonkird *et al.*, 2008; Xia *et al.*, 2010; Wang *et al.*, 2011). UAE allows the extraction solvent to penetrate cell walls, and the bubbles produced by acoustic cavitation aid in the disruption of the cell wall and the release of the targeted compounds (Wu *et al.*, 2001). UAE has been used on numerous occasions to extract isoflavones from soybeans, soy foods and from different matrixes, such as peanuts, *Trifolium pretense, Puerariae radix, Pueraria lobata, Radix astragali* and *Glycyrrhizae radix* (Rostagno *et al.*, 2002, 2003; He *et al.*, 2005; Lee and Lin, 2007; Xu and He, 2007). However, optimization of UAE based methods has not been conducted without minor objections. For example, Rostagno *et al.* (2003) have used UAE in the extraction four isoflavone derivatives (daidzin, glycitin, genistin and malonyl genistin) from freeze-dried ground soybeans. When compared with other methods, UAE improved extraction efficiency of soy isoflavones and also reduced extraction time. However, this method was dependent on the volume of solvent, temperature and length of extraction time; optimum conditions were 50% ethanol at 60 °C using UAE for 20 min.

High-power ultrasonication (HPU) method To date, HPU is the newest method that researchers tend to use for extraction of phytonutrient compounds. Pananun *et al.* (2012) have shown the effect of HPU on extraction of soybean isoflavones and components. Isoflavones from defatted soybean flakes were extracted using a bench scale HPU system at 20 kHz and varying amplitudes (18–54 μm) for 1 and 3 min (Figure 10.11). Aqueous acetonitrile and aqueous ethanol-based solvents were evaluated for extraction at samples-to-solvent ratios of 0.1 : 1 and 0.2 : 1. The non-sonication control extraction was mixed with a magnetic stirrer for 2 h. Preliminary data indicated 1.2–1.5 times more genistein recovery at 1 and 3 min sonication compared to the control; conversely, total phenolic decreased. The genistein recovery was lower at higher sonication levels. RSA also decreased to 40% for HPU-assisted extractions. Total isoflavone recovery in HPU-assisted extractions increased from 600 to 5813 μg/g. The concentration of major isoflavone components genistein, daidzein and glycitein also increased by 10-fold. HPU for 3 min reduced the average particle size of treated soy flakes from 530 to 60 μm.

Table 10.4 summarizes some of the most popular methods for extraction of isoflavones used by various researchers found in peer-reviewed literature during the past decade. The extraction time used by different researchers varied between 20 min and 6 h. In most published studies on soybean, extractions have been carried out directly without defatting. However, several researchers have defatted soybean prior

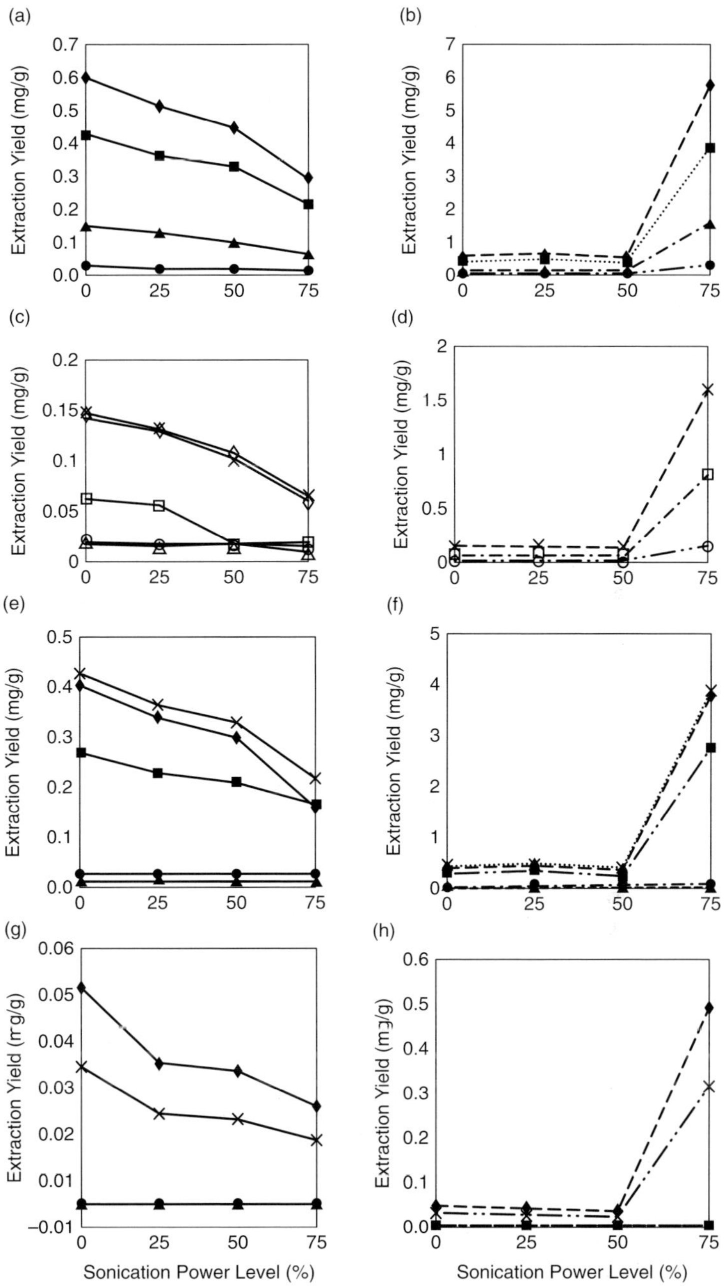

Figure 10.11 Isoflavone components, mg/g dry extract, as affected by high-power ultrasonication at 0.1 : 1 solid-solvent ratio with ACN59, various power levels, and extraction times: 1 min sonication (solid lines, left), and 3 min sonication (broken lines, right). Symbol keys: (a) and (b) –♦–total isoflavone, –■–total genistein, –▲–total daidzein and –✕–total glycitein; (c) and (d) –✕–total daidzein, –+–daidzein, –□–malonyldaidzin, –△–acetyldaidzin and –○–daidzein; (e) and (f) –✕–total genistein, –♦–genistein, –■–malonylglycitin, –●–genistein, and –▲–acetylgenistin; (g) and (h) –✕–total glycitein, –♦–glycitein, –■–malonylglycitin, –●–glycitein and –▲–acetylglycitin. *Source:* Adapted from Pananun *et al.*, 2012. Reproduced with permission from Elsevier

Table 10.4 Summary of commonly deployed procedures used by various authors for extraction of isoflavones soybean samples

Serial #	Extraction procedure	Best solvent[a]	Publication year	Reference
1	Two grams of different food samples were extracted with four different acidified solvents 53% ACN, 53% MeOH, 53% EtOH and 53% acetone. The mixture was stirred at room temperature for 2 h	53% ACN	2002	Murphy *et al.*
2	Soy meal was extracted with acidified ACN (58%) by shaking sample for 2 h at RT	One solvent	2004	Lee *et al.*
3	The authors used a high pressure hot water process to extract five isoflavones from detffated soy flakes An experimental design was adopted to optimize extraction conditions, and five isoflavones were purified. The optimum conditions were determined as 110 °C and 641 psig over 2.3 h of extraction	One solvent	2004	Li-Hsun *et al.*
4	Comparison of four different sample preparation (extraction and hydrolysis) procedures with three different solvents (80% EtOH, 80% acidified EtOH, and 80% MeOH) was carried out at various temperature (60–100 °C) for different time intervals (30–240 min)	80% EtOH containing 1M HCl	2004	Penalvo *et al.*
5	Freeze dried soybeans were extracted with pressurized liquid extractor (PLE) with different proportions of (30–80%) of aqueous EtOH and MeOH solvent mixtures at different temperature, pressures, solid-to-solvent ratios. Optimization of PLE conditions are described	70% EtOH	2004	Rostagno *et al.*
6	Comparison of different extraction conditions (extraction time, temperature, pressure, cycles, solvents) and techniques (PLE,PLE + sonication, sonication, and Soxhlet)	90% MeOH	2004 and 2005	Klejdus *et al.*
7	Defatted soy samples were extracted with 80% ACN, 80% MeOH and 80% EtOH by stirring and sonicating samples. The authors suggest replicate extraction is essential for optimum extraction. Significant decrease in isoflavone yields were obtained with one extraction cycle.	Similar yields with all three solvents	2005	Achouri *et al.*
8	Ground manokin soybeans (2 g) were extracted with 12 ml of six different extraction solvents (83% ACN, 83% acidified ACN, 80% MeOH, 80% acidified MeOH, 58% ACN, and 58% acidified ACN). Extractions of isoflavones were carried out at RT for 2 hrs.	58% ACN	2005	Lin and Giusti

Table 10.4 (*Continued*)

Serial #	Extraction procedure	Best solvent[a]	Publication year	Reference
9	The authors systematically compared three commonly used extraction solvents or solvent mixtures (acetonitrile: water 58: 42, % v/v, ethanol: water 70: 30, % v/v, methanol: water 90: 10, % v/v) and identified increased extraction efficiencies with dimethyl sulfoxide: ethanol: water (5:70: 25, % v/v/v). In addition, authors carried out comparison between six commonly used extraction techniques (shaking, vortexing, sonication, stirring, Soxhlet and pressurized liquid extraction (PLE)) and found that PLE provided optimum efficiency recoveries.	dimethyl sulfoxide:EtOH: water (5:70: 25, %v/v/v)	2007	Luthria *et al.*
10	The authors used ultrasound-assisted extraction procedure. The extraction protocol consisted of extracting 0.25 g of the freeze-dried sample with 25mL of 50% EtOH at 60°C in an ultrasonic bath for 20 min.	50% EtOH	2007	Rostagno *et al.*
11	The authors used n-butanol/water, two phase solvent system for the extraction of isoflavones from the stem of *Pueraria lobata* (Willd.) followed by alumina column purification and recrystallization	1:1 (v/v)n-butanol:water	2007	Xu and He
12	The authors compared extraction yields of isoflavones from soybean cake by solvent and supercritical carbon dioxide and studied the conversion of isoflavone glucosides to the biologically active aglycone by employing β-glucosidase.	supercritical carbon dioxide	2008	Kao *et al.*
13	The authors extract the formononetin and biochanin-A from chickpeas with PLE was achieved using Hydromatrix as a dispersant agent, methanol/water (50:50), a temperature of 90 °C, and three cycles by compare with methanol/water (75:25)-for solvent extraction were obtained for the extraction of daidzin, genistin, and formononetin from lentils.	MeOH/water (50:50)	2012	Delgado-Zamarreño *et al.*

*[a] ACN, Acetonitrile; EtOH, ethanol; MeOH, methanol.

acetone–petroleum ether (3 : 1) and then in ethanol–chloroform (1 : 1). Bands are detected with appropriate chromogenic sprays or with a UV lamp at 366 nm (Pratt and Birac, 1979). Lapcik *et al.* (1998a) stated that diethyl ether extract chromatographed on a silica plate developed three times in dichloromethane–methanol (95 : 5, v/v) gave the following rate: daidzein 0.20, genistein 0.30, formononetin 0.55 and biochanin A 0.75, respectively.

Gas chromatography (GC) GC analysis is performed on silylated isoflavones (Naim *et al.*, 1974). Isoflavones, together with other flavonoid aglycones, have been separated into well-resolved sharp and symmetrical peaks by a rapid and sensitive capillary column GC method (Koupai-Abyazani *et al.*, 1992). An improved GC method for the analysis of daidzein and genistein has been described by many researchers (Liggins *et al.*, 1998). Parthasarathi and Fenner (1999) used GC-MS in selected ion mode to develop a simple analytical method for routine quantification of the isoflavones daidzein and genistein in food using synthetic glucosides daidzein and genistein as internal standards, combined with the food prior to extraction. In this method daidzein and formonotetin are liberated from their respective glycosides by a hydrolytic enzyme from *Aspergillus niger* in aqueous buffer.

UV spectrophotometric assay Isoflavones have characteristic UV absorption spectra with two absorption maxima in the ranges 245–275 nm and 300–330 nm. The second band at the higher wavelength has a weaker relative intensity (Wu *et al.*, 2004). This method identifies soy isoflavone aglycones and their conjugates (glycosides, glycoside acetylates and glycoside malonates) along with their MS (Wu *et al.*, 2004a,Otieno *et al.*, 2007, Maul *et al.*, 2008). Furthermore, the absorption is affected by the nature of the solvent and pH. Moreover, the possibility of interference by UV-absorbing substances such as protein, nucleic acids and amino acids should be considered. This is a rather cumbersome and difficult task. Therefore, the suitability of UV assay depends on the material to be analysed.

High-performance liquid chromatography (HPLC) Murphy (1981) reported the analysis of genistein, daidzin and their aglycones and coumestrol in toasted, defatted soy flakes by HPLC without the use of external standards. Eldridge (1982a, 1982b) reported analysis of soybean and soy products using HPLC with an external standard method. Similarly, Ha *et al.* (1992) used C18 HPLC to analyse extract from defatted soybean. A linear gradient with methanol and detection with UV 280 nm were used for elution and quantification. Wang and Murphy (1994a) have analysed isoflavones in commercial soy food by HPLC using an external standard method. In contrast, Song *et al.* (1998) extracted isoflavones from soybean and soy food using an acetronitrile–HCl–water mixture and separated 12 forms of isoflavones by HPLC and quantitated them using isoflavones standards and an internal standard 2,4,4′-trihydroxyl benzoin (THB).

Ultra high-pressure/performance liquid chromatography (UHPLC) The development of chromatography has led to the reduction in the size of the packing materials used to make HPLC columns (Jason *et al.*, 2007). The increase in the backpressure required has led to this method being referred to as ultra high-pressure liquid chromatography (UHPLC) when the column backpressure exceeds 10 000 psi (1700 bar). Until recently, columns packed with sub-2-μm materials have generally fitted into two classes, either short (less than 5 cm) columns designed for use on traditional HPLC systems at pressures less than 5000 psi (350 bar), or capillary columns (inner diameters less than 100 μm). A new ultra high-pressure liquid chromatography (UV-UPLC™) method was developed for the rapid and reliable determination of total aglycones in soybeans (daidzein, glycitein and genistein) after enzymatic hydrolysis applying *Helix pomatia* digestive juice. Capitalizing on the enhanced performance of UPLC™, aglycones were separated within only 3 min, with a total run-time of 8 min until the next injection (Fiechter *et al.*, 2013).

10.6 Isoflavones: metabolism and bioavailability

The bioavailability of isoflavones has been shown to be influenced by their chemical form in foods (generally glycoside conjugates), susceptibility to degradation, the microbial flora of the consumer and by the food matrix. Bioavailability of isoflavonoids may depend to some extent upon interaction with other dietary components (Birt *et al.*, 2001). Isoflavones are plentiful in soya and soya-derivative products such as dietary supplements. The range of different dietary soya-based supplements available through chemists, health-food stores and supermarkets has grown many times over in recent years in Western countries (Nurmi *et al.*, 2002). The bioavailability of isoflavones has been investigated using glycosylated pure compounds or aglycone pure compounds (Setchell *et al.*, 2001; Bloedon *et al.*, 2002; Busby *et al.*, 2002) or single soya-based foods (Richelle *et al.*, 2002; Vergne *et al.*, 2007).

The metabolism of isoflavones in animals and humans is complex and is a combination of mammalian and gut microbial processes. Furthermore, there is a vast amount of individual variability in the metabolism of isoflavones. Individual differences in gut microflora, intestinal transit time and genetic polymorphisms are all likely to contribute to this variability (Duffy *et al.*, 2007). During digestive and absorptive processes, isoflavones often undergo metabolic transformations. In some individuals, daidzein can be converted by the intestinal microflora to the metabolite equol or to *O*-desmethylangolensin, and genistein to *P*-ethyl phenol. Currently, it still remains essential to understand whether blood, serum and urine levels are similar following consumption of a known dose of isoflavones, which are present in different food matrices (De Pascual-Teresa *et al.*, 2006).

Several researchers stated that aglycone forms of isoflavones are transported from the intestine to the blood or they are further metabolized directly in the intestine. Degradation of isoflavones occurs in the liver, where they are conjugated with glucuronic acid and to a lesser degree with sulfates. They are excreted from the body in urine or bile. Most daidzein and genistein is eliminated from the body within 24 h (Axelson *et al.*, 1982; Setchell *et al.*, 2001). Additionally, Franke *et al.* (2009) reported a good correlation between peak concentrations of plasma daidzein and genistein and their concentrations in urine in the first 24 h following soy consumption.

In blood serum, the highest levels of isoflavones are reached within 2–8 h after consumption. After administration of 125 g of boiled soy, the highest total level of daidzein was about 500 nmol/l. Adlercreutz *et al.* (1993) examined isoflavone concentrations in relation to regional differences in food. In serum samples of Japanese men, the average concentrations amounted to 107 nmol/l of daidzein and 276 nmol/l of genistein (maximum values were 900 nmol/l for daidzein and 2400 nmol/l for genistein).

10.7 Isoflavones: health benefits

The structure of isoflavone is similar to the endogenous oestrogen 17β-oestrodiol, as shown in Figure 10.13. Research in several areas of health care has shown that consumption of isoflavones may play a role in lowering risk for disease. Isoflavones can prevent disease on several fronts related to lowering cancer risk (Wu *et al.*, 1996, Cline and Hughes, 1998), heart disease prevention (Rimbach *et al.*, 2008), bone mass density increase to prevent osteoporosis (Arjmandi *et al.*, 1996, Zhang *et al.*, 2007), protection against prostate problems (Nagata *et al.*, 2007) and the reduction of post-menopausal syndromes in women (Knight *et al.*, 1996; Adlercreutz and Mazur, 1997; Somekawa *et al.*, 2001; Zhang *et al.*, 2005). Due to the purported beneficial effects of soy isoflavones, the use of soy products has become popular (Chang, 2002). The following list of potential health benefits are attributed to isoflavones.

Ease menopause symptoms Recent studies have found that soy isoflavones can reduce menopause symptoms such as hot flushes and increase bone density in women. Indeed, many menopausal and post-menopausal health problems may result from a lack of isoflavones in the typical Western diet. Although study results are not entirely consistent, isoflavones from soy or red clover may be helpful for symptoms of menopause in women who consume a typical Western diet (Adlercreutz and Mazur, 1997; Somekawa *et al.*, 2001; Zhang *et al.*, 2005; Concetta *et al.*, 2009). Consequently, many menopausal women use phyto-oestrogens to maintain their bone mass because they are unlikely to cause the undesirable effects associated with steroid

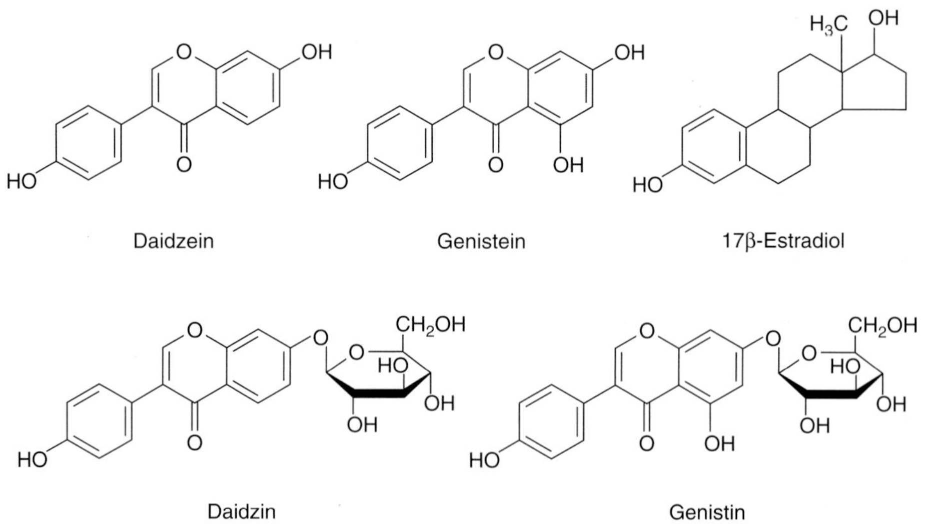

Figure 10.13 Chemical structures of isoflavones and 17β-estradiol. *Source:* Kurie *et al.*, 2003. Reproduced with permission from Elsevier

hormones (Messina, 2002). Fifty-one women finished a 12-week clinical study which showed that isoflavone can relieve menopausal symptoms. In women receiving 60 mg isoflavones daily, hot flushes and night sweats were reduced by 57% and 43%, respectively (Cheng *et al.*, 2007).

Isoflavones improve bone health Soy isoflavones that occur naturally have been shown to act as selective oestrogen receptor modulators with beneficial effects on bone similar to raloxifene (Henderson *et al.*, 1993; Brezinski and Debi, 1999). The relationships between soybean isoflavones and bone tissue have been studied for less than decade. Data from several animal studies have demonstrated that soy isoflavones had bone-conserving effects by retaining bone mass following ovariectomy (Bone *et al.*, 2000). A possible role for soy isoflavones in modifying human bone mass has been suggested. Henderson *et al.* (1993) found that soy protein supplements enriched in isoflavones attenuated bone loss in postmenopausal and perimenopausal women. Some *in vitro* studies have suggested that isoflavones had biphasic effects – bone formation and bone resorption (Delmas *et al.*, 2000). Epidemiological studies indicate that women who have high soy food consumption have a lower risk of osteoporosis. This is forwarded as the reason why people in China and Japan very rarely have osteoporosis, despite their low consumption of dairy products, whereas in Europe and North America the contrary happens. Unlike oestrogen, which helps prevent the destruction of bone, evidence suggests that isoflavones may also support the creation of new bone. Additional studies are not entirely consistent, but evidence suggests that genistein and other soy isoflavones can help prevent osteoporosis. However, random control trials on the effect of soy isoflavones on osteoporosis are conflicting, possibly due to the varying content of the soy isoflavones intake, trial duration and sample size. Nonetheless, a meta-analysis by Wei *et al.* (2012) found that soy isoflavones significantly increased bone mineral density by 54% and decreased levels of the bone resorption marker urinary deoxypyridinoline by 23% compared to baseline in women. Using a random effects model, the effect of isoflavones on bone mineral density regarding menopausal status and isoflavone dose revealed higher weighted mean difference changes were found in postmenopausal women and an isoflavone dose above 75 mg/d.

Reduce heart disease risk Soy isoflavones also seem to reduce cardiovascular disease risk via several distinct mechanisms. Isoflavones inhibit the growth of cells that form artery-clogging plaque. Blood clots usually form in affected arteries, which can lead to a heart attack. Recent studies showed that soybean products with a high content of isoflavones decrease low-density lipoprotein oxidation in the hyperlipidaemic population (Jenkins *et al.*, 2002), which can prevent cardiovascular disease. Furthermore, a review of 38 controlled studies on soy and heart disease concluded that soy is definitely effective for improving cholesterol profile. There is some evidence that isoflavones are the active ingredients in soy responsible for improving cholesterol profile (Rimbach *et al.*, 2008).

Cancer prevention The benefits of soy isoflavones go beyond reducing long-term cancer risk. Several mechanisms of isoflavones have been suggested for the inhibition of carcinogenesis. Naturally competitive activity to oestrogen was considered in oestrogen-related cancer prevention (Adlercreutz *et al.*, 1995). Hosokawa *et al.* (1990)

have shown that isoflavones binding to oestrogen receptors (ERs) is related to inhibition of the cell cycle, whereas other independent effects are also present that interact with inhibition of the cell cycle in the prevention of cancer. Likewise, there are many proposed mechanisms for the therapeutic effects of isoflavones, including inhibition of protein tyrosine kinase, binding to oestrogen receptors (although soy's inhibition of cancer cell growth does not seem to be entirely oestrogen dependent), inhibition of production of reactive oxygen species (Wei *et al.*, 1995) and induction of DNA strand breakage resulting in apoptosis or cell death (Barnes *et al.*, 1995). The findings from two recent large prospective clinical studies have indicated a strong association between soy food intake and decreased risk of death or cancer recurrence in breast cancer survivors (Shu *et al.*, 2009)

Protect against prostate problems Eating isoflavone-rich products may protect against enlargement of the male prostate gland. Studies show isoflavones slowed prostate cancer growth and caused prostate cancer cells to die. Isoflavones act against cancer cells in a way similar to many common cancer-treating drugs (Nagata *et al.*, 2007).

References

Achouri, A., Boye, J.I. and Belanger, D. (2005). Soybean isoflavones: efficacy of extraction conditions and effect of food type on extractability. *Food Research International*, 38, 1199–1204.

Adlercreutz, H., Fotsis, T., Lampe, J. *et al.* (1993). Quantitative determination of lignans and isoflavonoids in plasma of omnivorous and vegetarian women by isotope dilution gas chromatography–mass spectrometry. *Scandinavian Journal of Clinical Laboratory Investigations*, 53, 5–18.

Adlercreutz, H., Godlin, B.R., Gorbach, S.L. *et al.* (1995). Soybean phytooestrogen intake an cancer risk. *Nutrition and Cancer*, 125, 757S–770S.

Adlercreutz, H. and Mazur, W. (1997). Phyto-ooestrogens and Western diseases. *Annals of Medicine*, 29, 95–120.

Alexandrakis, M.G., Kyriakou, D.S., Kempuraj, D. *et al.* (2003). The isoflavone genistein inhibits proliferation and increases histamine content in human leukemic mast cells. *Allergy and Asthma Proceedings*, 24, 373–377.

Anderson, J.J.B. and Carner, S.C. (1997). The effects of phytooestrogens on bones. *Nutrition Research*, 17, 1617–1632.

Arjmandi, B.H., Alekel, L., Hollis, B.W. *et al.* (1996). Dietary soybean protein prevents bone loss in an ovariectomized rat model of osteoporosis. *Journal of Nutrition*, 126, 161–167.

Axelson, M., Kirk, D., Farrant, R. *et al.* (1996). The identification of the weak ooestrogen equol [7-hydroxy-3-(4'-hydroxyphenyl)chroman] in human urine. *Biochemical Journal*, 201, 353–357.

Beninger, C.W., Hosfield, G.L. (2003). Antioxidant activity extracts, condensed tannin fractions, and pure flavonoids from *Phaseolus vulgaris* L. seed coat colour genotypes. *Journal of Agricultural and Food Chemistry*, 51, 7879–7883.

Barbosa, A.C.L., Lajolo, F.M. and Genovese, M.I. (2006). Influence of temperature pH and ionic strength on the production of isoflavone-rich soy protein isolates. *Food Chemistry*, 98, 757–766.

Barnes, S. (2010). The biochemistry, chemistry and physiology of the isoflavones in soybeans and their food products. *Lymphatic Research and Biology*, 8, 89–98.

Barnes, S., Kirk, M. and Coward, L. (1994). Isoflavones and their conjugates in soy foods: extraction conditions and analysis by HPLC mass spectrometry. *Journal of Agricultural and Food Chemistry*, 42, 2466–2474.

Barnes, S., Peterson, T.G. and Coward, L. (1995). Rationale for the use of genistein-containing soy matrices in chemoprevention trials for breast and prostate cancer. *Journal of Cell Biochemistry Supplement*, 22, 181–187.

Bhandari, P., Kumar, N., Singh, B. and Kaul, V.K. (2008). Simultaneous determination of sugars and picrosides in *Picrorhiza* species using ultrasonic extraction and high-performance liquid chromatography with evaporative light scattering detection. *Journal of Chromatography A*, 1194, 257–261.

Birt, D.F., Hendrich, S. and Wang, W. (2001). Dietary agents in cancer prevention: Flavonoids and isoflavonoids. *Pharmacology & Therapeutics*, 90, 157–177.

Bloedon, L.T., Jeffcoat, A.R. and Lopaczynski, W. (2002). Safety and pharmacokinetics of purified soy isoflavones: Single-dose administration to postmenopausal women. *American Journal of Clinical Nutrition*, 76, 1126–1137.

Bone, H.G., Greenspan, S.L. and McKeever, C. (2000). Alendronate and oestrogen effects in postmenopausal women with low bone mineral density alendronate/oestrogen study group. *Journal of Clinical Endocrinology and Metabolism*, 85 (2), 720–726.

Boonkird, S., Phisalaphong, C. and Phisalaphong, M. (2008). Ultrasound assisted extraction of capsaicinoids from *Capsicum frutescens* on a lab- and pilot-plant scale. *Ultrasonics Sonochemistry*, 15, 1075–1079.

Brezinski, A. and Debi, A. (1999). Phytooestrogens: the 'natural' selective oestrogen receptor modulators. *European Journal of Obstetrics & Gynecology and Reproductive Biology*, 85, 47–51.

Busby, M.G., Jeffcoat, A.R. and Bloedon, L.T. (2002). Clinical characteristics and pharmacokinetics of purified soy isoflavones: single-dose administration to healthy men. *American Journal of Clinical Nutrition*, 75, 126–136.

Chacko, B.K., Chandler, R.T., D'Alessandro, T.L. *et al.* (2007). Anti-inflammatory effects of isoflavones are dependent on flow and human endothelial cell PPARc. *Journal of Nutrition*, 137, 351–356.

Chandra, A. and Nair, M.G. (1996). Supercritical carbon dioxide extraction of daidzein and genistein from soybean products. *Phytochemical Analysis*, 7, 259–262.

Chang, S.K.C. (2002). Isoflavones from soybeans and soy foods,.in *Functional Foods, Biochemical and Processing Aspects*, Vol. 2 (eds G. Mazza, M. Le Maguer and J. Shi). CRC Press, Boca Raton, FL, pp. 39–69.

Chen, F., Sun, Y.Z., Zhao, G.H. *et al.* (2007). Optimization of ultrasound-assisted extraction of anthocyanins in red raspberries and identification of anthocyanins in extract using high performance liquid chromatography-mass spectrometry. *Ultrasonics Sonochemistry*, 14, 767–778.

Cheng, G., Wilczek, B., Warner, M., Gustafsson, J.A. and Landgren, B.M. (2007). Isoflavone treatment for acute menopausal symptoms. *Menopause*, 14 (3 Pt 1), 468–473.

Choi, Y.B. and Kim, K.S. (2005). Purification of isoflavone from soybean hypocotyls using various resins. *Korean Journal of Environmental Health*, 31 (3), 221–226.

Chung, H., Hogan, S., Zhang, L., Rainey, K. and Zhou, K. (2008). Characterization and comparison of antioxidant properties and bioactive components of Virginia soybeans. *Journal of Agricultural and Food Chemistry*, 56, 11515–11519.

Chung, M.J., Kang, A.Y., Lee, K.M. *et al.* (2006). Water soluble genistein glycoside isoflavone up-regulate antioxidant metallothionein expression and scavenge free radicals. *Journal of Agricultural of Food Chemistry*, 54, 3819–3826.

Chun, J., Kim, G.M., Lee, K.W. *et al.* (2007). Conversion of isoflavone glucosides to aglycones in soy milk by fermentation with lactic acid bacteria. *Journal of Food Science*, 72, M39–M44.

Cline, J.M. and Hughes, C.L., Jr. (1998). Phytochemicals for the prevention of breast and endometrial cancer, in *Biological and Hormonal Therapies of Cancer* (eds K.A. Foon and H.B. Muss). Kluwer Academic Publishers, Boston, pp. 107–134.

Concetta, B., Brunella, C., Raffaella, G. *et al.* (2009). Content of phytooestrogens in soy-based dietary supplements. *Food Chemistry*, 115, 1389–1392.

Coward, L., Barnes, N.C., Setchell, K.D.R. and Barnes, S. (1993). Genistein, daidzein, and their b-glycoside conjugates: Antitumor isoflavones in soybean foods from American and Asian diets. *Journal of Agricultural and Food Chemistry*, 41, 1961–1967.

Coward, L., Smith, M., Kirk, M. and Barnes, S. (1998). Chemical modification of isoflavones in soyfoods during cooking and processing. *The American Journal of Clinical Nutrition*, 68 (6), 1486–1491.

Deavours, B.E. and Dixon, R.A. (2005). Metabolic engineering of isoflavonoid biosynthesis in alfalfa. *Plant Physiology*, 138, 2245–2259.

Delgado-Zamarreño, M.M., Pérez-Martín, L., Bustamante-Rangel, M. and Carabias-Martínez, R. (2012). Pressurized liquid extraction as a sample preparation method for the analysis of isoflavones in pulses. *Analytical and Bioanalytical Chemistry*, 404 (2), 361–366.

Delmas, P.D., Eastell, R., Garnero, P., Seibel, M.J. and Stepan, J. (2000). The use of biochemical markers of bone turnover in osteoporosis. Committee of Scientific Advisors of the International Osteoporosis Foundation. *Osteoporosis International*, 11 (Suppl), S2–S17.

De Pascual-Teresa, S., Hallund, J., Talbot, D. *et al.* (2006). Absorption of isoflavones in humans: Effects of food matrix and processing. *The Journal of Nutritional Biochemistry*, 17, 257–264.

Dewick, P.M (1993). Isoflavonoids, in *The Flavonoids: Advances in Research Since 1986* (ed. J.B. Harborne). Chapman & Hall, London, pp. 117–238.

Duffy, C., Perez, K. and Partridge, A. (2007). Implications of phytooestrogen intake for breast cancer. CA Cancer *J. Clin.* 57 (5), 260–277.

Eldridge, A.C. (1982a). Determination of isoflavones in soybean flours, protein concentrate and isolates. *J. Agric Food Chem*, 30, 353–355.

Eldridge, A.C. (1982b). High perfomance liquid chromatography separation of soybean isoflavones and their glycosides. *Journal of Chomatography*, 234, 494–496.

Eldridge, A.C., Kwolek, W.F. (1983). Soybean isoflavones: effect of environment and variety on composition. *Journal of Agricultural and Food Chemistry*, 31, 394–396.

Esaki, H., Kawakishi, S., Morimitsu, Y. and Osawa, T. (1999). New potent antioxidative *o*-dihydroxyisoflavones in fermented Japanese soybean products. *Bioscience, Biotechnology and Biochemistry*, 63, 1637–1639.

Fedeniuk, R.W. and Shand, P.J. (1998). Theory and methodology of antibiotic extraction from biomatrices. *Journal of Chromatography A*, 812 (1–2), 3–15.

Fiechter, G., Opacak, I., Raba, B. and Mayer, H.K. (2013). A new ultra-high pressure liquid chromatography method for the determination of total isoflavone aglycones after enzymatic hydrolysis: Application to analyze isoflavone levels in soybean cultivars. *Food Research International*, 50 (2), 586–592.

Franke, A.A., Halm, B.M., Kakazu, K., Li, X. and Custer, L.J. (2009). Phytooestrogenic isoflavonoids in epidemiologic and clinical research. *Drug Testing and Analysis*, 1 (1), 14–21.

Ha, E.Y.W., Morr, C.V. and Seo, A. (1992). Isoflavone aglycone and volatile organic compounds in soybeans: Effects of soaking treatments. *Journal of Food Science*, 57, 414–426.

Hanasaki, Y., Ogawa, S. and Fukui, S. (1994). The correlation between active oxygen scavenging and antioxidative effects of flavonoids. *Free Radical Biology and Medicine*, 16, 845–850.

He, J., Zhao, Z., Shi, Z. *et al.* (2005). Analysis of isoflavone daidzein in *Puerariae radix* with micelle-mediated extraction and preconcentration. *Journal of Agricultural and Food Chemistry*, 53, 518–523.

Hennion, M.C. (1999). Solid-phase extraction: Method development, sorbents, and coupling with liquid chromatography. *Journal of Chromatography A*, 856 (1–2), 3–54.

Henderson, B.E., Ross, R.K. and Pike, M.C. (1993). Hormonal chemoprevention of cancer in women. *Science*, 259, 633–638.

Hoeck, J.A., Fehr, W.R., Murphy, P.A. and Welke, G.A. (2000). Influence of genotype and environment on isoflavone contents of soybean. *Crop Science*, 40, 48–51.

Hosokawa, N., Hosokawa, Y., Sakai, T. *et al.* (1990). Inhibitory effect of quercetin on the synthesis of a possibly cell-cycle-related 17-kDa protein, in human colon cancer cells. *International Journal of Cancer*, 45, 1119–1124.

Huang, H., Liang, H. and Kwok, K.C. (2006). Effect of thermal processing on genistein, daidzein and glycitein content in soy milk. *Journal of the Science of Food and Agriculture*, 86, 1110–1114.

Hwang, K.T., Jung, S.T., Lee, G.D. *et al.* (2002). Controlling molecular weight and degree of deacetylation of chitosan by response surface methodology. *Journal of Agricultural and Food Chemistry*, 50 (7), 1876–1882.

Jackson, C.J.C., Dini, J.P., Lavandier, C. *et al.* (2002). Effects of processing on the content and composition of isoflavones during manufacturing of soy beverage and tofu. *Process Biochemistry*, 37, 1117–1123.

Jason, A.A., Todd, D.M. and Luis, A. Col. (2007). Ultrahigh-pressure liquid chromatography using a 1-mm id column packed with 1.5-μm porous particles. *Journal of Separation Science*, 30, 1207–1213.

Jenkins, D.J., Kendall, C.W., Jackson, C.J. *et al.* (2002). Effects of high- and low-isoflavone soyfoods on blood lipids, oxidized LDL, homocysteine, and blood pressure in hyperlipidemic men and women. *American Jpurnal of Clinical Nutrition*, 76, 365–372.

Jenkins, D.J.A., Kendall, C.W.C., Vidgen, E. and Mehling, C.C (2000).The effect on serum lipids and oxidized low-density lipoprotein of supplementing self-selected low-fat diets with soluble-fiber, soy, and vegetable protein foods. *Metabolism*, 49, 67–72.

Kao, T.H., Chien, J.T. and Chen, B.H. (2008). Extraction yield of isoflavones from soybean cake as affected by solvent and supercritical carbon dioxide. *Food Chemistry*, 107, 1728–1736.

Kao, T.H., Lu, Y.F., Hiseh, H.C., and Chen, B.H. (2004). Stability of isoflavone glucosides during processing of soy milk and tofu. *Food Research International*, 37, 891–900.

Kaufman, P.B., Duke, J.A., Brielmann, H., Boik, J. and Hoyt, J.E. (1997). A comprehensive survey of leguminous plants as sources of the isoflavones, genistein and daidzein: Implications for human nutrition and health. *Journal of Alternate Complementary Medicine*, 3, 7–22.

Knight, D.C., Wall, P.L. and Eden, J.A (1996). A review of phytooestrogens and their effects in relation to menopausal symptoms. *Australian Journal of Nutrition and Dietetics*, 53, 5–11.

Kim, E.M., Lee, K.J. and Chee, K.M. (2004). Comparison in isoflavone contents between soybean and soybean sprouts of various soybean cultivars. *Korean Journal Nutrition*, 37, 45–51.

Kim, J.A., Hong, S.B., Jung, W.S. *et al.* (2007).Comparison of isoflavones composition in seed, embryo, cotyledon and seed coat of cooked-with-rice and vegetable soybean (*Glycine max* L.) varieties. *Food Chemistry*, 102, 738–744.

Kim, J.T., Cha, D.S., Lee, G.D. *et al.* (2002). Process optimization of sweet potato pulp-based biodegradable plastics using response surface methodology. *Journal of Applied Polymer Science*, 83 (2), 423–434.

Kim, S.L., Kim, H.B., Chi, H.Y. *et al.* (2005). Variation of anthocyanins and isoflavones between yellow-cotyledon and green-cotyledon seeds of black soybean. *Food Science and Biotechnology*, 14, 778–782.

Kitamura, K., Igita, K., Kikuchi, A., Kudou, S. and Okubo, K. (1991). Low isoflavone content in early maturing cultivars, so-called summer-type soybeans (*Glycine max* (L.) Merrill). *Japanese Journal of Breeding*, 41, 651–654.

Klejdus, B., Mikelova, R., Adam, V. *et al.* (2004). Liquid chromatographic-mass spectrophotometric determination of genistin and daidzin in soybean food samples after accelerated solvent extraction with modified content of extraction cell. *Analytica Chimica Acta*, 517, 1–11.

Klejdus, B., Mikelova, R., Petrlova, J. *et al.* (2005).Evaluation of isoflavone aglycon and glycoside distribution in soy plants and soybeans by fast column high-performance liquid chromatography coupled with a diode-array detector. *Journal of Agricultural and Food Chemistry*, 53, 5848–5852.

Knight, D.C., Wall, P.L. and Eden, J.A. (1996). A review of phytooestrogens and their effects in relation to menopausal symptoms. *Australian Journal of Nutrition and Dietetics*, 53, 5–11.

Koupai-Abyazani, M.R., Creaser, C.S. and Stehpenson, G.R. (1992). Separation and identification of flavone, flavonol, isoflavone and flavanone aglycones by capillary column gas chromatography. *Phytochemical Analysis*, 3, 80–84.

Kudou, S., Fleury, Y., Welti, D. *et al.* (1991). Malonyl isoflavone glycosides in soybean seeds (*Glycine max* MERRILL). *Journal of Agricultural and Biological Chemistry*, 55 (9), 2227–2233.

Kurie, M., Shizuo, N. and Hiroyuki, K. (2003). Determination of daidzein and genistein in soybean foods by automated on-line in-tube solid-phase microextraction coupled to high-performance liquid chromatography. *Journal of Chromatography A*, 986, 169–177.

Kuo, L.C., Cheng, W.Y., Wu, R.Y., Huang, C.J. and Lee, K.T. (2006). Hydrolysis of black soybean isoflavone glycosides by *Bacillus subtilis natto*. *Applied Microbiology and Biotechnology*, 73, 314–320.

Lapcik, O., Hill, M., Hampl, R., Wahala, K. and Adlercreulz, H. (1998a). Identification of isoflavonoids in beer. *Steroids*, 63, 14–20.

Lee, M.H. and Lin, C.C. (2007). Comparison of techniques for extraction of isoflavones from the root of *Radix puerariae*: Ultrasonic and pressurized solvent extractions. *Food Chemistry*, 105 (1), 223–228.

Lee, S.J., Ahn, J.K., Tran, D.K. *et al.* (2007b). Comparison of isoflavone concen trations in soybean (*Glycine max* (L.) Merrill) sprouts grown under two different light conditions. *Journal of Agricultural and Food Chemistry*. 55: 9415–9421.

Lee, S.J., Ahn, J.K., Kim, S.H. *et al.* (2003). Variation in isoflavone of soybean cultivars with location and storage duration. *Journal of Agriculture and Food Chemistry*, 51, 3382–3389.

Lee, J.H., Renita, M., Fioritto, R.J. *et al.* (2004). Isoflavone characterization and antioxidant activity of Ohio soybeans. *Journal of Agricultural and Food Chemistry*, 52, 2647–2651.

Li, H.B. and Chen, F. (2005a). Preparative isolation and purification of phillyrin from the medicinal plant *Forsythia suspensa* by high-speed countercurrent chromatography. *Journal of Chromatography A*, 1083, 102–105.

Li, H.B. and Chen, F. (2005b). Simultaneous separation and purification of five bioactive coumarins from the Chinese medicinal plant *Cnidium monnieri* by high-speed countercurrent chromatography. *Journal of Separation Science*, 28, 268–272.

Liggins, J., Bluck, L.J.C., Coward, W.A. and Bingham, S.A. (1998). Extraction and quantification of daidzein and genistein in food. *Analytical Biochemistry*, 264, 1–7.

Li-Hsun, C., Ya-Chuan, C. and Chieh-Ming, C. (2004). Extracting and purifying isoflavones from defatted soybean flakes using superheated water at elevated pressures. *Food Chemistry*, 84, 279–285.

Li, S., Zhu, R.H., Zhong, M. *et al.* (2010). Effects of ultrasonic-assistant extraction parameters on total flavones yield of *Selaginella doederleinii* and its antioxidant activity. *Journal of Medicinal Plant Research*, 4, 1743–1750.

Lin, F. and Giusti, M.M. (2005). Effects of solvent polarity and acidity on the extraction efficiency of isoflavones from soybeans (*Glycine max*). *Journal of Agricultural and Food Chemistry*, 53, 3795–3800.

Liu, J., Chang, S.K. and Wiesenborn, D. (2005). Antioxidant properties of soybean isoflavone extract and tofu in vitro and in vivo. *Journal of Agricultural of Food Chemistry*, 53, 2333–2340.

Luthria, D.L., Biswas, R. and Natarajan, S.S. (2007). Comparison of extraction solvents and techniques used for the assay of isoflavones from soybeans. *Food Chemistry*, 105, 325–333.

Matsuura, M., Obata, A. and Fukushima, D. (1989). Objectionable flavour of soy milk developed during the soaking of soybeans and its control. *Journal of Food Science*, 54 (3), 602–605.

Matsuura, M., Sasaki, J. and Murao, S. (1995). Studies on β-glucosidases from soybeans that hydrolyse daidzin and genistin: Isolation and characterization of an isozyme. *Bioscience, Biotechnology and Biochemistry, Tokyo*, 59 (9), 1623–1627.

Maul, R., Schebb, N.H. and Kulling, S.E. (2008). Application of LC and GC hyphenated with mass spectrometry as tool for characterization of unknown derivatives of isoflavonoids. *Analytical and Bioanalytical Chemistry*, 391, 239–250.

Mazur, W.M., Duke, J.A., Wahala, K., Rasku, S. and Adlercreutz, H. (1998). Isoflavonoids and lignans in legumes: Nutritional and health aspects in humans. *The Journal of Nutritional Biochemistry*, 9, 193–200.

McCue, P. and Kalidas, S. (2004). Health benefits of soy isoflavonoids and strategies for enhancements: a review. *Critical Reviews in Food Science and Nutrition*, 44, 361–367.

Messina, M. (1995). Modern applications for an ancient bean: Soybeans and the prevention and treatment of chronic disease. *Journal of Nutrition*, 125, 567S–569S.

Messina, M.J. (2002). Soy foods and soybean isoflavones and menopausal health. *Nutrition in Clinical Care*, 5 (6), 272–282.

Morales-de la Peña, M., Salvia-Trujillo, L., Rojas-Graü, M.A. and Martín-Belloso, O. (2010). Isoflavone profile of a high intensity pulsed electric field or thermally treated fruit juice-soy milk beverage stored under refrigeration. *Innovative Food Science and Emerging Technologies*, 11, 604–610.

Murphy, P.A. (1981). Separation of genistein, daidzein and their aglucones, and coumestrol by gradient high-performance liquid chromatography. *Journal of Chromatography*, 211, 166–169.

Murphy, P.A., Song, T., Buseman, G. *et al.* (1999). Isoflavones in retail and institutional soy foods. *Journal of Agricultural and Food Chemistry*, 47, 2697–2704.

Murphy, P.A., Barua, K. and Hauck, C.C. (2002). Solvent extraction selection in the determination of isoflavones in soy foods. *Journal of Chromatography B*, 777, 129–138.

Nagata, Y., Sonoda, T., Mori, M. *et al.* (2007). Dietary isoflavones may protect against prostate cancer in Japanese men. *Journal of Nutrition*, 137, 1974–1979.

Naim, M., Gestetner, B., Zilkah, S., Birk, Y. and Bondi, A. (1974). Soybean isoflavones. characterization, determination and antifungal activity. *Journal of Agricultural Chemistry*, 24, 1174–1177.

Nurmi, T., Mazur, W., Heinonen, S., Kokkonen, J. and Adlercreutz, H. (2002). Isoflavone content of the soy based supplements. *Journal of Pharmaceutical and Biomedical Analysis*, 28, 1–11.

Otieno, D.O., Ashton, J.F. and Shan, N.P. (2007). Isoflavone phytooestrogen degradation in fermented soy milk with selected β-glucosidase producing *L. acidophilus* strains during storage at different temperatures. *International Journal of Food Microbiology*, 115, 79–88.

Otieno, D.O., Rose, H. and Shah, N.P. (2007). Profiling and quantification of isoflavones in soy milk from soy protein isolate using extracted ion chromatography and positive ion fragmentation techniques. *Food Chemistry*, 105, 1642–1651.

Pananun, T., Montalbo-Lomboy, M., Noomhorm, A., Grewell, D. and Lamsal, B. (2012). High-power ultrasonication-assisted extraction of soybean isoflavones and effect of toasting. *LWT – Food Science and Technology*, 47, 199–207.

Parthasarathi, G. and Fenner, G.P. (1999). Improved method for gas chromatographic analysis of genistein and daizein from soybean (*Glycine max*) seeds. *Journal of Agricultural and Food Chemistry*, 47, 3455–3456.

Pedersen-Bjergaard, S., Rasmussen, K.E. and Halvorsen, T.G. (2000). Liquid–liquid extraction procedures for sample enrichment in capillary zone electrophoresis. *Journal of Chromatography A*, 902 (1), 91–105.

Penalvo, J.L., Nurmi, T. and Adlercreutz, H.A. (2004). Simplified HPLC method for total isoflavones in soy products. *Food Chemistry*, 87, 297–305.

Phommalth, S., Jeong, Y.S., Kim, Y.H. and Hwang, Y.H. (2008). Isoflavone composition within each structural part of soybean seeds and sprouts. *Journal of Crop Science and Biotechnology*, 11 (1), 57-62.

Ribeiro, M.L., Mandarino, J.M.G., Carrão-Panizzi, M.C. *et al.* (2007). Isoflavone content and β-glucosidase activity in soybean cultivars of different maturity groups. *Journal of Food Composition and Analysis*, 20, 19–24.

Richelle, M., Pridmore-Merten, S., Bodenstab, S., Enslen, M. and Offord, E.A. (2002). Hydrolysis of isoflavone glycosides to aglycones by beta-glycosidase does not alter plasma and urine isoflavone pharmacokinetics in postmenopausal women. *The Journal of Nutrition*, 132, 2587–2592.

Riedl, K.M., Zhang, Y.C., Schwartz, S.J. and Vodovotz, Y. (2005). Optimizing dough proofing conditions to enhance isoflavone aglycones in soy bread. *Journal of Agricultural and Food Chemistry*, 53, 8253–8258.

Rimbach, G., Boesch-Saadatmandi, C., Frank, J. *et al.* (2008). Dietary isoflavones in the prevention of cardiovascular disease – A molecular perspective. *Food and Chemical Toxicology*, 46, 1308–1319.

Rolfe, B.G. (1988). Flavones and isoflavones as inducing substances of legume nodulation. *Biofactors*, 1, 3–10.

Rostagno, M.A., Araujo, J.M.A. and Sandi, D. (2002). Supercritical fluid extraction of isoflavones from soybean flour. *Food Chemistry*, 78, 111–117.

Rostagno, M.A., Miguel, P., Carmelo, G. and Barroso, C.G. (2003). Ultrasound-assisted extraction of soy isoflavones. *Journal of Chromatography A*, 1012, 119–128.

Rostagno, M.A., Palma, M. and Barroso, C.G. (2004). Pressurized liquid extraction of isoflavones from soybeans. *Analytica Chimica Acta*, 522, 169–177.

Rostagno, M.A., Palma, M. and Barroso, C.G. (2005). Solid-phase extraction of isoflavones. *Journal of Chromatography A*, 1076, 110–117.

Rostagno, M.A., Palma, M. and Barroso, C.G. (2007). Ultrasound-assisted extraction of isoflavones from soy beverages blended with fruit juices. *Analytica Chimica Acta*, 597, 265–272.

Rostagno, M.A., Villares, A., Guillamon, E., Garcia-Lafuente, A. and Martinez, J.A. (2009). Sample preparation for the analysis of isoflavones from soybeans and soy foods. *Journal of Chromatography A*, 1216, 2–29.

Sakai, T., Kikuchi, A., Shimada, H. *et al.* (2005). Evaluation of isoflavone contents and compositions of soybean seed and its relation with seeding time. *Japanese Journal of Crop Science*, 74, 156–164.

Scheiber, M.D., Liu, J.H., Subbiah, M.T.R., Rebar, R.W. and Setchell, K.D.R. (2001). Dietary inclusion of whole soy foods results in significant reductions in clinical risk factors for osteoporosis and cardiovascular disease in normal postmenopausal women. *Menopause*, 8, 384–392.

Seguin, P., Bodo, R. and Al-Tawaha, A.M. (2007). Soybean isoflavones: Factors affecting concentrations in seeds, in *Advances in Medicinal Plant Research* (eds S.N. Acharya, and J.E. Thomas). Research Signpost, Trivandrum, Kerala, India, pp. 65–80.

Seguin, P., Zheng, W., Smith, D.L. and Deng, W. (2004). Isoflavone content of soybean cultivars grown in eastern Canada. *Journal of the Science Food and Agriculture*, 84, 1327–1332.

Setchell, K.D., Brown, N.M., Desai, P. *et al.* (2001). Bioavailability of pure isoflavones in healthy humans and analysis of commercial soy isoflavone supplements. *The Journal of Nutrition*, 131, 1362S–1375S.

Setchell, K.D. and Cole, S.J. (2003). Variations in isoflavone levels in soy foods and soy protein isolates and issues related to isoflavone databases and food labelling. *Journal of Agriculture and Food Chemistry*, 51, 4146–4155.

Seung, Y.C., Yu, N.L. and Hyun, J.P. (2009). Optimization of ethanol extraction and further purification of isoflavones from soybean sprout cotyledon. *Food Chemistry*, 117, 312–317.

Shu, X.O., Zheng, Y., Cai, H. *et al.* (2009). Soy food intake and breast cancer survival. *JAMA*, 302 (22), 2437–2443.

Simonne, A.H., Smith, M., Weaver, D.B. *et al.* (2000). Retention and changes of soy isoflavones and carotenoids in immature soybean seeds (Edamame) during processing. *Journal of Agricultural and Food Chemistry*, 48, 6061–6069.

Siviengkhek, P., Yeon-Shin, J., Yong-Hoon, K. and Young-Hyun, H. (2008). Isoflavone composition within each structural part of soybean seeds and sprouts. *Journal of Crop Science and Biotechnology*, 11, 57–62.

Somekawa, Y., Chiguchi, M., Ishibashi, T. and Aso, T. (2001). Soy intake related to menopausal symptoms, serum lipids, and bone mineral density in postmenopausal Japanese women. *Obstetrics and Gynecology*, 97 (1), 109–115.

Song, T., Barua, K., Buseman, G. and Murphy, P.A. (1998). Soy isoflavones analysis: Quality control and a new internal standard. *America Journal of Clinical Nutrition*, 68, 1474–1479.

Steiner, C., Peters, W.H.M., Gallagher, E.P. *et al.* (2007). Genistein protects human mammary epithelial cells from benzo(a)pyrene-7,8-dihydrodiol-9,10- epoxide and 4-hydroxy-2-nonenal genotoxicity by modulating the glutathione/glutathione S-transferase system. *Carcinogenesis*, 28, 738–748.

Suqin, S., Alison, M., Duncan, R.Y. *et al.* (2009). Tracking isoflavones: From soybean to soy flour, soy protein isolates to functional soy bread. *Journal of Functional Foods*, 1, 119 – 127.

Sun-Joo, L., Philippe, S., Joung-Jin, K. *et al.* (2010). Isoflavones in Korean soybeans differing in seed coat and cotyledon colour. *Journal of Food Composition and Analysis*, 23, 160–165.

Synder, H.E. and Kwon, T.W. (1987). Oriental soy food products, in *Soybean Utilization*, Chapter 7. Van Nostrand Reinhold, New York, pp. 218–241.

Terigar, B.G., Balasubramanian, S., Boldor, D. *et al.* (2010). Continuous microwave-assisted isoflavone extraction system: Design and performance evaluation. *Bioresource Technology*, 101 (7), 2466–2471.

Tsukamoto, C., Shimada, S., Igita, K. *et al.* (1995). Factors affecting isoflavone content in soybean seeds: Changes in isoflavones, saponins, and composition of fatty acids at different temperatures during seed development. *Journal of Agricultural and Food Chemistry*, 43, 1184–1192.

Udgata, J.R. and Naik, S.N. (2006). Soybean isoflavones: Remadial nutraceuticals in Indian perspective. *Journal of Scientific and Industrial Research*, 66, 11–18.

USDA (2008). USDA Database for the Isoflavone Content of Selected Foods, 2.0. US Department of Agriculture. http://www.ars.usda.gov/is/pr/2008/080923.htm [accessed 25 July 2013].

Uzzan, M. and Labuza, T.P. (2004). Critical issues in R&D of soy isoflavone-enriched foods and dietary supplements. *Journal of Food Science*, 69, 77–86.

Vergne, S., Titier, K., Bernard, V. (2007). Bioavailability and urinary excretion of isoflavones in humans: Effects of soy-based supplements formulation and equol production. *Journal of Pharmaceutical and Biomedical Analysis*, 43, 1488–1494.

Wan, H.B. and Wong, M.K. (1996). Minimization of solvent consumption in pesticide residue analysis. *Journal of Chromatography A*, 754, 43–47.

Wang, B.F., Wang, J.S., Lu, J.F., Kao, T.H. and Chen, B.H. (2009). Antiproliferation effect and mechanism of prostate cancer cell lines as affected by isoflavones from soybean cake. *Journal of Agricultural of Food Chemistry*, 57, 2221–2232.

Wang, C., Ma, Q., Pagadala, S., Sherrard, M.S. and Krishnan, P.G. (1998). Changes of isoflavones during processing of soy protein isolates. *Journal of American Oil Chemists' Society*, 75, 337–341.

Wang, C., Sherrard, M., Pagadala, S., Wixon, R., Scott, R.A. (2000). Isoflavone content among maturity group 0 to II soybeans. *Journal of America Oil Chemistry Society*, 77, 483–487.

Wang, G., Kuan, S.S., Francis, O.J., Ware, G.M., and Carman, A.S. (1990). A simplified HPLC method for the determination of phytooestrogens in soybean and its processed products. *Journal of Agricultural and Food Chemistry*, 38, 185–190.

Wang, H.J. and Murphy, P.A. (1994a). Isoflavone composition of the American and Japanese soybeans in Iowa: Effects of variety, crop year, and location. *Journal of Agricultural and Food Chemistry*, 42: 1674–1677.

Wang, H.J. and Murphy, P.A. (1994b). Isoflavone content in commercial soybean foods. *Journal of Agricultural and Food Chemistry*, 42, 1666–1673.

Wang, H.J. and Murphy, P.A. (1996). Mass balance study of isoflavones during soybean processing. *Journal of Agricultural and Food Chemistry*, 44, 2377–2383.

Wang, L. and Weller, C.L. (2006). Recent advances in extraction of nutraceuticals from plants. *Trends in Food Science and Technology*, 17, 300–312.

Wang, Y., Hu, Y.C., Wang, J.H. *et al.* (2011). Ultrasound-assisted solvent extraction of swainsonine from *Oxytropis ochrocephala* Bunge. *Journal of Medicinal Plants Research*, 5, 890–894.

Wei, H., Bowen, R. and Cai, Q. (1995). Antioxidant and antipromotional effects of the soybean isoflavone genistein. *Proceedings of the Society for Experimental Biology and Medicine*, 208, 124–130.

Wei, P., Liu, M., Chen, Y. and Chen, D.P. (2012). Systematic review of soy isoflavone supplements on osteoporosis in women. *Asian Pacific Journal of Tropical Medicine*, 5 (3),243–248.

Wu, A.H., Horn-Ross, P.L., Nomura, A.M. *et al.* (1996). Tofu and risk of breast cancer in Asian-Americans. *Cancer Epidemiology, Biomarkers and Prevention*, 5, 901–906.

Wu, J.Y., Lin, L.D. and Chau, F.T. (2001). Ultrasound-assisted extraction of ginseng saponins from ginseng roots and cultured ginseng cells. *Ultrasonics Sonochemistry*, 8, 347–352.

Wu, Q., Wang, M., Sciarappa, W.J. and Simon, J.E. (2004a). LC/UV/ESI-MS analysis of isoflavones in edamame and tofu soybeans. *Journal of Agricultural and Food Chemistry*, 52, 2763–2769.

Wu, Q., Wang, M. and Simon, J.E. (2004b). Analytical methods to determine phytooestrogenic compounds. *Journal of Chromatography B*, 812, 325–355.

Xia, E.Q., Song, Y., Ai, X.X. *et al.* (2010). A new high performance liquid chromatographic method for the determination and distribution of linalool in *Michelia alba*. *Molecules*, 15, 4890–4897.

Xu, H.N. and He, C.H. (2007). Extraction of isoflavones from stem of *Pueraria lobata* (Willd.) Ohwi using *n*-butanol/water two-phase solvent system and separation of daidzein. *Separation and Purification Technology*, 56, 85–89.

Zhang, E.J., Ng, K.M and Luo, K.Q. (2007). Extraction and purification of isoflavones from soybeans and characterization of their oestrogenic activities. *Journal of Agricultural and Food Chemistry*, 55, 6940–6950.

Zhang, M., Xie, X., Lee, A.H. and Binns, C.W. (2004a). Soy and isoflavone intake are associated with reduced risk of ovarian cancer in southeast China. *Nutrition and Cancer*, 49, 125–130.

Zhang, X., Shu, X.O., Li, H. *et al.* (2005). Prospective cohort study of soy food consumption and risk of bone fracture among postmenopausal women. *Archives of Internal Medicine*, 165 (16), 1890–1895.

Zhang, Y.C., Albrecht, D., Bomser, J., Schwartz, S.J. and Vodovotz, Y. (2003). Isoflavone profile and biological activity of soy bread. *Journal of Agricultural and Food Chemistry*, 51, 7611–7616.

Zhang, Y.C., Lee, J.H., Vodovotz, Y. and Schwartz, S.J. (2004b). Changes in distribution of isoflavones and beta-glucosidase activity during soy bread proofing and baking. *Cereal Chemistry*, 81, 741–745.

III

Processing Effects on the Functional Components during Product Development

11 Thermal and Non-thermal Processing of Functional Foods

Jiraporn Sripinyowanich Jongyingcharoen[1] and Imran Ahmad[2]
[1]*Faculty of Engineering, King Mongkut's Institute of Technology Ladkrabang, Bangkok, Thailand*
[2]*Asian Institute of Technology, Pathum Thani Thailand*

11.1 Introduction

Processing is the set of methods and techniques used to transform raw materials into products. Since prehistoric times, crude processing of food materials including fermenting, sun drying, salting, smoking and various types of cooking have been used to preserve foodstuffs and make them edible. Primarily, the concept of food processing involves sterilization of foodstuffs. Food processing has been developed to inactivate pathogens, toxins and detrimental constituents so that the processed foods can meet safety and shelf-stability requirements. Nowadays, beyond the traditional requirements, there is much more emphasis on informatively labelled, high-quality and value-added foods that are convenient to use (Awuah *et al.*, 2007). The need for foods that are beneficial to health has increased concern about the effects of processing on the functional components of the food products. A number of health-conscious consumers try to eat more raw foods. However, many foods are available only when they are processed and they need to be processed to make them safe for consumption.

In general, food processing can be divided into two main types: thermal and non-thermal processing. Thermal processing is the most common and traditional technique because of its ability to inactivate microorganisms and spoilage enzymes (Rawson *et al.*, 2011a). However, it is recognized that heat treatment, especially under severe conditions, may induce chemical and physical changes, form toxic compounds and/or reduce the bioavailability of some nutrients. An adverse effect on the organoleptic properties of foods caused by thermal processing has also been reported.

Functional Foods and Dietary Supplements: Processing Effects and Health Benefits, First Edition.
Edited by Athapol Noomhorm, Imran Ahmad and Anil Kumar Anal.

Therefore, milder processing techniques including novel thermal, minimal thermal and non-thermal processing has become the new trend. These processing techniques are claimed to provide food of high quality and with improved functionality. Mostly, they are also more cost efficient and environmentally friendly compared to conventional thermal processing techniques. This chapter aims to provide a critical review of the effects of thermal, novel thermal, minimal thermal and non-thermal processing on the functional components of processed food.

11.2 Thermal processing

The thermal processing technique employs high temperatures to provide foods with various product options. It persists as the most widely used technique for ensuring microbiological safety and prolonging the shelf life of foods. However, the functional benefits of thermally processed foods is still doubtful as thermal treatment causes considerable changes in the quality and nutritional attributes of foods. Both beneficial and adverse effects of thermal processing on the functional components of foods depending on food material type and processing method and condition have been reported as summarized in Table 11.1.

Although some desirable changes may be obtained during thermal processing, the rather severe conditions (harsh temperature for an extended period of time) triggers chemical reactions, loss of nutrients and changes in organoleptic properties. Vitamins are among the most sensitive components in foods to be affected by heat treatment. Heat-sensitive vitamins include fat-soluble vitamins A (in the presence of oxygen), D, E and β-carotene, and water-soluble vitamins C (ascorbic acid), B_1 (thiamine), B_2 (riboflavin) in an acid environment, nicotinic acid, pantothenic acid and biotin C (Ryley and Kajda, 1994). Vitamin C, among others, presents the largest loss during heating (Awuah *et al.*, 2007). Its loss tends to follow consecutive first-order reactions, that is a rapid oxygen-dependent reaction proceeding until oxygen is depleted, followed by anaerobic degradation (Rawson *et al.*, 2011a). Carotenoid isomerization is also induced by heat or oxygen. However, it has been reported that cis-isomers of carotenoids have greater antioxidant capacity than their parent compounds (Zepka and Mercadante, 2009). Polyphenolic compounds are also present in a wide range of diets. A class of phenolic compounds easily found in plant produce is the anthocyanins. They are water-soluble pigments that confer the bright red, blue and purple colours of fruits and vegetables and are sensitive to high-temperature treatment. Degradation of anthocyanins eventually leads to brown pigments in the thermally processed products (Cavalcanti *et al.*, 2011; Rawson *et al.*, 2011a). It is well known that anthocyanin degradation is attributed to indirect oxidation of phenolic quinines generated by polyphenoloxidase (PPO) and peroxidase (POD), which are antinutritional enzymes (Rawson *et al.*, 2011a).

Maillard reactions, a complex series of reactions between proteins and reducing sugars via Amadori rearrangements, are also triggered by heat treatment. These reactions cause protein damage and loss of amino acids, especially lysine, an essential amino acid in the diet (Awuah *et al.*, 2007). However, it has been suggested that Maillard reaction products from coffee roasting are the prevailing antioxidants present in dark roasted coffee brew extracts (Liu and Kitts, 2011). The mechanisms of the antioxidant action associated with the Maillard reaction products involve both a hydrogen atom transfer mechanism and a single electron transfer mechanism.

Table 11.1 Effects of thermal processing on functional components of food products

Food	Type	Processing conditions[a]	Parameters affected[b]	References
Acai (*Euterpe oleracea*) Acai (*Euterpe precatoria*)	Puree Puree	t: 1–60; T: 80	(↔) Non-anthocyanin polyphenolic compounds (↓) Anthocyanin	Pacheco-Palencia *et al.*, 2009
Bean (pinto bean, black bean, yellow soybean and black soybean)	Seed	(a) Boiling; t: 90 (b) Pressure boiling; t: 10; P: 103 (c) Steaming; t: 70 (d) Pressure steaming; t: 60; P: 103	(↓) Total phenolics (↓) Total saponins (↓) Phytic acid	Xu and Chang, 2011
Black soybean (*Glycine max* L. Merrill)	Seed	Roasting; t: 26–34; T: 150–250	(↑) Antioxidant capacity (↑) Total phenolics (↑) Maillard reaction products	Kim *et al.*, 2011
Cashew apple	Clarified juice	t: 300; T: 88–121	(↓) Vitamin C (↑) 5-hydroxymethylfurfural (5-HMF)	Damasceno *et al.*, 2008
Cashew apple	Juice	t: 60–240; T: 60–90	(↓) Xanthophylls (↑) Cis-isomers of carotenoids (↓) Total carotenoids	Zepka and Mercadante, 2009
Chickpea (*Cicer arietinum* L.)	Seed	(a) Boiling; t: 90; T: 100 (b) Autoclaving; t: 35; T: 121; P: 15 lbs pressure	(↓) Antinutrient activity (trypsin inhibitor, haemagglutinin activity, tannins, phytic acid, saponin) (↓) Vitamin B (↓) Minerals	Alajaji and El-Adawy, 2006
Cladodes (*Opuntia ficus indica*)	Young stem	Boiling; t: 20	(↓) Vitamin C (↓) Total polyphenols (↓) Total antioxidant capacity	Ramírez-Moreno *et al.*, 2013
Cowpea	Seed	(a) Soaking in sodium bicarbonate solutions; t: 120–360 (b) Cooking; t: 20–60 (c) Autoclaving; t: 10–30; T: 121; P: 2.175	(↓) Polyphenols (↓) Tannin (↓) Phytic acid	Avanza *et al.*, 2013
Durian	Juice	Drying; T: 88–130	(↓) Flavor volatile	Chin *et al.*, 2010
Grain (wheat, buckwheat, oats and corn)	Sprout and seedling	Autoclaving; t: 20; T: 121; P: 15 lbs pressure	(↑) Total phenolics (↑) Antioxidant capacity	Randhir *et al.*, 2008
Jackfruit	Bulb slice	Drying; T: 50–70	(↓) Total carotenoids	Saxena *et al.*, 2012

(*continued*)

Table 11.1 (*Continued*)

Food	Type	Processing conditions[a]	Parameters affected[b]	References
Mango	Fruit	Hot water treatment; t: 75; T: 46.1	(↔) Gallic acid (↔) Total hydrolysable tannins (↔) Antioxidant capacity	Kim *et al.*, 2007
Mango	Fruit	Hot water treatment; t: 75–110; T: 46.1	(↓) Gallic acid (↓) Gallotannins (↓) Total soluble phenolics (↔) Antioxidant capacity	Kim *et al.*, 2009
Mango	Fruit	Hot water dipping; t: 30–75; T: 46–50	(↔) Total carotenoids (↔) Ascorbic acid	Djioua *et al.*, 2009
Mango	Slice	Drying; t: 1200; T: 60	(↓) Total carotenoids	Chen *et al.*, 2007
Mango	Puree	t: 16; T: 85–93	(↓) Vitamin A (↓) Polyphenoloxidase (PPO) (↔) Residual peroxidase (POD)	Vasquez-Caicedo *et al.*, 2007
Pineapple	Juice	t: 80; T: 55–95	(↑) Hydroxymethylfurfural (HMF) (↓) Carotenoid	Rattanathanalerk *et al.*, 2009
Pink guava	Puree	Drying; t: 240–360; T: 43.79–86.21	(↓) Lycopene (↓) Lipophilic antioxidant capacity	Kong *et al.*, 2010
Pumpkin	Puree	t: 0–120; T: 60–100	(↓) β-carotene	Dutta *et al.*, 2006
Tamarillo tree	Nectar	Pasteurization; t: 10; T: 80–95 (a) Degassed (b) Not degassed	 (↔) Ascorbic acid (↓) Dehydroascorbic acid (↔) Total carotenoids (↓) Ascorbic acid (↓) Dehydroascorbic acid (↔) Total carotenoids	Mertz *et al.*, 2010
Tomato	Puree	Pasteurization; t: 0.67; T: 98	(↑) Folates (↓) Ascorbic acid (↓) Total phenolics (↔) Carotenoids	Pérez-Conesa *et al.*, 2009
Tomato	Puree	(a) Pasteurization; t: 1–10; T: 60–90 (b) Sterilization; t: 1.5–3; T: 117	(↔) Total lycopene (↓) Total lycopene	Knockaert *et al.*, 2012

[a]t, Processing time (min); T, temperature (°C); P, pressure (kPa).
[b](↓) decreased level; (↑) increased level; (↔) neither increase nor decrease in the level.
Source: Adapted from Rawson *et al.*, 2011a with permission from Elsevier.

11.3 Novel thermal processing

Novel thermal processing techniques are mostly designated for the novel heating alternatives that offer quicker heating rates and hence can minimize nutrient degradation. Table 11.2 presents the effects of these techniques on the functional components of food products. Such techniques include, but are not limited to, ohmic, radio frequency (RF) and microwave (MW) heating. These three heating methods are electroheating. Ohmic heating is direct electroheating where electrical current is applied directly to the food while MW and RF heating are indirect electroheating where the electrical energy is firstly converted to electromagnetic radiation that subsequently generates heat within a product (Marra *et al.,* 2009). Electromagnetic heating transfers energy from its radiation source directly and volumetrically into the food without heating up the heat transfer surface of the processing equipment.

These novel heating methods have various applications in food processing such as cooking, thawing, drying and pasteurization. They operate at a frequency range of 50–60 Hz for ohmic heating, 10–60 MHz for RF heating and 1–3 GHz for MW heating. However, RF applications are restricted to 13.56, 27.12 and 40.68 MHz for industrial, scientific and medical purposes, respectively (Awuah *et al.,* 2007; Marra *et al.,* 2009). The frequencies of 915 and 2450 MHz are also permitted for industrial microwave applications, and only 2450 MHz is generally operated in domestic microwave ovens.

Ionic depolarization and dipole rotation are the two mechanisms involved in dielectric heating. During the ionic depolarization, positive ions in a food material move towards negative regions of an alternating electric field applied to the material and negative ions move towards positive regions of the electric field. The ionic mechanism is essentially electric resistance heating as found in ohmic heating where the field polarity changes at much lower frequencies as compared to the other two electroheating methods. Irrespective of the frequency, the continued reversal of polarity in the electrical field leads to the oscillation of ions forwards and backwards in the material, the net effect of this being the internal generation of heat within the material by friction. The other mechanism of heating is the movement of dipolar molecules such as water in the material. Besides the ion movement, the dipoles attempt to align themselves appropriately with the changing polarity of the electrical field, resulting in friction between molecules that leads to heat generation. In general, RF frequency range has a dominant heating mechanism of ionic depolarization while MW frequency range has both ionic depolarization and dipole rotation as the dominant heating mechanism (Marra *et al.,* 2009). Therefore, RF is more appropriate for materials with a regular shape, large dimensions and a high loss factor. On the other hand, MW is better adapted to compact materials with complex shapes and a low loss factor (Awuah *et al.,* 2007).

A comparative study on the thermal degradation kinetics of nutrients in orange juice heated by the three novel thermal methods and a conventional thermal process (heating in a shaker water bath) was conducted by Vikram *et al.* (2005). It was concluded that the destruction of vitamin C was influenced by the heating method and processing temperature. Uncontrollable temperature generated during microwave heating led to the highest degradation of vitamin C while ohmic heating gave the highest vitamin retention at all temperatures. The temperature profile and vitamin C degradation for these studied methods are presented in Figure 11.1 and Figure 11.2, respectively.

Table 11.2 Effects of novel thermal processing on functional components of food products

Food	Type	Processing conditions[a]	Parameters affected[b]	References
Ohmic heating				
Acerola	Pulp	F: 60; t: 0–90; T: 75–90	(↓) Monomeric anthocyanins	Mercali *et al.*, 2013
Apple and peach	Chunky fruit dessert	t: 45; T: 105	(↓) 5-HMF and furfural (↓) Ascorbic acid	Louarme and Billaud, 2012
Blueberry	Pulp	F: 60; t: 2; T: 90	(↓) Anthocyanins	Sarkis *et al.*, 2013
Grape	Juice	t: 5–25; T: 60–90; Voltage gradient: 20–40 V/cm	(↓) Polyphenoloxidase (PPO) activity	İçïer *et al.*, 2008
Radio frequency heating				
Apple (Golden delicious)	Fruit derivatives	E: 4.0–6.9; F: 27.12; t: 3; T: 52–98	(↓) PPO activity (↓) lipoxygenase (LOX) activity	Manzocco *et al.*, 2008
Mustard (*Sinapis alba*)	Seed	F: 13.5; T: 112	(↓) Isothiocyanate (↔) Glucosinolate (↔) Total polyphenols (↔) Free radical scavenging activity	Ildikó *et al.*, 2006
Microwave heating				
Chickpea (*Cicer arietinum* L.)	Seed	F: 2450; t: 15	(↓) Antinutrient activity (trypsin inhibitor, haemagglutinin activity, tannins, phytic acid, saponin) (↓) Vitamin B (↓) Minerals	Alajaji and El-Adawy, 2006
Citrus (Thompson navel, mandarin and lemon)	Peel	F: 2450; P: 100–600; t: 8.75–79	(↑) Phenolics for thompson navel peel (↓) Phenolics for mandarin and lemon peels	Ghanem *et al.*, 2012
Citrus mandarin pomace	Powder	F: 2450; P: 125–500; t: 5–15	(↑) Antioxidant capacity (↑) Flavonol, flavonone and flavonol (↑) Free fraction of phenolic acids (↓) Bound fraction of phenolic acids	Hayat *et al.*, 2010
Green coconut	Liquid	F: 2450; T: 52.5–92.9	(↓) PPO activity (↓) POD activity	Matsui *et al.*, 2008
Orange	Juice	F: 2450; t: 0.5–10; T: 60–85	(↓) Total carotenoids	Fratianni *et al.*, 2010

[a]E, Electric field (kV); F, frequency (Hz for ohmic heating and MHz for RF and MW heating); P, power (W); t, exposure time (min); T, temperature (°C).
[b](↓) decreased level; (↑) increased level; (↔) neither increase nor decrease in the level.

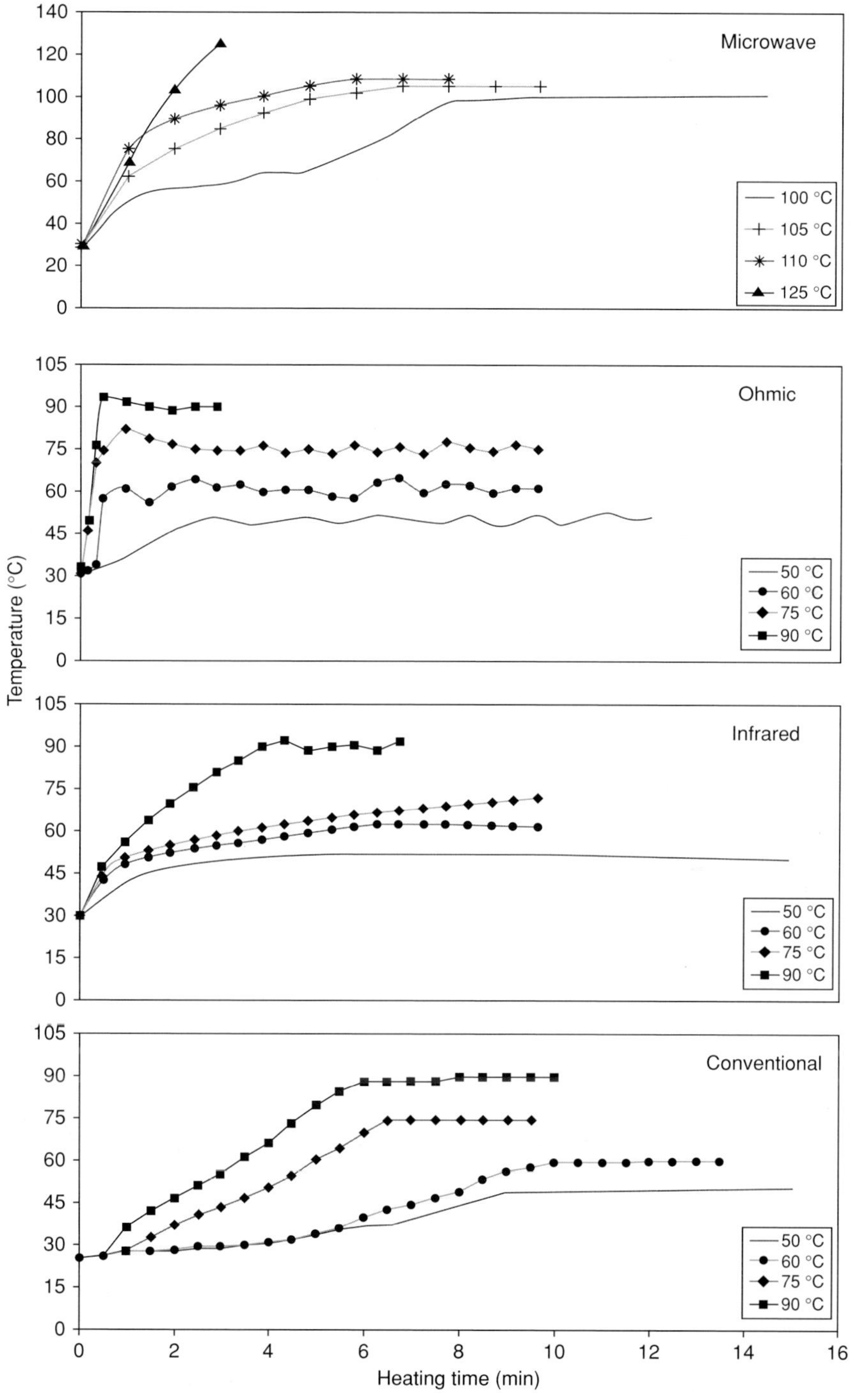

Figure 11.1 Temperature profiles during the heating of orange juice by the novel thermal heating methods as compared to the conventional heating method at different temperatures. *Source:* Vikram *et al.*, 2005. Reproduced with permission from Elsevier

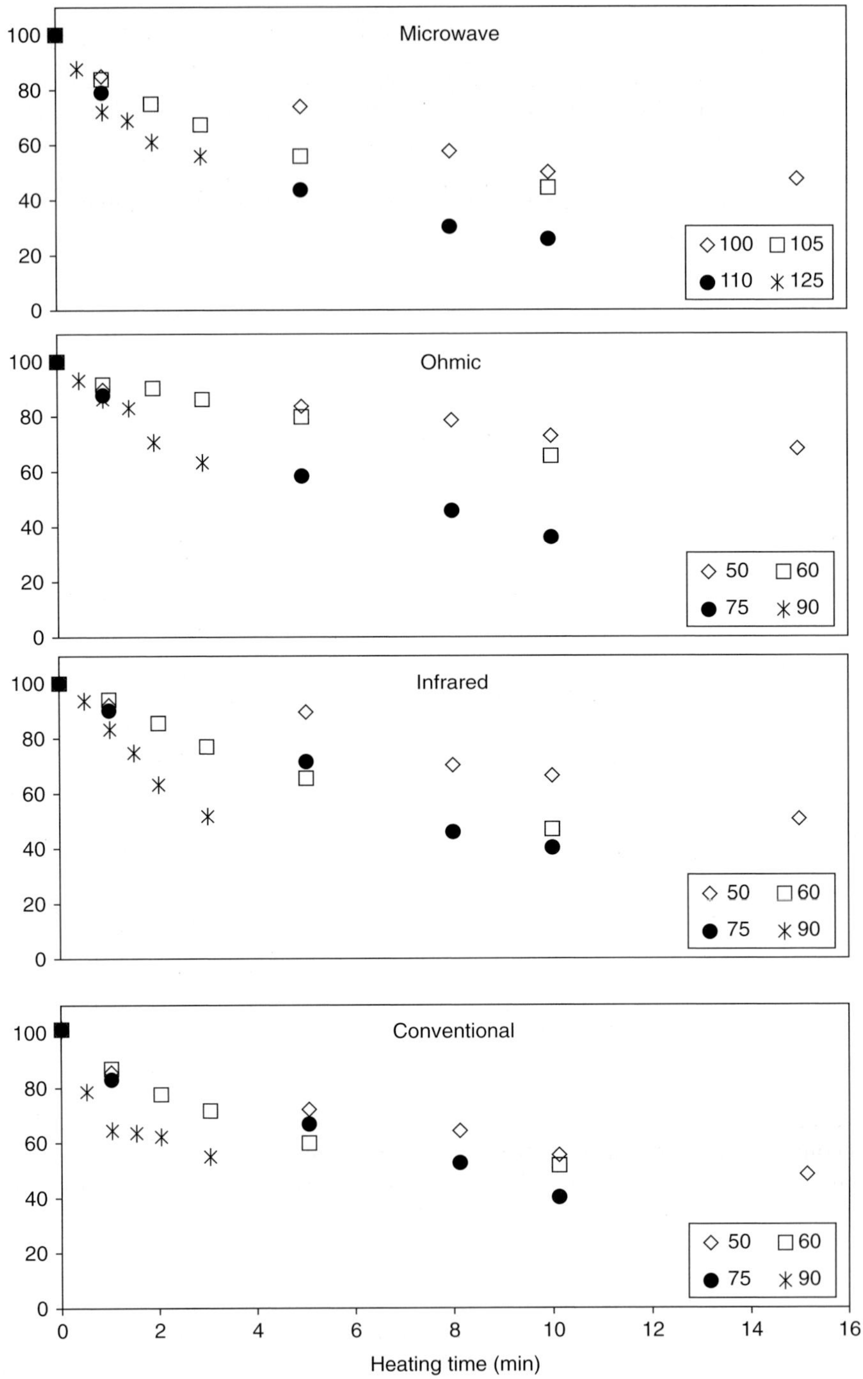

Figure 11.2 Vitamin C retention during heating by the novel thermal heating methods as compared to the conventional heating method at different temperatures. *Source:* Vikram *et al.*, 2005. Reproduced with permission from Elsevier

11.4 Minimal thermal and non-thermal processing

Recent developments in food processing operations involve technologies that avoid the deleterious effects of heat on the organoleptic properties and nutrients of foods. Promising methods include minimal thermal and non-thermal processing which can be conducted at ambient or slightly above-ambient temperature. Recent alternative or novel minimal-thermal and non-thermal processing methods are being examined to produce safe and better quality food products. These methods include, but are not limited to, ultrasound, high hydrostatic pressure, radiation and pulsed electric field processing. They may replace conventional thermal processes in certain applications and are particularly beneficial for thermally sensitive products.

11.4.1 Ultrasound processing

Ultrasound refers to sound waves at a frequency above the threshold of human hearing (20 kHz to 10 MHz). The major effects of ultrasound on liquid systems is contributed by cavitation phenomena, which is the physical processes that create, enlarge and implode micro-bubbles of gases dissolved in a liquid medium by the compression and decompression of the molecules that constitute the medium (Soria and Villamiel, 2010; Pingret *et al.*, 2013). The implosion of the cavitation bubble creates a transitory hot spot with elevated localized temperature (5000 K) and pressure (1000 atm) (Pingret *et al.*, 2013). As a result, the chemical reactivity is accelerated into the medium. Highly reactive free radicals ($H_2O \rightarrow H + \cdot OH$) are generated and may react with and modify other molecules (Soria and Villamiel, 2010). Besides the chemical effects, the cavitation phenomena also generate extreme physical forces including shear forces, micro-jets, shock waves and turbulence (Chandrapala *et al.*, 2012). Some forms of force such as vibration, heating and physical agitation are also generated by ultrasound in the absence of acoustic cavitation (Chandrapala *et al.*, 2012). Both the chemical and physical effects of ultrasound are useful in many food processing applications such as emulsification, homogenization, filtration, crystallization, hydrolysis, extraction and enzyme and microbial inactivation.

To date, there are many studies on the applications of ultrasound related to food processing. Impacts of this technology on the quality and property parameters of food products have been reviewed by many researchers (Soria and Villamiel, 2010; Chandrapala *et al.*, 2012; Pingret *et al.*, 2013). It is observed that ultrasonic conditions including frequency, amplitude of the wave, power and intensity considerably affect the process (Table 11.3). Optimized ultrasound processing causes less alterations in food components than conventional thermal treatments.

Many reports are available on the degradation of ascorbic acid in sonicated foods. Ascorbic acid is known to be an effective antioxidant protecting cells from damage induced by free radicals. However, it is thermolabile and highly sensitive to various processing conditions. Adekunte *et al.* (2010) reviewed that ascorbic acid degradation during sonication is mainly due to sonochemical reactions and the extreme physical conditions generated by the cavitation phenomena. Hydrogen ions (H^+), free radicals (O^-, OH^-, HO_2^-) and hydrogen peroxide (H_2O_2) are formed by sonolysis of water molecules and acoustic cavitation (Adekunte *et al.*, 2010; Pingret *et al.*, 2013). The radicals generally accumulate in the surface of the cavitation bubble and are responsible for the degradation of ascorbic acid. However, a different finding was reported

Table 11.5 Effects of radiation processing on functional components of food products

Food	Type	Processing conditions[a]	Parameters affected[b]	References
Blueberry	Fruit	S: UV-C; D: 0–4; t: 1–15; T: 20	(↑) Total anthocyanins (↔) Total phenolics	Perkins-Veazie *et al.*, 2008
Broccoli (*Brassica oleracea* var. *Italica*)	Floret	S: UV-C; D: 8	(↑) Total phenolics (↑) Ascorbic acid (↑) Antioxidant capacity	Lemoine *et al.*, 2007
Chestnut (*Castanea sativa* Mill.)	Nut	S: Electron beams; D: 0–6	(↔) Organic acids (oxalic, quinic, malic, ascorbic, citric and fumaric acids)	Carocho *et al.*, 2013
Fenugreek	Seed	S: Gamma rays (^{60}Co, 10 Gy/min); D: 0–10	(↑) Phenol	Chatterjee *et al.*, 2009
Fruits (pineapple, banana and guava)	Fresh cut	S: UV-C; D: 2.158×10^{-3}; t: 0–30; T: room	(↑) Polyphenols (↑) Flavonoids (↓) Vitamin C	Alothman *et al.*, 2009b
Green gram and garden pea	Seed sprout	S: Gamma rays (^{60}Co, 36 Gy/min); D: 1–2; T: 0–4	(↔) Vitamin C (↔) Total carotenoids	Hajare *et al.*, 2007
Green onion (*Allium wakegi*)	Fresh cut	S: Gamma rays (^{60}Co, 0.8 Gy/min); D: 1.2	(↑) Polyphenols (↓) Ascorbic acid	Jimenez *et al.*, 2011
Legume (pea, cowpea, lentil, kidney bean and chickpea)	Seed	S: Gamma rays; D: 0–10; T: room	(↓) Phytic acid (↓) Tannins	El-Niely, 2007

Mango	Fresh cut	S: UV-C; t: 0–30	(↑) Phenolics (↑) Flavonoids (↓) β-carotene (↓) Ascorbic acid	González-Aguilar *et al.*, 2007
Mango (*Mangifera indica* L.)	Fruit	S: Electron beams; D: 1–3.1	(↑) Flavonols (↔) Total phenolics (↔) Carotenoids	Reyes and Cisneros-Zevallos, 2007
Starfruit	Juice	S: UV-C; D: 2.158×10^{-3}; t: 0–60; T: room	(↑) 1,1-diphenyl-2-picrylhydrazyl (DPPH) inhibition (↑) Total phenols (↑) Flavonols and flavonoids (↑) Antioxidant capacity (↓) Ascorbic acid	Bhat *et al.*, 2011a
Strawberry	Fruit	S: UV-C; D: 0.43–4.30; t: 1–10	(↑) Antioxidant capacity (↑) Anthocyanins (↑) Phenolics	Erkan *et al.*, 2008
Velvet bean (*Mucuna pruriens*)	Seed	S: Gamma rays (^{60}Co, 6.5 kGy/h); D: 2.5–30; T: room	(↑) Phenolics (↑) Tannins (↓) Phytic acid	Bhat *et al.*, 2007

[a]S, Radiation source; D, dose (kGy for gamma rays and electron beams and kJ/m^2 for UV-C); t, exposure time (min); T, temperature (°C).
[b](↓) decreased level; (↑) increased level; (↔) neither increase nor decrease in the level.

their possible antioxidant activities and potential health benefits to reduce cardio-cerebrovascular diseases and cancer mortality (Hertog *et al.,* 1997).

11.7 Pulsed electric field processing

Pulsed electric field (PEF) technology is recognized as a non-thermal technology for food processing capable of inactivating microorganisms and enzymes and retaining health-related compounds concurrently. The PEF process is commonly applied to liquid foods; the effects of this processing technique on the nutritional attributes of processed foods are shown in Table 11.6. It involves the application of a series of short, high-voltage pulses (20–80 kV/cm) to a liquid food flowing between two electrodes that confine a treatment zone in the PEF chamber (Alkhafaji and Farid, 2007). Typically, PEF is applied at high field strength in food processing. High-intensity PEF (HIPEF) can be applied using exponentially decaying, square wave, bipolar or oscillatory pulses.

The mechanism of PEF causing microorganism inactivation is known as electroporation of cells (Alkhafaji and Farid, 2007; Huang *et al.,* 2012). PEF causes local instabilities and tension in the cell membrane attributable to electromechanical compression and facilitates the formation of pores in the membrane (Huang *et al.,* 2012). As shown in Figure 11.3, the plasma membranes of cells become permeable to small molecules after being exposed to an electric field. The permeation then causes swelling and the eventual rupture of the cell membrane (Vega-Mercado *et al.,* 1997). A review by Moritz *et al.* (2012) found that the effect of PEF on proteins could entail: polarization of the protein molecule, dissociation of non-covalently bound protein subunits involved in quaternary structure, changes in the protein conformation so that hydrophobic amino acids or sulfhydryl groups are exposed, attraction of polarized structures by electrostatic forces and hydrophobic interactions or covalent bonds of forming aggregates.

Studies have shown that the inactivation of enzymes by PEF treatment could depend on the sensitivity of the enzymes to this treatment. The most common discussed enzymes are polyphenoloxidase (PPO) and peroxidase. These enzymes catalyse oxidation of phenolic compounds and cause enzymatic browning leading to colour changes of foods (Bi *et al.,* 2013).

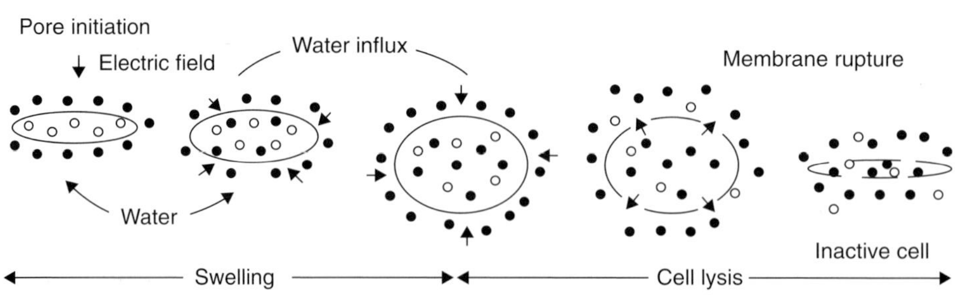

Figure 11.3 Mechanism of cell inactivation. *Source:* Vega-Mercado *et al.,* 1997. Reproduced with permission from Elsevier

Table 11.6 Effects of pulsed electric field processing on functional components of food products

Food	Type	Processing conditions[a]	Parameters affected[b]	References
Apple	Juice	E: 20–40; t: 25–100; T: 23–50	(↓) Residual activity of polyphenoloxidase (PPO) and peroxidase (POD)	Riener *et al.*, 2008
Apple	Juice	M: monopolar; E: 0–35; F: 16; w: 0.2–2; t: 75; T: 21–42	(↑) Ferric reducing antioxidant power (FRAP) (↑) Oxygen radical absorbance capacity (ORAC) (↔) 1,1-diphenyl-2-picrylhydrazyl (DPPH) (↓) Vitamin C (↓) Total phenols (↓) Residual activity of PPO and POD	Bi *et al.*, 2013
Fruit (orange, kiwi and pineapple blend) juice-soymilk mixture	Beverage	M: bipolar; E: 35; F: 200; w: 4; t: 800–1400; T: 32	(↔) Total isoflavone	Morales-de la Peña *et al.*, 2010
Fruit (orange, kiwi and pineapple blend) juice-soymilk mixture	Beverage	M: bipolar; E: 35; F: 200; w: 4; t: 800; T: 32	(↑) Total phenolic compounds (↓) Carotenoids	Morales-de la Peña *et al.*, 2011a
Fruit (orange, kiwi and pineapple blend) juice-soymilk mixture	Beverage	M: bipolar; E: 35; F: 200; w: 4; t: 800; T: 32	(↑) Fe and Zn (↓) Elaidic and linoleic acid	Morales-de la Peña *et al.*, 2011b
Fruit (orange, kiwi and pineapple blend) juice-soymilk mixture	Beverage	M: bipolar; E: 35; F: 200; w: 4; t: 800; T: 32 M: bipolar; E: 35; F: 200; w: 4; t: 1400; T: 32	(↑) Val (↔) Arg, Pro, Glu, Asp, Ala, Ser, Phe, Leu, Lys, Thr, Tyr, Met, Gly, Hys and Ile (↑) Arg, Ala and Met (↓) Glu, Gly, Tyr, Val, Leu, Phe, Lys and Ile	Morales-de la Peña *et al.*, 2012
Gazpacho	Cold vegetable soup	M: monopolar and bipolar; E: 15–35; F: 50–450; w: 2–10; t: 100–1000; T: <35	(↔) Antioxidant capacity (↓) Vitamin C	Elez-Martínez and Martín-Belloso, 2007
Orange	Juice	E: 25–40; t: 30–340	(↓) Total carotenoids (↓) Vitamin A	Cortés *et al.*, 2006
Orange	Juice	M: monopolar and bipolar; E: 15–35; F: 50–450; w: 2–10; t: 100–1000; T: <35	(↔) Antioxidant capacity (↓) Vitamin C	Elez-Martínez and Martín-Belloso, 2007
Orange	Juice	M: bipolar; E: 35; F: 800; w: 4; t: 750; T:, 50	(↔) Total carotenoid (↔) Flavanone (↔) Vitamin A	Plaza *et al.*, 2011

(continued)

Table 11.6 (*Continued*)

Food	Type	Processing conditions[a]	Parameters affected[b]	References
Orange juice-milk mixture	Beverage	M: bipolar; E: 15–40; w: 2.5; t: 40–700	(↓) Ascorbic acid	Zulueta *et al.*, 2010
Orange juice-milk mixture fortified with water-soluble vitamins (biotin, folic acid, pantothenic acid and riboflavin and angiotensin-I-converting enzyme (ACE) inhibitory peptides)	Beverage	M: bipolar; E: 15–40; w: 2.5; t: 0–700; T: <55	(↔) Vitamins (↔) ACE inhibitory activity	Rivas *et al.*, 2007
Strawberry	Juice	M: bipolar; E: 35; F: 100; w: 4; t: 1700; W: <35	(↓) Browning index (↓) 5-(hydroxymethyl)-2-furfural (HMF)	Aguiló-Aguayo *et al.*, 2009
Strawberry	Juice	M: monopolar and bipolar; E: 35; F: 50–250; w: 1–7; t: 1000; T: <40	(↓) Vitamin C (↓) Anthocyanins (↓) Antioxidant capacity	Odriozola-Serrano *et al.*, 2009a
Tomato	Juice	M: monopolar and bipolar; E: 35; F: 50–250; w: 1–7; t: 1000–2000; T: <35	(↓) Relative residual activity of POD	Aguiló-Aguayo *et al.*, 2008
Tomato	Juice	M: bipolar; E: 35; F: 100; w: 4; t: 1500; T: <40	(↑) Lycopene (↔) Antioxidant capability (↔) Total phenolic compounds (↓) Vitamin C	Odriozola-Serrano *et al.*, 2008
Tomato	Juice	M: bipolar; E: 35; F: 100; w: 4; t: 1500; T: <40	(↑) Some carotenoids (lycopene, β-carotene and phytofluence) (↔) Phenolic compounds	Odriozola-Serrano *et al.*, 2009b
Tomato	Fruit	M: monopolar; E: 0.4–2; F: 0.1; w: 4	(↑) Polyphenol (↑) Carotenoid	Vallverdú-Queralt *et al.*, 2013
Watermelon	Juice	M: monopolar and bipolar; E: 30–35; F: 50–250; w: 1–7; t: 50–2050; T: <40	(↑) Lycopene (↑) Antioxidant capacity (↓) Vitamin C	Oms-Oliu *et al.*, 2009
Watermelon	Juice	M: monopolar and bipolar; E: 35; F: 50–250; w: 1–7; t: 1000; T: <35	(↓) Relative residual activity of POD	Aguiló-Aguayo *et al.*, 2010

[a] M, Pulse mode; E, electric field strength (kV/cm); F, pulse frequency (Hz); w, pause width (μs); t, treatment time (μs); T, temperature (°C).
[b] (↓) decreased level; (↑) increased level; (↔) neither increase nor decrease in the level.

11.8 Conclusions and future trends

Food processing technologies whether thermal, novel thermal, minimal-thermal or non-thermal can affect the levels of health-related phytochemicals in foods either beneficially or adversely. The degradation mechanisms of phytochemicals are rather complex and sometimes unknown. Degradation by thermal processing may be mainly attributed to heat damage while the degradation by alternative processing methods could be caused by various mechanisms and may lead to the production of some functional substances. It is considered that phytochemical alteration is entirely dependent on the type and the conditions of processing. Applying the correct type and conditions for processing will result in the maximum retention of health-related components in the processed food. Recently, there has been an increased interest in food processing techniques that can deliver food safety while simultaneously fulfilling the demand for nutritious food that has improved properties and quality. Several technologies, especially novel thermal and non-thermal processing, are considered as alternatives for developing new products with unique bioactivity and functionality. However, the applicability of these technologies needs much further investigation and more research is required to optimize the process for nutritional retention in the food products. Hybrid systems of thermal and non-thermal processing also have considerable potential for the increased retention of phytochemicals in foods.

References

Adekunte, A.O., Tiwari, B.K., Cullen, P.J., Scannell, A.G.M. and O'Donnell, C.P. (2010). Effect of sonication on colour, ascorbic acid and yeast inactivation in tomato juice. *Food Chemistry*, 122, 500–507.

Aguiló-Aguayo, I., Odriozolo-Serrano, I., Quintão-Teixeira, J. and Martín-Belloso, O. (2008). Inactivation of tomato juice peroxidase by high-intensity pulsed electric fields as affected by process conditions. *Food Chemistry*, 107, 949–955.

Aguiló-Aguayo, I., Oms-Oliu, G., Soliva-Fortuny, R. and Martín-Belloso, O. (2009). Flavour retention and related enzyme activities during storage of strawberry juices processed by high-intensity pulsed electric fields or heat. *Food Chemistry*, 116, 59–65.

Aguiló-Aguayo, I., Soliva-Fortuny, R. and Martín-Belloso, O. (2010). Impact of high-intensity pulsed electric field variables affecting peroxidase and lipoxygenase activities of watermelon juice. *LWT – Food Science and Technology*, 43, 897–902.

Alajaji, S.A. and El-Adawy, T.A. (2006). Nutritional composition of chickpea (*Cicer arietinum* L.) as affected by microwave cooking and other traditional cooking methods. *Journal of Food Composition and Analysis*, 19, 806–812.

Alkhafaji, S.R. and Farid, M. (2007). An investigation on pulsed electric fields technology using new treatment chamber design. *Innovative Food Science and Emerging Technologies*, 8, 205–212.

Alothman, M., Bhat, R. and Karim, A.A. (2009a). Effects of radiation processing on phytochemicals and antioxidants in plant produce. *Trends in Food Science and Technology*, 20, 201–212.

Alothman, M., Bhat, R. and Karim, A.A. (2009b). UV radiation-induced changes of antioxidant capacity of fresh-cut tropical fruits. *Innovative Food Science and Emerging Technologies*, 10, 512–516.

Anese, M., Mirolo, G., Beraldo, P. and Lippe, G. (2013). Effect of ultrasound treatments of tomato pulp on microstructure and lycopene in vitro bioaccessibility. *Food Chemistry*, 136, 458–463.

Avanza, M., Acevedo, B., Chaves, M. and Añón, M. (2013). Nutritional and anti-nutritional components of four cowpea varieties under thermal treatments: Principal component analysis. *LWT – Food Science and Technology*, 51, 148–157.

Awuah, G.B., Ramaswamy, H.S. and Economides, A. (2007). Thermal processing and quality: Principles and overview. *Chemical Engineering and Processing*, 46, 584–602.

Baron, A., Dénes, J.M. and Durier, C. (2006). High-pressure treatment of cloudy apple juice. *LWT*, 39, 1005–1013.

Bhat, R., Ameran, S.B., Voon, H.C., Karim, A.A. and Tze, L.M. (2011a). Quality attributes of starfruit (*Averrhoa carambola* L.) juice treated with ultraviolet radiation. *Food Chemistry*, 127, 641–644.

Bhat, R., Kamaruddin, N.S.B.C., Min-Tze, L. and Karim, A.A. (2011b). Sonication improves kasturi lime (*Citrus microcarpa*) juice quality. *Ultrasonics Sonochemistry*, 18, 1295–1300.

Bhat, R., Sridhar, K.R. and Tomita-Yokotani, K. (2007). Effect of ionizing radiation on antinutritional features of velvet bean seeds (*Mucuna pruriens*). *Food Chemistry*, 103, 860–866.

Bi, X., Liu, F., Rao, L. *et al.* (2013). Effects of electric field strength and pulse rise time on physicochemical and sensory properties of apple juice by pulsed electric field. *Innovative Food Science and Emerging Technologies*, 17, 85–92.

Briones-Labarca, V., Muñoz, C. and Maureira, H. (2011a). Effect of high hydrostatic pressure on antioxidant capacity, mineral and starch bioaccessibility of a non conventional food: *Prosopis chilensis* seed. *Food Research International*, 44, 875–883.

Briones-Labarca, V., Venegas-Cubillos, G., Ortiz-Portilla, S., Chacana-Ojeda, M. and Maureira, H. (2011b). Effects of high hydrostatic pressure (HHP) on bioaccessibility, as well as antioxidant activity, mineral and starch contents in Granny Smith apple. *Food Chemistry*, 128, 520–529.

Buzrul, S. (2012). High hydrostatic pressure treatment of beer and wine: A review. *Innovative Food Science and Emerging Technologies*, 13, 1–12.

Caminiti, I.M., Noci, F., Muñoz, A. *et al.* (2011). Impact of selected combinations of non-thermal processing technologies on the quality of an apple and cranberry juice blend. *Food Chemistry*, 124, 1387–1392.

Cao, S., Hu, Z. and Pang, B. (2010). Optimization of postharvest ultrasonic treatment of strawberry fruit. *Postharvest Biology and Technology*, 55, 150–153.

Carbonell-Capella, J.M., Barba, F.J., Esteve, M.J. and Frígola, A. (2013). High pressure processing of fruit juice mixture sweetened with *Stevia rebaudiana* Bertoni: Optimal retention of physical and nutritional quality. *Innovative Food Science and Emerging Technologies*, http://dx.doi.org/10.1016/j.ifset.2013.01.011.

Carocho, M., Barros, L., Antonio, A.L. *et al.* (2013). Analysis of organic acids in electron beam irradiated chestnuts (*Castanea sativa* Mill.): Effects of radiation dose and storage time. *Food and Chemical Toxicology*, 55, 348–352.

Cavalcanti, R.N., Santos, D.T. and Meireles, M.A.A. (2011). Non-thermal stabilization mechanisms of anthocyanins in model and food systems-An overview. *Food Research International*, 44, 499–509.

Chandrapala, J., Oliver, C., Kentish, S. and Ashokkumar, M. (2012). Ultrasonics in food processing – Food quality assurance and food safety. *Trends in Food Science and Technology*, 26, 88–98.

Chatterjee, S., Adhikari, S., Gupta, S., Variyar, P.S. and Sharma, A. (2009). Estimation of aroma precursors in radiation processed fenugreek. *Food Chemistry*, 115, 1102–1107.

Chen, J.P., Tai, C.Y. and Chen, B.H. (2007). Effects of different drying treatments on the stability of carotenoids in Taiwanese mango (*Mangifera indica* L.). *Food Chemistry*, 100, 1005–1010.

Chin, S., Nazimah, S.A.H., Quek, S. *et al.* (2010). Effect of thermal processing and storage condition on the flavour stability of spray dried durian powder. *LWT – Food Science and Technology*, 43, 856–861.

Clariana, M., Valverde, J., Wijngaard, H., Mullen, A.M. and Marcos, B. (2011). High pressure processing of swede (*Brassica napus*): Impact on quality properties. *Innovative Food Science and Emerging Technologies*, 12, 85–92.

Considine, K.M., Kelly, A.L., Fitzgerald, G.F., Hill, C. and Sleator, R.D. (2008). High-pressure processing – effects on microbial food safety and food quality. *FEMS Microbiology Letter*, 281, 1–9.

Cortés, C., Esteve, M.J., Rodrigo, D., Torregrosa, F. and Frígola. (2006). Changes of colour and carotenoids contents during high intensity pulsed electric field treatment in orange juices. *Food and Chemical Toxicology*, 44, 1932–1939.

Crawford, L.M. and Ruff, E.H. (1996). A review of the safety of cold pasteurization through irradiation. *Food Control*, 7, 87–97.

Damasceno, L.F., Fernandes, F.A.N., Magalhães, M.M.A. and Brito, E.S. (2008). Non-enzymatic browning in clarified cashew apple juice during thermal treatment: Kinetics and process control. *Food Chemistry*, 106, 172–179.

Djioua, T., Charles, F., Lopez-Lauri, F. *et al.* (2009). Improving the storage of minimally processed mangoes (*Mangifera indica* L.) by hot water treatments. *Post Harvest Biology and Technology*, 52, 221–226.

Doblado, R., Frías, J. and Vidal-Valverde, C. (2007). Changes in vitamin C content and antioxidant capacity of raw and germinated cowpea (*Vigna sinensis* var. *carilla*) seeds induced by high pressure treatment. *Food Chemistry*, 101, 918–923.

Dutta, D., Dutta, A., Raychudhuri, U. and Chakraborty, R. (2006). Rheological characteristics and thermal degradation kinetics of beta-carotene in pumpkin puree. *Journal of Food Engineering*, 76, 538–546.

El-Niely, H.F.G. (2007). Effect of radiation processing on antinutrients, in-vitro protein digestibility and protein efficiency ratio bioassay of legume seeds. *Radiation Physics and Chemistry*, 76, 1050–1057.

Elez-Martínez, P. and Martín-Belloso, O. (2007). Effects of high intensity pulsed electric field processing conditions on vitamin C and antioxidant capacity of orange juice and *gazpacho,* a cold vegetable soup. *Food Chemistry*, 102, 201–209.

Erkan, M., Wang, S.Y. and Wang, C.Y. (2008). Effect of UV treatment on antioxidant capacity, antioxidant enzyme activity and decay in strawberry fruit. *Postharvest Biology and Technology*, 48, 163–171.

Farkas, J. (2006). Irradiation for better foods. *Trends in Food Science and Technology*, 17, 148–152.

Fratianni, A., Cinquanta, L. and Panfili, G. (2010). Degradation of carotenoids in orange juice during microwave heating. *LWT – Food Science and Technology*, 43, 867–871.

Gamboa-Santos, J., Soria, A.C., Pérez-Mateos, M. *et al.* (2013). Vitamin C content and sensorial properties of dehydrated carrots blanched conventionally or by ultrasound. *Food Chemistry*, 136, 782–788.

Ghanem, N., Mihoubi, D., Kechaou, N. and Mihoubi, N.B. (2012). Microwave dehydration of three citrus peel cultivars: Effect on water and oil retention capacities, color, shrinkage and total phenols content. *Industrial Crops and Products*, 40, 167–177.

Gómez-López, V.M., Orsolani, L., Martínez-Yépez, A. and Tapia, M.S. (2010). Microbiological and sensory quality of sonicated calcium-added orange juice. *LWT – Food Science and Technology*, 43, 808–813.

González-Aguilar, G.A., Villegas-Ochoa, M.A., Martínez-Téllez, M.A., Gardea, A.A. and Ayala-Zavala, J.F. (2007). Improving antioxidant capacity of fresh-cut mangoes treated with UV-C. *Journal of Food Science*, 72, S197–S202.

Hajare, S.N., Saroj, S.D., Dhokane, V.S., Shashidhar, R. and Bandekar, J.R. (2007). Effect of radiation processing on nutritional and sensory quality of minimally processed green gram and garden pea sprouts. *Radiation Physics and Chemistry*, 76, 1642–1649.

Hayat, K., Zhang, X., Farooq, U. *et al.* (2010). Effect of microwave treatment on phenolic content and antioxidant activity of citrus mandarin pomace. *Food Chemistry*, 123, 423–429.

Hertog, M.G.L., Sweetnam, P.M., Fehily, A.M., Elwood, P.C. and Kromhout, D. (1997). Antioxidant flavonols and ischaemic heart disease in a Welsh population of men – the Caerphilly study. *American Journal of Clinical Nutrition*, 65, 1489–1494.

Hu, J.L., Nie, S.P. and Xie, M.Y. (2013). High pressure homogenization increases antioxidant capacity and short-chain fatty acid yield of polysaccharide from seeds of *Plantago asiatica* L. *Food Chemistry*, 138, 2338–2345.

Huang, K., Tian, H., Gai, L. and Wang, J. (2012). A review of kinetic models for inactivating microorganisms and enzymes by pulsed electric field processing. *Journal of Food Engineering*, 111, 191–207.

Huang, W., Bi, X., Zhang, X. *et al.* (2013). Comparative study of enzymes, phenolics, carotenoids and color of apricot nectars treated by high hydrostatic pressure and high temperature short time. *Innovative Food Science and Emerging Technologies*, http://dx.doi.org/10.1016/j.ifset.2013.01.001 [accessed 25 July 2013].

Hugas, M., Garriga, M. and Monfort, J.M. (2002). New mild technologies in meat processing: high pressure as a model technology. *Meat Science*, 62, 359–371.

İçïer, F., Yildiz, H. and Baysal, T. (2008). Polyphenoloxidase deactivation kinetics during ohmic heating of grape juice. *Journal of Food Engineering*, 85, 410–417.

Igual, M., Sampedro, F., Martínez-Navarrete, N. and Fan, X. (2013). Combined osmodehydration and high pressure processing on the enzyme stability and antioxidant capacity of a grape fruit jam. *Journal of Food Engineering*, 114, 514–521.

Ildikó, S.G., Klára, K.A., Marianna, T.M. *et al.* (2006). The effect of radio frequency heat treatment on nutritional and colloid-chemical properties of different white mustard (*Sinapis alba* L.) varieties. *Innovative Food Science and Emerging Technologies*, 7, 74–79.

Jimenez, L., Alarcón, E., Trevithick-Sutton, C., Gandhi, N. and Scaiano, J.C. (2011). Effect of γ-radiation on green onion DNA integrity: Role of ascorbic acid and polyphenols against nucleic acid damage. *Food Chemistry*, 128, 735–741.

Keenan, D.F., Brunton, N.P., Gormley, T.R. *et al.* (2010). Effect of thermal and high hydrostatic pressure processing on antioxidant activity and colour of fruit smoothies. *Innovative Food Science and Emerging Technologies*, 11, 551–556.

Keenan, D.F., Rößle, C., Gormley, R., Butler, F. and Brunton, N.P. (2012b). Effect of high hydrostatic pressure and thermal processing on the nutritional quality and enzyme activity of fruit smoothies. *LWT – Food Science and Technology*, 45, 50–57.

Kim, H.G., Kim, G.W., Oh, H. *et al.* (2011). Influence of roasting on the antioxidant activity of small black soybean (*Glycine max* L. Merrill. *LWT – Food Science and Technology*, 44, 992–998.

Kim, Y., Brecht, J.K. and Talcott, S.T. (2007). Antioxidant phytochemical and fruit quality changes in mango (*Mangifera indica* L.) following hot water immersion and controlled atmosphere storage. *Food Chemistry*, 105, 1327–1334.

Kim, Y., Lounds-Singleton, A.J. and Talcott, S.T. (2009). Antioxidant phytochemical and quality changes associated with hot water immersion treatment mangos (*Mangifera indica* L.). *Food Chemistry*, 115, 989–993.

Knockaert, G., Pulissery, S.K., Colle, I. *et al.* (2012). Lycopene degradation, isomerization and *in vitro* bioaccessibility in high pressure homogenized tomato puree containing oil: Effect of additional thermal and high pressure processing. *Food Chemistry*, 135, 1290–1297.

Kong, K.W., Ismail, A., Tan, C.P. and Rajab, N.F. (2010). Optimization of oven drying conditions for lycopene content and lipophilic antioxidant capacity in a by-product of the pink guava puree industry using response surface methodology. *LWT – Food Science and Technology*, 43, 729–735.

Lemoine, M.L., Civello, P.M., Martnez, G.A. and Chaves, A.R. (2007). Influence of postharvest UV-C treatment on refrigerated storage of minimally processed broccoli (*Brassica oleracea* var. *Italica*). *Journal of the Science of Food and Agriculture*, 87, 1132–1139.

Liu, Y. and Kitts, D.D. (2011). Confirmation that the Maillard reaction is the principle contributor to the antioxidant capacity of coffee brews. *Food Research International*, 44, 2418–2424.

López-Fandiño, R. (2006). High pressure-induced changes in milk proteins and possible applications in dairy technology. *International Dairy Journal*, 16, 1119–1131.

Louarme, L. and Billaud, C. (2012). Evaluation of ascorbic and sugar degradation products during fruit dessert processing under conventional or ohmic heating treatment. *LWT—Food Science and Technology*, 49, 184–187.

Manzocco, L., Anese, M. and Nicoli, M.C. (2008). Radiofrequency inactivation of oxidative food enzymes in model systems. *Food Research International*, 41, 1044–1049.

Marra, F., Zhang, L. and Lyng, J.G. (2009). Radio frequency treatment of foods: Review of recent advances. *Journal of Food Engineering*, 91, 497–508.

Matsui, K.N., Gut, J.A.W., de Oliveira, P.V. and Tadini, C.C. (2008). Inactivation kinetics of polyphenol oxidase and peroxidase in green coconut water by microwave processing. *Journal of Food Engineering*, 88, 169–176.

McInerney, J.K., Seccafien, C.A., Stewart, C.M. and Bird, A.R. (2007). Effects of high pressure processing on antioxidant activity and total carotenoid content and availability, in vegetables. *Innovative Food Science and Emerging Technologies*, 8, 543–548.

Mercali, G.D., Jaeschke, D.P., Tessaro, I.C. and Marczak, L.D.F. (2013). Degradation kinetics of anthocyanins in acerola pulp: Comparison between ohmic and conventional heat treatment. *Food Chemistry*, 136, 853–857.

Mertz, C., Brat, P., Caris-Veyrat, C. and Gunata, Z. (2010). Characterization and thermal lability of carotenoids and vitamin C of tamarillo fruit (*Solanum betaceum* Cav.). *Food Chemistry*, 119, 653–659.

Moltó-Puigmartí, C., Permanyer, M., Castellote, A.I. and López-Sabater, M.C. (2011). Effects of pasteurization and high-pressure processing on vitamin C, tocopherols and fatty acids in mature human milk. *Food Chemistry*, 124, 697–702.

Morales-de la Peña, M., Salvia-Trujillo, L., Rojas-Graü, M.A. and Martín-Belloso, O. (2010). Isoflavone profile of a high intensity pulsed electric field or thermally treated fruit juice-soymilk beverage stored under refrigeration. *Innovative Food Science and Emerging Technologies*, 11, 604–610.

Morales-de la Peña, M., Salvia-Trujillo, L., Rojas-Graü, M.A. and Martín-Belloso, O. (2011a). Changes on phenolic and carotenoid composition of high intensity pulsed electric field and thermally treated fruit juice-soymilk beverages during refrigerated storage. *Food Chemistry*, 129, 982–990.

Morales-de la Peña, M., Salvia-Trujillo, L., Rojas-Graü, M.A. and Martín-Belloso, O. (2011b). Impact of high intensity pulsed electric fields or heat treatments on the fatty acid and mineral profiles of a fruit juice-soymilk beverage during storage. *Food Control*, 22, 1975–1983.

Morales-de la Peña, M., Salvia-Trujillo, L., Garde-Cerdán, T., Rojas-Graü, M.A. and Martín-Belloso, O. (2012). High intensity pulsed electric fields or thermal treatments effects on the amino acid profile of a fruit juice-soymilk beverage during refrigeration storage. *Innovative Food Science and Emerging Technologies*, 16, 47–53.

Moritz, J., Balasa, A., Jaeger, H., Meneses, N. and Knorr, D. (2012). Investigating the potential of polyphenol oxidase as a temperature-time-indicator for pulsed electric field treatment. *Food Control*, 26, 1–5.

Nuñez-Mancilla, Y., Pérez-Won, M., Uribe, E., Vega-Gálvez, A. and Scala, K.D. (2013). Osmotic dehydration under high hydrostatic pressure: Effects on antioxidant activity, total phenolics compounds, vitamin C and colour of strawberry (*Fragaria vesca*). *LWT – Food Science and Technology*, 52, 151–156.

Odriozola-Serrano, I., Soliva-Fortuny, R. and Martín-Belloso, O. (2008). Changes of health-related compounds throughout cold storage of tomato juice stabilized by thermal or high intensity pulsed electric field treatments. *Innovative Food Science and Emerging Technologies*, 9, 272–279.

Odriozola-Serrano, I., Soliva-Fortuny, R. and Martín-Belloso, O. (2009a). Impact of high-intensity pulsed electric fields variables on vitamin C, anthocyanins and antioxidant capacity of strawberry juice. *LWT – Food Science and Technology*, 42, 93–100.

Odriozola-Serrano, I., Soliva-Fortuny, R., Hernández-Jover, T. and Martín-Belloso, O. (2009b). Carotenoid and phenolic profile of tomato juices processed by high intensity pulsed electric fields compared with conventional thermal treatments. *Food Chemistry*, 112, 258–266.

Oms-Oliu, G., Odriozola-Serrano, I., Soliva-Fortuny, R. and Martín-Belloso, O. (2009). Effects of high-intensity pulsed electric field processing conditions on lycopene, vitamin C and antioxidant capacity of watermelon juice. *Food Chemistry*, 115, 1312–1319.

Otero, L. and Sanz, P.D. (2003). Modelling heat transfer in high pressure food processing: A review. *Innovative Food Science and Emerging Technologies*, 4, 121–134.

Pacheco-Palencia, L.A., Duncan, C.E. and Talcott, S.T. (2009). Phytochemical composition and thermal stability of two commercial açai species, *Euterpe oleracea* and *Euterpe precatoria. Food Chemistry*, 115, 1199–1205.

Patras, A., Brunton, N.P., Pieve, S.D. and Butler, F. (2009a). Impact of high pressure processing on total antioxidant activity, phenolic, ascorbic acid, anthocyanin content and colour of strawberry and blackberry purées. *Innovative Food Science and Emerging Technologies*, 10, 308–313.

Patras, A., Brunton, N., Pieve, S.D., Butler, F. and Downey, G. (2009b). Effect of thermal and high pressure processing on antioxidant activity and instrumental colour of tomato and carrot purées. *Innovative Food Science and Emerging Technologies*, 10, 16–22.

Pérez-Conesa, D., García-Alonso, J., García-Valverde, V. *et al.* (2009). Changes in bioactive compounds and antioxidant activity during homogenization and thermal processing of tomato puree. *Innovative Food Science and Emerging Technologies*, 10, 179–188.

Perkins-Veazie, P., Collins, J.K. and Howard, L. (2008). Blueberry fruit response to postharvest application of ultraviolet radiation. *Postharvest Biology and Technology*, 47, 280–285.

Pingret, D., Fabiano-Tixier, A.S. and Chemat, F. (2013). Degradation during application of ultrasound in food processing: A review. *Food Control*, 31, 593–606.

Plaza, L., Sánchez-Moreno, C., de Ancos, B. *et al.* (2011). Carotenoid and flavanone content during refrigerated storage of orange juice processed by high-pressure, pulsed electric fields and low pasteurization. *LWT – Food Science and Technology*, 44, 834–839.

Ramírez-Moreno, E., Córdoba-Díaz, D. and Sánchez-Mata, M.D.C. (2013). Effect of boiling on nutritional, antioxidant and physicochemical characteristics in cladodes (*Opuntia ficus indica*). *LWT – Food Science and Technology*, 51, 296–302.

Randhir, R., Kwon, Y.I. and Shetty, K. (2008). Effect of thermal processing on phenolics, antioxidant activity and health-relevant functionality of select grain sprouts and seedlings. *Innovative Food Science and Emerging Technologies*, 9, 355–364.

Rattanathanalerk, M., Chiewchan, N. and Srichumpoung, W. (2009). Effect of thermal processing on the quality loss of pineapple juice. *Journal of Food Engineering*, 66, 259–265.

Rawson, A., Patras, A., Tiwari, B.K. *et al.* (2011a). Effect of thermal and non thermal processing technologies on the bioactive content of exotic fruits and their products: Review of recent advances. *Food Research International*, 44, 1875–1887.

Rawson, A., Tiwari, B.K., Tuohy, M.G., O'Donnell, C.P. and Brunton, N. (2011b). Effect of ultrasound and blanching pretreatments on polyacetylene and carotenoid content of hot air and freeze dried carrot discs. *Ultrasonics Sonochemistry*, 18, 1172–1179.

Rawson, A. Tiwari, B.K., Patras, A. *et al.* (2011c). Effect of thermosonication on bioactive compounds in watermelon juice. *Food Research International*, 44, 1168–1173.

Rendueles, E., Omer, M.K., Alvseike, O. *et al.* (2011). Microbiological food safety assessment of high hydrostatic pressure processing: A review. *LWT – Food Science and Technology*, 44, 1251–1260.

Reyes, L.F. and Cisneros-Zevallos, L. (2007). Electron-beam ionizing radiation stress effects on mango fruit (*Mangifera indica* L.) antioxidant constituents before and during postharvest storage. *Journal of Agriculture and Food Chemistry*, 55, 6132–6139.

Riener, J., Noci, F., Cronin, D.A., Morgan, D.J. and Lyng, J.G. (2008). Combined effect of temperature and pulsed electric fields on apple juice peroxidase and polyphenoloxidase inactivation. *Food Chemistry*, 109, 402–407.

Rivas, A., Rodrigo, D., Company, B., Sampedro, F. and Rodrigo, M. (2007). Effects of pulsed electric fields on water-soluble vitamins and ACE inhibitory peptides added to a mixed orange juice and milk beverage. *Food Chemistry*, 104, 1550–1559.

Roldán-Marín, E., Sánchez-Moreno, C., Lloría, R., de Ancos, B. and Cano, M.P. (2009). Onion high-pressure processing: Flavonol content and antioxidant activity. *LWT – Food Science and Technology*, 42, 835–841.

Ryley, J. and Kajda, P. (1994). Vitamins in thermal processing. *Food Chemistry*, 49, 119–129.

Sarkis, J.R., Jaeschke, D.P., Tessaro, I.C. and Marczak, L.D.F. (2013). Effects of ohmic and conventional heating on anthocyanin degradation during the processing of blueberry pulp. *LWT – Food Science and Technology*, 51, 79–85.

Saxena, A., Maity, T., Raju, P.S. and Bawa, A.S. (2012). Degradation kinetics of colour and total carotenoids in jackfruit (*Artocarpus heterophyllus*) bulb slices during hot air drying. *Food and Bioprocess Technology*, 5, 672–679.

Serra, X., Sárraga, C., Grèbol, N. *et al.* (2007). High pressure applied to frozen ham at different process stages. 1. Effect on the final physicochemical parameter and on the antioxidant and proteolytic enzyme activities of dry-cured ham. *Meat Science*, 75, 12–20.

Soria, A.C. and Villamiel, M. (2010). Effect of ultrasound on the technological properties and bioactivity of food: a review. *Trends in Food Science and Technology*, 21, 323–331.

Stojanovic, J. and Silva, J.L. (2007). Influence of osmotic concentration, continuous high frequency ultrasound and dehydration on antioxidants, color and chemical properties of rabbiteye blueberries. *Food Chemistry*, 101, 898–906.

Tiwari, B.K., O'Donnell, C.P., Patras, A. and Cullen, P.J. (2008). Anthocyanin and ascorbic acid degradation in sonicated strawberry juice. *Journal of Agricultural and Food Chemistry*, 56, 10071–10077.

Tokuşoğlu, Ö, Alpas, H. and Bozoğlu, F. (2010). High hydrostatic pressure effects on mold flora, citrinin mycotoxin, hydroxytyrosol, oleuropein phenolics and antioxidant activity of black table olives. *Innovative Food Science and Emerging Technologies*, 11, 250–258.

Tiwari, B.K., O'Donnell, C.P. and Cullen, P.J. (2009). Effect of sonication on retention of anthocyanins in blackberry juice. *Journal of Food Engineering*, 93, 166–171.

Vallverdú-Queralt, A., Oms-Oliu, G., Odriozola-Serrano, I. *et al.* (2013). Metabolite profiling of phenolic and carotenoid contents in tomatoes after moderate-intensity pulsed electric field treatments. *Food Chemistry*, 136, 199–205.

Varela-Santos, E., Ochoa-Martinez, A., Tobilo-Munizaga, G. *et al.* (2012). Effect of high hydrostatic pressure (HHP) processing on physicochemical properties, bioactive compounds and shelf-life of pomegranate juice. *Innovative Food Science and Emerging Technologies*, 13, 13–22.

Vasquez-Caicedo, A.L., Schilling, S., Carle, R. and Neidhart, S. (2007). Effects of thermal processing and fruit matrix on β-carotene stability and enzyme inactivation during transformation of mangoes into puree and nectar. *Food Chemistry*, 102, 1172–1186.

Vega-Gálvez, A., Miranda, M., Aranda, M. *et al.* (2011). Effect of high hydrostatic pressure on functional properties and quality characteristics of Aloe vera gel (*Aloe barbadensis* Miller). *Food Chemistry*, 129, 1060–1065.

Vega-Mercado, H., Martín-Belloso, O., Qin, B.L. *et al.* (1997). Non-thermal food preservation: Pulsed electric fields. *Trends in Food Science and Technology*, 8, 151–157.

Vikram, V.B., Ramesh, M.N. and Prapulla, S.G. (2005). Thermal degradation kinetics of nutrients in orange juice heated by electromagnetic and conventional methods. *Journal of Food Engineering*, 69, 31–40.

Xu, B. and Chang, S.K.C. (2011). Reduction of antiproliferative capacities, cell-based antioxidant capacities and phytochemical contents of common beans and soybeans upon thermal processing. *Food Chemistry*, 129, 974–981.

Zepka, L.Q. and Mercadante, A.Z. (2009). Degradation compounds of carotenoids formed during heating of a simulated cashew apple juice. *Food Chemistry*, 117, 28–34.

Zulueta, A., Esteve, M.J. and Frígola, A. (2010). Ascorbic acid in orange juice-milk beverage treated by high intensity pulsed electric fields and its stability during storage. *Innovative Food Science and Emerging Technologies*, 11, 84–90.

12 Changes of Properties and Functional Components of Extruded Foods

Vilai Rungsardthong
King Mongkut's University of Technology North Bangkok, Bangkok, Thailand

12.1 Introduction

Food extrusion is a process in which food ingredients are forced to flow, under one or several conditions of mixing, heating and shear, through a die that forms and/or puff-dries the ingredients (Rossen and Miller, 1973). Extrusion is a unique form in food and feed processing because of the conditions used to transform the raw materials. Normal moisture levels used are relatively low compared to conventional processing, in the range of 10–40% on a wet weight basis (Guy, 2001). Extrusion is a continuous cooking, mixing and shaping process with high production capacity, versatility and low cost per product unit, yielding high product quality as well as being environmentally friendly with low process effluents (Colonna *et al.*, 1984; Guy, 2001). In the extruder, the food mix is mechanically cooked at a high temperature, usually in the range 100–180 °C, under pressure and shear stress that are generated in the screw-barrel, and the residence time is usually only 20–40 s (Riaz, 2000).

The machine which forces the mix through the die is an extruder, and the mix is known as the extrudate. The extruder consists of a large, rotating screw tightly fitting within a stationary barrel, at the end of which is the die. The duration of time that the extrudate is in the extruder is the residence time. Food extruders can perform one or several functions simultaneously during the processing of food or feed such as mixing, grinding, shearing, degassing ingredient, homogenization, starch gelatinization, protein texturization, enzyme inactivation, pasteurization and sterilization, thermal cooking, shaping products, puffing, agglomerating ingredients and dehydration (Riaz, 2000).

Functional Foods and Dietary Supplements: Processing Effects and Health Benefits, First Edition.
Edited by Athapol Noomhorm, Imran Ahmad and Anil Kumar Anal.

as starch gelatinization, protein denaturation, complex formation between amylose and lipid, and degradation reactions of vitamins, pigments, etc. (Ilo and Berghofer, 1999). Product quality can vary considerably depending on the extruder type, screw configuration, feed moisture and temperature in the barrel session, screw speed and feed rate (Ding *et al.*, 2005). There are many studies on the effect of extrusion conditions such as feed rate, feed moisture content, screw speed and barrel temperature on the physicochemical properties, those are bulk density, expansion, water absorption index and water solubility index of extruded snack foods (Sacchetti *et al.*, 2004; Ding *et al.*, 2005; Thymi *et al.*, 2005; Stojceska *et al.*, 2008). It is generally accepted that the degree of gelatinization and molecular degradation of starch will increase with an increase in barrel temperature. The increase in barrel temperature creates a higher vapour pressure in the dough resulting in more flashing of moisture as the product exits the die and, consequently, greater expansion occurs. The changes in expansion ratios were closely linked to the extent of macromolecular degradation of the amylopectin component in corn starch (Tang and Ding, 1994).

Thongkum *et al.* (2010) used broken rice (Chainat variety) for the extrusion of a rice snack. The increase of feed moisture content led to a sharp decrease of extrudate expansion at all barrel temperatures (Table 12.1 and Figure 12.1). The results agree with many works reported previously that moisture content was found to be the main factor affecting extrudate expansion and bulk density (Faubion and Hoseney, 1982; Launay and Lisch, 1983; Fletcher *et al.*, 1985; Ilo *et al.*, 1999). The high dependence of bulk density and expansion on moisture content resulted from its influence on the elasticity characteristics of the starch-based material. The increase of moisture content during extrusion could lead to a change in the amylopectin molecular structure of the material, thus reducing melt elasticity, decreasing expansion and increasing bulk density of the extrudate (Ding *et al.*, 2005; Thymi *et al.*, 2005). The increase of feed moisture from 16 to 17% significantly increased the water absorption index (WAI) of the rice extrudate as shown in Figure 12.1a (Thongkum *et al.*, 2010). These findings

Table 12.1 Effect of barrel temperature (zone 3) and feed moisture content (MC) on expansion ratio and bulk density of extruded rice snack

Feed MC (%)	Barrel temperature zone 3 (°C)	Expansion ratio	Bulk density (g/cm^3)
14	140	3.28 ± 0.08^{f}	0.12 ± 0.01^{a}
	160	3.13 ± 0.11^{d}	0.13 ± 0.01^{ab}
	180	3.25 ± 0.12^{ef}	0.12 ± 0.00^{a}
15	140	3.12 ± 0.06^{d}	0.12 ± 0.01^{a}
	160	3.14 ± 0.11^{d}	0.12 ± 0.01^{a}
	180	3.19 ± 0.07^{de}	0.13 ± 0.01^{ab}
16	140	3.01 ± 0.10^{bc}	0.15 ± 0.00^{c}
	160	2.94 ± 0.09^{b}	0.15 ± 0.01^{c}
	180	3.04 ± 0.11^{c}	0.14 ± 0.01^{bc}
17	140	2.80 ± 0.08^{a}	0.21 ± 0.02^{f}
	160	2.85 ± 0.08^{a}	0.19 ± 0.01^{e}
	180	2.83 ± 0.09^{a}	0.17 ± 0.01^{d}

Note: Barrel temperature of zone 1 : 2 was fixed at 100 °C and 120 °C, respectively.
Means in the same column followed by a different letter indicate significant difference ($p < 0.05$).

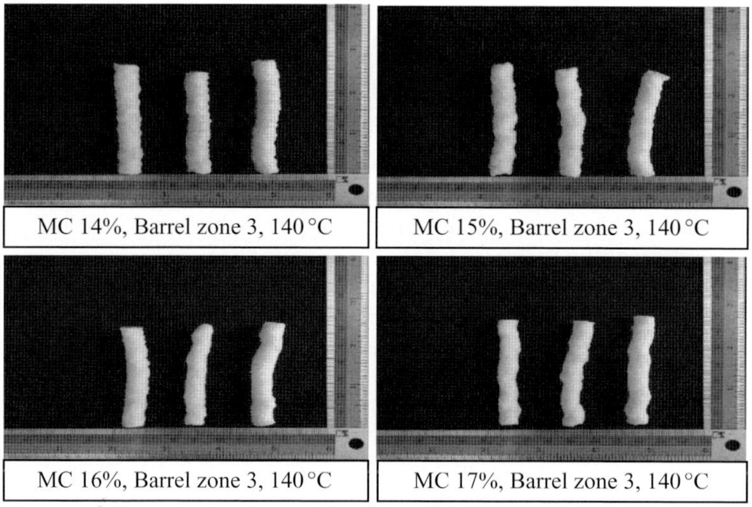

Figure 12.1 Appearance of rice snack extruded from broken rice with different percentage feed moisture content (% MC), feeder speed at 30 rpm, screw speed of 180 rpm and barrel temperature zone 1 : 2 : 3 at 100 : 120 : 140 °C. For colour details, see the colour plates section

correlated to the experiments of Owusu-Ansah *et al.* (1983), Pinnavaia and Pizzirani (1998), Ding *et al.* (2005) and Tang and Ding (1994).

Barrel temperature and feed moisture have the greatest effect on gelatinization. Maximum gelatinization is found at high moisture and low temperature or vice versa (Lawton *et al.*, 1972). The WAI generally increases with decreased temperature, due to increased dextrinization (Sacchetti *et al.*, 2004). The decrease in the WAI might be related to the degradation of starch that causes a reduction in the water-holding capacity of the molecules as a result of decreases in the molecular size. A decrease in the water solubility index (WSI) was observed with the increase of feed moisture content as shown in Figure 12.2b (Thongkum *et al.*, 2010). Increasing barrel temperature from 140 to 160 °C, led to an increase of WSI at 14 and 15%, while a decrease of

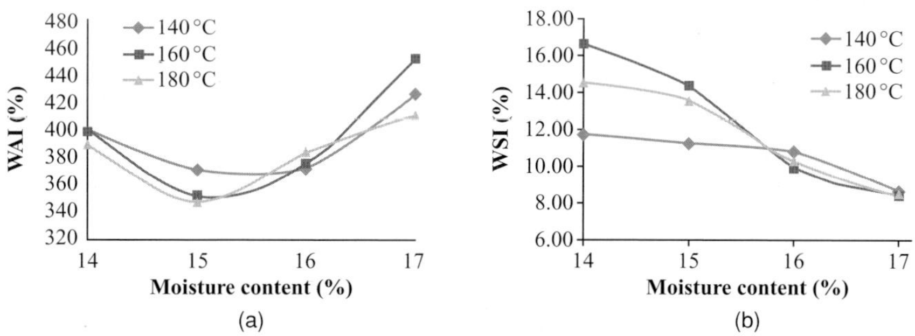

Figure 12.2 (a) Water absorption index (WAI) and (b) water solubility (WSI) of extruded rice snack at different feed moisture and zone 3 barrel temperature

WSI was revealed when barrel temperature was increased to 180 °C, possibly due the molecular weight of complex formed and the decrease in the solubility index (Altan *et al.*, 2009).

Weerapong (2004) investigated the use of rice flour from four Thai cultivars with different amylose content and different sizes of rice flour particles on the physico-chemical properties of the rice snack. The results showed that rice flour with a higher amylose content gave a product with a lower expansion ratio and a higher bulk density. A decrease in the size of rice flour particles gave a higher expansion ratio and a lower bulk density of the snack.

Lopkulkiaert *et al.* (2008) investigated the effects of extrusion conditions on the expansion and oil adsorption of a snack obtained by frying extruded pellet. The raw materials used were cassava starch and wheat flour mixed at the ratio of 75 : 25. Three frying parameters – pellet moisture content (3–5%, 8–10%, 13–15%), frying temperature (160, 180, 200 °C) and time (20, 40, 60 s) – were initially studied using a response surface methodology (RSM) design and full factorial 3 × 3. The results showed that the oil absorption of the snacks increased with increased frying time and temperature, and moisture content of the pellet (Figure 12.3 and Table 12.2). The highest

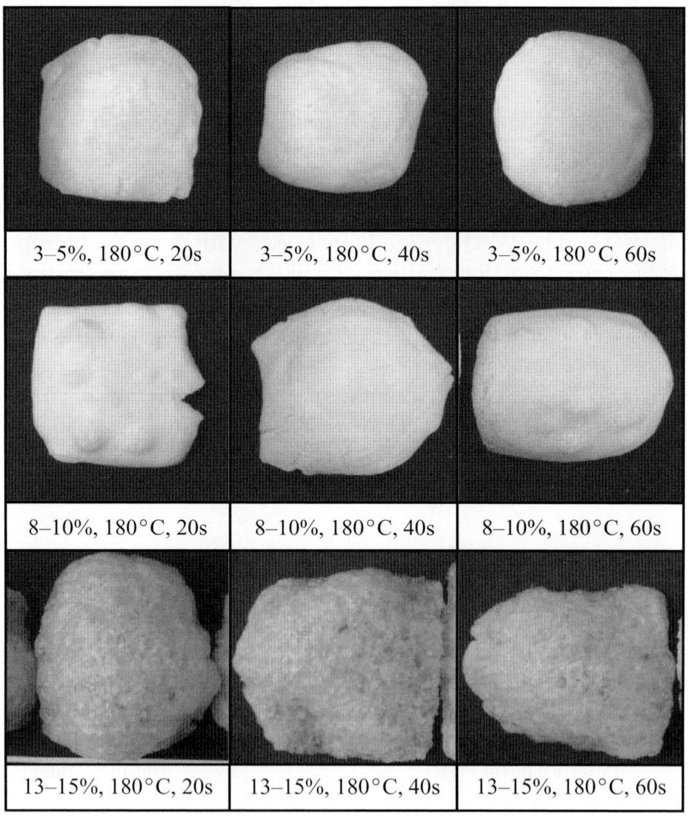

Figure 12.3 Appearance of snack after frying the extruded pellet which were dried to different percentage of moisture content at 180 °C for 20, 40 and 60 s. For colour details, see the colour plates section

Table 12.2 Oil absorption (%) of snack from extruded pellet dried to different percentage of moisture content (% MC) and fried at different time and temperature

	3–5% MC			8–10% MC			13–15% MC		
Temp	20S	40S	60S	20S	40S	60S	20S	40S	60S
160 °C	$13.40 \pm 0.78^{a}_{ns}$	14.35 ± 1.47^{a}	18.05 ± 3.17^{a}	$15.82 \pm 1.27^{a}_{ns}$	18.90 ± 3.04^{a}	18.17 ± 0.59^{a}	$17.02 \pm 0.19^{a}_{ns}$	18.94 ± 2.51^{a}	19.54 ± 0.78^{a}
180 °C	$15.89 \pm 0.75^{a}_{ns}$	16.68 ± 0.09^{a}	20.11 ± 3.16^{a}	$21.41 \pm 1.83^{b}_{ns}$	20.61 ± 0.28^{a}	20.92 ± 1.52^{a}	$21.73 \pm 0.40^{b}_{ns}$	21.24 ± 1.57^{a}	21.59 ± 0.89^{a}
200 °C	$20.64 \pm 0.47^{b}_{a}$	$25.25 \pm 0.93^{b}_{b}$	$29.34 \pm 0.02^{b}_{c}$	$23.81 \pm 0.06^{b}_{a}$	$27.18 \pm 0.36^{b}_{b}$	$29.06 \pm 0.09^{b}_{c}$	$24.47 \pm 0.09^{c}_{a}$	$29.01 \pm 0.41^{b}_{b}$	$29.57 \pm 1.10^{b}_{b}$

Means in the same column and row followed by the same letter are not significantly different at $p < 0.05$.

oil absorption, 29.57%, was found in pellets with 13–15% moisture content, fried at 200 °C for 60 s. The authors chose the optimum pellet frying conditions for a further study: drying the extruded pellet to 8–10% moisture content and frying at 180 °C for 20 s. RSM analysis showed that oil absorption increased with increased flour-mix moisture, screw speed and die temperature. Figures 12.4 and 12.5 show the appearance and the air bubble of the snacks after frying the extruded pellet at different conditions. The fried snacks showed higher oil absorption and expansion ratio with the increased degree of pellet gelatinization.

12.3 Protein-rich extruded foods

Several studies have been carried out to fortify cereal with high protein, high lysine material to improve the nutritional balance of the extruded snacks. Chickpeas have a high lysine content (1.4%) and can be a good protein enhancer when combined with cereal proteins, which are low in lysine (Ainsworth *et al.*, 2007). Brewers spent grain (BSG), the main by-product of the brewing industry, is a rich source of dietary fibre, protein and phenolic compounds has been considered as an adjunct to human food (Laufenberg *et al.*, 2003; Mussatto *et al.*, 2006; Santos *et al.*, 2003). Ainsworth and coworkers (2007) investigated the effects of adding BSG, as a fibre source, on the selected physical and nutritional properties of a chickpea-based extruded snack product. The chickpea snack was extruded from the following formulation (%, w/w, wet basis): chickpea flour (30), maize flour (30), oat flour (20), corn starch (15) onion powder (5), and BSG (0–30, of the maize flour). The extrusion was carried out using a twin-screw extruder, at screw speeds of 100, 200 and 300 rpm, with a feed rate of 42 kg/h (wb). Both the feed and second zone of the barrel were maintained at 80 °C, while the final zone was controlled at 110 °C. The moisture content of the feed was 11.8% (wb). The replacement of the maize flour with BSG significantly ($p < 0.05$) increased the crude protein, as well as the crude fat and fibre content of the samples compared to the samples without BSG. Similarly to the other studies, a decrease in expansion was observed at the increased levels of BSG replacement. An increase in screw speed tended to increase the WAI because there was higher gelatinization or mechanical destruction of the starch molecules in the samples, which increased their water-holding capacity (Colonna *et al.*, 1989). Neither changing screw speed nor the addition of BSG to the feed showed any significant effect on the phenolic compounds or the total antioxidant capacity of the samples. However, a reduction in the total phenolics of extruded oat cereals by 24–46% was reported by Viscidi *et al.* (2004). Higher screw speeds led to increased protein digestibility values *in vitro* in the sample with no BSG addition. The thermal process applied during the extrusion of the chickpea-based snack did not reduce the phytic acid in the study.

Soybeans contain a high content of various important nutrients including protein, oil and several bioactive compounds such as isoflavones, phytosterols and oligosaccharides (Shao *et al.*, 2009). Although isoflavones have a weak oestrogenic property, they show beneficial effects on human health such as reducing the risk of cardiovascular, haemolytic and carcinogenic diseases (Klein *et al.*, 1995; Lee *et al.*, 2008). Defatted soybean meal (DSM) from soybean oil processing contains more than 40% protein. Soy protein is highly nutritious, inexpensive and widely used in many food products such as meat, dairy, cereal products and snack food (Qi *et al.*, 1997).

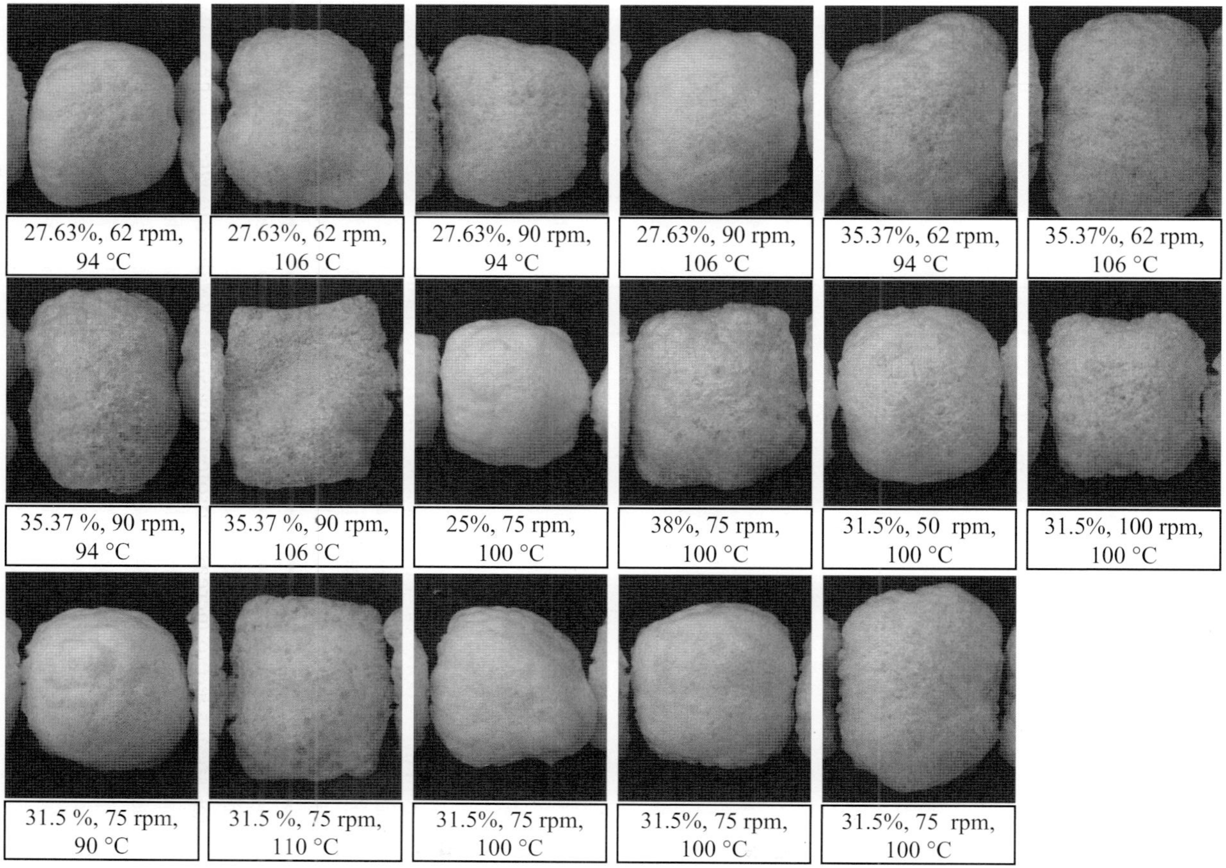

Figure 12.4 Appearance of snack after frying the pellet extruded with different percentage of feed moisture content, screw speed and zone 3 barrel temperature. The pellet from all extrusion conditions were dried to about 8–10% moisture content and fried at 180 °C for 20 s. For colour details, see the colour plates section

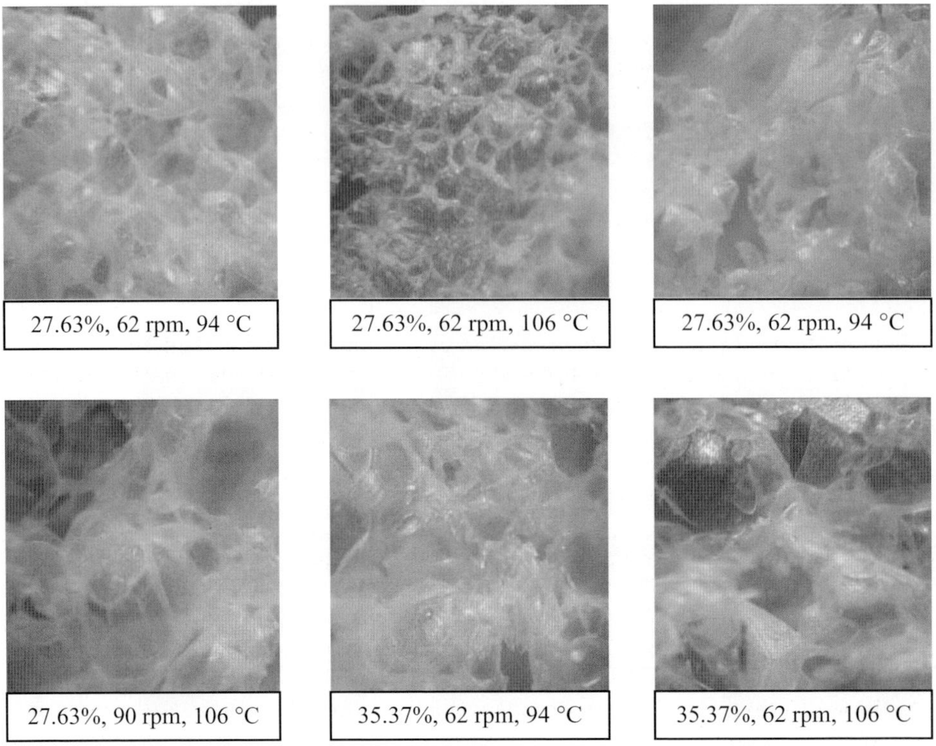

Figure 12.5 Stereomicrograph of air bubbles in the fried snack from the pellet extruded with different percentage of feed moisture content, screw speed and zone 3 barrel temperature ($\times$ 10.5). For colour details, see the colour plates section

There are many reports on the efficiency of the extrusion process in improving product digestibility and removing antinutrients at the same time (Abd El-Hady and Habiba, 2003). Extrusion significantly improved the protein digestibility of faba, kidney beans and pea seed, compared with dehulling, soaking and germination (Alonso *et al.,* 1998, 2000). The extrusion process increased *in vitro* protein digestibility (IVPD) in lupin seed, hardened chickpeas and a maize–lima bean flour blend, and flaxseed (Milán-Carillo *et al.,* 2002; Rémond *et al.,* 2003; Pérez-Navarrete *et al.,* 2006; Wang *et al.,* 2008). Singh *et al.* (2007) has reviewed the effects of processing on the nutritional properties of the extruded foods. It can be concluded that mild extrusion conditions, such as high moisture content, low residence time and low temperature, can improve the nutritional properties of the foods. A higher retention of amino acids and vitamins as well as better protein and starch digestibility were observed. An increase in the soluble dietary fibre (SDF) content, a decrease in lipid oxidation and an improved absorption of minerals were reported (Singh *et al.,* 2007).

Flaxseed (*Linum usitatissimum*) has been used as a hot functional food in North America recently (Wang *et al.,* 2008). Flaxseed can be a good nutrition source for animals (Rees *et al.,* 2001; Basmacioğlu *et al.,* 2003). It contains approximately 40% oil, 30% dietary fibre, 20% protein, 6% moisture and 4% ash (Oomah and Mazza,

1998). Flaxseed protein was found to decrease plasma cholesterol in rats (Bhathena *et al.*, 2002) and was more protective than soy protein against hypertriglyceridaemia and steatosis of liver (Bhathena *et al.*, 2003). However, the presence of antinutritional components, such as antivitamin B_6 and cyanogenic glycoside, limits the use of flaxseed (Oomah *et al.*, 1992). Wang *et al.* (2008) found that extrusion cooking of flaxseed using a twin-screw extruder could improve IVPD in two respects. First, denaturation of protein occurs when the thermal denaturation temperature is reached. The denaturation of flaxseed protein varied between 66 °C and 117 °C depending on the cultivars and processing conditions (Oomah *et al.*, 2006). Second, the cyanogenic glycoside in flaxseed transforms into hydrogen cyanide at high temperature (Feng *et al.*, 2003).

Fortification with milk protein such as whey protein in significant amounts tends to reduce expansion, an important textural parameter of the extruded snack (Lue *et al.*, 1991; Akdogan, 1996; Guha *et al.*, 1997). Martinez-Serna and Villota (1992) reported a 30% decrease in the expansion ratio of an extruded snack due to changes in viscoelasticity during extrusion. The adverse effects such as decreased expansion and increased bulk density have limited the amount of added whey protein to less than 100 g/kg product. The addition of small amounts of proteins from milk raffinate and non-fat dry milk with less than 50 g/kg could improve the textural properties of the starch-based extruded product (Martinez-Serna and Villota, 1992). Onwulata *et al.* (2001) improved the nutrition of a snack product by co-extrusion of wheat bran dietary fibre and milk proteins (casein, whey protein concentrate or whey protein isolate) with corn meal flour using a twin-screw extruder, under high shear and high temperature conditions. Co-extrusion of corn-based products and fibre led to the reduction of specific mechanical energy (SME) with increased expansion and breaking strength of the extruded snacks. The addition of fibre at 125 g/kg resulted in increased expansion and breaking strength, while adding whey protein alone at a concentration of 250 g/kg, reduced expansion and water absorption properties. However, the incorporation of wheat bran fibre at 125 g/kg significantly reversed the effect and improved expansion (Onwulata *et al.*, 2001). There was a significant interaction between protein and fibre ($P < 0.05$). The amount of fibre added resulted in increased shear, which increased temperature (Hsieh *et al.*, 1989), reduced viscoelasticity and decreased SME.

The effects of raw material composition and process conditions such as chicken meat, feed moisture content, screw speed and extrusion temperature on a high-protein corn-based snack were examined by Rungsardthong *et al.* (1998). The authors mixed dry chicken meat with the corn-based snack by using a single-screw extruder. Highly acceptable products were achieved when the temperature of zone 1 : 2 : 3 was 120 : 70 : 180 °C with a die diameter of 3 mm and a feed moisture content of 14%. The increase in dry chicken meat, and consequently the protein content, significantly decreased the expansion ratio of the extrudate compared to the formula without added meat (5.89% protein content) as shown in Figure 12.6. Products supplemented with chicken meat giving up to 12.5% added protein content showed a bulk density of 0.45 g/cm^3, water absorption at 505% and an expansion ratio of 3.26. The products 100 g contained 374.10 kcal of energy. The snacks dusted with spicy barbecue flavour were highly accepted in terms of appearance, taste and texture in a consumer test conducted with 150 panelists aged between 10 and 20 years old.

Some processed cheeses and cheese analogues are also made by extrusion. Cheddar cheese extruded at a temperature of 80 °C had a lower moisture content and

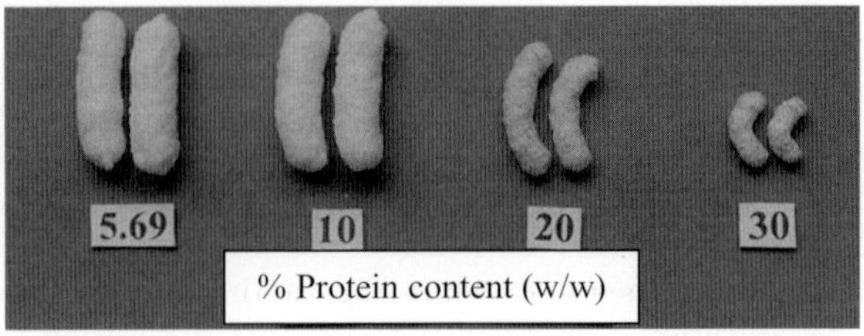

Figure 12.6 Extruded snacks supplemented with dry chicken meat at different percentage of protein content (w/w). For colour details, see the colour plates section

was firmer and chewier than other extruded cheddar cheese produced under different conditions (Adhikari *et al.*, 2009). The authors concluded that processed cheeses that were extruded at lower temperatures with lower moisture levels might be better suited for manufacturing using extrusion technology. According to Zuber *et al.* (1987), an extrudate mean residence time of about 100 s can produce 'processed cheeses or cheese analogues of varying texture (spreadable to sliceable)'.

12.4 Fibre-rich extruded foods

Dietary fibre is defined as 'the edible, polymeric plant tissue resistant to digestion and absorption in the human small intestine with complete or partial fermentation in the large intestine' (AACC, 2001). Dietary fibre includes polysaccharides, oligosaccharides, lignin and associated plant substances. It is classified into insoluble and soluble fibre fractions, based on water solubility properties (Tungland and Meyer, 2002). The insoluble fibres are composed of cellulose, hemicellulose and lignin, which stimulate an increase in faecal bulk and reduced transit time of faeces through the large intestine (Rodŕiquez *et al.*, 2006). Soluble fibres include pectins, β-glucans and galactomannan gums that can help lower blood cholesterol and regulate blood glucose levels. The exact mechanism for delaying the glycaemic response in the blood is still debated; however, many possible hypotheses have been discussed, such as an increased viscosity slowing enzyme efficacy, delaying gastric emptying or preventing bile salt reabsorption from the small intestine (Jenkins *et al.*, 1978; Mäkeläinen *et al.*, 2007; Gunness and Gidley, 2010).

The addition of dietary fibre in the extruded snacks often leads to decreased expansion volumes, higher density and a less crispy texture, so they are less preferred by consumers (Lue *et al.*, 1991). However, soluble dietary fibre usually indicates higher expansion volumes and affects the bulk density of extruded products less than insoluble dietary fibre (IDF) such as cereal bran fibre (Blake, 2006). Treatments of IDF prior to extrusion can significantly improve its expansion and textural properties and thus increase its application potential in human nutrition (Robin *et al.*, 2012).

Non-traditional cereal flours, such as amaranth, buckwheat or millet, were used to reduce the glycaemic index of extruded breakfast cereals by Brennan *et al.* (2012). The products using these cereal flours exhibited a higher bulk and product density, indicated a similar expansion ratio, and a significant reduction in readily digestible carbohydrates and slowly digestible carbohydrates. The breakfast cereal mix extruded from the wheat flour and white flour replaced with dietary fibre at 5% to

15% resulted in significant reduction of 'the rate and extent of carbohydrate hydrolysis of the extruded products' which increased the level of slowly digested carbohydrates and reduced the level of quickly digested carbohydrates (Brennan *et al.*, 2008).

Many food processing industries produce large quantities of by-products. The by-products cause a major disposal problem for the food industry. However, these by-products still contain many nutrients that are beneficial to health such as protein, dietary fibre, antioxidants, essential amino acids and minerals. They are promising sources of compounds that can be used for nutrition (Schieber *et al.*, 2001). Altan and Maskan (2012) intensively reviewed the development of extruded foods by utilizing food industry by-products. Fruits and vegetables have drawn much attention as a source of functionally active ingredients because they are rich in dietary fibre and phytochemicals such as polyphenols, carotenoids and ascorbic acid. They can also serve as functional components to improve hydration and/or oil holding capacity, viscosity, texture and sensory chacteristics of the extruded food products (Elleuch *et al.*, 2011). Peel from fruits such as apple, mango, orange, peach and pear contained more than 30% fibre by dry weight (Grigelmo-Miguel and Martin-Belloso, 1999). Fresh mango peel contains various valuable functional compounds such as polyphenols, carotenoids and dietary fibres (Ajila *et al.*, 2007). In addition, mango peel powder (Nam Dok Mai variety) contained 50.95% dietary fibre by dry weight and 95.11 mg antioxidant as gallic acid per gram of sample of total polyphenol. One gram of mango peel powder exhibits a 1.5 times greater capacity than 200 mg vitamin E in inhibition of lipid oxidation and 3.5 times greater 2,2-diphenyl-1-picryhydrazyl (DPPH) scavenging potential compared to 50 mg of vitamin E (Chanjarujit *et al.*, 2008).

The addition of whey protein to the snack at 25% to corn, rice and potato flour resulted in an increase of fibre and protein content (Onwulata *et al.*, 2001). A number of researchers have used fruits and vegetable by-products such as apple, pear, orange, peach, cherry, artichoke, asparagus, onion, carrot pomace and potato peel (Camire *et al.*, 1997; Grigelmo-Miguel and Martin-Belloso, 1999; Ng *et al.*, 1999; Nawirska and Kwasnievska, 2005) as sources of dietary fibre supplements in food. Sugar beet fibre added to extruded snacks in significant amounts (>100 g/kg) increased structural strength but reduced expansion, which is one of the important snack characteristics (Hsieh *et al.*, 1989).

Ralet *et al.* (1991) reported the use of extrusion to solubilize pectic substances from sugar-beet pulp by-products. Ng *et al.* (1999) found that extrusion cooking of onion waste increased the solubility of pectic substances and hemicellulose, accompanied by an increase in swelling of the cell-wall materials. Similar results were obtained from the extrusion of orange pulp to modify the properties of the fibre components (Larrea *et al.*, 2005). The orange pulp contained 9.27% of total carbohydrate and a high content of total dietary fibre (TDF, 74.87%), consisting of significant contents of both IDF (54.81%) and SDF (20.06%). Response surface methodology was used following a central rotational composite, experimental design. The extrusion conditions were: barrel temperature 83, 100, 125, 150 and 167 °C; moisture content 22, 25, 30, 35 and 38%; and screw speed 126, 140, 160, 180 and 194 rpm; with feed rate maintained at 70 g/min (dry matter). The authors reported that TDF content in orange pulps decreased with higher barrel temperatures and lower moisture contents with the screw speed fixed at 160 rpm. In addition, IDF content decreased with higher barrel temperatures and lower moisture contents, when the screw speed was at the highest value (194 rpm). However, the lowest values for IDF were observed when the moisture was fixed at 30%, with a barrel temperature higher than 150 °C and a longer residence time (screw speed lower than 140 rpm). When the barrel temperature was fixed at 125 °C, the lowest values for IDF were obtained with longer times of residence and higher moisture contents. The authors discussed that under these conditions of adequate residence time, the solubilization of the fibre component is assured due to the effect of barrel temperature. The redistribution of IDF as SDF during the extrusion process results in a reduction of IDF levels as reported previously for the extrusion of fibre from pea hull (Ralet *et al.*, 1993), wheat flour and bran (Wang *et al.*, 1993) and blends of wheat and barley (Fornal *et al.*, 1987). This effect was explained as a result of the breakage of covalent and non-covalent linkages between carbohydrates and proteins associated with the fibre, leading to small molecule fragments, which would be more soluble (Larrea *et al.*, 2005).

Dried and milled cauliflower by-products at levels of 5–20% were added to ready-to-eat snacks by Stojceska *et al.* (2008). The process conditions were set as follows: water feed between 9 and 11%, screw speeds of 250, 300 and 350 rpm and two barrel temperatures in two zones of 80 °C at the feed entry and 120 °C at the die exit. They found that the addition of cauliflower by-product yielded a snack with lower expansion. Extrusion processing significantly ($p < 0.0001$) increased total phenolic compounds (all levels of cauliflower) and total antioxidant capacity (0% and 10% cauliflower levels) while the level of protein *in vitro* digestibility was decreased significantly ($p < 0.001$). Incorporation of dietary fibre in the extruded snack led to reduced expansion volume of the products. Phenolic compounds are the main functional compound contributing to changes of antioxidant capacity (Dykes and Rooney, 2007; Reyes *et al.*, 2007). The authors discussed that the high temperature, water-stress and wounding (Reyes *et al.*, 2007) could induce the synthesis of enzymes in the metabolic pathway that are responsible for the production of phenolic compounds (Saltveit, 1998).

Kordkerd *et al.* (2010) reported the extrusion of a corn-based snack containing fibre sources from food processing by-products including defatted soybean meal (DSM), germinated brown rice residue (GBR) and mango peel fibre (MPF). GBR (Figure 12.7) contains many nutritional components such as dietary fibre, vitamin, mineral, phytic acid, essential amino acid and γ-aminobutyric acid (GABA). GABA, the inhibitory neurotransmitter, can prevent hypertension and Alzheimer's disease. The amount of GABA in regular brown rice is about 10 times the amount in white rice (Jeon *et al.*, 2003). Total dietary fibre of DSM, GBR and MPF was 16.22%, 5.36%

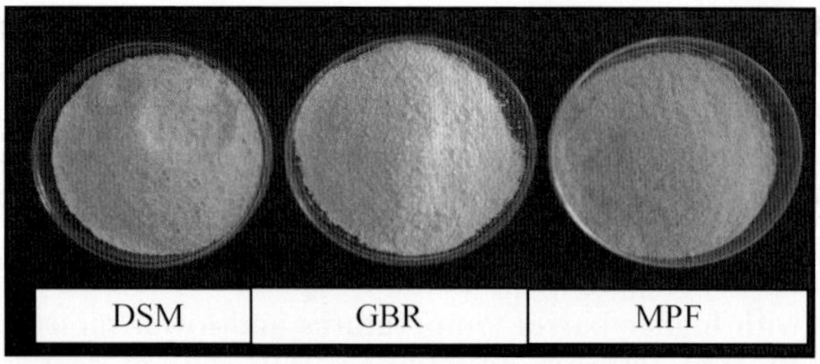

Figure 12.7 Fibre sources from food processing by products: defatted soybean meal (DSM), germinated brown rice meal (GBR) and mango peel fibre (MPF). For colour details, see the colour plates section

Table 12.3 Chemical compositions (g/100 g dry weight basis) of defatted soybean meal, germinated brown rice residue and mango peel fibre

Composition (%)	DSM	GBR	MPF
Moisture	3.71 ± 0.03	8.53 ± 0.09	8.27 ± 0.05
Fat	1.27 ± 0.08	4.28 ± 0.07	3.38 ± 0.06
Protein	45.14 ± 0.09	44.27 ± 0.12	5.68 ± 0.08
Ash	5.95 ± 0.03	1.88 ± 0.01	2.86 ± 0.04
Carbohydrate	47.73 ± 0.05	41.04 ± 0.07	79.82 ± 0.05
IDF	11.46 ± 0.18	2.82 ± 0.23	41.94 ± 0.27
SDF	4.76 ± 0.20	2.54 ± 0.34	22.79 ± 0.13
TDF	16.22 ± 0.16	5.36 ± 0.23	64.73 ± 0.18
Carbohydrate – TDF	26.71 ± 0.09	33.48 ± 0.27	14.58 ± 0.23

and 64.73%, respectively (Table 12.3). The addition of DSM, GBR and MPF significantly affected expansion ratio (ER) and TDF of the extrudate. The addition of MPF showed a more significant effect on the ER and TDF of the extruded product than using the other two fibre sources. Study by RSM indicated that ER of the extrudates decreased with an increase of moisture content and barrel temperature zone 3 (Figure 12.8 and Figure 12.9). The low moisture content in feed may restrict the flow of material and increase shearing rate and residence time, which might increase the degree of gelatinization and expansion (Chinnaswamy and Hanna, 1990). A decreased ER at temperatures higher than 150 °C was observed, which was probably due to the increase of dextrinization and weakening of structure (Mendoça *et al.*, 2000). An increase in both moisture content and barrel temperature led to an increase of WAI and decreasing WSI. The results agree with many earlier studies (Sacchetti *et al.*, 2004; Ding *et al.*, 2005; Altan *et al.*, 2009; Thongkum *et al.*, 2010). Increasing screw speed

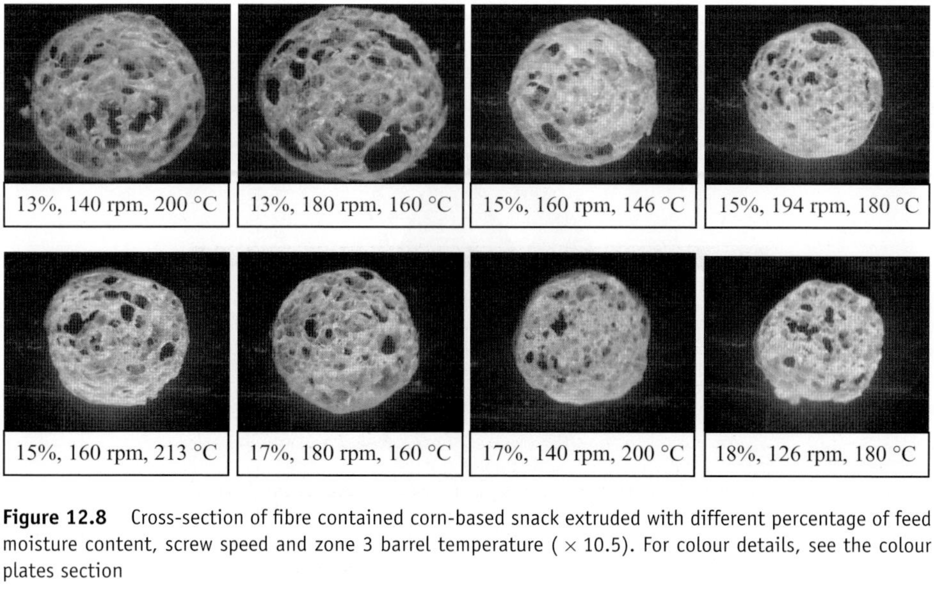

Figure 12.8 Cross-section of fibre contained corn-based snack extruded with different percentage of feed moisture content, screw speed and zone 3 barrel temperature (× 10.5). For colour details, see the colour plates section

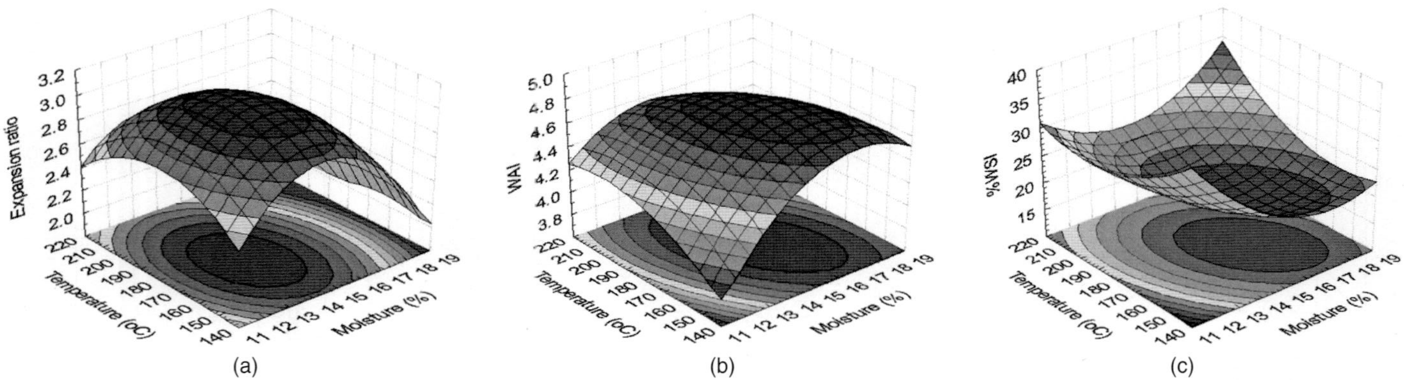

Figure 12.9 RSM on the effects of percentage feed moisture content and barrel temperature of zone 3 on expansion ratio (a), water absorption index (b) and water solubility index (c) of the extruded fiber contained corn based sracks with screw speed 160 rpm. For colour details, see the colour plates section

resulted in an increased shear rate. TDF content (Figure 12.10) decreased with higher barrel temperature and low moisture content, probably due to heat and moisture solubilizing and degrading pectin substances, leading to a decrease in fibre content (Larrea *et al.*, 2005; Stojceska *et al.*, 2008). Total polyphenol content and antioxidant activity was reduced with a higher barrel temperature of zone 3.

A number of studies have investigated the antioxidant and health promoting effects of phenolic compounds contained in grapes and wine, particularly in relation to cardiovascular disease (Scalbert *et al.*, 2005). Grape pomace also has a high dietary fibre content (Valiente *et al.*, 1995) and could be used as a potential source for dietary-rich supplements (Martín-Carrón *et al.*, 2000). Altan *et al.* (2008) extruded barley-grape pomace using a twin-screw extruder and characterized the extrudate properties in order to determine the optimum processing conditions. It was found that after a critical temperature, which depends both on the starch type and moisture content, expansion decreased with temperature, probably due to excessive softening and potential structural degradation of the starch melt, which became unable to withstand the high vapour pressure and then collapsed (Kokini *et al.*, 1992). Similarly, Colonna *et al.* (1989) also reported that a decrease in the expansion of a starchy product at higher temperatures resulted from the increased dextrinization and weakening of the structure. An increase of bulk density was observed with increasing fibre content in grape pomace. The presence of fibre particles tended to rupture the cell walls before the gas bubbles could expand to their full potential (Lue *et al.*, 1991). A similar influence of fibre has been reported for extrusion of yellow corn with wheat and oat fibre, corn meal and sugar beet fibre (Hsieh *et al.*, 1989; Lue *et al.*, 1991; Jin *et al.*, 1994; Chang *et al.*, 1998; Yanniotis *et al.*, 2007; Kordkerd *et al.*, 2010).

Oat bran, which is a by-product of oat processing, is a good source of dietary fibre. Oat bran has been reported to show many health benefits such as lowering cholesterol levels (Chen *et al.*, 2006), blood glucose levels (Tapola *et al.*, 2005), coronary heart disease (Berg *et al.*, 2003) and blood pressure. The SDF of oat bran was considered to play a major role in these health benefits (Zhang *et al.*, 2011). The bioactivities of dietary fibre from oat are related to its (1→3) /(1→4) chemical bond ratio, viscosity and molecular weight (Ripsin *et al.*, 1992; Wood, 2004), which are affected by the oat processing methods before they are consumed. Zhang *et al.* (2009) reported that extrusion treatment could change the distribution of the molecular weight and the ratio of the (1→3) and (1→4) chemical bonds in oat bran SDF. In 2011, Zhang and coworkers investigated the effects of extrusion processing on the functionality and physicochemical properties of SDF from oat bran. They found that SDF in extruded oat bran showed higher yields (14.2%) compared to the untreated oat bran. The extrusion at high temperature (140 °C) could increase the solubility and the extractability of SDF from oat bran. The result coincides with Gualberto *et al.* (1997) who found a decrease in the content of ISF and an increase of SDF during extrusion cooking of cereal bran. SDF from the extruded oat bran was found to have a higher mean particle diameter (1718.19 nm), peak temperature ($T_p = 69.0\,^{\circ}C$), solubility, swelling capacity, solvent retention capacity, foam ability, apparent viscosity and lower flow behavior index than those of SDF in untreated oat bran. The extrusion process improved the functional properties of SDF from the oat bran.

Okara (soy pulp), a by-product of tofu and soy milk, contained more than 20% protein, 50% dietary fibre (Watanabe and Kishi, 1984) and about 10% isoflavones (Wang and Murphy (1996). It was used to enrich the dietary fibre and isoflavone content of

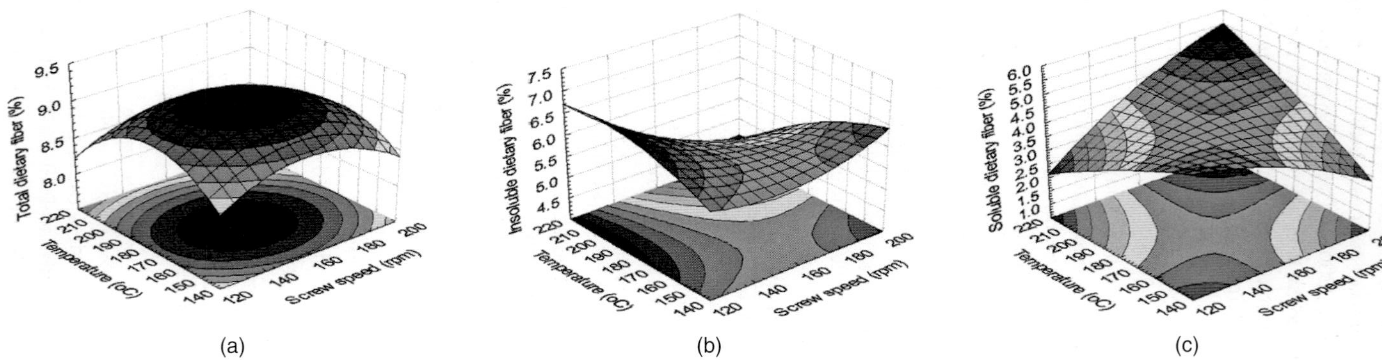

Figure 12.10 RSM on the effects of screw speed and barrel temperature of zone 3 on total dietary fiber (a), insoluble dietary fiber (b) and soluble dietary fiber (c) of the extruded fiber contained corn based snacks with percentage feed moisture content at 13%. For colour details, see the colour plates section

extruded cereal products (Rinaldi *et al.*, 2000). The radial ER of the extruded product decreased with the increased fibre content from the okara. The results agreed with Jin *et al.* (1995) who studied the effects of soy fibre and screw speed on the physical structure and microstructure of corn meal extrudate. They suggested that increasing fibre content caused thickening of the cell walls and decreased cell air in the microstructure of the extrudates, resulting in decreased radial expansion. The decreasing trends of the radial ER could be explained by the breaking down of the component into smaller particles, thus reducing the extensibility of the cell walls and the premature rupture of the cells in the extrudate microstructure (Harper, 1991). Rinaldi and coworkers (2000) also reported that the breaking strength of the extruded snack increased as radial ER decreased. Total dietary fibre of the extruded food increased after heat processing, which was due to the formation of resistant starch during the cooling of the product (Englyst *et al.*, 1992). The IDF of the extruded products decreased while the SDF increased after extrusion when compared to the non-extruded samples. The results were consistent with Wang *et al.* (1993) and Ralet *et al.* (1991) who studied the supplement of dietary fibre from other sources such as fruit and vegetables. However, total isoflavone contents of the extruded products were 3–22% lower ($p < 0.05$) than those of the non-extruded samples. The decrease may be due to the degradation of the isoflavone compounds resulting from the heat and shear generated by the extrusion process (Rinaldi *et al.*, 2000).

12.5 Changes to polyphenolic compounds, vitamins and other functional components during food extrusion

Functional compounds in food and food products play a major role in human protection against many chronic and degenerative diseases (Van Dokkum *et al.*, 2008). Fruits and vegetables are considered as a major source of polyphenols, vitamins and antioxidants while grains are potential sources of functional components, especially phenolic acids (Brennan *et al.*, 2011). However, most of these components are lost due to their sensitivity during processing conditions (Riaz *et al.*, 2009).

Korus *et al.* (2007) reported a significant decrease in polyphenol content and antioxidant activity of the common bean (*Phaseolus vulgaris* L.) during extrusion. A significant decrease in ß-carotene and anthocyanin for both yellow and orange sweet potatoes after extrusion was reported by Shih *et al.* (2009). El-Hady and Habiba (2003) investigated the influences of extrusion conditions such as barrel temperature and feed moisture on total phenol content of whole meal of peas, chickpeas, faba and kidney beans. They reported a significant decrease in total phenol in the extrudates. This decrease was affected by both temperature and moisture. Most of the functional components are temperature sensitive and barrel temperature shows a significant effect on the stability of these components. However, increases of the functional components in extruded products were also reported: ferulic acid content was increased by three times in extruded cereal grains (Zieliński *et al.*, 2001); and an increase in total phenolic compounds after extrusion cooking of sweet potato (Shih *et al.*, 2009) and cereals in combination with cauliflower by-products (Stojceska *et al.*, 2008). A significant increase in free/bound phenolic acid during extrusion of buckwheat was discussed by Zieliński *et al.* (2006). They indicated that the increase of the phenolic compounds could be due to the increased release of these functional compounds from the cell wall matrix during extrusion. Brennan *et al.* (2011) have reviewed the effects of extrusion on bioactive compounds, such as phenolic compounds, anthocyanins and isoflavones, and their antioxidant activity. They have also discussed the factors affecting the levels and stability of the compounds during extrusion.

Extrusion cooking also has a significant effect on the stability of vitamins in extruded foods. There are extensive reviews on the stability of vitamins during extrusion (Camire *et al.,* 1990; Cheftel, 1986; Killeit, 1994; Riaz *et al.,* 2009). Tiwari and Cummins (2009) investigated the decrease of fat-soluble vitamins E and A after extrusion at high temperature and short time. Similarly, Zieliński *et al.* (2001) observed a significant decrease (63–94%) in tocopherol and tocotrienols content of extruded cereal. They also reported a profound decrease (about 63%) of the vitamin E content of buckwheat during extrusion cooking (Zieliński *et al.,* 2006). Both α-tocopherol and α-tocotrienol, the active forms of vitamin E, are least resistant to temperature compared to other forms (Zieliński *et al.,* 2001).

12.6 Noodle, pasta and pasta-like product

12.6.1 Rice noodle

The manufacturing method for the production of rice noodle in Asia is generally a conventional process which is a long, non-continuous process that involves high energy consumption and high production loss; it is also subject to hygiene problems (Cruz, 1959; Chen and Luh, 1980; Li and Luh, 1980; Umali, 1980; Wongchaithong, 1998). Rice noodle, also known as rice vermicelli or beehoon, is one of popular type of noodle consumed in Asia and exported to western countries. Broken rice is usually soaked overnight, followed by milling, and pre-gelatinized by steaming (Wongchaithong, 1998; Fu, 2008). The filtered rice cake, with a moisture content of about 40%, is extruded to form small cylindrical pellets (Figure 12.11a) and subsequently steamed to partially gelatinize the starch granules. They are then extruded into noodle strands with a die diameter around 0.6 mm (Figure 12.11b) and hung on canes and dried slowly. Direct extrusion of rice vermicelli from rice flour has been reported (Khandker *et al.,* 1986; Yeh *et al.,* 1991; Yeh and Jaw, 1999; Charutigon *et al.,* 2008).

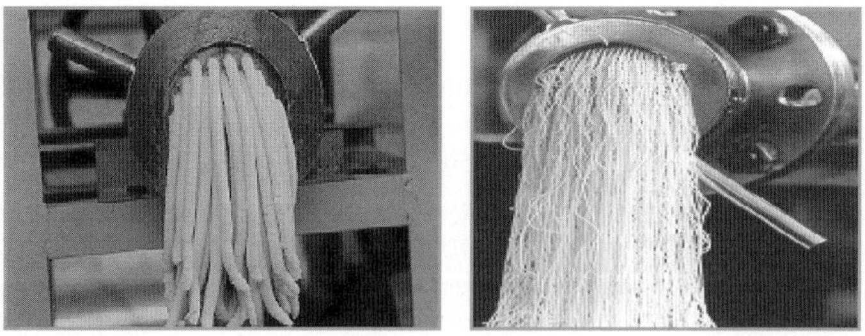
(a) (b)

Figure 12.11 Extrusion of rice cake (a) and after pregelatinized by steaming (b) in most conventional method for rice vermicelli production. *Source:* Yoenyongbuddhagal, S. (2002). The effects of processing condition on ricevermicelli quality, Dissertation No. PH-02-2, Food Engineering and Bioprocess Technology Program, School of Environment, Resources and Development, Asian Institute of Technology, Thailand, 140pp. For colour details, see the colour plates section

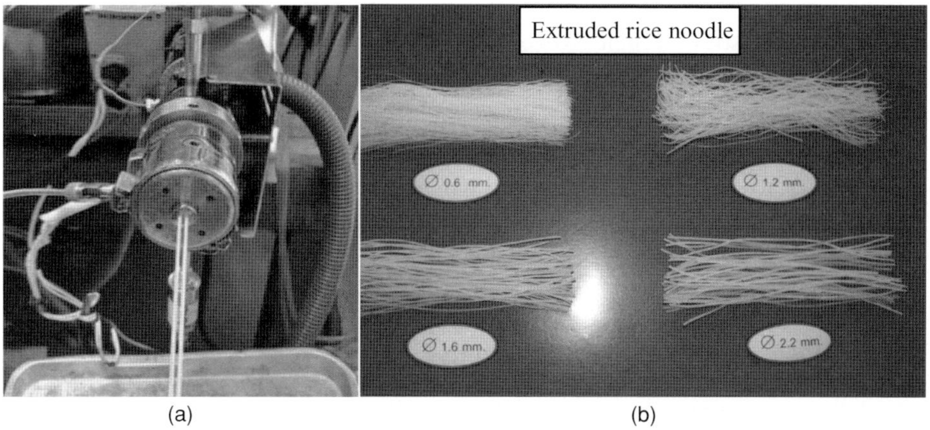

Figure 12.12 Direct extrusion of rice noodle from rice flour using a Laboratory single screw extruder (a) and the rice noodles extruded through die with different diameter (b). For colour details, see the colour plates section

Native flour or starches are generally not resistant to the high temperatures and high-shear processing involved in the extrusion process, which results in low-quality rice noodles (Atwell *et al.*, 1988). Rice noodles are judged by their uniformity, whiteness, low cooking loss, retention of shape or firmness, and non-sticking when cooked (Cruz, 1959; Umali, 1980; Yoenyongbuddhagal and Noomhorm, 2002). Sometimes the extruded noodles are subjected to surface gelatinization in boiling water or steam to improve their stability and texture (Juliano and Sakurai, 1985). Figure 12.12 shows the extrusion of rice noodle and different diameter size of the product obtained by using a laboratory single-screw extruder (Brabender 19/20 DN Model Do-Corder DCE 330, Germany). The surface of extruded rice noodle is comparatively smoother than those of commercial products prepared by conventional processes (Figure 12.13).

Charutigon *et al.* (2008) reported the extrusion of rice vermicelli (diameter about 0.6 mm) from rice flour mixed with cross-linked modified starch and emulsifier at 95 : 4 : 1 with the extrusion temperature of zone 1 : 2 : 3 set at 90 : 100 : 100 °C respectively, with screw speed 30 rpm and feeder speed, 50 rpm. The rice noodle was white and had good shape retention but stuck together after cooking. The breakdown

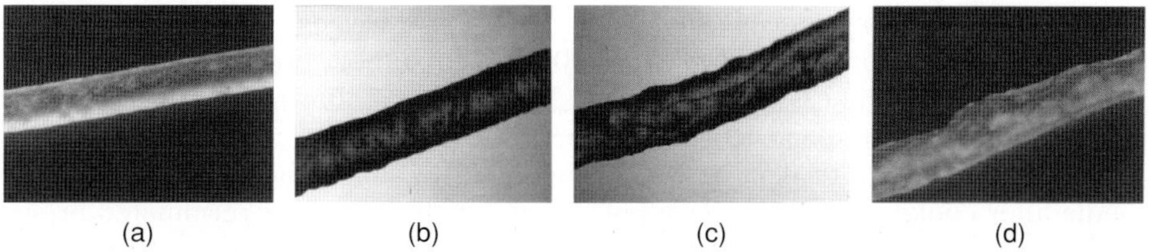

Figure 12.13 Microscopic observation of rice noodle (diameter 0.6 mm) surface prepared by direct extrusion cooking (a) and commercial products prepared by conventional process (b-d). *Source:* Adapted from Charutigon *et al.*, 2008. For colour details, see the colour plates section

of the starch granules and formation of dextrins and short-chain polymers during processing results in sticky dough (Atwell *et al.*, 1988). Monoglyceride at 1% (w/w) and cross-linked modified starch at 4% (w/w) were added to the rice flour to decrease the noodle stickiness and improve the noodle texture when cooked. Monoglyceride can form water-insoluble complexes with amylose, prevent leaching of amylose during gelatinization, inhibit swelling of starch granules heated in water, reduce the water-binding capacity of starch resulting in reduced stickiness and cooking weight (Eliasson and Krog, 1985; Donnelly and Ponte, 2000). Similar phenomena for wheat and potato starch were also reported by Eliasson and Krog (1985). Cross-linking reinforces the hydrogen bonds in the granule with chemical bonds that act as bridges between the starch molecules. As a result, cross-linked starches are generally resistant to high temperature and high shear, resulting in lowered breakdown, and improved viscosity and textural properties of the blend (Langan, 1986; Yook *et al.*, 1993). Sensory evaluation showed that the acceptance of the extruded rice vermicelli was not significantly different from three other commercial products.

The increase of barrel temperature tended to increase percentage cooking weight and reduce percentage cooking loss of the rice vermicelli (Charutigon *et al.*, 2008). The extent of cooking loss depends mainly on the degree of starch gelatinization and the strength of the gel network-like structure of the noodles (Khandker *et al.*, 1986; Wang *et al.*, 1999). Surface gelatinization of traditional extruded noodles has been shown to be critical for hot-water stability of the noodles (Resmini *et al.*, 1979).

The cooking time of the extruded rice vermicelli developed by Charutigon *et al.* (2008) was about 2 min (AACC, 1995). Five grams (5 cm long) of rice vermicelli were placed in 300 ml of boiling water in a 500 ml beaker. The time required for the opaque part of the strand to be gelatinized was considered as the cooking time. Rungsardthong *et al.* (2007) reported the use of cassava flour, modified starch and guar gum mixed into rice flour to produce instant rice vermicelli which cooked when boiling water was poured over and kept in the cup for about 3 min. Instant rice vermicelli extruded from rice flour and cassava flour at 75 : 25 had a good appearance with a smooth surface without air bubbles. The rice flour mixed with modified cassava (substituted type) and guar gum could reduce the gelatinization temperature of the rice flour. The cooked noodle exhibited acceptable properties as instant vermicelli products such as good stability and good texture, similar to commercial products, after pouring with hot water, standing for 3 minutes and tested by sensory evaluation.

Flat-shape rice noodles, known as ‘Seng Lek’ (in Thai), is another popular type of rice noodle for local consumption and export. The production of flat-shape rice noodle generally consists of soaking broken rice, wet milling, steaming, drying, retrogradation and drying process. Flat-shape rice noodle was extruded using a single-screw extruder by Tanapatjiranon *et al.* (2011). The authors prepared the rice noodle from rice flour and cassava starch (75 : 25) using the following conditions: screw speed 30 rpm; feeder speed 50 rpm; temperature of zone 1 : 2 : 3 as 90 : 100 : 100 °C with die aperture size of 0.65 × 3 mm. Figure 12.14 shows the the flat-shape rice noodle after cooking. The noodle supplemented with fibre from germinated brown rice meal or GBR had high dietary fibre and protein content derived from GBR, which contained 48.82% protein and 5.41% dietary fibre. Tensile strength of the noodle decreased with the increase of GBR. The addition of GBR up to 15% to the noodle exhibited a non-significant difference in terms of ‘cookness’, texture, taste, cohesiveness and overall acceptance by sensory evaluation compared to

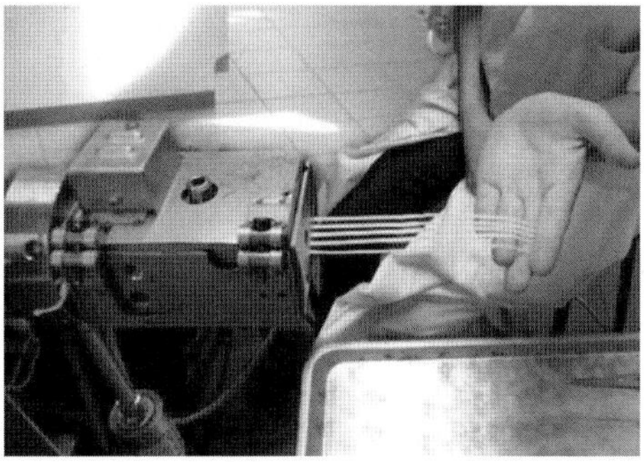

Figure 12.14 Direct extrusion of rice noodle (flat type) from rice flour using a laboratory single screw extruder (Brabender 19/20 DN Model Do-Corder DCE 330, Germany). For colour details, see the colour plates section

noodles made from rice flour and cassava starch. Cookness refered to how well the noodle was cooked. A well-cooked noodle strand meant that all the opaque part of the strand became gelatinized after cooking. Similar trends in decreasing tensile strength and hardness were observed with the noodle extruded from rice flour, cassava starch and fibre source from cassava pulp, which is a by-product from a cassava starch production plant.

Macaroni-like rice noodles were prepared by extrusion of rice (*Oryza sativa* L.) flour (Rungsardthong *et al.*, 2004). The effects of process variables (initial moisture content, incubation temperature and time, and extrusion temperature) on extruded rice noodle properties (appearance, cooking time, cooking weight, cooking loss, degree of gelatinization and hardness) were evaluated. The initial moisture content of rice flour at 30% with incubation at 30 °C for 5 h and barrel temperature of first zone : second zone at 50 : 60 °C gave product with a good appearance and cooking quality. Drying noodles at temperatures higher than 40 °C and longer than 45 min caused cracking of the products. Cooking time, cooking weight and cooking loss of the noodles produced at optimum conditions were 3.5 min, 199.91 g and 2.35%, respectively. The degree of gelatinization of extrudate was 71% whereas hardness of the cooked noodles was 8657 g (Table 12.4). However, rice noodles extruded at 30% had a firmer

Table 12.4 Properties of macaroni-like rice noodles extruded at initial moisture content 30 and 35% and different barrel temperatures

Feed moisture content (%)	Barrel temperature zone 1 : 2 (°C)	Degree of gelatinization (%)	Cooking time (min)	Cooking weight (%)	Cooking loss (%)	Hardness (g)
30	50 : 60	71.4[a]	3.50[a]	199[a]	2.35[a]	8657[c]
	60 : 60	76.8[b]	3.50[a]	190[a]	3.08[b]	7607[b]
35	50 : 60	75.9[b]	4.50[b]	255[b]	4.51[c]	4345[a]
	60 : 60	76.4[b]	4.75[b]	256[b]	4.94[c]	4586[a]

Means in the same column followed by the same letter are not significantly different at $p < 0.05$ by Duncan's multiple range test.
Source: Taungwilai *et al.*, 2008.

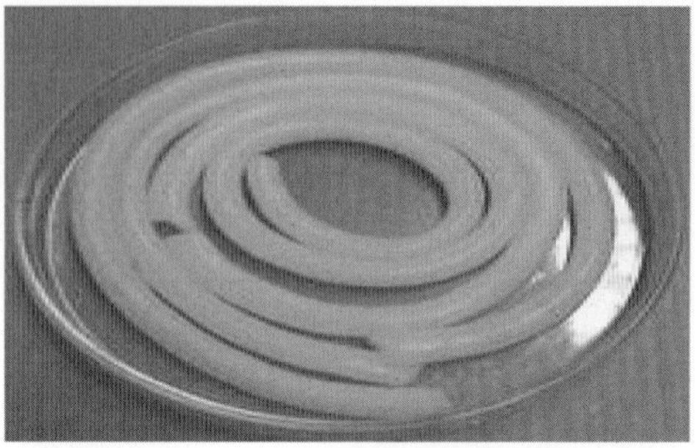

Figure 12.15 Extruded macaroni-like rice noodle after cooking in boiling water for 3.5 min. For colour details, see the colour plates section

texture with lower cooking weight than those extruded at 35%. The colour of the products tended to be white rather than yellowish like commercial macaroni from durum wheat (Figure 12.15).

Organic jasmine rice had a low amylose cotntent and was hard to process into noodles. Thongkum *et al.* (2008) reported the use of potato starch and sweet potato, which contain amylose contents of 29.11 and 17.46%, respectively, mixed with the jasmine rice flour (amylose 16.84%). The spaghetti-like product extruded from the flour mix exhibited a firmer texture compared to the product from the jasmine rice flour only. A spaghetti-like product obtained from Jasmine rice flour and sweet potato flour at 45 : 25 mixing ratio extruded through a 1.4-mm diameterdie, had a cooking loss of 16.4% and gelatinization at 77.9%. The increase of white egg protein up to 15% reduced the cooking loss to 9.28% compared to 7.06% when gluten was used at 15%. The products from the mixture of jasmine rice flour and sweet potato flour mixed supplemented with wheat gluten at 15% gained high acceptance in sensory evaluation.

12.6.2 Clear glass noodle

Clear glass noodle is another noodle which is translucent and has an elastic texture after cooking. Mung bean starch is the major raw material used in the production of clear glass noodles. There are some investigations on the potential use of legume starches such as red bean starch, pegionpea starch, tapioca starch, and edible canna starch (Lii and Chang, 1981; Singh *et al.*, 1989; Kasemsuwan *et al.*, 1998; Charnsri *et al.*, 2005). However, the production of the glass noodles reported followed a conventional method which is a non-continuous and long process. Rungsardthong *et al.* (2006) has formed the edible canna starch into clear glass noodles by using a single-screw extruder with die diameter of 0.6 mm. They investigated the effects of feed moisture content (30, 35 and 40%) and barrel temperature of the extrusion process on the cooking quality of the noodle. The optimum barrel temperature in producing the clear noodle product from edible canna, Japanese green, starch by extrusion process was barrel temperature zone 1 : 2 : 3 at 70 : 70 : 100 °C. The cooking time, cooking weight, cooking loss of the clear glass noodle extruded from canna starch (Figure 12.16) were 2.22 min, 326% and 11.7% repectively while those of the noodle extruded from mung bean starch were 3.3 min, 368% and 6.01%, respectively.

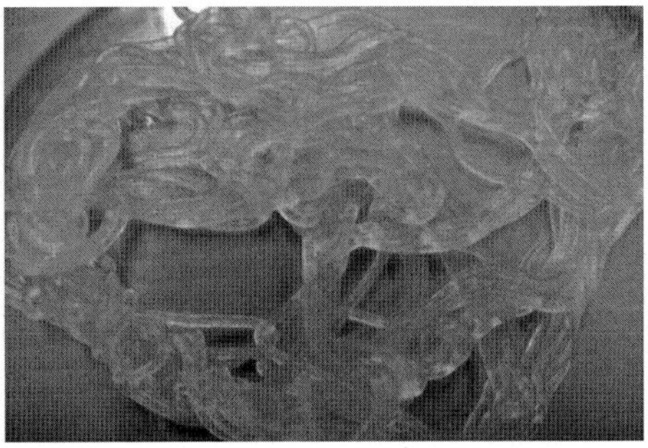

Figure 12.16 Cooked clear glass noodle made from edible canna starch (Japanese Green) using a laboratory single screw with feed moisture content at 30%, barrel temperature of zone 1: 2: 3 at 70: 70: 100 °C, feeder and screw speed at 50 rpm and 30 rpm respectively. For colour details, see the colour plates section

12.6.3 Wheat noodle

Fried instant noodles are made by frying gelatinized noodles, leading to a high oil uptake in the noodle. Jotikasthira *et al.* (2011) reported on the use of extrusion to produce an instant wheat noodle instead of using a conventional frying method. The main ingredients were wheat flour 99.7%, salt 1.5%, sodium carbonate 0.2% and propylene glycol alginate 0.3%. Propylene glycol alginate (PGA) was used to improve the texture of the extruded noodle. The effects of processing conditions studied were: feed moisture content at 25–33%, barrel temperature of zone 1, 60–100 °C, zone 2, 80–120 °C, and zone 3, 80–120 °C with screw speed 20–50 rpm and die diameter 0.6 mm. Cooking time and cooking loss of the wheat noodle prepared by Jotikasthira *et al.* (2011) was not affected by the barrel temperature, 80–100 °C. Figure 12.17 shows the

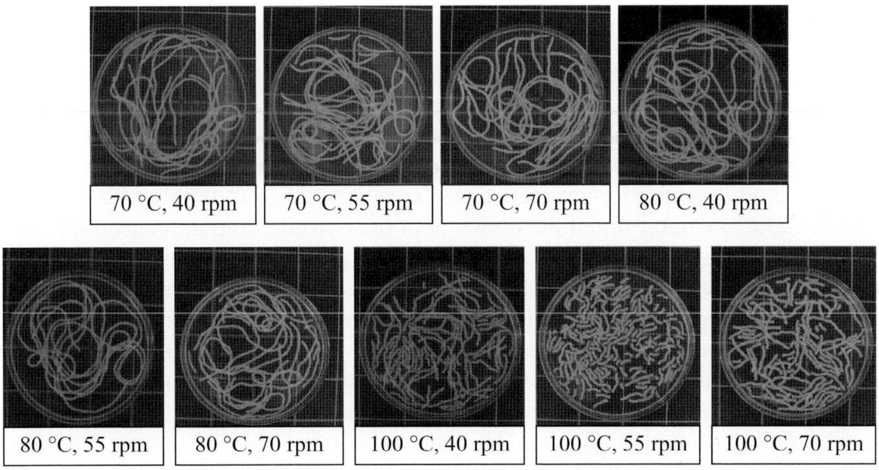

Figure 12.17 Instant wheat noodle, extruded with different barrel temperature of zone 3 and screw speed, after pouring boiling water and kept for 4 minute. For colour details, see the colour plates section

Table 12.5 Effects of zone 3 barrel temperature and screw speed on cooking quality of instant wheat noodle extruded at feed moisture content of 30%, barrel temperature of zone 1 : 2 at 100 : 120 °C, feeder screw screw at 50 rpm

	Cooking time	Cooking weight	Cooking loss
Barrel temp of zone 3 (°C)			
70	3.67^{ns}	239^{a}	6.01^{ns}
80	3.67^{ns}	246^{a}	6.03^{ns}
100	3.42^{ns}	281^{b}	5.18^{ns}
Screw speed (rpm)			
40	3.92^{b}	247^{a}	6.51^{b}
55	3.5^{a}	266^{b}	5.94^{ab}
70	3.33^{a}	252^{a}	4.77^{a}

Means in the same column followed by the same letter are not significantly different at $p < 0.05$.
ns: not significantly different at $p < 0.05$.

stability of the noodle strand after it was poured with boiling water and kept for 4 min. Table 12.5 shows the effects of zone 3 barrel temperature and screw speed on cooking quality of instant wheat noodle extruded at a feed moisture content of 30% with the feeder screw at 50 rpm. Good product quality was obtained using a flour mix with a feed moisture content of 30%, barrel temperature of zone 1, 100 °C, zone 2, 120 °C and zone 3, 80 °C with screw speed 55 rpm (Rungsardthong *et al.*, 2008). The product obtained showed cooking time, cooking weight, cooking loss, hardness and tensile strength at 3.30 min, 254%, 5.29%, 3919 g and 8.06 g, respectively. The extruded noodle contained almost no fat, whereas the commercial instant noodle produced using a conventional frying method contained about 20% fat. Sensory evaluation showed that the extruded instant wheat noodle was not significantly different from the commercial fried instant noodle in terms of colour, cookness, texture and overall liking.

12.6.4 Pasta products and pasta-like products

Pasta is a staple food product that is typically produced from a mixture of durum semolina and water. It is widely consumed in Western countries, and total world pasta production is increasing yearly. Abecassis *et al.* (1994) investigated the effects of experimental parameters (hydration, temperature and shearing) on the pasta-making process and on the quality characteristics of spaghetti. They found that the rotational speed of the screw determined the flow rate of the extruder and influenced the extrusion speed. The average specific mechanical energy transferred to the product for pasta extrusion was about 70 kJ/kg, but it could vary in a 1:5 ratio according to the extruding conditions, especially dough hydration and dough temperature, which both determine dough viscosity. Production factors were found to have little influence on the colour of pasta; however, they did affect the cooking quality. An excessive increase of pasta temperature during extrusion appeared to be the main factor in the degradation of cooking quality. Therefore, a control of pasta temperature at the die was proposed as the simplest method to guarantee the quality of finished products. Wang *et al.* (1999) reported that decreasing the barrel temperature led to increased cooking time, firmness and stickiness of the pasta-like product from pea flour. They reported that the degree of gelatinization increased with decreasing screw speed due to the increase in residence time.

Gluten is considered to be the most significant factor related to the firm structure, elasticity and chewability of pasta (Dexter and Matsuo, 1978; Matsuo *et al.,* 1972; Sozer, 2009). Glutenin and gliadin form gluten when water is added to the durum wheat semolina and the dough is mixed mechanically. The protein compound, gluten, forms a kind of mesh in the structure of the dough and traps the starch grains and prevents the pasta from turning into polenta during cooking (Matsuo and Irvine, 1970). Some humans are not tolerant to wheat gluten and show a specific disorder of intestinal absorption (Hamer, 2005). To prevent wheat gluten allergy, dietary pasta products are now made from different kinds of cereal grains, for example gluten-free pasta made without wheat from rice and legumes, which helps a small but significant portion of the population who cannot tolerate wheat gluten (Kruger *et al.,* 1996; Pszczola, 2000). However, ordinary pasta produced with durum wheat semolina shows better quality attributes (low cooking loss, firm pasta structure, lower adhesiveness, etc.) than pasta made from gluten-free starch such as rice pasta (Sozer, 2009).

A pasta-like product was extruded from pea flour by Wang *et al.* (1999). The authors suggested that an increase in moisture content caused a reduction in mass temperature within the extruder barrel resulting in an increase in dough viscosity. The degree of gelatinization and the WAI of the pasta were also increased due to an increase in both granule swelling and amylose leaching. Product characteristics included increased moisture content, decreased brightness, bulk density, cooking loss and stickiness while increased cooking time and firmness were observed. Wang *et al.* (1999) concluded that decreasing the barrel temperature led to increased cooking time, firmness and stickiness of the pasta-like product from pea flour.

Rice pasta and noodles are also gaining popularity in Europe as an alternative to wheat pasta due to their high digestibility, bland taste and the absence of gluten (Kadan *et al.,* 2003). However, rice pasta tends to have a soft texture because of the lack of gluten (Sozer, 2009). Lai (2001) tried to improve the textural properties of the rice pasta by pre-gelatinizing the rice flour before forming the pasta and another alternative was the gelatinization of the extruded-pasta surface during drying. Many approaches have been taken for the replacement of gluten in gluten-free starch-based products. These include the use of appropriate substitute ingredients – i.e. modified starch, pre-gelatinized rice flour, emulsifiers and protein – suitable for creating a cohesive structure that can overcome the absence of gluten (Chillo *et al.,* 2007; Lai, 2001; Sozer, 2009). Sozer (2009) investigated the rheological properties of rice pasta dough supplemented with substitute ingredients including guar gum, egg white and casein.

Spaghetti-like rice pasta was prepared from rice flour with an amylose content of 33.1% by Sereewat *et al.* (2013). Cooking properties and sensory acceptability of the spaghetti-like product were investigated. The substitution of rice flour with DSM at 90 : 10 increased protein content from 6.28 to 10.69 g/100 g pasta, and resulted in a more yellowish product with greater hardness of the cooked spaghetti strand compared to the product extruded from rice flour only. The addition of cross-linked modified starch (rice flour : DSM : Elastitex 3 at 86 : 10 : 4) improved the texture of the cooked rice pasta (Figure 12.18). Sensory evaluation showed that rice spaghetti made from rice flour, DSM and the modified starch at the given ratio was comparable to commercial spaghetti made from durum semolina.

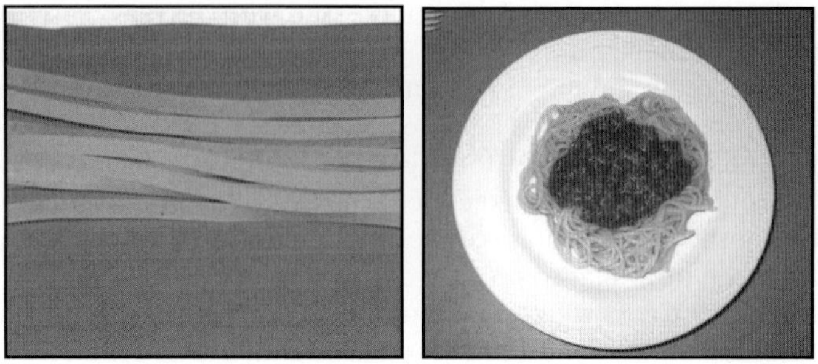

(a) (b)

Figure 12.18 Rice spaghetti extruded from rice flour substituted with DSM and Elastitex 3 at 10 and 4 g/100 g flour mix (a) and cooked rice spaghetti with meat sauce on the top (b). For colour details, see the colour plates section

Rice spaghetti was prepared from rice flour, DSM and modified starch (ester type, Perfectamill A.C.) at 3% following Seerewat *et al.* (2013) and supplemented with dietary fibre and antioxidant from durian fibre (Mulmud, 2010). The formula with durian fibre at 7.5% showed no significant difference compared to that without fibre added. The product had cooking time 11 min, cooking weight 240%, cooking loss 10.2%, and tensile strength 13.2 g, hardness 2936 N, and chewiness 947 g. The product exhibited the increase of TDF from 8.13 to 20.9% and antioxidant capacity (IC_{50}) from 344 to 91 mg with the supplement of durian fibre at 7.5%.

12.7 Summary

Extrusion is a promising technology which provides simultaneous mixing, cooking and texturization of different food products under the shearing effects of screws that generate thermal energy. Extrusion cooking processes generally need short processing times, can cook starchy materials efficiently and lead to highly productive and flexible processes. Food processing by-products are potentially good sources for providing the health benefits associated with non-nutrient compounds such as dietary fibre, antioxidants and phenolic compounds. The results from several studies indicate that it is possibile to produce extruded products as well as pasta or pasta-like products from blends of by-products with different cereals. Extrusion cooking can lead to both improvements and decreases in the functional properties of the extruded food products. Additional research is required for a deeper understanding of the impact of extrusion processing parameters on various food components beneficial to health.

References

AACC (American Association of Cereal Chemists) (1995). *Approved Methods*. Association of Cereal Chemists, St Paul, Minnesota.

AACC (American Association of Cereal Chemists) (2001) The definition of dietary fibre. Report of the dietary fibre definition committee to the Board of Directors of the AACC. *Cereal Foods World*, 46 (3), 112–126.

Abd El-Hady, E.A., and Habiba, R.A. (2003). Effect of soaking and extrusion conditions on antinutrients and protein digestibility of legume seeds. *Lebensmittel-Wissenchaft u-Technologie*, 36, 285–293.

Abecassis, J., Abbou, R., Chaurand, M., Morel, M.-H. and Vernoux, P. (1994). Influence of extrusion conditions on extrusion speed, temperature, and pressure in the extruder and on pasta quality. *Cereal Chemistry*, 71(3), 247–253.

Adhikari, K., Cole, A., Grün, I. *et al.* (2009) Physical and sensory characteristics of processed cheeses manufactured by extrusion technology. *Journal of the Science of Food and Agriculture*, 89 (9), 1428–1433.

Ainsworth, P., İbanoğlu, Ş., Plunkett, A., İbanoğlu, E. and Stojceska, V. (2007). Effect of brewers spent grain addition and screw speed on the selected physical and nutritional properties of an extruded snack. *Journal of Food Engineering*, 81, 702–709.

Ajila, C.M., Bhat, S.G. and Prasada Rao, U.J.S. (2007). Valuable components of raw and ripe peels from two Indian mango varieties. *Food Chemistry*, 102, 1006–1011.

Akdogan, H. (1996). Pressure, torque and energy responses of a twin screw extruder at high moisture contents. *Food Research International*, 29, 423–429.

Alonso, R., Aguirre, A. and Marzo, F. (2000). Effects of extrusion and traditional processing methods on protein and antinutrients and IVPD of protein and starch in faba and kidney beans. *Food Chemistry*, 68, 159–165.

Alonso, R., Orúe, E. and Marzo, F. (1998). Effects of extrusion and conventional processing methods on protein and antinutritional factor contents in pea seeds. *Food Chemistry*, 63 (4), 505–512.

Altan, A. and Maskan, M. (2012). Development of extruded foods by utilizing food industry by-product. In Altan, A. and Maskan, M. (Eds.), *Advances in food extrusion technology*. CRC Press. Boca Raton, London, New York.

Altan, A., McCarthy, K.L. and Maskan, M. (2009). Effect of extrusion cooking on functional properties and *in vitro* starch digestibility of barley-based extrudates from fruit and vegetable by-products. *Journal of Food Science*, 74, 77–86.

Altan, A., McCarthy, K.L. and Maskan, M. (2008). Twin-screw extrusion of barley-grape pomace blends extrudate characteristics and determination of optimum processing conditions. *Journal of Food Engineering*, 89, 24–32.

Atwell, W.A., Hood, L.F., Lineback, D.R., Varriano-Marston, E. and Zobel, H.F. (1988). The terminology associated with basic starch phenomena. *Cereal Foods World*, 33, 306–311.

Basmacioğlu, H., Çabuk, M., Ünal, K. *et al.* (2003). Effects of dietary fish oil and flaxseed on chloresterol and fatty acid composition of egg yolk and blood parameters of laying hens. *South African Journal of Animal Science*, 33 (4), 266–273.

Berg, A., König, D., Deibert, P. *et al.* (2003). Effect of an oat bran enriched diet on the atherogenic lipid profile in patients with an increased coronary heart disease risk. *Annals of Nutrition and Metabolism*, 47, 306–311.

Bhathena, S.J., Ali, A.A., Haudenschild, C. *et al.* (2003). Dietary flaxseed meal is more protective than soy protein concentrate against hypertriglyceridemia and steatosis of the liver in an animal model of obesity. *Journal of the American College of Nutrition*, 22 (2), 157–164.

Bhathena, S.J., Ali, A.A., Mohamed, A.I., Hansen, C.T. and Velasquez, M.T. (2002). Differential effects of dietary flaxseed protein and soy protein on plasma triglyceride and uric acid levels in animal models. *Journal of Nutritional Biochemistry*, 13, 684–689.

Blake, O. (2006). Effect of molecular and supramolecular characteristics of selected dietary fibres on extrusion expansion. PhD Dissertation. Purdue University, West Lafayette, IN.

Brennan, C., Brennan, M., Derbyshire, E. and Tiwari, B.K. (2011). Effects of extrusion on the polyphenols, vitamins and antioxidant activity of foods. *Trends in Food Science and Technology*, 22, 570–575.

Brennan, M.A., Menard, C., Roudaut, G. and Brennan, C.S. (2012). Amaranth, millet and buckwheat flours affect the physical properties of extruded breakfast cereals and modulates their potential glycaemic impact. *Starch/Stärke*, 64, 392–398.

Brennan, M.A., Monro, J.A. and Brennan, C.S. (2008). Effect of inclusion of soluble and insoluble fibres into extruded breakfast cereal products made with reverse screw configuration. *International Journal of Food Science and Technology*, 43, 2278–2288.

Camire, M.E. (2001). Extrusion and nutritional quality, in *Extrusion Cooking: Technologies and Applications* (ed. R. Guy). Woodhead Publishing, Cambridge, UK.

Camire, M.E., Camire, A. and Krumhar, K. (1990). Chemical and nutritional changes in foods during extrusion. *Critical Reviews in Food Science and Nutrition*, 29 (1), 35–57.

Camire, M.E., Violette, D., Dougherty, M.P. and McLaughlin, M.A. (1997). Potato peel dietary fibre composition: effects of peeling and extrusion cooking processes. *Journal of Agricultural and Food Chemistry*, 45, 1404–1408.

Chang, Y.K., Silva, M.R., Gutkoski, L.C., Sebio, L. and Da Silva, M.A.A.P. (1998). Development of extruded snacks using jatobá (*Hymenaea stigonocarpa* Mart). flour and cassava starch blends. *Journal of the Science of Food and Agriculture*, 78, 59–66.

Chanjarujit, W., Seangsawang, T., Keaprajuk, K. and Pinsirodom, P. (2008). Characterization of antioxidant and dietary fibre prepared from mango peels and its effect on bread qualities. *Food*, 38(3), 241–253.

Charnsri, R., Puttanlek, C., Rungsardthong, V. and Uttapap, D. (2005). Characteristics of clear noodles prepared from edible canna starches. *Journal of Food Science*, 70 (5), 337–342.

Charutigon, C., Jitpupakdree, J., Namsree, P. and Rungsardthong, V. (2008). Effects of processing conditions and the use of modified starch and monoglyceride on some properties of extruded rice vermicelli. *LWT – Food Science and Technology*, 41 (4), 642–651.

Cheftel, J.C. (1986). Nutritional effects of extrusion cooking. *Food Chemistry*, 20 (4), 263–283.

Chen, J., He, J., Wildman, R.P., Reynolds, K. and Streiffer, W. (2006). A randomized controlled trial of dietary fibre intake on serum lipids. *European Journal of Clinical Nutrition*, 60, 62–68.

Chen, S. Y. and Luh, B. S. (1980). Chemical, physical and cooking properties of rice vermicelli, in *Proceedings of the 18th Rice Technology Working Group*. Texas A&M University, College Station, TX, pp. 65–66.

Chessari, C.J. and Sellahewa, J.N. (2001). Effective process control, in *Extrusion Cooking: Technologies and Applications* (ed. R. Guy). Woodhead Publishing, Cambridge, UK.

Chillo, S., Laverse, J., Falcone, P.M. and Del Nobile, M.A. (2007). Effect of carboxymethylcellulose and pregelatinized corn starch on the quality of maranthus spaghetti. *Journal of Food Engineering*, 83, 492–500.

Chinnaswamy, R. and Hanna, M.A. (1990). Relationship between viscosity and expansion properties of various extrusion-cooked grain components. *Food Hydrocolloids*, 3, 423–434.

Colonna, P., Doublier, J.L., Melcion, J.P., de Monredon, F. and Mercier, C. (1984). Extrusion cooking and drum drying of wheat starch. I. Physical and macromolecular modifications. *Cereal Chemistry*, 61, 538–543.

Colonna, P., Tayeb, J. and Mercier, C. (1989). Extrusion cooking of starch and starchy products, in *Extrusion Cooking* (eds C. Mercier, P. Linko and J.M. Harper). American Association of Cereal Chemists Inc., St Paul, MN, pp. 247–319.

Cruz, F. R. (1959). A study of bihon industries in Bulacan and its vicinity. BSc Thesis. College of Home Economics, University of the Philippines, Quezon City, Philippines.

Dexter, J. E. and Matsuo, R. (1978). The effect of gluten protein fractions on pasta dough rheology and spaghetti making quality. *Cereal Chemistry*, 55, 44–57.

Ding, Q.B., Ainsworth, P., Tucker, G. and Marson, H. (2005). The effect of extrusion conditions on the physicochemical properties and sensory characteristics of rice-expanded snacks. *Journal of Food Engineering*, 66, 283–289.

Dinkins, J. (2000). Belief and attitudes of Americans towards their diet. *Nutrition Insight*, 19, 1–2.

Donelly, B.J. and Ponte, J.G., Jr. (2000). Pasta: Raw materials and processing, in *Handbook of Cereal Science and Technology* (eds K. Kulp and J.G. Ponte). Marcel Dekker, Inc., New York, Basel.

Dykes, L. and Rooney, L.W. (2007). Phenolic compounds in cereal grains and their health benefits. *Cereal Foods World*, 52 (3), 105–111.

El-Hady, E.A.A. and Habiba, R.A. (2003). Effect of soaking and extrusion conditions on antinutrients and protein digestibility of legume seeds. *Lebensmittel-Wissenschaft and Technologie*, 36 (3), 285–293.

Eliasson, A.-C. and Krog, N. (1985). Physical properties of amylose–monoglyceride complexes. *Journal of Cereal Science*, 3, 239–246.

Elleuch, M., Bedigian, D., Roiseux, O. *et al.* (2011). Dietary fibre and fibre rich by-products of food processing: Characterization, technological functionality and commercial applications: A review. *Food Chemistry*, 124, 411–421.

Englyst, H.N., Kingman, S.M. and Cummings, J.H. (1992). Classification and measurement of nutritionally important starch fractions. *European Journal of Clinical Nutrition*, 46, S33–S50.

Faubion, J.M. and Hoseney, R.C. (1982). High-temperature short-time extrusion cooking of wheat starch and flour. I. Effect of moisture and flour type on extrudate properties. *Cereal Chemistry*, 59, 529–533.

Feng, D., Shen, Y. and Chavez, E.R. (2003). Effectiveness of different processing methods in reducing hydrogen cyanide content of flaxseed. *Journal of the Science of Food and Agriculture*, 83, 836–841.

Fletcher, S.I., Richmonnd, P. and Smith, A.C. (1985). An experimental study of twin-screw extrusion cooking of maize grits. *Journal of Food Engineering*, 4, 291–312.

Fornal, L., Soral-Smietana, M. and Szpenelowski, J. (1987). Chemical characteristics and physico-chemical properties of the extruded mixtures of cereal starches. *Starch/Stärke*, 39, 75–82.

Fu, B. X. (2008). Asian noodles: History, classification, raw materials and processing. *Food Research International*, 41, 888–902.

Grigelmo-Miguel, N. and Martin-Belloso, O. (1999). Comparison of dietary fibre from by-products of processing fruits and greens and from cereals. *LWT – Food Science and Technology*, 32, 503–508.

Gu, L., House, S.E., Rooney, L.W. and Prior, R.L. (2008). Sorghum extrusion increased bioavailability of catechins in weanling pigs. *Journal of Agricultural and Food Chemistry*, 56 (4), 1283–1288.

Gualberto, D., Bergman, C., Kazemzadeh, M. and Weber, C. (1997). Effect of extrusion processing on the soluble and insoluble fibre and phytic acid contents of cereal brans. *Plant Foods for Human Nutrition*, 51, 187–198.

Guha, M., Ali, S.Z. and Bhattacharaya, S. (1997). Twin-screw extrusion of rice flour without a die-effect of barrel temperature and screw speed on extrusion and extrudate characteristics. *Journal of Food Engineering*, 32, 251–267.

Gunness, P. and Gidley, M.J. (2010). Mechanisms underlying the cholesterol-lowering properties of soluble dietary fibre polysaccharides. *Food and Functioning*, 1 (2), 149–155.

Guy, R. (2001). Raw materials for extrusion cooking, in *Extrusion Cooking: Technologies and Applications* (ed. R. Guy). Woodhead Publishing, Cambridge, UK.

Hamer, R.J. (2005). Coeliac disease: Background and biochemical aspects. *Biotechnology Advances*, 23, 401–408.

Harper, J.M. (1991) *Extrusion of Food*, Vol. 2. CRC Press Inc., Boca Raton, FL.

Harper, J.M. (1978). Food extrusion. *Critical Reviews in Food Science and Nutrition*, 11 (2), 155–215.

Hsieh, F., Mulvaney, S. J., Huff, H. E., Lue, S. and Brent, J., Jr. (1989). Effect of dietary fibre and screw speed on some extrusion processing and product variables. *Lebensmittel-Wissenschaft und-Technologie*, 22, 204–207.

Ilo, S. and Berghofer, E. (1999). Kinetics of colour change during extrusion cooking of maize grits. *Journal of Food Engineering*, 39, 73–80.

Iqbal, A., Khalil, I.A., Ateeq, N. and Kahn, M.S. (2006). Nutritional quality of important food legumes. *Food Chemistry*, 97, 331–335.

Jenkins, D.J.A., Wolever, T.M., Leeds, A.R. *et al.* (1978). Dietary fibres, fibre analogues and glucose tolerance: importance of viscosity. *British Medical Journal*, 1 (6124), 1392–1394.

Jeon, T.I., Hwang, S.G., Lim, B.O. and Park, D.K. (2003). Extracts of *Phellinus linteus* grown on germinated brown rice suppress liver damage induced by carbon tetrachloride in rats. *Biotechnology Letters*, 25 (24), 2093–2096.

Jin, Z., Hsieh, F. and Huff, H.E. (1994). Extrusion cooking of corn meal with soy fibre, salt and sugar. *Cereal Chemistry*, 71, 227–234.

Jin, Z., Hsieh, F. and Huff, H.E. (1995). Effects of soy fibre, salt, sugar and screw speed on physical properties and microstructure of corn meal extrudate. *Journal of Cereal Science*, 22, 185–194.

Jotikasthira, P. S., Khaokham, N., Puttanlek, C., Uttapap, D. and Rungsardthong, V. (2011) Effects of extrusion conditions on quality of instant wheat noodle. 2011 European Federation of Food Science and Technology Annual Meeting. Process–Structure–Function Relationships, 9–11 November 2011. Technische Universitat Berlin, Berlin, Germany.

Juliano, B. O. and Sakurai, J. (1985). Miscellaneous rice products, in *Rice Chemistry and Technology* (ed. B. O. Juliano). American Association of Cereal Chemists, St Paul, MN, pp. 569–618.

Kadan, R.S., Bryant, R.J. and Pepperman, A.B. (2003). Functional properties of extruded rice flour. *Journal of Food Science*, 68, 1669–1672.

Kasemsuwan, T., Bailey, T. and Jane, J. (1998). Preparation of clear glass noodles with mixtures of tapioca and high-amylose starches. *Carbohydrate Polymers*, 32, 301–312.

Khandker, A.K., de Mosqueda, M.B., del Rosario, R.R. and Juliano, B.O. (1986). Factors affecting properties of rice noodles prepared with an extruder. *ASEAN Food Journal*, 2 (1), 31–35.

Killeit, U. (1994). Vitamin retention in extrusion cooking. *Food Chemistry*, 49 (2), 149–155.

Klein, B.P., Perry, A.K. and Adair, N. (1995). Incorporating soy proteins into baked products for use in clinical studies. *American Journal of Clinical Nutrition*, 125, 666–674.

Kokini, J.L., Chang, C.N. and Lai, L.S. (1992). The role of rheological properties on extrudate expansion, in *Food Extrusion Science and Technology* (eds J.L. Kokini, C.T. Ho and M.V. Karwe). Marcel Dekker Inc., New York, pp. 631–652.

Kordkerd, S., Wanlapa, S., Uttapap, D., Puttanlek, C. and Rungsardthong, V. (2010) Extrusion of fibre-supplemented snacks using food processing by-products. 5th International Conference on Innovations in Food and Bioprocess Technology, 7–9 December, 2010. Asian Institute of Technology, Bangkok, Thailand.

Korus, J., Gumul, D. and Czechowska, K. (2007). Effect of extrusion on the phenolic composition and antioxidant activity of dry beans of *Phaseolus vulgaris* L. *Food Technology and Biotechnology*, 45 (2), 139–146.

Kruger, J.E., Matsuo, R.B. and Dick, W.J. (1996). *Pasta and Noodle Technology*. American Association of Cereal Chemists, USA, St Paul, MN.

Lai, H. M. (2001). Effects of rice properties and emulsifiers on the quality of rice pasta. *Journal of the Science of Food and Agriculture*, 82, 203–216.

Langan, R.E. (1986). Food industry, in *Modified Starches: Properties and Use* (ed. O.B. Wurzburg). CRC Press, Boca Baton, FL, pp. 199–212.

Launay, B. and Lisch, J.M. (1983). Twin-screw extrusion cooking of starches: Flow behavior of starch pastes, expansion and mechanical properties of extrudates, *Journal of Food Engineering*, 2, 259–280.

Larrea, M.A., Chang, Y.K. and Martínez Bustos, F. (2005). Effect of some operational extrusion parameters on the constituents of orange pulp. *Food Chemistry*, 89, 301–308.

Laufenberg, G., Kunz, B. and Nystroem, M. (2003). Transformation of vegetable waste into value added products: (A). the upgrading concept, (B). practical implementations. *Bioresource Technology*, 87, 167–198.

Launay, B. and Lisch, L.M. (1983). Twin-screw extrusion cooking of starches: Flow behaviour of starch pastes, expansion and mechanical properties of extrudates. *Journal of Food Engineering*, 52, 1746–1747.

Lawton, B.T., Henderson, G.A. and Derlatke, E.J. (1972). The effects of extruder variables on the gelatinization of corn starch. *Canadian Journal of Chemical Engineering*, 50, 168–171.

Lee, S.J., Kim, J.J., Moon, H.I. *et al.* (2008) Analysis of isoflavones and phenolic compounds in Korean soybean [*Glycine max* (L.). Merrill] seeds of different seed weights. *Journal of Agricultural and Food Chemistry*, 56, 2751–2758.

Li, C.F. and Luh, B.S. (1980). Rice snack foods, in *Rice: Production and Utilization* (ed. B.S. Luh). AVI Publishing. Co. Inc., Westport, CT, pp. 690–711.

Lii, C.Y. and Chang, S.M. (1981). Characterization of red bean (*Phaseolus radiatus* var. Aurea) starch and its noodle quality. *Journal of Food Science*, 46, 78–81.

Lopkulkiaert, W., Siriwong, N., Uttapap, D. and Rungsardthong, V. (2008) Effects of frying parameters on some properties of snacks from fried extruded pellets. Proceeding of the 10th National Conference on Graduate Research, 11–12 September 2008. Sukhothai Thammathirat Open University, Bangkok, Thailand, pp. 1–11.

Lue, S., Hsieh, F. and Huff, H.E. (1991). Extrusion cooking of corn meal and sugar beet fibre: Effects on expansion properties, starch gelatinization and dietary fibre content. *Cereal Chemistry*, 68, 227–234.

Lusas, E.W. and Riaz, M.N. (1994). An introduction to extruders and extrusion principles. *Extrusion Communiqué*, 7 (4), 9.

Mäkeläinen, H., Anttila, H., Sihvonenm, J. *et al.* (2007). The effect of beta-glucan on the glycemic and insulin index. *European Journal of Clinical Nutrition*, 61 (6), 779–785.

Martín-Carrón, N., Saura-Calixto, F. and Goñi, I. (2000). Effects of dietary fibre- and polyphenol-rich grape products on lipidaemia and nutritional parameters in rats. *Journal of the Science of Food and Agriculture*, 80, 1183–1188.

Martinez-Serna and Villota, R. (1992). Reactivity, functionality and extrusion performance of native and chemically modified whey, in *Food Extrusion Science and Technology* (eds J.L. Kokini, C. Ho and M.V. Karwe). Marcel Dekker, Inc., New York, pp. 387–414.

Matsuo, R.R. and Irvine, G.N. (1970). Effect of gluten on the cooking quality of spaghetti. *Cereal Chemistry*, 47, 173–180.

Matsuo, R.R., Bradley, J.W. and Irvine, G.N. (1972). Effect of protein content on the cooking quality of spaghetti. *Cereal Chemistry*, 49, 707–711.

Mendoça, S., Grossmann, M.V.E. and Verhé, R. (2000). Corn bran as a fibre source in expanded snacks. *Lebensmittel.-Wissenschaft und.-Technologie*, 33, 283–297.

Mercier, C., Linko, P. and Harper, J.M. (1989). *Extrusion Cooking*. American Association of Cereal Chemists, St Paul, MN.

Milán-Carillo, J., Reyes-Moreno, C., Camacho-Hernández, I.L. and Rouzaud-Sandez, O. (2002). Optimization of extrusion process to transform hardened chickpeas (*Cicer arietinum* L.). into a useful product. *Journal of the Science of Food and Agriculture*, 82, 1718–1728.

Mulmud, W. (2010). Product development of spaghetti-like rice noodles supplement with dietary fibre and antioxidant from durians peel powder by extrusion process. Special

Singh, J., Dartois, A. and Kaur, L. (2010) Starch digestibility in food matrix: a review. *Trends in Food Science and Technology*, 21 (4), 168–180.

Singh, S., Gamlath, S. and Wakeling, L. (2007). Nutritional aspects of food extrusion: a review. *International Journal of Food Science and Technology*, 42 (8), 916–929.

Singh, U., Voraputhaporn, W., Rao, P.V. and Jambunathan, R. (1989). Physico-chemical characteristics of pigeonpea and mung bean starches and their noodle quality. *Journal of Food Science*, 54, 1293–1297.

Sozer, N. (2009). Rheological properties of rice pasta dough supplemented with proteins and gums. *Food Hydrocolloids*, 23, 849–855.

Stojceska, V., Ainsworth, P., Plunkett, A. and Ibanoglu., S. (2008). Cauliflower by-products as a new source of dietary fibre, antioxidants and proteins in cereal based ready-to-eat expanded snacks. *Journal of Food Engineering*, 87, 554–563.

Tanapatjiranon, T., Chanjareon, P., Julasavake, S. and Rungsardthong, V. (2011) Product development of rice noodles supplemented with dietary fibre from food processing by-products by extrusion process. Special project in Agro-Industrial Technology Program. Department of Agro-Industrial Technology, Faculty of Applied Science, King Mongkut's University of Technology North Bangkok, Thailand, 118pp.

Tang, J. and Ding, X.L. (1994). Relationship between functional properties and macromolecular modifications of extruded corn starch. *Cereal Chemistry*, 71 (4), 364–369.

Tapola, N., Karvonen, H., Niskanen, L., Mikola, M. and Sarkkinen, E. (2005). Glycemic responses of oat bran products in type 2 diabet patients. *Nutrition, Metabolism and Cardiovascular Diseases*, 15 (4), 255–261.

Thongkum, T., Uttapap, D., Puttanlek, C. and Rungsardthong, V. (2010). Effect of storage time of paddy rice on expansion of rice snack. International Conference on Agriculture and Agro-Industry 2010. 'Food, Health and Trade'. 19–20 November 2010. Mae Fah Luang University, Chiang Rai, Thailand. p. 56.

Thongkum, T., Wutthisilanon, S. and Suttiniam, T. (2008). Development of spaghetti-like pasta from organic Jasmine rice by extrusion process. Special project in Agro-Industrial Technology Program. Dept. of Agro-Industrial Technology, Faculty of Applied Science, King Mongkut's University of Technology North Bangkok, Thailand. 158pp.

Thymi, S., Krokida, M.K., Pappa, A. and Maroulis, Z.B. (2005). Structural properties of extruded corn starch. *Journal of Food Engineering*, 68 (4), 519–526.

Tiwari, U. and Cummins, E. (2009). Nutritional importance and effect of processing on tocols in cereals. *Trends in Food Science and Technology*, 20 (11–12), 511–520.

Tungland, B. and Meyer, D. (2002). Non-digestible oligo- and polysaccharides (dietary fibre): Their physiology and role in human health and food. *Comprehensive Reviews in Food Science and Food Safety*, 1(3), 90–109.

Turgeon, S.L. and Rioux, L.-E. (2011). Food matrix impact on macronutrients nutritional properties. *Food Hydrocolloids*, 25, 1915–1924.

Umali, J.G. (1980). Physico-chemical properties of milled rice in relation to quality characteristics of noodles (bihon). MS Thesis. University of the Philippines, Los Baños, Laguna, Philippines.

Valiente, C., Arrigoni, E., Esteban, R.M. and Amado, R. (1995). Grape pomace as a potential food fibre. *Journal of Food Science*, 60, 818–820.

Van Dokkum, W., Frølich, W., Saltmarsh, M. and Gee, J. (2008). The health effects of bioactive plant components in food: results and opinions of the EU Cost 926 action. *Nutrition Bulletin*, 33 (2), 133–139.

Viscidi, K.A., Dougherty, M.P., Briggs, J. and Camire, M.E. (2004). Complex phenolic compounds reduce lipid oxidation in extruded oat cereals. *LWT – Food Science and Technology*, 37, 789–796.

Wang, H.J. and Murphy, P.A. (1996). Mass balance study of isoflavones during soybean processing. *Journal of Agricultural and Food Chemistry*, 44, 2377–2383.

Wang, N., Bhirud, P.R., Solsulski, F.W. and Tyler, R.T. (1999). Pasta like product from pea flour by twin screw extruder. *Journal of Food Science*, 64 (4), 671–678.

Wang, W.M., Klopfenstein, C.F. and Ponte, J.G. (1993). Effects of twin-screw extrusion on the physical properties of dietary fibre and other components of whole wheat and wheat bran on the baking quality of the wheat bran. *Cereal Chemistry*, 70, 707–711.

Wang, Y., Li, D., Wang, L-J. *et al.* (2008). Optimization of extrusion of flaxseeds for *in vitro* protein digestibility analysis using response surface methodology. *Journal of Food Engineering*, 85, 59–64.

Watanabe, T. and Kishi, A. (1984). Current ways of using and processing soybeans, in The Book of Soybeans. Japan Publications Inc., *Tokyo*, pp. 31–38.

Weerapong, P. (2004). Effects of amylose content and storage condition of various rice varieties on physicochemical properties of extrudates. MSc Dissertation. Kasetsart University, Bangkok, Thailand, 109pp.

Wongchaithong, W. (1998). Clean technology in 'Pra Atit' rice vermicelli factory. *Journal of Industrial Technology*, 48, 111–113.

Wood, P.J. (2004). Relationships between solution properties of cerel beta-glucans and physiological effects – a review. *Trends in Food Science and Technology*, 15, 313–320.

Yanniotis, S., Petraki, A. and Soumpasi, E. (2007). Effect of pectin and wheat fibres on quality attributes of extruded corn starch. *Journal of Food Engineering*, 80, 594–599.

Yeh, A.I. and Jaw, Y.M. (1999). Effect of feed rate screw speed on operating characteristic and extrudate properties during single-screw extrusion cooking of rice flour. *Cereal Chemistry*, 76 (2), 236–241.

Yeh, A.-I., Hsiu, W.H. and Shen, J.S. (1991). Some characteristics in extrusion-cooking of rice noodle by a twin-screw extruder. *Journal of Chinese Agricultural Chemistry Society*, 29, 340–351.

Yoenyongbuddhagal, S. (2002). The effects of processing condition on ricevermicelli quality, Dissertation No. PH-02-2, Food Engineering and Bioprocess Technology Program, School of Environment, Resources and Development, Asian Institute of Technology, Thailand, 140pp.

Yoenyongbuddhagal, S. and Noomhorm, A. (2002). Effect of raw material preparation on rice vermicelli quality. *Starch/Stärke*, 54, 534–539.

Yook, C., Pek, U.H. and Park, K.H. (1993). Gelatinization and retrogradation characteristics of hydroxypropylated and cross-linked rices. *Journal of Food Science*, 58, 405–407.

Zhang, M., Bai, X. and Zhang, Z. (2011). Extrusion process improves the functionality of soluble dietry fibre in oat bran. *Journal of Cereal Science*, 54, 98–103.

Zhang, M., Liang, Y., Pei, Y., Gao, W.W. and Zhang, Z.S. (2009). Effect of process on physicochemical properties of oat bran soluble dietary fibre. *Journal of Food Science*, 74, C628-C636.

Zieliński, H., Kozlowska, H. and Lewczuk, B. (2001). Bioactive compounds in the cereal grains before and after hydrothermal processing. *Innovative Food Science and Emerging Technologies*, 2 (3), 159–169.

Zieliński, H., Michalska, A., Piskula, M.K. and Kozlowska, H. (2006). Antioxidants in thermally treated buckwheat groats. *Molecular Nutrition and Food Research*, 50 (9), 824–832.

Zuber, F., Mégard, D., and Cheftel, J.C. (1987). Continuous emulsification and gelation of dairy ingredients by HTST extrusion cooking: Production of processed cheeses. *International Journal of Food Science and Technology*, 22 (6), 607–626.

13 Recent Advances in Applications of Encapsulation Technology for the Bioprotection of Phytonutrients in Complex Food Systems

Alisha Tuladhar and Anil Kumar Anal
Food Engineering and Bioprocess Technology, Asian Institute of Technology, Pathum Thani, Thailand

13.1 Introduction

Plants contain numerous bioactive compounds such as lipids, flavours, vitamins, polyphenols, flavonoids, fragrances, pigments and minerals. There is a rapidly growing interest in the role of plant secondary metabolites in food and their potential effects on human health (Adom and Liu, 2002; Wang and Weller, 2006). Recent advances in the food and nutrition sciences support the concept that diet has a significant role in the modulation of various functions in the body. There is an increasing amount of scientific evidence to support the beneficial effects of several nutraceuticals including antioxidants, vitamins, minerals, fatty acids, probiotics and other dietary supplements. The functionality of these ingredients is based on bioactive components, which may be contained naturally in the product but usually require formulation by appropriate technologies in order to optimize the desired beneficial properties (Acosta, 2009). Because of the limited understanding of bioavailability and delivery systems in nutritional science, dietary supplements are taken in excessive amounts or delivered to unwanted sites. Thus, the processing technologies applied have to focus

Functional Foods and Dietary Supplements: Processing Effects and Health Benefits, First Edition.
Edited by Athapol Noomhorm, Imran Ahmad and Anil Kumar Anal.

on two aspects: (i) maximally retaining the bioactivity during the processing and storage of the formulated product; and (ii) delivering the desired bioactive compounds to the target sites in the body.

It is believed that delivering the phytochemicals including antioxidants, polyphenolic compounds, vitamins and, unsaturated fatty acids directly into the small and large intestines, is beneficial to those individuals with gastrointestinal inflammatory disorders, such as ulcerative colitis and Crohn's disease (Friedman *et al.*, 1997; Dillard and German, 2000). It has been found that the intake of such nutrients does not reach the minimum recommended value to achieve these health benefits due to people's dieting habits. By definition, a colonic delivery system should retard the release of these functional components in the stomach and small intestine but allow complete release in the colon. The fact that such a system will be exposed to a diverse range of gastrointestinal conditions during passage through the gut makes colonic delivery via the oral route a challenging proposition.

Microencapsulation can be used to improve the stability of active compounds in the biological environment, to mediate their biodistribution and to improve their loading, targeting, transport, release and interaction with biological barriers. In a broad sense, encapsulation can be used for many applications in food technology, including stabilizing core materials, controlling oxidative reactions, providing sustained or controlled release (both temporal and time-controlled release), masking flavours, colours or odours, extending shelf life and protecting components against nutritional loss (Gibbs *et al.,* 1999; Gouin, 2004; Anal and Singh, 2007; Acosta, 2009). Encapsulation of these bioactive compounds enhances their stability in gastric fluids and controls their release in intestinal fluids. Microencapsulation is a technology of entrapping some active materials or ingredients (core material) into a sealed matrix (coating material), which can release their contents at controlled rates under specific conditions. The term 'controlled release' means releasing the core material at the right speed and at the right place under specific conditions (Desai and Park, 2005; Anal, 2008; Murano, 1998).

13.2 Encapsulation technology in complex food systems

Many encapsulation procedures have been proposed but to adapt them universally for bioactive food components to incorporate into complex food systems is still a challenge. Different encapsulation approaches are needed to entrap and thus to preserve the particular molecular characteristics (e.g. molecular weight, polarity, solubility, etc.) of each bioactive compound (Champagene and Fustier, 2007; Augustin and Hemar, 2009).

The encapsulating and coating materials chosen for a particular application depends on the physical and chemical properties of the core materials as well as the method used for capsule formation. These materials must be non-reactive with the core materials, biocompatible and biodegradable. Coating materials, which are basically film-forming materials, can be selected from a wide variety of natural or synthetic polymers, depending on the material to be coated and the characteristics desired in the final encapsulated products. The composition of the coating material is the main determinant of the functional properties of the microcapsules and of how it may be used to improve the performance of a particular ingredient (Goud *et al.*, 2005). An ideal coating material in food applications should exhibit the following characteristics:

- good rheological properties and easy to work with during encapsulation;
- increase ability to disperse or emulsify the core materials and stabilize the emulsion or particles produced;
- non-reactivity either physically or chemically with the materials to be encapsulated both during processing and on prolonged storage;
- ability to seal and hold the core materials within its structure during processing and storage;
- ability to release completely the solvent used during the processes of encapsulation under drying conditions;
- ability to provide maximum protection to the active material against environmental conditions (e.g. heat, oxygen, light, humidity);
- either soluble in physiological environment or biodegradable by enzymatic reaction;
- biocompatible; and
- inexpensive and of food grade status.

13.3 Encapsulation techniques

Brief descriptions of the various methods of encapsulation and the release mechanisms of the encapsulated core materials from the beads, microcapsules, microspheres, nanocapsules, nanospehres and emulsions are provided in the following sections (Gutcho, 1976; Goud *et al.*, 2005).

13.3.1 Air suspension or fluidized bed coating

This method, known as the Wurster process or fluidized bed coating involves dispersing solid particulate core materials in a supporting airstream and spray-coating the suspended materials. The design of the chamber and its operating parameters affect the recirculation flow of particles through the coating zone of the chamber, where a coating material, usually a polymer solution, is sprayed onto the fluidized particles. The cyclic process is repeated till the desired coat thickness is obtained. In fluidized-bed coating microencapsulation, solid particles are suspended by high-velocity air in a chamber with controlled temperature and humidity, where the coating material is atomized, so the major steps of this technique are coating material, fluidization of core material and coating of the core material (Desai and Park, 2005). The choice for matrix molecule is broader than for traditional spray drying; they may be fats, proteins and carbohydrate and may be applied to the sensitive core as well. The core is always solid.

The diverse fluidized-air suspension methods are top-spray, bottom spray and tangential spray. For top-spray, the coating solution is sprayed from above onto the randomly fluidized particles where the air is passed through the bed of core particles to suspend them in the air. In contrast, bottom spray uses the same inlet side for the coating solution and the air.

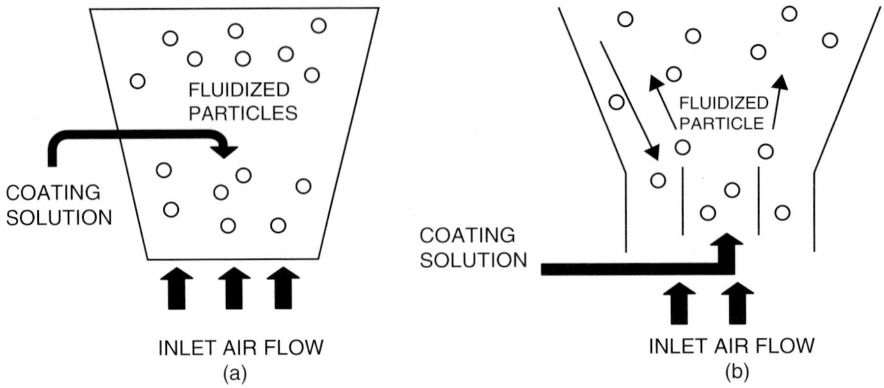

Figure 13.1 (a) Top spray fluidized-bed coating; (b) bottom spray fluidized bed coating. *Source:* Desai & Park, 2005. Reproduced with permission from Taylor & Francis

Aqueous solutions of hydrocolloids such as gums and proteins, ethanolic solutions of synthetic polymers and melted fats or waxes have all been used as coating formulations in the fluidized bed microencapsulation process. A number of food ingredients have been encapsulated by fluidized bed coating, such as ascorbic acid, acidulants for processed meat and leavening agents (Figure 13.1).

13.3.2 Spray drying

Spray drying is the most commonly used microencapsulation technique in the food industry (Anal and Singh, 2007; Champagene and Fustier, 2007; Gharsallaoui *et al.*, 2007). The process is relatively simple and easily converts liquids to powders and protects volatile compounds against degradation and oxidation (Gouin, 2004). Consequently, spray drying has been used to encapsulate a variety of substances, for example, flavours, vitamins and fish oils (Gibbs *et al.*, 1999).

The principal steps of the process involve preparation and homogenization of the dispersion, atomization of the dispersion and subsequent dehydration of the atomized particles (Figure 13.2). The dispersant is prepared by mixing the core material into a liquid coating material. This mixture is homogenized and sprayed into a hot chamber whereby water is evaporated off the surface of the atomized particles to produce capsules (Dziezak, 1988; Watanabe *et al.*, 2002). A cyclone separator, separates the capsules, which are subsequently collected.

The stability of capsules prepared using spray drying is a consequence of the chemical and physical properties of the coating and core materials, atomization and drying conditions such as solid content of the dryer and processing temperature. The functionality of the wall material is particularly important and the most effective materials will have high solubility in water, low viscosity at high concentrations and have effective emulsifying and film forming properties (Goubet *et al.*, 1998; Bomben *et al.*, 1973). If solubility in water is limited, capsules will adopt a matrix-type structure whereby small particles of the core material are embedded throughout a coating material matrix. Often, the core material is incompletely covered, allowing exposure to the environment. Even under a high viscosity interface during the atomization

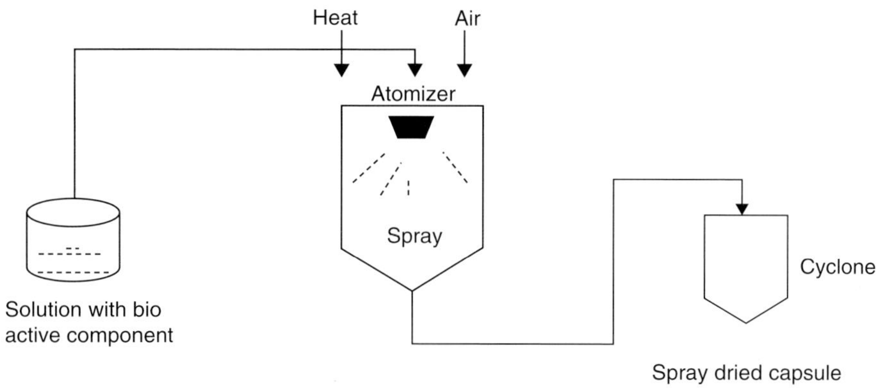

Figure 13.2 Schematic presentation of the spray drying procedure

process, the formation of bulky and elongated droplets is seen, which adversely affects the drying rate (Rosenberg, 1990).

Spray drying is widely used in the food industry due to the many advantages offered by the method (Gibbs *et al.,* 1999; Madene *et al.,* 2006). The chief advantages are the relatively low process cost and flexibility, allowing various coating materials to be used, and adaptability to commonly used equipment. The particles are of good quality and offer good stability and retention to volatile substances. In terms of large-scale production, spray drying can be operated in continuous mode allowing effortless incorporation into many industrial processes. Furthermore, the method is suitable for heat-labile substances as core materials are exposed to lower temperatures (Dziezak, 1988; Gibbs *et al.,* 1999; Madene *et al.,* 2006).

Spray drying is, however, limited to liquid feeds and therefore coating materials must be water soluble and have a low viscosity at high concentrations (Madene *et al.,* 2006). Typical shell materials include gum acacia, maltodextrin and hydrophobic modified starches. Whey proteins and alginate have also been used; however, the solubility in water is much reduced requiring a greater volume of water to be evaporated. Therefore, the use of less soluble compounds as coating materials can be tedious and increase processing costs. For example, mesquite gum has been shown to impart better stability to oil–water emulsions and provide higher encapsulation efficiencies than gum acacia. Soybean soluble polysaccharide proved to be an advanced emulsifier over gum arabic for retaining microencapsulated ethyl butyrate during spray drying (Yoshii *et al.,* 2001).

13.3.3 Spray chilling or spray cooling

Spray chilling is a simple technique where the coating wall solidifies around the core when the mixture is atomized into cooled or chilled air, depending on the usage of polymeric or lipid wall materials. The coating material generally uses fat or stearin having 45–122 °C as their melting point, along with hard monoacylglycerols and diacylglycerols with melting points of 45–65 °C (Taylor, 1983). It is the least expensive encapsulation technology designed for a number of organic and inorganic salts in addition to textural ingredients, enzymes, flavour and further functional ingredients to improve heat stability and delay release in wet environments.

In contrast to spray drying, spray chilling does not involve evaporation (i.e. no mass transfer); hence the coating solidifies to perfect spheres that make free-flowing powders. This technique is in demand mostly for encapsulating water-soluble core materials, water-soluble vitamins and enzymes (Lamb, 1987).

13.3.4 Extrusion

Extrusions is used exclusively for encapsulation of volatile and unstable flavours in glassy carbohydrate matrices (Benczédi and Blake, 1999; Benczédi and Bouquerand, 2001). In general, it works on a low temperature entrapping method, forcing a core material in a molten carbohydrate mass through a chain of dies into a bath of dehydrated liquid. When the coating material comes in contact with the liquid it hardens forming an encapsulation matrix, which is then isolated, dried and sized (Shahidi and Han, 1993) (Figure 13.3). The pressure and temperature engaged are generally 100 psi and 115 °C (Reineccius, 1989).

Having the advantage of long shelf life imparted, usually for oxidation-prone flavour compounds, product can be kept for 1–2 years without any substantial

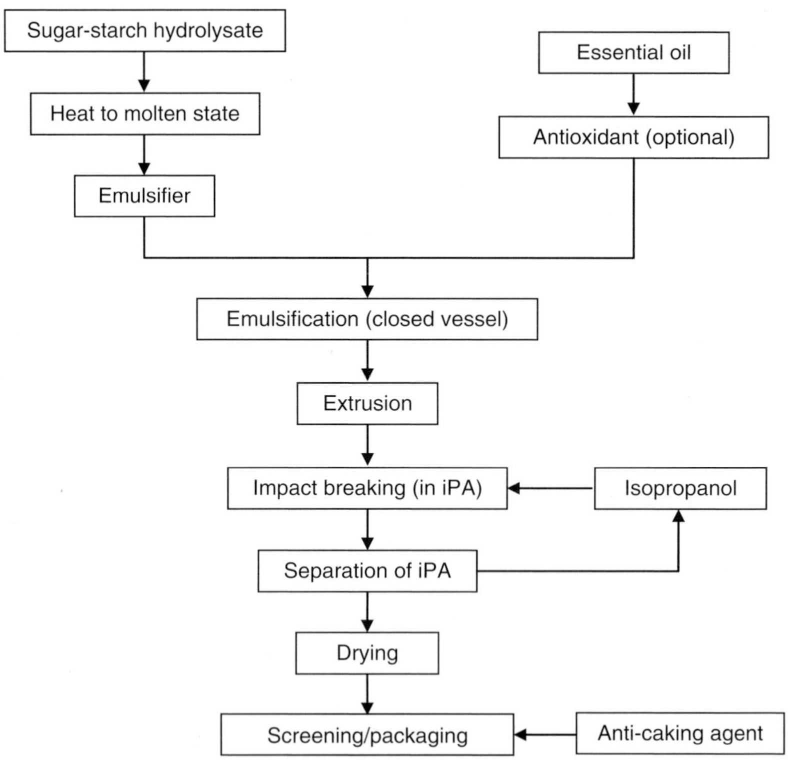

Figure 13.3 Flow diagram representation of encapsulation of flavoured food by the extrusion method. *Source:* Desai & Park, 2005. Reproduced with permission from Taylor & Francis

degradation (Jones, 1998; Deazarn, 1995). This can be accounted for by the slow diffusivity of atmospheric gases through the hydrophilic glassy matrix.

One of the major drawbacks of this technology is the relatively larger particles produced by extrusion, which range from 500 to 1000 μm.

13.3.5 Ionotropic gelation

Ionotropic gelation is a simple microencapsulation method, and can be used to enhance the shelf life and controlled release of the bioactive compounds (Anal *et al.*, 2003; Anal and Stevens, 2005; Anal and Singh, 2007). Typically, ionotropic gelation is performed with alginate and makes use of the gelation of this hydrocolloid in the presence of divalent metal ions. The major steps of ionotropic gelation are mixing together the wall material and the core material and adding drops of the mixture into a solution containing calcium ions, whereby gelation occurs through a reaction between alginate and the ion solution. The hardened capsules are subsequently collected and dried. The mechanism of gelation includes the addition of ions, such as calcium or sodium chloride, which shields electrostatic charges on the surface of proteins allowing the molecules to move closer (Figure 13.4). As a result, molecules can aggregate due to the absence of electrostatic repulsion and gelation can occur.

The major advantage of ionotropic gelation is that capsules are easily prepared in aqueous solutions at room temperature, enabling the method to be used for heat-labile materials. The drawbacks of this method include very low payload, unacceptable cost-in-use, large capsule size, a limited range of wall materials and an undesirable amount of substantial polymers to be incorporated into the foods. To improve this technique, hydrophobically modified starch, epimerized alginate and polyelectrolyte-based multilayer microcapsules can be used to increase the payload.

13.3.6 Coacervation

Coacervation is the process by which colloidal particles are separated from solution and deposited around a core material. Coacervation is typically used for the

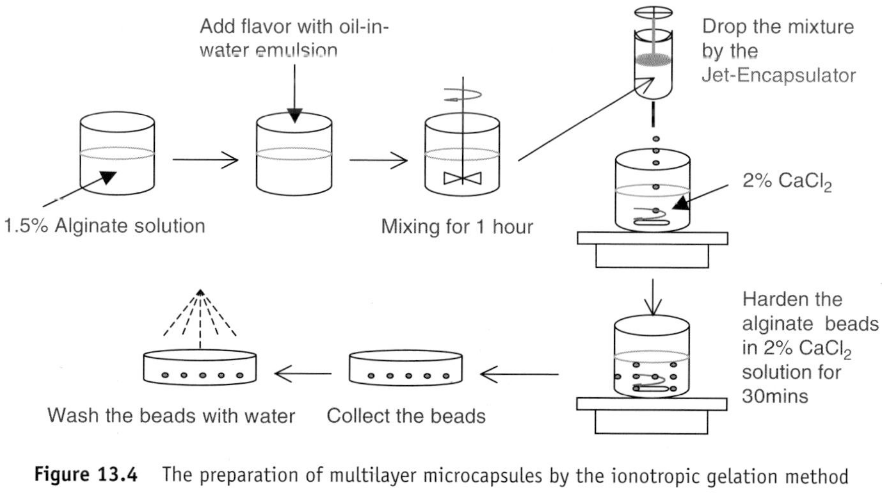

Figure 13.4 The preparation of multilayer microcapsules by the ionotropic gelation method

encapsulation of flavours, lipid-soluble vitamins and phytochemicals, and certain enzymes. Coacervation can be simple or complex. Simple coacervation involves the use of only one hydrocolloid, whereas complex coacervation uses two or more polymers. The coacervation process consists of three principle steps – phase separation, deposition and solidification. In the initial step, the coating material, usually consisting of one or more polymers, undergoes a phase separation to form a coacervate. Core materials are suspended or emulsified in the same reaction medium and as the particles coalesce, a decrease in surface area occurs. The decreased surface area of the coating particles prompts a decrease in total free interfacial energy of the system, which in turn favours coacervate nuclei adsorption on to the core material surface (Madene *et al.*, 2006). As a result, a uniform layer of coacervate forms around core particles. In the final step, solidification of the coating material is achieved by cross-linking using chemical, thermal or enzymatic methods. Microcapsules are then collected by filtration or centrifugation before being dried.

The major advantages of using coacervation techniques are achieving very high pay loads (up to 99%) and excellent controlled release (Gouin, 2004). The process has also been adapted to allow room temperature processing which is particularly useful for the encapsulation of heat sensitive ingredients.

The most well understood coacervation system is the gelatin-gum acacia system (Arneodo, 1996; Jegat and Taverdet, 2001). Other systems under study include gliadin, heparin-gelatin, carrageenan, chitosan, soy protein, polyvinyl alcohol, gelatin-carboxymethylcellulose, starch, β-lactoglobulin-gum acacia, and guar/dextran. These systems have shown very good encapsulation properties.

13.3.7 Liposome entrapment

Formed by the self-assembly of phospholipid molecules in an aqueous environment, liposome entrapment has been mostly used in pharmaceutical applications and has only recently been practised in the food industry. The liposome can enclose either water- or lipid-soluble materials. The resulting closed sphere encapsulates water-soluble bioactive compounds within a central aqueous compartment or lipid-soluble bioactive ingredients within the bilayer membrane (Figure 13.5). Alternatively, lipid soluble compounds may be complexed with other polymers (e.g. cyclodextrin) and subsequently encapsulated within the liposome aqueous compartment.

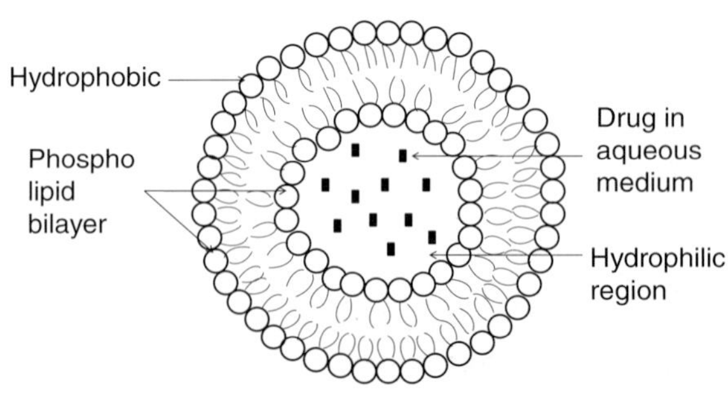

Figure 13.5 The structure of liposome

The major steps of this technique are microfluidization, ultrasonication and reverse-phase evaporation. Permeability, stability, surface activity and affinity vary with different sizes and lipid compositions. In the food industry, large unilamellar vesicles (LUV) are the most suitable liposomes because of their high encapsulation efficiency.

Liposomes have attractive biological properties. They:

- are biocompatible;
- can entrap hydrophilic bioactive compounds in their internal compartment and hydrophobic ones (or compounds) into the membrane;
- protect the incorporated bioactive materials from the inactivating effect of external conditions without causing undesirable side reactions;
- provide a unique opportunity to deliver the active ingredient into the cells or even inside individual cellular compartments; and
- can be easily have their size, charge and surface properties changed by adding new ingredients to the lipid mixture before liposome preparation and/or by varying the preparation methods.

Enzymes encapsulated in liposomes can be delivered to specific parts of the foodstuff. This property improves cheese production as encapsulated flavour-producing enzymes are able to concentrate in the curd during cheese formation.

The use of bromelain loaded with liposomes has shown improved stability of the enzymes during processing (Gregoriadis, 1987). Kirby *et al.* (1998) showed a process to stabilize vitamin C in the inner core of liposomes. Liposomes can also release their contents at a particular temperature. The major problems of using this technique include the cost-in-use, which can be unacceptable if scaling up the microencapsulation process. Liposomes are kept in dilute aqueous suspension, which creates difficulties during large-scale production, storage and shipping.

13.3.8 Inclusion complexation

Inclusion complexation is the entrapment of smaller molecules inside the hollow cavity of a larger molecule (Hedges and McBride, 1999; Madene *et al.*, 2006). Relatively few food-appropriate molecules exist with such cavities; however, cyclodextrins are commonly used in the food industry (Figure 13.6). Cyclodextrins are typically used as coating molecules and are formed by the enzymatic hydrolysis of starch molecules (Pagington, 1986). Glycosyl transferase cleaves starch molecules to form linear fragments which are then joined to form circular structures with hollow cavities inside (Gouin, 2004).

Cyclodextrins then form inclusion complexes with compounds that are small enough to fit inside the cavity. While the internal diameter varies among cyclodextrins, the typical diameter is 5–8 Å which is large enough to hold 6–17 molecules of water. Small molecules may displace the water, forming thermodynamically stable complexes (Figure 13.7). The inner cavity is typically hydrophobic and core molecules are stabilized inside the cavity by Van der Waals forces, hydrogen bonding or entropy-driven hydrophobic interactions (Dziezak, 1988).

Molecular inclusion is typically used to encapsulate unstable, high added value products, for example flavours, aromas, vitamins and minerals. The process produces

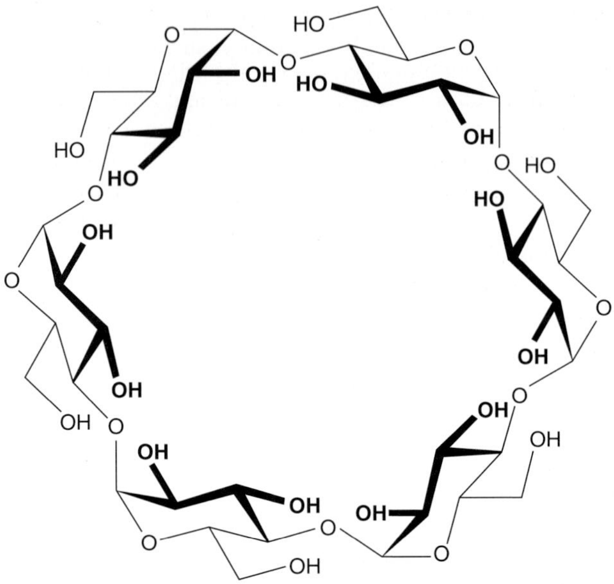

Figure 13.6 The structure of the cyodextrin molecule. *Source:* Madene *et al.*, 2006. Reproduced with permission from John Wiley & Sons

unique release characteristics whereby core materials may be displaced by more favourable substrates. For example, compounds found in the mouth have been shown to be favourable substrates for cyclodextrins, which allows unique flavour bursts to occur (Pagington, 1986 cited in Gouin, 2004). Furthermore, microcapsules formed using molecular inclusion may be resistant to high temperature ($<200\,^{\circ}$C) and chemical degradation (Hedges and McBride, 1999).

A major limitation to molecular inclusion technology is the low payload and relative high cost of cyclodextrin. Gouin (2004) reported that a maximum theoretical payload of 11% (w/w) is possible with molecular inclusion, although other sources have reported up to 15% (w/w) inclusion for artificial flavours (Heath and Reineccius, 1985). In addition, Madene *et al.* (2006) stated that the cost of cyclodextrin would never fall below \$6 per kg, which further reduces the economic viability of the method. Lastly, the use of β-cyclodextrins in the food industry is limited by regulatory requirements.

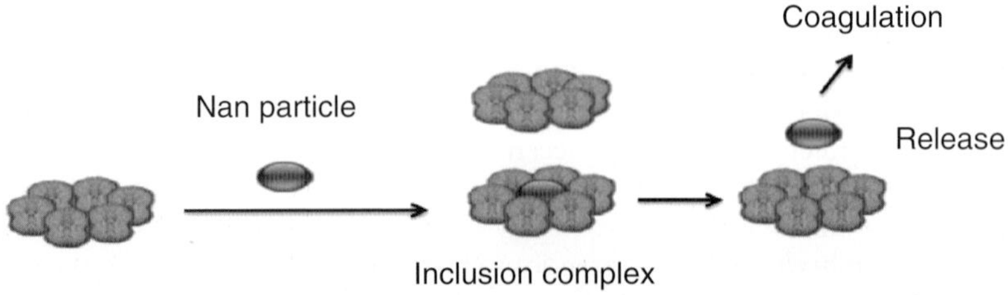

Figure 13.7 General overview of the molecular inclusion process

13.4 Encapsulation in polymer systems

Encapsulation of bioactive compounds from plant sources in a biodegradable polymer matrix has a number of advantages. Once entrapped or encapsulated in matrix beads or in microcapsules, the cells are easier to handle than in a suspension or slurry (Holzapfel *et al.,* 2001). Cryoprotective and osmoprotective components can be incorporated into the matrix, enhancing the stability of the bioactive compounds during processing and storage. Finally, once the matrix beads or microcapsules have been dried, a further surface coating can be applied. This outer layer can be used to alter the aesthetic and sensory properties of the product and may also be functional, providing an extra level of protection to the cells. In addition, the coating layer can have desirable dissolution properties, which permit delayed release of the cells or release upon, for example, a change in pH.

Various polymer systems have been used to encapsulate bioactive compounds to protect and enhance physical stability during downstream processing conditions, including pH, heat and pressure. Microcapsule or bead systems using various biopolymers are very easy to prepare on a laboratory scale, and any ingredients can be encapsulated, whether it is hydrophilic, hydrophobic, liquid or viscous oil, a solid, etc. However, scaling up the process is very difficult and processing costs are very high. Moreover, most of the conventionally produced microcapsules (e.g. calcium alginate beads or microcapsules), tend to be very porous, which allows quick and easy diffusion of water and other fluids in and out of the matrix. Spherical polymer beads with diameters ranging from 0.3 to 3.0 mm and immobilizing active biomass are produced using extrusion or emulsification techniques, by thermal (k-carrageenan, gellan, agarose, gelatin) or ionotropic (alginate, chitosan) gelation of the droplets. Some of these systems are discussed in more detail in the following sections.

13.4.1 Encapsulation of bioactive compounds in carbohydrates

Carbohydrates are used extensively in encapsulation of food ingredients as wall materials or as carriers (Anal and Stevens, 2005; Anal and Singh, 2007). The ability of carbohydrates such as starches, maltodextrins, corn syrup solids, gum arabic, alginates, chitosan and carageenan to bind flavours is advantageous because of their diversity, low cost and abundant use in foods and makes them the preferred choice for encapsulation. These materials also have the properties that are desirable in encapsulation technology, such as good solubility and low viscosity with high solid content. Polysaccharides with gelling properties could stabilize emulsions undergoing flocculation and coalescence (Dalgleish, 2006).

Starch and starch-based ingredients are widely used in the food industry to retain and protect volatile compounds. They can be used as carriers for aroma encapsulation, fat replacers and stabilizers in emulsion (Smelik, 1991; Yamada *et al.,* 1995). Starch granules are able to form complex and potentially useful porous spheres when spray dried with small amounts of bonding agents such as proteins or wide ranges of water-soluble polysaccharides (Zeller *et al.,* 1999). Starch granules treated with amylase can produce highly porous structures. The development of porosity in foods during drying depends on the composition, moisture level, particle size and drying methods. Hot air-drying causes shrinkage due to transportation of liquid water while freeze-drying produces porous structures due to transport of water vapour only (Marousis and Saravacos, 1990). Amylose is able to form inclusion complexes with a wide spectrum of ligand molecules, for instance with flavour and other bioactive compounds (Kuge and Taeko, 1968; Solms, 1986; Escher *et al.*, 2000). Starch is a dietary component and hence, has an important role in colonic physiology and functions and has a potential protective role against colorectal cancer (Cassidy *et al.*, 1994). Resistant starch, is the starch that is not digested by pancreatic amylases in the small intestine and reaches the colon, where it can be fermented by human and animal gut microflora. The fermentation of carbohydrates by anaerobic bacteria produces short-chain fatty acids and lowers the pH in the lumen (Kleessen *et al.*, 1997; Le Blay *et al.*, 1999). Resistant starch can be used to ensure the passage of bioactive compounds from the food to the large intestine (Crittenden *et al.*, 2001).

Maltodextrins are formed by partially hydrolysing the starch by acids or enzymes. They are able to form matrices that are important in making wall systems. Maltodextrins provide good oxidative stability to encapsulated oil but exhibit poor emulsifying capacity, emulsion stability and low oil retention (Kenyon, 1995).

13.4.2 Encapsulation of bioactive compounds in gum arabic

Gum arabic is one of the materials used most often to encapsulate flavour. Its solubility, low viscosity, emulsification characteristics and its good retention of volatile compounds make it very versatile for most encapsulating methods (Madene *et al.*, 2006). Mixtures of gum arabic and maltodextrins have shown promise as high solid carriers to encapsulate cardamom oil by spray drying (Sankarikutty *et al.*, 1988). When a mixture of ethyl propionate, ethyl butyrate, orange oil, cinnamic aldehyde and benzaldehyde was encapsulated in a blend of gum arabic and maltodextrins, a general trend towards an increase in retention was observed when the gum arabic fraction increased (Reineccius, 1991). The spray-dried particles, made from the mixtures of gum arabic and maltodextrins are typically 10–200 μm in size and with about 80% of entrapped flavours in the particles. Apintanapong and Noomhorm (2003) used different ratios of gum arabic and maltodextrins to obtain the appropriate wall materials to encapsulate 2-acetyl-1-pyrroline by the spray drying method. They found that the ratio of 70 : 30 of gum arabic and maltodextins has the best encapsulation efficiency. Beristain and Vernon-Carter (1995) noted that a blend of 60% gum arabic and 40% mesquite gum encapsulated 94% of orange peel oil.

13.4.3 Encapsulation of bioactive compounds in alginate systems

Alginic acid, a natural polymer, is a polyuronic acid extracted from seaweeds and composed of various proportions of 1–4 linked β-D-mannuronic (M) and α-L-guluronic (G) acids. These residues are present in various proportions depending on the source of the alginic acid. Alginic acid and its salts are block copolymers contain both MM and GG homopolymer blocks and mixed blocks containing irregular sequences of M and G units. The binding of divalent cations and the subsequent gel formation is dependent on the composition and arrangement of the blocks of residues

(Gemeiner *et al.*, 1994). The GG blocks have preferential binding sites for divalent counter-ions, such as Ca^{2+}, and the bound ions interact with other GG blocks to form linkages that lead to gel formation. Upon addition of sodium alginate solution to a calcium solution, interfacial polymerization is instantaneous, with precipitation of calcium alginate followed by a more gradual gelation of the interior as calcium ions permeate through the alginate systems. The size of the beads is generally dependent on the viscosity of the polymer solution, the diameter of the orifice and the distance between the outlet and the coagulation solution (Anal *et al.*, 2003; Anal and Stevens, 2005). Alginates are compatible with almost all encapsulation procedures including spray drying, extrusion and emulsification–gelation methods. Champagne (2000) developed a slightly more complex design to produce up to 50 kg/h of wet alginate beads. The process involves atomizing a solution of alginate from a spinning disk onto a rotating vortex bowl containing a recirculating calcium chloride solution. The beads are hardened upon contact with the solution in the rotating vortex bowl and discharged into a large container underneath when the vortex reaches the edge of the bowl. The calcium chloride solution from the container is continuously recycled to the vortex bowl. Various researchers (Sheu and Marshall, 1993; Chandramouli *et al.*, 2004; Lee *et al.*, 2004b) have studied factors affecting bead preparation, such as concentrations of alginate and $CaCl_2$, and timing of hardening of the beads during encapsulation of probiotics and other bioactive compounds.

13.4.4 Encapsulation of bioactive compounds in chitosan

The biopolymer chitosan, the *N*-deacetylated product of the polysaccharide chitin, is gaining importance in the food and pharmaceutical field because of its unique polymeric cationic character, good biocompatibility, non-toxicity and biodegradability.

Chitosan can be isolated from crustacean shells, insect cuticles and the membranes of fungi. The properties of chitosan vary with its source. The chitin and chitosan refer not to specific compounds but to two types of copolymers, containing the two monomer residues anhydro-*N*-acetyl-D-glucosamine and anhydro-D-glucosamine. Chitin is a polymer of b-(1–4)-2-acetamido-2-deoxy-D-glucopyranose and is one of the most abundant organic materials on earth, next to cellulose and murein, which is the main structural polymer of the bacterial cell wall. In order to achieve sufficient stability, chitosan gel beads and microspheres can be ionically cross-linked with polyphosphates (Anal and Stevens, 2005) and alginic acid (Anal *et al.*, 2003) to withstand low pH, as in the stomach. Chitosan is also a well-known dietary food additive. It is of special interest for the sustained and targeted release of bioactive compounds, such as vitamin C (Desai and Park, 2005). The mixture of chitosan and vitamin C was cross-linked with tripolyphosphate and spray dried to obtain the chitosan microspheres. Vitamin C encapsulated in chitosan microspheres of different surface morphology, loading efficiency and zeta potential with controlled-release property, could be obtained by varying the manufacturing parameters (inlet temperature, flow rate) and using the different molecular weight and concentration of chitosan. Microencapsulation of vitamin C in this type of polymeric matrix improves application and enhances stability during the manufacture of functional foods and beverages, and improves its gastrointestinal passage.

13.4.5 Encapsulation of bioactive compounds in proteins

Proteins possess high binding properties for flavour compounds (Landy *et al.*, 1995). The most commonly used proteins for encapsulating bioactive components in food are milk proteins and gelatin. Landy *et al.* (1995) also reported that retention of ethyl butyrate and ethyl caprylate was affected by the concentration of wall solids, initial ester load and by ester and wall type.

The use of dairy proteins for microencapsulation has been widely studied due to their well-known functional properties (Moreau and Rosenberg, 1993; Rosenberg and Lee, 1993; Young *et al.*, 1993; Rosenberg and Sheu, 1996; Keogh and O'Kennedy, 1999; Lee and Rosenberg, 2000a; Chen and Subirade, 2007). A large variety of dairy proteins are available on a commercial scale including casein, whey proteins, whey protein isolates and specific fractions such as β-lactoglobulin, α-lactalbumin and lactoferrin.

Whey is the soluble fraction separated from the casein curd during cheese manufacture. It contains many proteins including β-lactoglobulin and α-lactalbumin. The use of whey as a microencapsulation agent has been well studied due to both its nutritional and functional properties, including its ability to form gels and emulsions (Moreau and Rosenberg, 1993; Rosenberg and Lee, 1993; Rosenberg and Sheu, 1996; Chen and Subirade, 2007).

Lee and Rosenberg (2000b) studied the effects of core-to-wall ratio for the microencapsulation of theophylline in whey proteins. Significant effects on microcapsules size, core content and core retention were observed. It was found that core retention and microcapsule size increased with increased core-to-wall ratio. However, regardless of core-to-wall ratio, release of bioactive compounds is governed by the same diffusion-driven phenomena.

As the wall matrix of microcapsules is designed to limit mass transfer between the core and the environment (Moreau and Rosenberg, 1999), it is important that core materials are non-porous to liquids and gases. Moreau and Rosenberg (1999) studied the porosity characteristics of whey protein and lactose spray-dried microcapsules using a gas displacement technique. The study suggested that microcapsules exhibited molecular-sieve-like characteristics which were affected by wall composition and core load. Walls consisting of whey protein isolate (WPI) only were more permeable to nitrogen than WPI walls containing lactose. Furthermore, the permeability of wall material to nitrogen was inversely affected by lactose concentration. Since oxygen has similar molecular dimensions to nitrogen, it was suggested that the results could be used to predict oxygen permeation in microcapsules especially where core material is prone to oxidation.

13.4.6 Encapsulation of bioactive compounds in proteins and polysaccharide mixtures

Alginate is a natural polysaccharide, extracted from brown seaweed and commonly used as a gelling agent and stabilizer in the food industry (Fennema, 1996). Chen and Subirade (2007) investigated the effect of preparation conditions on nutrient release of alginate–whey protein microspheres. WPI/alginate ratio, microsphere diameter, total polymer concentration and core material loading were investigated. Efficiency rates were above 80% for most microspheres apart from high and pure alginate microspheres. Findings suggested that WPI/alginate ratio, microsphere diameter and core material loading have a major impact on nutrient release. Furthermore, a WPI/alginate ratio of 8 : 2, core material loading of 1% in the initial aqueous phase and diameters close to 94 μm provided microcapsules that were protected from simulated gastric fluid (SGF, pH 1.2) and released core material to simulated intestinal fluid (SIF, pH 7.4).

Various researchers have investigated the use of chitosan as an encapsulating agent; however; fewer studies have looked at the use of whey proteins and chitosan as synergistic encapsulating agents. Chitosan is able to act as a stabilizer in the formed gel while WPI is a useful emulsifier (Laplante *et al.*, 2005). Chen and Subirade (2007) prepared nanoparticles made of chitosan and β-lactoglobulin (β-Lg). Uniform nanoparticles were prepared by ionic gelation and the pH and initial concentrations of native and denatured β-Lg were investigated. Particles prepared with native β-Lg were more resistant to gastric and pepsin degradation than those prepared with denatured β-Lg, and denatured β-Lg cross-linked with calcium ions. Particles were degraded in simulated intestinal conditions in the presence of pancreatin. While nanoparticles are significantly smaller (1–100 nm) than microcapsules, similar principles could be applied to encapsulate probiotic bacteria.

Di Pierro *et al.* (2006) studied the effect of protein concentration and enzymatic cross-linking on the stability of edible chitosan–whey films. Transglutaminase was used as a cross-linking agent and was found to increase the mechanical resistance and resistance to deformability of the films. Cross-linked films were also found to have reduced oxygen, carbon dioxide and water vapour permeability. The results of the investigation suggest that chitosan–whey films treated with transglutaminase may have a potential application as a microencapsulating agent for probiotics.

Carrageenan, a natural polymer extracted from seaweed, consists of alternating 1,3-linked *h*-D-galactose and 1,4-linked 3,6-anhydro-*a*-D-galactose units (Fennema, 1996). Depending on the source, three types of carrageenan exist – kappa (κ), lambda (λ) and (ι) iota – of which κ-carrageenan is most suitable for encapsulation purposes due to its gelling properties (Yi *et al.*, 2005).

Xanthan is an anionic long chain polysaccharide derived from fermentation of glucose or sucrose by the *Xanthomonas campestris* bacterium (Fennema, 1996). Interactions between xanthan and whey proteins are hydrophobic, driven by entropy changes and promoted by increasing temperature (Schmitt *et al.*, 1998). As temperature increases, denaturation of globular proteins exposes hydrophobic reactive sites and conformational changes in polysaccharide structure occur. Strands of hydrophobic polymers come into contact with polysaccharide strands allowing hydrophobic interactions to occur. Le Hanaff *et al.* (cited in Schmitt *et al.*, 1998) found that thc number of complexes between xanthan gum and whey proteins (protein : polysaccharide ratio 20 : 1, polymer concentration 1 wt%) was larger after heat treatment at 80 °C for 20 min.

13.4.7 Encapsulation with lipids

In many studies, the use of hydrophilic molecules as filling agents in walls of microcapsules was investigated (Lee and Rosenberg, 2001; Lee *et al.*, 2004b; Picot and Lacroix,

2004; Pongjanyakul *et al.*, 2004). The release of water-soluble phytochemicals from protein-based microcapsules has been reported to be relatively rapid and is influenced by the swelling of the capsule matrices in the aqueous medium (Lee and Rosenberg, 2001). In addition, research has suggested that cross-linking of protein-based microcapsules provides only limited inhibition of swelling.

Lee and Rosenberg (2001) investigated the use of different proportions of milk fat incorporated into protein-based microcapsule walls. Microcapsules were also cross-linked using glutareldahyde-saturated toluene. The core retention is proportionally related to wall composition and more specifically to wall lipid concentration. Results suggested that the lipid filler increased the resistance to diffusion of fluid through the wall matrix and prevented swelling of the microcapsule. Core release from the microcapsule was governed by diffusion-driven phenomena and was affected by dissolution medium, microcapsule size and composition.

Pongjanyakul *et al.* (2004) evaluated the use of glyceryl palmitostearate (GPS) and hydrophilic substances such as polyethylene glycol and gelucire 50/13 for encapsulating lysozyme. GPS is a mixture of mono-, di- and tri-glyceride esters of palmitic and stearic acids made from glycerin palmitic acid and stearic acid (Lee *et al.*, 2004b). It is typically used in the pharmaceutical industry as a tablet lubricant and a matrix for controlled drug release. Lysozyme was incorporated into GPS pellets by compression and melting methods and its subsequent *in vitro* release, amount (or concentration) and enzyme activity was evaluated. A SEM image of the surface of compression-prepared pellets indicated a porous structure which would allow the entry of water and the likely release of core material. Similar images of GPS pellets prepared simply by melting the material indicated a smoother, less porous surface which would effectively restrict water entry and preserve the core material.

In the same study (Pongjanyakul *et al.*, 2004), polyethylene glycol (PEG 4000) and gelucire 50/13 were added to manipulate the release characteristics of the pellets prepared by melting. The hydrophilic components had similar melting properties; however, gelucire had little effect on restricting pellet swelling. Conversely, polyethylene glycol showed good protection and therefore retention of enzymatic activity.

Polyethylene glycols are often added to the controlled release systems to reduce porosity of microcapsules and therefore affect drug release (Kim *et al.*, 2004). Bonny and Leuenberger (1993, cited in Pongjanyakul, *et al.*, 2004) defined critical porosity as the matrix porosity below which the core material is encapsulated by the matrix material. Above the critical porosity, a complex pore network is thought to be formed through the matrix. Therefore, GPS was a suitable matrix for controlled release of proteins and release rates could be slowed by inclusion of hydrophilic compounds.

Polyacyl glycerol monostearate (PGMS) fatty acid emulsifier is also commonly used as an encapsulating agent (Lee *et al.*, 2004a). Preparation of microcapsules involved the preparation of a viscous solution followed by spray drying and centrifugation. Lee *et al.* (2004a) found that the emulsifier effectively encapsulated water-soluble L-ascorbic acid with high efficiency (94.2%) with an optimal coating-to-core ratio of 5:1. Encapsulating efficiency decreased with increasing ratio of coating-to-core material, for example, 10:1, 15:1 and 20:1 (w/w). A limitation associated with using PGMS is that it is solid at room temperature and therefore requires heating prior to spray drying.

13.5 Controlled release of bioactive compounds from complex food systems

13.5.1 Release of core materials from the encapsulated particles

Microcapsules and microspheres can be engineered to gradually release their active ingredients. There are three primary mechanisms by which active agents can be released from a delivery system: diffusion, degradation and swelling followed by diffusion (Whateley, 1996; Brannon-Peppas, 1997). Any or all of these mechanisms may occur in a given delivery system.

Release by diffusion Diffusion occurs when a core substance or an active agent passes through the polymer that forms the controlled-release device. The diffusion can occur on a macroscopic scale – as through pores in the polymer matrix – or on a molecular level, by passing between polymer chains (Crank, 1975; Cussler, 1997). The major driving force which has greater influence is the vapour pressure of a volatile substance on each side of the matrix (Gibbs *et al.,* 1999). Food components that aren't soluble in the matrix will not enter the matrix, hence, not leading to diffusion irrespective of the pore size of the matrix (Reineccius, 1995).

There are two divergent mechanisms, static diffusion and convective diffusion. Static or molecular diffusion is the result of the random movement of molecules in stagnant fluids. In contrast, convective diffusion conveys elements of the fluid from one site to another along with the solutes. The rate of molecular diffusion is far superior to the rate of convective diffusion (Roos *et al.,* 2003).

For the diffusion-controlled systems described thus far, the delivery device is fundamentally stable in the biological environment and does not change its size either through swelling or degradation. It is also possible for a delivery system to be designed so that it is incapable of releasing its agent or agents until it is placed in an appropriate biological environment.

Release by degradation Delivery of the active compounds to the matrix could either be through diffusion, erosion or a combination of both. Heterogeneous degradation is confined to the thin layer at the surface, while homogeneous degradations are the consequences of wholesome degradation of the polymer matrix at a uniform rate.

Release by swelling This is the chief mechanism for releasing bioactive molecules when they are unable to diffuse through the polymer matrix to any significant extent. Swelling-controlled release systems are initially dry and, when placed in the body will absorb water or other body fluids and swell. The swelling increases the aqueous solvent content within the formulation as well as the polymer mesh size, enabling the core substances to diffuse through the swollen network into the external environment (Fan and Singh, 1989).

This release is accomplished only when the polymer swells. Because many of the potentially most useful pH-sensitive polymers swell at high pH values and collapse at low pH values, the triggered delivery of active ingredients occurs when environmental pH increases. Such materials are ideal for systems such as oral delivery, in which the active compound is not released at low pH values in the stomach but rather at high pH in the upper small intestine (Figure 13.8).

For the reservoir systems, the delivery rate can remain fairly constant. In this design, a reservoir – whether solid core, dilute solution or highly concentrated core solution within a polymer matrix – is surrounded by a film or membrane of a rate-controlling material. The only structure effectively limiting the release of the core substance is the polymer layer surrounding the reservoir. Since this polymer coating is essentially uniform and of a non-changing thickness, the diffusion rate of the active agent can be kept fairly stable throughout the lifetime of the delivery system.

13.5.2 Bioavailability

Bioavailability is defined as the degree to which bioactive molecules become available to the target tissue after administration. The particular amount of a bioactive compound given to the body and the percentage retained within the body can be different. To determine the ascorbate concentration found in humans, it is necessary to describe ascorbate availability. Humans can obtain ascorbate only exogenously. Even when the vitamin is taken in from an external source, it is not completely absorbed by the tissues. Taking pH value into account, encapsulation has to be achieved with an ingredient that is resistant to low pH and high temperature, so that the vitamin can pass unaffected through the stomach to its respective target (the intestine) where maximum absorption takes place. Over time, the target capsules or particles slowly disintegrate and the vitamin is safely absorbed by the tissues.

The schematic diagram (Figure 13.8) illustrates the procedure of nutritional involvement taking place in our body. Partial digestion of food in the oral cavity (pH 5–7), leads to food dissolution in the stomach at acidic conditions (pH 1–3), where it is stored for 1–4 h. Various enzymes such as pepsin act on the food to break down some proteins and carbohydrate. It then proceeds towards the duodenum where it is mixed with bile salts released by the gall bladder. In addition to the release of bile salts, a bicarbonate solution containing a cocktail of enzymes is also released in the duodenum increasing the pH to 6–7.5. The presence of small microvilli on the inner surface helps increase the surface area for nutrient absorption. Two mechanisms are responsible for nutrient absorption: active transport and passive transport.

For microencapsulation of probiotics, delivery of viable microbial cells into foods proceeding towards the targeted cells has become a topic of debate. Nevertheless, to overcome this problem, cultures that are encapsulated in alginate beads have shown an improved resilience to acid in the gastric environment and to bile salts (Kailasapathy and Masondole, 2005). When coated with the gel particles, the cells do not get released into the food when incorporated *in vitro* and *ex vivo*. Experimental studies showed that beads maintained their integrity in simulated stomach circumstances and subsequently release their load in the gastrointestinal tract. Microencapsulation can also serve to co-entrap prebiotics which are non-digestible food components enhancing the activity of bacteria in the gut. However, co-encapsulation with prebiotics has so far not proven better than glucose for enhancing the resilience of lactobacilli within gastrointestinal tracts (Iyer *et al.*, 2005). On the other hand, spray drying and fluidized coatings are the most accepted technique for the encapsulation of water-soluble

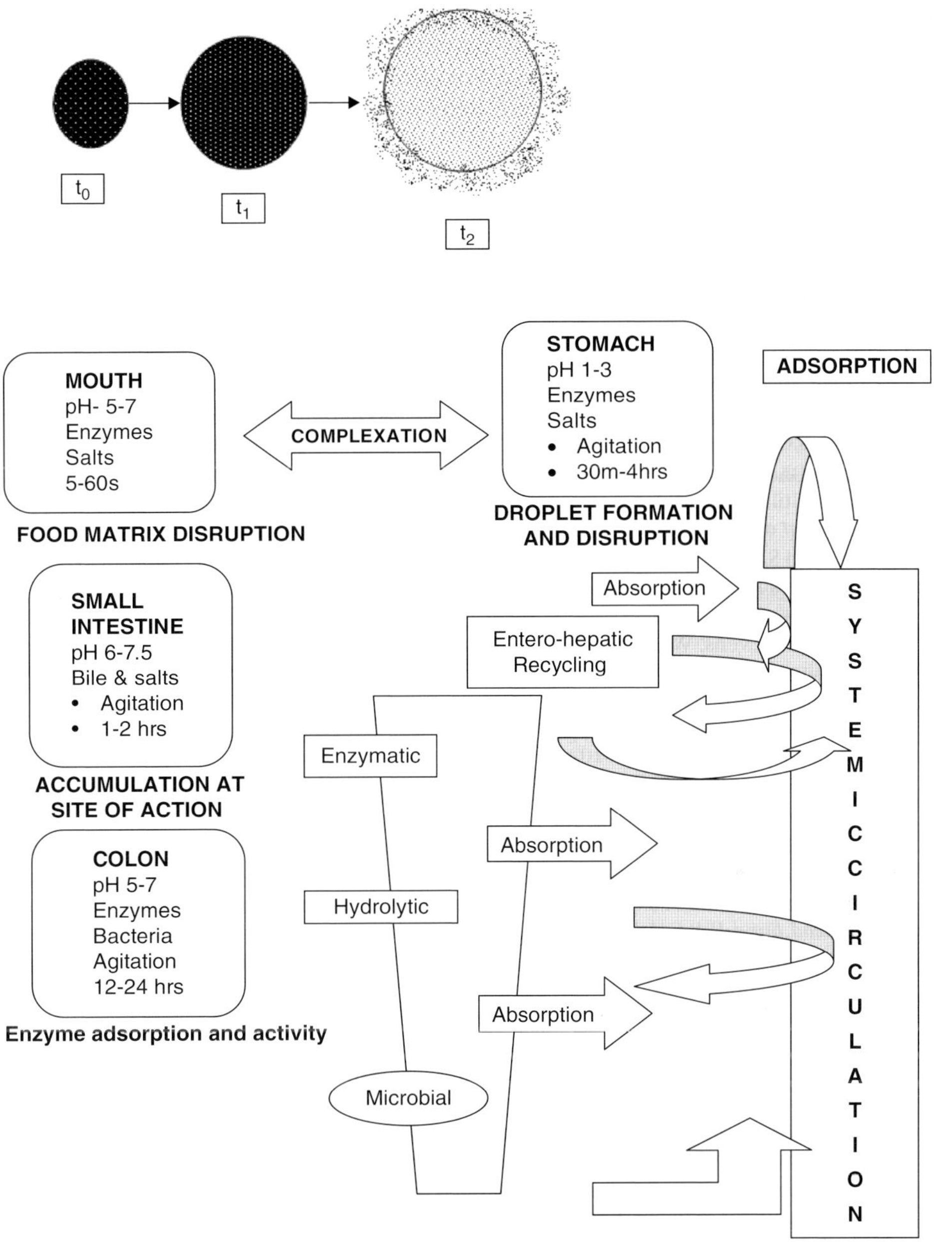

Figure 13.8 Representation of the complex physiochemical and physiological process that may occur during digestion, and absorption in the gastrointestinal tract

14.2 Food irradiation

Food irradiation uses energy emitted from ionizing radiation (Urbain, 1986), which is the propagation of energy through space that has the ability to penetrate into the food. It interacts with the atoms and molecules of food and food contaminants and causes ionization, which is a process in which one or more orbital electrons are removed from an atom, consequently inducing alterations to its chemical and biological properties.

Generally, ionization requires a certain minimum amount of radiation energy, which is absorbed by orbital electrons and raises their energy level from ground state to electronically excited state. When the electron absorbs sufficient energy, it may leave the atom and be free from the control of the nucleus. Thus, two separate bodies are formed: a free or unpaired electron with a negative electric charge and the residue of the atom – the ion – with a positive electric charge. From electromagnetic spectrum, radiation with a short wavelength (high frequency) – ultraviolet, X rays and gamma rays – has great energy (>4 eV) and is capable of causing ionization.

Commonly two techniques introduced for commercial food irradiation are gamma rays (electromagnetic radiation produced during the decay of certain radio-isotopes, e.g. cobalt-60 or caesium-137), and electron accelerators (which produce high-energy electron beams and accelerate them to very high speeds). The process of electron acceleration is non-nuclear but the degree of irradiation penetration is much less than that of gamma irradiation.

Food irradiation has many useful applications: sprouting inhibition in potatoes, onions and garlic; killing insects and parasites in cereal grains, dried beans, dried and fresh fruits, meat and seafood; delaying ripening and spoilage of fresh fruits and vegetables; extending the shelf life of perishable products like beef, poultry and seafood; eliminating pathogenic bacteria, fungal spores and viruses causing foodborne diseases; sterilizing herbs, dried vegetables, food prescribed for immunocompromised hospital patients and for astronauts during space flight (Crawford and Ruff, 1996). Absorbed dose, which refers to the mean quantity of energy transferred and absorbed by a mass of material, is a key factor determining the application of food irradiation. The SI unit for irradiation dose is the gray (Gy), which is equal to the absorption of 1 J/kg. The purposes of food irradiation at varying dose levels are summarized in Table 14.1.

Food irradiation has been approved as a safe and effective technology by many international authorities such as the World Health Organization (WHO), Food and Agriculture Organization (FAO), International Atomic Energy Agency (IAEA), Food and Drug Administration (FDA), US Department of Agriculture (USDA), US Department of Defense and the US Army and National Aeronautics and Space Administration. Many national authorities have endorsed the irradiation of various foods. In 1980 the Joint Expert Committee on Food Irradiation assembled by FAO, IAEA and WHO concluded that irradiation of any food commodity up to an overall average dose of 10 kGy presents no toxicological hazard and hence toxicological testing of foods is no longer required. WHO (1981) pronounced that irradiation up to 10 kGy introduces no special nutritional or microbiological problems in foods.

14.3 Chemical effects of food irradiation

As explained by Urbain (1986), incident ionizing irradiation transfers energy to the absorber and subsequently generates chemical changes in the molecules of the

Table 14.1 Application of food irradiation

Dose level	Purpose	Product examples
Low dose disinfestation/ delay in ripening (up to 1 kGy)	Inhibits the growth of sprouts on potatoes and other foods Kills insects and larvae that can be found in wheat, flour, fruits and vegetables after harvesting Slows the ripening process Kill certain harmful parasites associated with foods	Potatoes, onions, garlic, root ginger, bananas, mangoes and certain other non-citrus fruit, cereals and pulses, dehydrated vegetables, dried fish and meal, fresh pork
Medium dose pasteurization (1–10 kGy)	Dramatically reduces the number of or eliminates certain microbes and parasites that cause food to spoil Reduces or eliminates a number of pathogenic microorganisms	Fresh fish, strawberries, grapes, dehydrated vegetables, fresh or frozen seafood, raw or frozen poultry and meat
High dose sterilization (10–50 kGy)	Sterilizes food for a variety of uses, such as meals for hospital patients who suffer from immune disorders and can eat only bacteria-free foods Eliminates some disease-causing viruses Decontaminates certain food additives and ingredients	Meat, poultry, seafood and other food prepared for sterilized hospital diets, spices, enzyme preparations, natural gum

Source: Crawford & Ruff, 1996. Reproduced with permission from Pergamon.

absorber, which is usually food and food contaminants. Absorber atoms gaining energy without losing electrons become 'excited atoms', whereas, atoms that lose electrons turn into 'ions'. Both excited atoms and ions are unstable and chemically reactive because they contain abnormal amounts of energy. They can retain extra energy for a period of 10^{-8} s. Loss of the excitation energy may occur after emission of energy as a photon (fluorescence), internal conversion to heat, transfer to a neighbouring molecule or during a chemical reaction. Unstable atoms and ions can chemically react with the reactants that are identical with their own or a new entity, through isomerization, dissociation, electron transfer, abstraction (of hydrogen) and addition. The new products formed may be stable molecules or reactive entities as free radicals, which are atoms or molecules with one or more unpaired electrons available to form a chemical bond. Additional chemical changes are possible when the new molecules interact with themselves, with other molecules or with free radicals and this is termed an indirect effect of irradiation. Consequences of the chemical reactions induced by irradiation are called radiolytic products.

Water content in food and food contaminants such as bacteria plays an important role in the indirect effects of food irradiation. Irradiation of pure water yields a number of highly reactive chemicals such as hydroxyl radicals ($\cdot OH$), aqueous electrons (e^-), hydrogen atoms ($H\cdot$), H_2, H_2O_2, and H_3O^+. These products react with many substances dissolved in water. Likewise liquid water assists the movement of primary radiolytic products to interact with other substances and subsequently increases the indirect action of radiation. Thus, irradiation parameters affecting formation of radiolytic products are dose, dose rate, water content, temperature, oxygen and additives.

The direct and indirect effects of food irradiation cause chemical changes in food components and living microorganisms contaminating food, the elimination of which is the aim of irradiation. For low molecular carbohydrates in the solid state, the occurrence of physical changes in melting point, optical rotation and absorption spectra indicates that there has been a chemical change after irradiation. A number of radiolytic products are formed such as formaldehyde, acetaldehyde, acetone, acid derivatives, lactones, malonaldehyde and derived sugar (Diehl *et al.*, 1978). In aqueous solution, low molecular sugars undergo oxidative degradation through interaction with the radiolytic products of water. Irradiation possibly breaks the glycosidic bond of disaccharides and polysaccharides such as starch, pectin, cellulose and thus smaller carbohydrate units are released. Radiation degradation of starch is observed from changes of cooking quality, texture and the reduction of viscosity in starch, flour and foods mainly containing starch (Lee, 1959; Ananthaswamy *et al.*, 1970; Roushdi *et al.*, 1981; MacArther and D'Appolonia, 1984; Rao and Vakil, 1985; Wootton *et al.*, 1988; Sabularse *et al.*, 1991; Roy *et al.* 1991; Navanugraha and Grant, 1992; Sokhey and Chinnaswamy, 1993; Hayashi *et al.*, 1997; Bao *et al.*, 2001; Sirisoontaralak and Noomhorm, 2006). Irradiation of foods composed of sugars and amino acid leads to polymerization followed by a browning effect. The Maillard reaction is claimed as a major reaction causing the increased yellowness of irradiated flours and cereals (Chaudhry and Glew, 1973; Roushdi *et al.*, 1981; Wootton *et al.*, 1988; Roy *et al.*, 1991; Sabularse *et al.*, 1992; Sirisoontaralak and Noomhorm, 2006).

Amino acids undergo reductive deamination and decarboxylation and radiolytic products are formed such as NH_3, CO_2, H_2, methylamine, acetic acid and formaldehyde, whereas peptides experience main chain degradation and yield amide-like products. The presence of thiol or disulfide groups increases sensitivity to irradiation. For wet proteins, irradiation disturbs the secondary and tertiary structure of the protein which exposes reactive groups to the action of the radiolytic products of water. This causes protein denaturation, splitting protein into smaller units or causing aggregation. Changes in the primary structure also occur through deamination, decarboxylation and oxidation of –SH and aromatic groups (Urbain, 1986). Destruction of a number of amino acids, especially ring-structured amino acids, has been reported (Drake *et al.*, 1957).

In fatty acids, the preferential cleavage of the oxygen atom of the carbonyl group or the double bond of unsaturated fatty acids satisfies the electron deficiency. This leads to the formation of particular intermediate free radicals and ultimately to particular end products such as CO_2, CO, H_2, alkanes and aldehydes. In the presence of oxygen, the free radicals may form hydroperoxides, which yield a number of products including aldehydes. Cleavage of triglycerides favourably occurs at bonds near carbonyl groups and consequently free radicals are formed. Free radicals turn to stable end products by abstraction, dissociation, recombination, disproportionation and radical–molecular interaction. In the presence of oxygen during or after irradiation, radiation accelerates auto-oxidation of lipids through formation of hydroperoxides, aldehydes, ketones and oxidized fats (Urbain, 1986). Thus, irradiation of foods containing lipids in the absence of oxygen is recommended as well as maintaining oxygen-free conditions after irradiation.

Apart from major food components, radiolytic products generated by irradiation can either increase or decrease the amount of bioactive compounds in materials. Note that food material with a high water content responded to irradiation, which led to a high content of radiolytic products. Chemical effects of irradiation on bioactive compounds are discussed in subsequent sections.

14.4 Application of gamma irradiation and its effect on bioactive compounds

14.4.1 Herbs

Herbs in Asia have been used in traditional medicine for the treatment of chronic diseases (van Rossum *et al.*, 1998, Fukai *et al.*, 2002, Krishnaiah *et al.*, 2011) and are often used as spices to flavour some foods (Aljabre *et al.*, 2005). However, during harvest, process and transportation, herbs are susceptible to contamination by microorganisms. Microbial decontamination is required to improve their hygienic quality as well as to reduce economic loss. An irradiation dose between 5 and 30 kGy can completely inactivate microorganisms (Pérez *et al.*, 2007; Khattak *et al.*, 2008; Khattak and Simpson, 2010; Aouidi *et al.*, 2011; Chiang *et al.*, 2011). The dose required to treat each material depends on the radioresistance of the microorganisms. In food with a high moisture content, microorganisms are more sensitive to radiation because more radiolytic products are generated (Al-Bachir *et al.*, 2003; Aouidi *et al.*, 2011). However, excess radiolytic products can damage the chemical structures of some bioactive compounds resulting in the loss of biological activities, such as 2,3,5,4′-tetra-hydroxystilbene-2-0-glucoside (THSG) in Polygoni Multiflori Radix (Chiang *et al.*, 2011). The THSG content decreased when irradiation dose increased (Figure 14.1). This compound is effectively protects against myocardial ischaemia–reperfusion injury (Ye *et al.*, 2006). Similarly, Khattak and Simpson (2010) found that the antibacterial activity of *Glycyrrhiza glabra* root decreased after irraditation at 25 kGy. Thus, the optimum dose for prolonging the shelf life of herbs is not only elimination of microbes, but also maintaining or enhancing biological activities in the herbs.

The optimum irradiation dose to preserve and improve the scavenging activity of some herbs is shown in Table 14.2. Increasing the scavenging activity of the irradiated

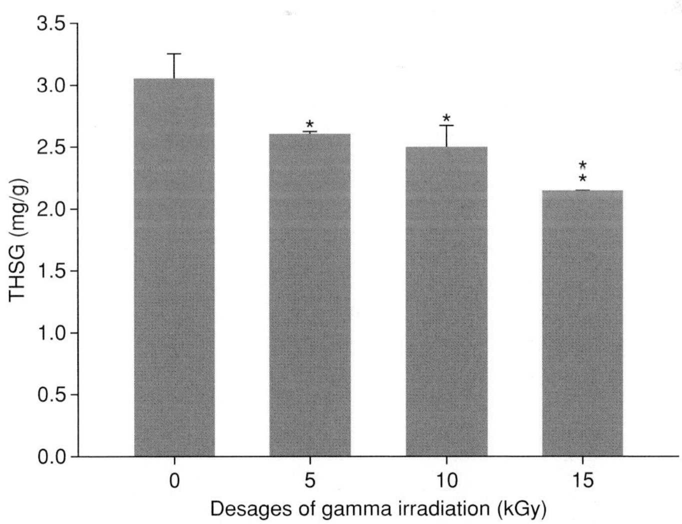

Figure 14.1 The 2,3,5,4′-tetra-hydroxystilbene-2-0-glucoside (THSH) contents in the methanol extracts of irradiated Polygoni Multiflori Radix. *Source:* Chiang *et al.*, 2011. Reproduced with permission from Elsevier

Table 14.2 The optimum irradiation dose for preserve and improve the scavenging activity of some herbs

Herbs	Main bioactive constituents	Benefits	Irradiation Dose (kGy)	Reference
Polygoni Multiflori Radix	2,3,5,4′-Tetra-hyproxystilben-2-*O*-glucoside	• Used for the treatment of liver diseases, anemia, hypopigmentary skin disease, prevention of hair-graying etc.	5	Chiang *et al.*, 2011
Nigella sativa seed	Thymoquinone, thymohycroquinone, dithymoquinone, thymol, carvacrol, migellicine, nigellone, nigellimine-*N*-oxide, nigellidine and α-hedrin	• Used for treatment of asthma, cough, bronchitis, headache, rheumatism, fever, kidney and liver disorder etc.	16	Khattak *et al.*, 2008
Glycyrrhiza glabra root	Glycyrrhizin, glycyrrhizinic acid, glabrin A&B, glycyrrhetol and glabrolide	• Give sweet taste for some food products. • Used for the treatment of sore throats, coughs, asthma, gastric ulcers, allergic reactions, eczema, rheumatism, arthritic and hepatitis and atopic dermatitis etc. • Antimicrobial	20	Khattak and Simpson, 2010
Olea europaea tree	Oleuropein, verbascoside, luteolin-7-glucoside and rutin	• Used for treatment of diabetes, cardiovascular diseases, viral and microbial infection	25	Aouidi *et al.*, 2011
Rosemary	Carnosic acid, carnosol, rosmanol, ep;I and iso-rosmanol, romadial and methyl carnosate, rosmarinic acid, caffeic acid and flavonoids	• Antibacterial and antimutagenic properties	30	Pérez *et al.*, 2007

Table 14.3 Total phenolics, ortho-diphenold and flavonoids contents in olive leaves presented in intact and powdered forms to gamma irradiation at different dose

Form of olive leaves	Dose (kGy)	Total phenolics content. (mg GAE $g^{-1\ DM}$)	*Ortho*-diphenols content (mg CAE/g ^{DM})	Flavonoids content (mg RE/g ^{DM})
Powder	0	53.05 ± 1.61^{ab}	9.46 ± 0.72^{a}	18.68 ± 0.27^{a}
	5	50.11 ± 1.56^{a}	8.19 ± 0.68^{b}	14.62 ± 0.96^{c}
	10	54.21 ± 1.44^{b}	11.57 ± 0.68^{c}	17.75 ± 0.29^{ab}
	15	50.66 ± 4.53^{ab}	10.05 ± 0.19^{a}	16.71 ± 1.09^{b}
	20	53.46 ± 3.37^{ab}	9.31 ± 0.20^{ab}	20.19 ± 1.13^{d}
	25	53.18 ± 2.02^{ab}	9.98 ± 1.52^{a}	20.16 ± 1.43^{d}
Intact olive leaves	0	63.98 ± 3.47^{a}	8.52 ± 2.91^{ab}	18.65 ± 0.44^{a}
	5	56.61 ± 1.39^{b}	7.47 ± 1.50^{ab}	15.03 ± 0.52^{a}
	10	59.12 ± 3.18^{ab}	9.03 ± 0.56^{ab}	16.05 ± 0.27^{a}
	15	60.96 ± 7.61^{ab}	10.20 ± 1.49^{a}	15.23 ± 2.23^{a}
	20	59.23 ± 2.93^{ab}	7.34 ± 1.94^{b}	18.07 ± 3.74^{a}
	25	62.09 ± 1.86^{ab}	7.82 ± 2.01^{ab}	18.11 ± 4.19^{a}

Means in the same column followed by different lower case superscripts are significantly different ($p < 0.05$).
GAE, gallic acid equivalents; CAE, caffeic acid equivalents; RE, rutin equivalents; DM, dry matter.
Source: Aouidi *et al.*, 2011. Reproduced with permission from Elsevier.

herbs was related to increasing phenolic compound content. Two mechanisms supported high levels of total phenolics: (i) degradation of larger phenolic compounds (e.g. tannins) into smaller ones (Variyar *et al.*, 1998) and (ii) induced formation of new compounds with higher antioxidant activity, such as found in the water-soluble quinine-type compounds in irradiated Lamiaceae herbs and dry rosemary leaf powder at a dose of 10 and 30 kGy, respectively (Calucci *et al.*, 2003; Pérez *et al.*, 2007). However, depolymerization of high molecular weight compounds and new compound formation were not observed in herbs with a low moisture content (Murcia *et al.*, 2004).

Herbs with a low moisture content still presented antioxidant content and activity equal to the non-irradiation treatment when irradiated at a high dose (Table 14.3), possibly be due to the low level of radiolytic product. Table 14.3 shows that altering the bioactive content also depended on herbs' characteristics; powder forms were altered more than original forms.

Although irradiation improved the health benefits of some herbs, irradiation of the polyethylene or polypropylene bag as well as the herb may play an important role because some components in plastic material – such as the phosphate stabilizer – were destroyed. Low molecular weight volatile compounds (e.g. 1,3-di-tert-butylbenzene) were released that may potentially be harmful to the consumer (Lee *et al.*, 2004).

14.4.2 Fruits and vegetables

Gamma irradiation has become an important technology in the fruit and vegetable industry because the tendency of consumers to want fresh food materials and unpasteurized products has been increased. In fresh fruits, firmness is the main property that affects its acceptance by consumers. Loss of firmness during maturation and storage occurs due to the degradation of pectin in the middle lamella and primary cell wall (Silva *et al.*, 2012). The major enzymes that responded to pectin degradation were polygalacturonase and pectinametilesterase (Singh and Dwivedi, 2008). Low-dose gamma irradiation (0.03–0.5 kGy) can inactivate these enzymes; therefore, the dose has been used to delay ripening of agricultural products (Uthairatanakij *et al.*, 2006). Patil *et al.* (2004) found that an irradiation dose at or below 0.2 kGy enhanced flavonone and terpenoid contents in 'Rio Red' grapefruit, particularly during storage at 10 °C for 35 days. Similarly, Hussain *et al.* (2010) found that antioxidant activity and anthocyanin content increased in peach (*Prunus persica Bausch,* Cv. Elberta) treated with gamma irradiation in the dose range 1.6–2.0 kGy as well as storage under refrigerated conditions (3 ± 1 °C, RH 80%). Note that irradiation not only delays ripening, but also enhances health promoting compounds in fresh fruits. The increase of antioxidant activity and the amount of bioactive compounds (e.g. phenolic compounds and anthocyanins, etc.) in the irradiated fresh fruits is due to: (i) the release of phenolic compounds from glycosidic compounds and the degradation of multimeric phenolic compounds to monomeric phenolic compounds by radiolytic products (Harrison and Were, 2007); and (ii) the increase in phenylalanine ammonia-lyase (PAL) activity during storage at low temperatures (3–10 °C, RH 80–95%) (Faragher, 1983; Oufedjikh *et al.,* 1996; Benoit *et al.,* 2000; Patil *et al.,* 2004; Hussain *et al.,* 2010). PAL is the main enzyme for the metabolism of phenols (Camm and Towers, 1973) and involves anthocyanin biosynthesis from phenylalanine (Cheng and Breen, 1991).

An irradiation dose between 3 and 12 kGy is able to break polysaccharide bonds in the cell wall (Figure 14.2) and leads to soft tissue (Nayak *et al.,* 2007). It has been used to increase the efficiency of extraction. Generally, flavonoids (e.g. quercetin and anthocyanins, etc.) are synthesized in the cytoplasm and vacuoles of plant cells (Markham *et al.,* 2000). Thus, degradation of the cell wall and vacuole of a plant cell affects leaching of flavonoids or other water-soluble compounds. Yang *et al.* (2012) found that the yield of quercetin (Figure 14.3a) and antioxidant activity (Figure 14.3b) of onion skin extract increased after irradiation at 10 kGy.

Ayed *et al.* (1999) found that irradiation inhibited the loss of anthocyanins in grape pomace extract, possibly due inhibition of an enzyme that has an influence on the stability of anthocyanins, such as anthocyanase, phenoloxidase and peroxidase (Constantinovici *et al.,* 2009). On the other hand, loss of anthocyanins was observed in irradiated juices, particularly monoglucoside forms (Figure 14.4) (Ailghourchi *et al.,* 2008). However, the yield of anthocyanins in juice or fruit extract might be improved by adding reducing agents (e.g. sodium metabisulfite) during extraction (Ayed *et al.,* 1999). Sulfur dioxide can react with the monomeric anthocyanin and form an uncharged anthocyanin sulfur dioxide complex (Langston, 1985).

14.4.3 Cereals

It is well known that insect damage and microbial growth are an important problem during cereals storage. Gamma irradiation in the dose range 0.1–5.0 kGy effectively kills insects and eliminates microorganisms from cereals. However, it induces a change of physicochemical properties. Generally, at dosages above 0.2 kGy, cereal grains had high water absorption, low cooking time and low flour paste viscosity (Sung, 2005; Sirisoontaralak and Noomhorm, 2006, 2007; Sung *et al.,* 2008). These

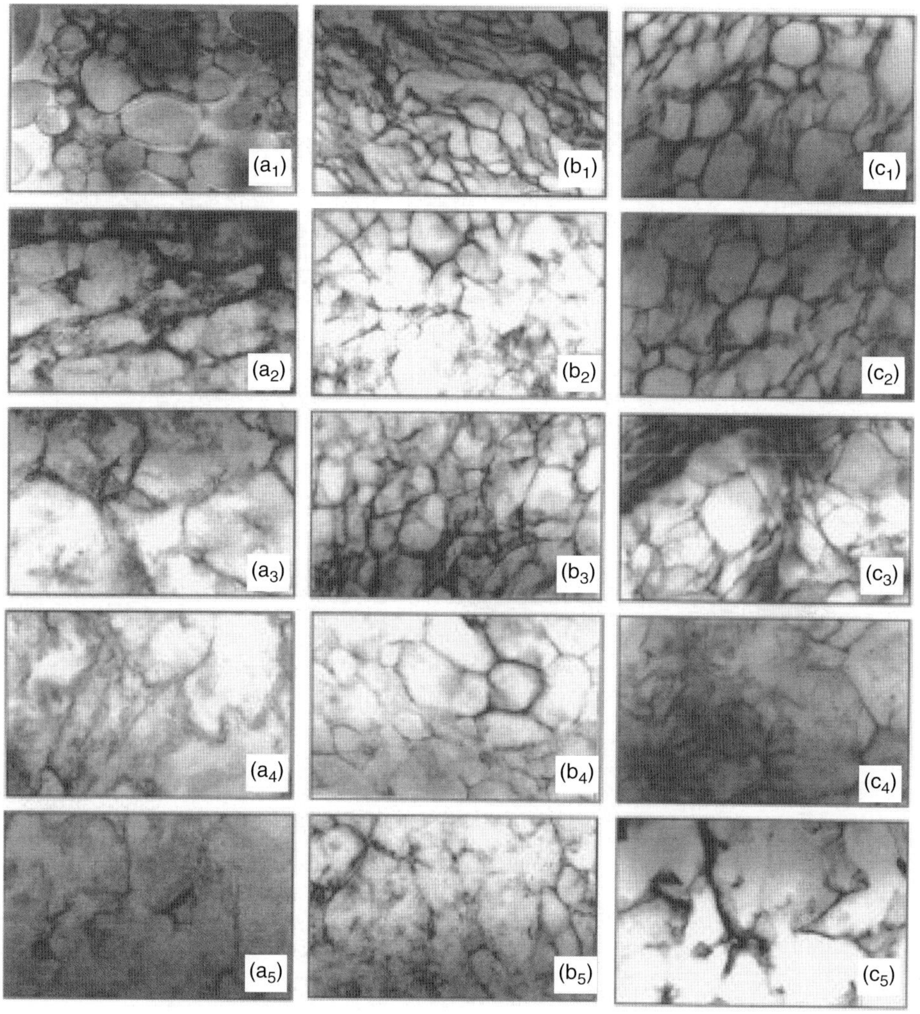

Figure 14.2 Photomicrographs of (a) potato, (b) carrot and (c) beetroot after gamma irradiation at different doses: 1 = 0 kGy, 2 = 3 kGy, 3 = 6 kGy, 4 = 9 kGy and 5 = 12 kGy. x400. *Source:* Nayak *et al.*, 2007. Reproduced with permission from Elsevier

properties may be suitable for some food products (e.g. noodle). Increasing resistant starch content was observed when the irradiation dose was above 10 kGy (Chung and Liu, 2010), which may benefit health.

Cereals contain not only starch but also a wide range of bioactive compounds, such as phenolic acids and flavonoids. Wheat grains irradiated at 0.1 kGy stimulated carotenoid biosynthesis and resulted in more carotenoid content than non-irradiated grains (Singh and Datta., 2011). Although the carotenoid content (0.60 μg/g) in the grain was still lower than that present in carrots, it indicated that gamma irradiation could be used to improve the health benefits of cereals. Kökselt *et al.* (1998) reported

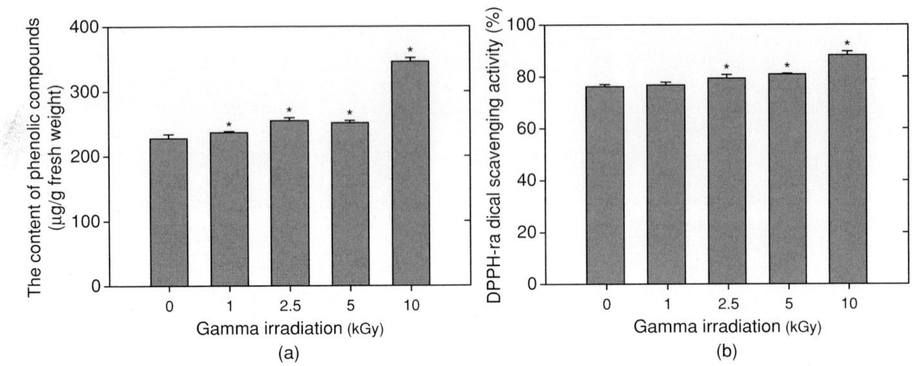

Figure 14.3 The properties of onion skin extracts after gamma irradiation in the dose range 0-10 kGy. (a) Total phenolic compound contents and (b) DPPH radical-scavenging activity. *Source:* Yang *et al.*, 2012. Reproduced with permission from Pergamon

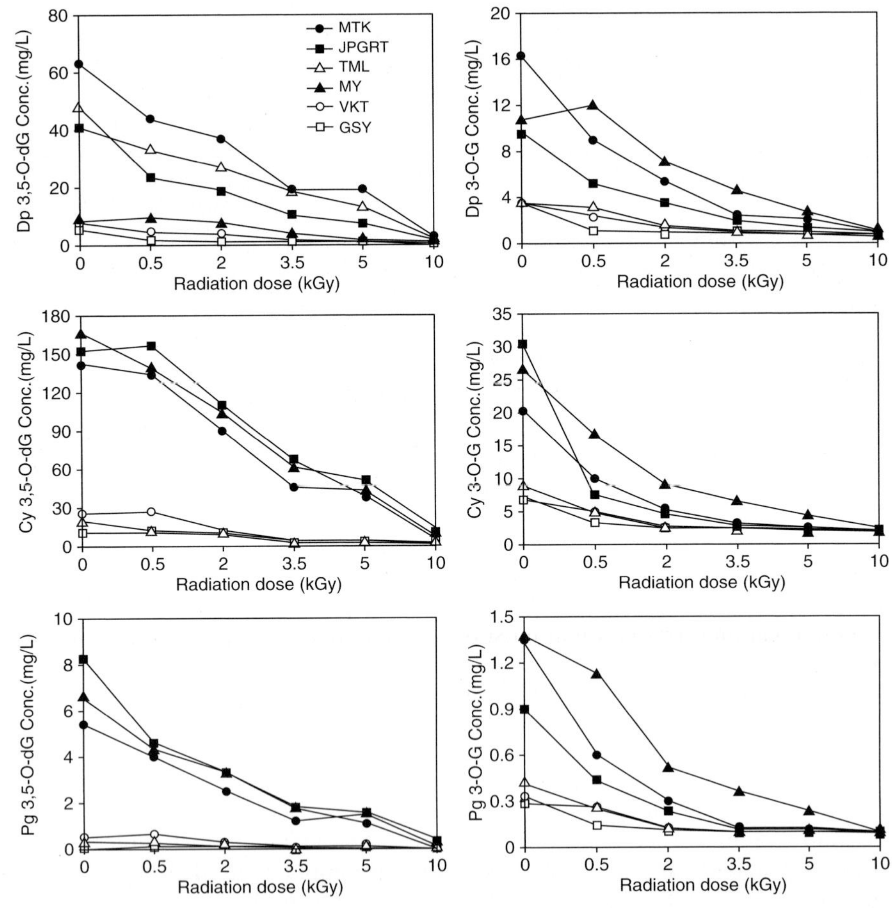

Figure 14.4 Evolution of the individual anthocyanin concentrations of pomegranate juices at different doses of irradiation. *Source:* Ailghourchi *et al.*, 2008. Reproduced with permission from Elseiver

Table 14.4 Effect of gamma irradiation on phenolic acids and anthocyanins in brown rice

	Phenolic acids[A]		Anthocyanins[B]	
Irradiation dose (kGy)	Black rice	Red rice	White rice	Black rice
0	381.6 ± 13.9^{b}	713.3 ± 14.2^{a}	417.5 ± 15.1^{a}	346.6 ± 8.4^{b}
2	314.8 ± 6.1^{c}	643.2 ± 9.5^{b}	430.4 ± 7.3^{a}	324.4 ± 5.7^{c}
4	332.2 ± 9.6^{c}	574.3 ± 22.2^{c}	382.7 ± 5.6^{b}	306.5 ± 3.7^{d}
6	268.9 ± 5.4^{d}	490.3 ± 10.1^{d}	250.4 ± 4.6^{d}	378.3 ± 10.6^{a}
8	423.3 ± 4.6^{a}	470.9 ± 9.6^{d}	353.3 ± 4.3^{c}	$312.5 \pm 9.6^{c,d}$
10	371.0 ± 9.4^{b}	558.8 ± 15.3^{c}	380.8 ± 9.1^{b}	261.5 ± 6.2^{e}

Means in the same column followed by different lower case superscripts are significantly different ($p < 0.05$).
[A]Total content of phenolic acids (ferulic acid, ρ-coumaric acid, and sinapinic acid) were expressed as ferulic acid equivalents mg/kg rice flour (dry basis).
[B]Total content of anthocyanins (cyanidin-3-glucoside and peonidin-3-glucoside) were expressed as cyanidin-3-glucoside equivalents mg/kg rice flour (dry basis).
Source: Zhu *et al.*, 2010. Reproduced with permission from Elsevier.

that rheological properties of dough from wheat flour reduced with increasing irradiation dosage greater than 5 kGy. Furthermore, a low irradiation dose (e.g. 0.002–0.016 kGy) induced seed or grain survival under mildly stressful conditions. Seeds or grains protected themselves from radiolytic products damage by producing detoxifying enzymes, namely superoxide dismutase, catalase and peroxidase (Zaka *et al.*, 2002; Kim *et al.*, 2004). These enzymes possess high antioxidant potential (Apel and Hirt, 2004). Treating cereal grains with a low dose of irradiation may be one method for preparing functional food or dietary supplements materials.

In rice (*Oryza sativa* L.), the major phenolic acids founds in the rice grain are ρ-coumaric acid, ferulic acid and sinapinic acid (Zhu, 2010). Coloured rice is thought to have high levels of anthocyanins (Escribano-Bailón *et al.*, 2004). Two anthocyanins have been identified in pigmented grain samples: cyanidin-3-*O*-β-glucoside and peonidin-3-*O*-β-glucoside (Abdel-Aal *et al.*, 2006; Yawadio *et al.*, 2007; Zhu *et al.*, 2010). Generally, parboiling and cooking reduced bioactive compound content and its biological activity in rice grains (Massaretto *et al.*, 2011). Loss of bioactive compound might be due to thermal decomposition and interaction with other components in the grains during heating (Walter *et al.*, 2013). Although, irradiation is a non-thermal process, radiolytic products could alter bioactive compound contents in rice grains, particularly white rice and rice with a red pericarp (Table 14.4). Zhu *et al.* (2010) showed that gamma-irradiation at most doses could decrease total phenolic acid and anthocyanins content of both red and white rice, whereas irradiation at 6 and 8 kGy increased total anthocyanins and phenolic acids in black rice, respectively.

14.4.4 Polysaccharide

It has been reported that some polysaccharides (e.g. chitosan and laminarin) possesses antimicrobial or antitumour activity (Srinvastava and Kulshŕestha, 1989; Miyanishi *et al.*, 2003; Wasser, 2003; Choi *et al.*, 2011). The biological activity of the polysaccharide depended on the molar mass, type and number of functional groups

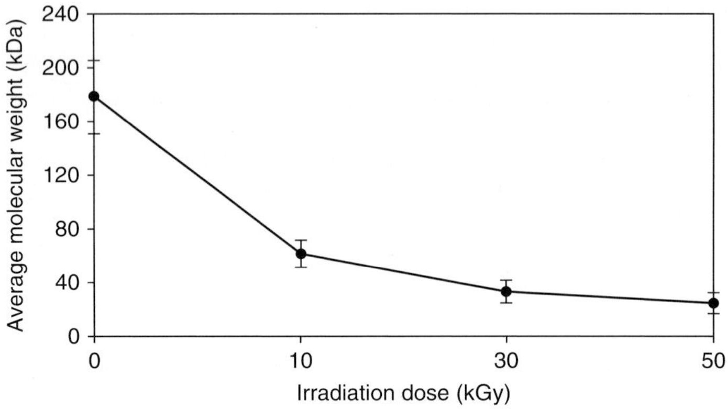

Figure 14.5 The effect of gamma irradiation on the molecular weight of β-glucan at dose of 0, 10, 30 and 50 kDa. *Source:* Byun *et al.*, 2008. Reproduced with permission from Pergamon

in the structure (Voegeli *et al.*, 1993; Qi, *et al.*, 2005; Choi *et al.* 2011). Low molecular weight polysaccharides had more biological activity than high molecular weight polysaccharides. Generally, enzymatic degradation (e.g. β-1,3 glucanase) is a widely used method for polysaccharide preparation (Miyanishi *et al.*, 2003), but it needs a long process time and is very expensive. Byun *et al.* (2008) found that the average molecular weight of β-glucan decreased as the irradiation dose increased (Figure 14.5). Similarly, Choi *et al.* (2011) and Feng *et al.* (2008) studied laminarin and chitosan, respectively. Thus, gamma irradiation could be used to prepare low molecular weight polysaccharide. As the process is simple, it is a better method when compared to using enzyme. Moreover, the low molecular weight polysaccharides produced had many carboxyl groups (Choi *et al.*, 2011) and high antioxidant activity (Figure 14.6).

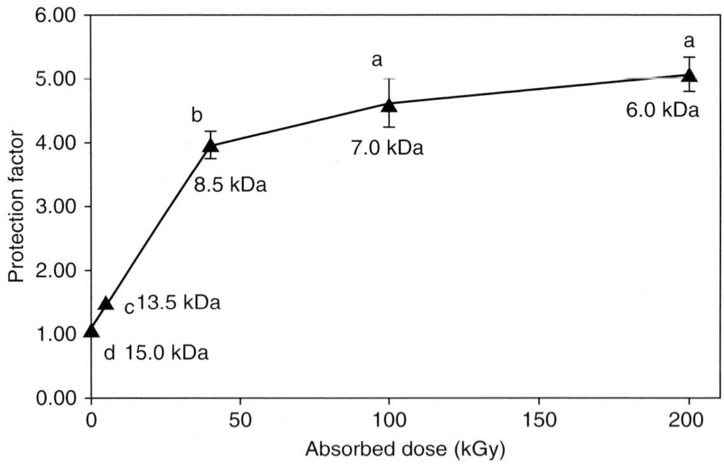

Figure 14.6 Protection factor of non-irradiated and gamma-irradiated laminarin measured at different absorbed doses by Rancimat test. *Source:* Choi *et al.*, 2011. Reproduced with permission from Elsevier

References

Abdel-Aal, E.S.M., Young, J.C. and Rabalski, I. (2006). Anthocyanin composition in black, blue, pink, purple and red cereal grains. *Journal of Agriculture and Food Chemistry*, 54, 4696–4706.

Abu-Tarboush, H.M., Al-Kahtani, H.A., Abou-Arab, A.A., Baijaber, A.S. and El-Mojadid, M.A. (1996). Sensory and microbial quality of chicken as affected by irradiation and post-irradiation on storage at 4°C. *Journal of Food Protection*, 60, 761–770.

Ailghourchi, H., Barzegar, M. and Abbasi, S. (2008). Effect of gamma irradiation on the stability of anthocyanins and shelf-life of various pomegranate juices. *Food Chemistry*, 110, 1036–1040.

Al-Bachir, M., Al-Adawi, M.A. and Asma, M. (2003). Synergetic effect of gamma irradiation and moisture content on decontamination of sewage sludge. *Bioresource Technology*, 62, 342–348.

Aljabre, S.H.M., Randhawa, M.A., Akhtar, N. *et al.* (2005). Atidermatophyte activity of ether extract of *Nigella sativa* and its active principle, thymoquinone. *Journal of Ethnopharmacology*, 101, 116–119.

Ananthaswamy, H.N., Vakil, U.K. and Sreenivasan, A. (1970). Effect of gamma irradiation on wheat starch and its components. *Journal of Food Science*, 35, 795.

Aouidi, F., Ayari, S., Ferhi, H., Rousson, S. and Hamdi, M. 2011. Gamma irradiation of air-dried olive leaves: Effective decontamination and impact on the antioxidative properties and on phenolic compounds. *Food Chemistry*, 127, 1105–1113.

Apel, K. and Hirt, H. (2004). Reactive oxygen species: Metabolism, oxidative stress, and signal transduction. *Annual Review of Plant Biology*, 55L, 373–399.

Ayed, N., Yu, H.-L. and Lacroix, M. (1999). Improvement of anthocyanin yield and shelf-life extension of grape pomace by gamma irradiation. *Food Research International*, 32, 539–543.

Bao, J., Shu, Q., Xia, Y., Bergman, C. and McClung, A. (2001). Effects of gamma irradiation on aspects of milled rice (*Oryza sativa*) end-use quality. *Journal of Food Quality*, 24, 327–336.

Beaulieu, M. Lacroix, M., Charbonneau, R., Laberge, I. and Gagnon, M. (1992). Effects of gamma irradiation dose rate on microbiological and physical quality of mushrooms (*Agaricus bisporus*). *Sciences des Aliments*, 12, 289–303.

Benoit, M.A., D'Aprano, G. and Lacroix, M. (2000). Effect of gamma irradiation on phenylalanine ammonia-lyase activity, total phenolic content, and respiration of mushroom (*Agaricus bisporus*). *Journal of Agricultural and Food Chemistry*, 48, 6312–6316.

Byun, E.H., Kim, J.H., Sung, N.Y. *et al.* (2008). Effects of gamma irradiation on the physical and structural properties of β-glucan. *Radiation Physics and Chemistry*, 77, 781–786.

Cai, Y.Z., Luo, Q., Sun, M. and Corke, H. (2004). Antioxidant activity and phenolic compounds of 112 traditional Chinese medicinal plants associated with anticancer. *Life Science*, 74, 2157–2184.

Calucci, L., Pinzino, C., Zandomeneghi, M., Capocchi, A., Ghiringhelli, S. and Saviozzi, F. (2003). Effects of γ-irradiation on the free radical and antioxidant contents in nine aromatic herbs and spices. *Journal of Agricultural and Food Chemistry*, 51, 927–934.

Camm, E.L. and Towers, G.H.N. (1973). Review article, phenylalanine ammonia-lyase. *Phytochemistry*, 12, 961–973.

Chaudhry, M.A. and Glew, G. (1973). The effect of ionizing radiations on some physical and chemical properties of Pakistani rice. *Journal of Food Technology*, 8, 295–303.

Cheng, G.W. and Breen, P.J. (1991). Activity of phenylalanine ammonia-lyase (PAL) and concentrations of anthocyanins and phenolics in developing strawberry fruit. *Journal of the American Society for Horticultural Science*, 116, 865–869.

Chiang, Y.C., Huang, G.J., Ho, Y.L. *et al.* (2011). Influence of gamma irradiation on microbial load and antioxidative characteristics of Polygoni Multiflori Radix. *Process Biochemistry*, 46, 777–782.

Choi, J.-i, Kim, H.J. and Lee, J.W. (2011). Structural feature an antioxidant activity of low molecular weight laminarin degraded by gamma irradiation. *Food Chemistry*, 129, 520–523.

Chung, H.J. and Liu, Q. (2010). Molecular structure and physicochemical properties of potato and bean starches as affected by gamma-irradiation. *International Journal of Biological Macromolecules*, 47, 214–222.

Constantinovici, M., Oancea, D. and Zaharescu, T. (2009). Gamma irradiation effect on the enzymatic activities of horseradish and apple peroxidases. *Radiation Physics and Chemistry*, 78, 33–36.

Crawford, L.M., and Ruff, E.H. (1996). A review of the safety of cold pasteurization through irradiation. *Food Control*, 7, 87–97.

Drake, M.P., Giffee, J.W., Johnson, D.J. and Koenig, V.L. (1957). Chemical effects of ionising radiation on proteins. I. Effect of gamma-radiation on amino acid content of insulin. *Journal of the American Chemical Society*, 79, 1395–1401.

Diehl, J.F., Adam, S., Delincee, H. and Jakubick, V. (1978). Radiolysis of carbohydrates and carbohydrate-containing foodstuffs. *Journal of Agriculture and Food Chemistry*, 26, 15.

Escribano-Bailón, M.T., Santos-Buelga, C. and Rivas-Gonzalo, J.C. (2004). Anthocyanins in cereals. *Journal of Chromatography A*, 1054, 129–141.

Faragher, J.D. (1983). Temperature regulation of anthocyanin accumulation in apple skins. *Journal of Experimental Botany*, 1291.

Feng, T., Du, Y., Li, J., Hu, Y. and Kennedy, J.F. (2008). Enhancement of antioxidant activity of chitosan by irradiation. *Carbohydrate Polymers*, 73, 126–132.

Fukai, T., Marumo, A., Kaitou, K. *et al.* (2002). Anti *Helicobacter pylori* flavonoids from Ilcorice extract. *Life Science*, 71, 1449–1463.

Harrison, K. and Were, L.M. (2007). Effect of gamma irradiation on total phenolic content yield and antioxidant capacity of almond skin extracts. *Food Chemistry*, 102, 932–937.

Hayashi, T., Takahashi, Y. and Todoriki, S. (1997). Low-energy electron effects on the sterility and viscosity of grains. *Journal of Food Science*, 62, 858–860.

Hussain, P.R., Wani, A.M., Meena, R.S. and Dar, M.A. (2010). Gamma irradiation induced enhancement of phenylalanine ammonia-lyase (PAL) and antioxidant activity in peach (*Prunus persica* Bausch, Cv. Elberta). *Radiation Physics and Chemistry*, 79, 982–989.

Khattak, K.F. and Simpson, T.J. (2010). Effect of gamma irradiation on the antimicrobial and free radical scavenging activities of *Glycyrrhiza glabra* root. *Radiation Physics and Chemistry*, 79, 507–512.

Khattak, K.F., Simpson, T.J. and Ihanullah. (2008). Effect of gamma irradiation on the extraction yield, total phenolic content and free radical-scavenging activity of *Nigella sativa* seed. *Food Chemistry*, 10, 967–972.

Kim, J.H., Baek, M.H., Chung, B.Y., Wi, S.G. and Kim, J.S. (2004). Alterations in the photosyntheitic pigments and antioxidant machineries of red pepper (*Capsicum annuum* L.) seedlings from gamma-irradiated seeds. *Journal of Plant Biology*, 47, 314–321.

Köksel, H., Sapirstein, H.D., Celikt, S. and Bushuk, W. (1998). Effects of gamma-irradiation of wheat on gluten proteins. *Journal of Cereal Science*, 28, 243–250.

Krishnaiah, D., Sarbatly, R. and Nithyanandam, R. (2011). A review of the antioxidant potential of medicinal plant species. *Food and Bioproducts Processing*, 89, 217–233.

Langston, M.S.K. (1985). Anthocyanin colorant from grape pomace. US Patent. No. 4. 400, 556.

Lee, C.C. (1959). The baking quality and maltose value of flour irradiated with CO^{60} gamma rays. *Cereal Chemistry*, 36, 70–77.

Lee, J.H., Sung, T.H., Lee, K.T. and Kim, M.R. (2004). Effect of gamma-irradiation on color, pungency, and volatiles of Korean red pepper powder. *Journal of Food Science*, 69, C585–C592.

Lefer, D.J. and Granger, D.N. (2000). Oxidative stress and cardiac disease. *American Journal of Medicine*, 109, 315–323.

MacArthur, L.A. and D'Appolonia, B.L. (1984). Gamma radiation of wheat. II. Effects of low-dosage radiations on starch properties. *Cereal Chemistry*, 61, 321–326.

Markham, K.R., Ryan, K.G., Gould, K.S. and Rickards, G.K. (2000). Cell wall sited flavonoids in lisianthus flower petals. *Phytochemistry*, 54, 681–687.

Massaretto, I.L., Alves, M.F.M., de Mira, N.V.M., Carmona, A.K. and Marquez, U.M.L. (2011). Phenolic compounds in raw and cooked rice (*Oryza sativa* L.) and their inhibitory effect on the activity of angiotensin I-converting enzyme. *Journal of Cereal Science*, 54, 236–240.

Miyanishi, N., Iwamoto, Y., Watanabe, E. and Oda, T. (2003). Induction of TNF-α production from human peripheral blood monocytes with β-1,3-glucan oligomer prepared from laminarin with β-1,3-glucanase from *Bacillus clausii* NM-1. *Journal of Bioscience and Bioengineering*, 95, 192–195.

Murcia, M.A., Egea, I. and Romojaro, J. (2004). Antioxidant evaluation in dessert spices compared with common food additives. Influence of irradiation procedure. *Journal of Agricultural and Food Chemistry*, 52, 1872–1881.

Navanugraha, U. and Grant, D.R. (1992). Effect of gamma irradiation on the cooking characteristics of wild rice (*Zizania aquatica* L.). *Food Research International*, 25, 199–202.

Nayak, C.A., Suguna, K., Narasimhamurthy, K. and Rastogi, N.K. (2007). Effect of gamma irradiation of histological and textural properties of carrot, potato and beetroot. *Journal of Food Engineering*, 79, 765–770.

Oufedjikh, H., Mahrouz, M., Amiot, M.J. and Lacroix, M. (1996). Effect of gamma irradiation on phenylalanine ammonialyase and phenolics compounds in Moroccan citrus elementina during storage, in *Proceedings of the 18th International Conference on Polyphenols*, vol. 2 (eds J. Vercauteren, C. Chèze, M.C. Dumon and J.F. Weber), 15–18 July, pp. 319–320.

Patil, B.S., Vanamala, J. and Hallman, G. (2004). Irradiation and storage influence on bioactive components and quality of early and late season 'Rio Red' grapefruit (*Citrus paradise* Macf.). *Postharvest Biology and Technology*, 34, 53–64.

Pérez, M.B., Calderón, N.L. and Croci, C.A. (2007). Radiation-induced enhancement of antioxidant activity in extracts of rosemary (*Rosmarinus officinalis* L.). *Food Chemistry*, 104, 585–592.

Qi, H., Zhao, T., Zhang, Q., Li, Z. and Zhao, Z. (2005). Antioxidant activity of different molecular weight sulfated polydaccharides from *Ulva pertusa* Kjellm (Chlorophyta). *Journal of Applied Phycology*, 17, 527–534.

Rahman, A., Rahman, M.M., Mominul, I.S. *et al.* (2008). Free radical scavenging activity and phenolic content of *Cassia sophera* L. *African Journal of Biotechnology*, 7, 1591–1593.

Rao, V.S. and Vakil, U.K. (1985). Effects of gamma irradiation on cooking quality and sensory attributes of four legumes. *Journal of Food Science*, 50, 372–375, 378.

van Rossum, T.G., Vulto, A.G., de Man, R.A., Brouwer, J.T. and Schalm, S.W. (1998). Review article, glycyrrhizin as a potential treatment of chronic hepatitis C. *Alimentary Pharmacology & Therapeutics*, 12, 199–205.

Roushdi, M., Harras, A., El-Meligi, A. and Bassim, M. (1981). Effect of high doses of gamma rays on corn grains. I. Influence on the chemical composition of whole grains and the technological process of starch and by-product isolation. *Cereal Chemistry*, 58, 110–112.

Roy, M.K., Ghosh, S.K. and Chatterjee, S.R. (1991). Gamma irradiation of rice grains. *Journal of Food Science and Technology*, 28, 337–340.

Sabularse, V.C., Liuzzo, J.A., Rao, R.M. and Grodner, R.M. (1991). Cooking quality of brown rice as influenced by gamma irradiation, variety and storage. *Journal of Food Science*, 56, 96–98, 108.

Sabularse, V.C., Liuzzo, J.A., Rao, R.M. and Grodner, R.M. (1992). Physicochemical characteristics of brown rice as influenced by gamma irradiation. *Journal of Food Science*, 57, 143–145.

Sies, H. (1986). Biochemistry of oxidative stress. *Angewandte Chemie International*, 25, 1058–1071. [Edition in English]

Silva, J.M., Villar, H.P. and Pimentel, R.M.M. (2012). Structure of the cell wall of mango after application of ionizing radiation. *Radiation Physics and Chemistry*, 81, 1770–1775.

Singh, B. and Datta, P.S. (2011). Effect of low dose gamma irradiation on plant and grain nutrition of wheat. *Radiation Physics and Chemistry*, 79, 819–825.

Singh, P. and Dwivedi, U.N. (2008). Purification and characterization of multiple forms of polygalacturonase from mango (*Mangifera indica* cv. Dashehari) fruit. *Food Chemistry*, 111, 345–349.

Sirisoontaralak, P. and Noomhorm, A. (2006). Changes to physicochemical properties and aroma of irradiated rice. *Journal of Stored Products Research*, 42, 264–276.

Sirisoontaralak, P. and Noomhorm, A. (2007). Changes in physicochemical and sensory-properties of irradiated rice during storage. *Journal of Stored Products Research*, 43, 282–289.

Sokhey, A.S. and Chinnaswamy, R. (1993). Chemical and molecular properties of irradiated starch extrudates. *Cereal Chemistry*, 70, 260–268.

Srinvastava, R. and Kulshŕestha, D.K. (1989). Bioactive polysaccharides from plants. *Phytochemistry*, 28, 2877–2883.

Sung, W.C. (2005). Effect of gamma irradiation on rice and its food products. *Radiation Physics and Chemistry*, 73, 224–228.

Sung, W.C., Hong, M.C. and Chang, T.S. (2008). Effects of storage and gamma irradiation on (*japonica*) waxy rice. *Radiation Physics and Chemistry*, 77, 92–97.

Tanaka, M., Kuei, C.W., Nagashima, Y. and Taguchi, T. (1988). Application of antioxidative maillard reaction products from histidine and glucose to sardine products. *Nippon Suisan Gakkaishi*, 54, 1409–1414.

Urbain, W.M. (1986). *Food Irradiation.* Academic Press, Inc., Orlando, FL.

Uthairatanakij, A., Jitareerat, P. and Kanlavanarat, S. (2006). Effects of irradiation on quality attributes of two cultivars of mango. *Acta Horticulture*, 712, 885–892.

Variyar, P.S., Bandyopadhyay, C. and Thomas, P. (1998). Effect of γ-irradiation on the phenolic acid of some Indian spices. International *Journal of Food Science and Technology*, 33, 533–537.

Voegeli, R., Meier, J. and Doppler, S. (1993). Defence strategies against reactive oxygen species-*in vitro* models. *International Journal of Cosmetic Science*, 15, 153–161.

WHO (1981). Wholesomeness of irradiated food. WHO Technical Report 659. Joint FAO/IAEA/WHO Expert Committee.

Walter, M., Marchesan, E., Massoni, P.F.S. *et al.* (2013). Antioxidant properties of rice grains with light brown, red and black paricarp colors and the effect of processing. *Food Research International*, 50, 698–703.

Wasser, S. (2003). Medicinal mushrooms as a source of antitumor and immunomodulating polysaccharides. *Applied Microbiology and Biotechnology*, 60, 258–274.

Winston, J.C. (1999). Health-promoting properties of common herbs. *The American Journal of Clinical Nutrition*, 70, 491–499.

Wootton, M., Djojonegoro, H. and Driscoll, R. (1988). The effect of gamma irradiation on the quality of Australian rice. *Journal of Cereal Science*, 7, 309–315.

Yang, E.I., Lee, E.M., Kim, Y.S. and Cheng, B.Y. (2012). The role of gamma irradiation on the extraction of phenolic compounds in onion (*Allium cepa* L.). *Radiation Physics and Chemistry*, 81, 1025–1028.

Yawadio, R., Tanimori, S. and Morita, N. (2007). Identification of phenolic compounds isolated from pigmented rices and their aldose reductase inhibitory activities. *Food Chemistry*, 101, 1616–1625.

Ye, S., Tang, L., Xu, J., Liu, Q. and Wang, J. (2006). Postconditioning's protection of THSG on cardiac ischemia-reperfusion injury and mechanism. *Journal Huazhong Universcity Science Technology Medical Sciences*, 26, 13–16.

Zaka, R., Vandecasteele, C.M. and Misset, M.T. (2002). Effects of low chronic dose of ionizing radiation on antioxidant enzymes and G_6PDH activities in *Stipa capillata* (Poaceae). *Journal of Experimental Botany*, 53, 1979–1987.

Zhu, F., Cai, Y.Z., Bao, J. and Corke, H. (2010). Effect of γ-irradiation on phenolic compounds in rice grain. *Food Chemistry*, 120, 74–77.

15 Nanoparticles and Nanoemulsions

Anges Teo[1], Kelvin K.T. Goh[1] and Sung Je Lee[2]

[1]*Institute of Food, Nutrition and Human Health, Massey University, Palmerston North, New Zealand*

[2]*Institute of Food, Nutrition and Human Health, Massey University, Auckland, New Zealand*

15.1 Introduction

Nanotechnology is starting to emerge in the food industry with many potential applications especially in the arena of functional foods. The US National Science and Technology Council (2006) defined nanotechnology as matter with dimensions of 1 to 100 nm. Materials that are nanoscale size exhibit physicochemical properties that are different from large particles and that can potentially be used to improve or modify the nutritional, sensorial and structural properties of food products. Particularly, nanotechnology can lead to the advancement of a delivery system for encapsulated bioactive food ingredients or nutraceuticals by enhancing their aqueous solubility, bioavailability and absorption. A number of different nano-sized carrier (or nano-delivery) systems have been extensively studied in many scientific disciplines for their applications in a variety of fields, such as pharmaceutical, cosmetic and food industries. These include nano-liposomes, nano-cochleates, micelles, dendrimers, nanoemulsions and other nanoparticles (Zuidam and Shimoni, 2010; Tiwari and Takhistov, 2012). Among them, nanoemulsions are of particular interest as they have many useful applications in the food industry.

As in conventional emulsions, nanoemulsions are colloidal dispersions of two immiscible liquids, normally oil and water, in which one phase is dispersed in another, but they contain smaller particles than conventional emulsions (Tiwari and Takhistov, 2012). Consequently, nanoemulsions are thought to have better stability and functional properties such as optical clarity, high kinetic stability and increased bioavailability of encapsulated components. Nanoemulsions can be created using various emulsification methods, such as high pressure homogenization, solvent displacement/evaporation or phase inversions (Tadros *et al.*, 2004; Solans *et al.*, 2005; Anton

Functional Foods and Dietary Supplements: Processing Effects and Health Benefits, First Edition.
Edited by Athapol Noomhorm, Imran Ahmad and Anil Kumar Anal.

et al., 2008; Lee and McClements, 2010; McClements and Rao, 2011). The formation and stability of nanoemulsions also depend on the emulsion formulation and composition used to produce them (McClements and Rao, 2011; Qian and McClements, 2011). Several characterization techniques used in determining the properties of conventional emulsions are also commonly used to analyze nanoemulsions to provide an understanding of their properties, functions and behaviours under various conditions (e.g. pH, ionic strength, thermal treatment, etc.), including their size, size distribution, shape, electrical charge and turbidity.

This chapter provides an overview of the current development of nanoemulsions in the food industry including the materials, methods and techniques used to prepare and characterize them. Some potential food applications of nanotechnology in food systems and their potential health effects are also reviewed in this chapter.

15.2 Nanotechnology in foods: nanoparticles versus nanoemulsions

15.2.1 Nanoparticles

Nanoparticles are very small particles in the size range 10–100 nm (Tiwari and Takhistov, 2012). An advantage of nanoparticles is their ability to remain stable against aggregation and gravitational separation (McClements, 2012). Also, suspended nanoparticles form transparent or translucent emulsions that can be used in clear beverages without affecting their visual appearance (Wooster *et al.*, 2008; McClements and Rao, 2011). In addition, bioactives delivered via nanoparticles have increased bioavailability due to enhanced adsorption and uptake of encapsulated bioactives in the small intestines (Hu *et al.*, 2009; Tiwari and Takhistove, 2012). Most bioactive compounds are poorly soluble in aqueous solution and are sensitive to degradation when exposed to the environmental conditions such as oxygen, light and temperature. The encapsulation of bioactive compounds via nanoparticles, which potentially improves their stability, can lead to the development of new functional foods with the ultimate aim to enhance human health.

Nanoparticles can be designed and assembled in diverse structural forms with different physicochemical properties depending on the materials and methods used. These include nano-liposomes, nano-cochleates, micelles, nanoemulsions, solid lipid nanoparticles (SLN) and coacervates (Onwulata, 2012; Tiwari and Takhistove, 2012). For example, nano-liposomes are lipid bilayer vesicles in the nanometer range formed by self-assembly of phospholipids enclosing an aqueous compartment. Micelles are formed in aqueous solution by self-assembly of small molecule surfactants with an inner hydrophobic core and a protective hydrophilic shell. In the case of reverse micelles, the structure consists of an inner hydrophilic core surrounded by a hydrophobic group orienting toward the continuous oil phase. Solid lipid nanoparticles are lipid particles consisting of high melting point triglycerides that can remain solid at room temperature but melt at higher temperature. Thus they are being used as lipid carriers to encapsulate more sensitive materials inside the solid lipid matrix. Oil-in-water (O/W) nanoemulsions are submicron emulsions used to encapsulate and deliver lipophilic components in foods. They tend to be transparent or translucent and have good stability to gravitational separation. Some of these delivery systems based on nanotechnology and their characteristics are listed in Table 15.1. The rest of the chapter is focused mainly on nanoemulsions.

Table 15.1 Types of nano-based delivery systems and their characteristics (Zuidam and Shimoni, 2010; Onwulata, 2012; Tiwari and Takhistove, 2012)

Types	Characteristics	Structure/size
Nano-liposomes • Small vesicles surrounded by lipid bilayer • Consist of phospholipids and cholesterol	Uses • Encapsulation of lipophilic and hydrophilic compounds • Control release of materials Limitations • Physical instability and chemical degradation	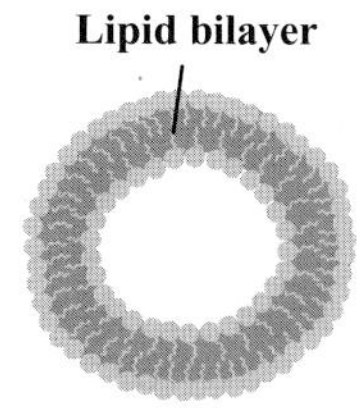 10–300 nm
Nano-cochleates • Small vesicles surrounded by solid lipid bilayer • Consist of phosphatidylserine, cholesterol and calcium	Uses • Encapsulation of lipophilic and hydrophilic compounds • Increase mechanical stability and protection of encapsulated materials Limitations • Expensive	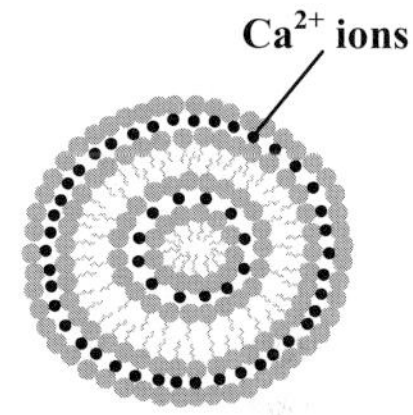 50–500 nm
Micelles • Consist of surfactant molecules with a hydrophobic core and a hydrophilic shell	Uses • Encapsulation of amphiphilic and lipophilic compounds Limitations • Large amount of surfactants used to produce them	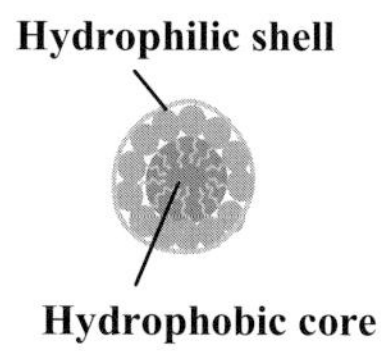 <100 nm
Nanoemulsions • Colloidal dispersion of two immiscible liquids (usually oil and water) with submicron size	Uses • Encapsulation of lipophilic compounds Limitations • Thermodynamically unstable	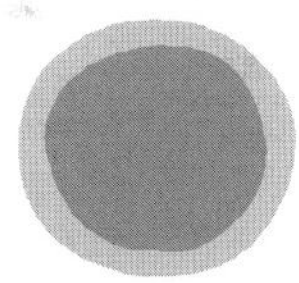 10–100 nm
Lipid nanoparticles • Consist of a solid lipid core	Uses • Increase stability of lipophilic compounds • Control release of materials Limitations • Fat crystallization; difficult to control	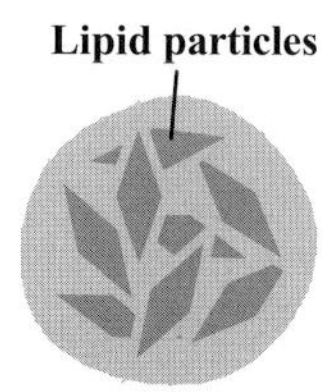 100–200 nm
Coacervates • Biopolymer complexes of two oppositely charged protein and/ or polysaccharides via electrostatic interactions	Uses • Encapsulation of small lipophilic molecules e.g. flavour oils • Control release of materials Limitations • Expensive; complex	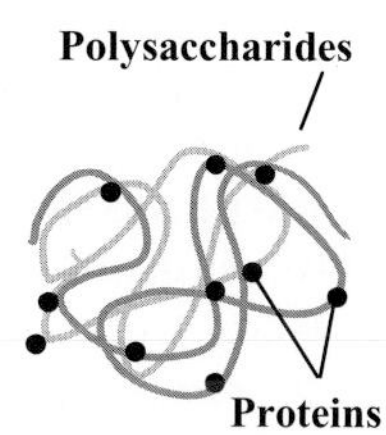 10–600 nm

15.2.2 Definition: conventional emulsions, nanoemulsions and microemulsions

There has been some controversy in the literature over the terminology for emulsions that have different droplet sizes. First and foremost, it is useful to describe some characteristics of the various emulsion systems. Most conventional emulsions contain large droplets of radii larger than 1000 nm and appear opaque or turbid. They are thermodynamically unstable and the phases separate readily over time (McClements, 1999; McClements and Rao, 2011). Similarly, nanoemulsions are also thermodynamically unstable but they contain markedly smaller particles with high kinetic stability and appear transparent or translucent (Tadros *et al.*, 2004; McClements and Rao, 2011; Solans and Solé, 2012). However, the size range of nanoemulsion particles reported in the literature varies from 10 to 100 nm up to 600 nm (Tadros *et al.*, 2004; Solans *et al.*, 2005; Gutiérrez *et al.*, 2008; Lee and McClements, 2010; McClements and Rao, 2011). There is no clear size cut-off for nanoemulsions because the physicochemical properties of an emulsion do not change drastically when the droplet size is reduced to the nanometer range (McClements, 2012; Solans and Solé, 2012). However, differences in some physical properties are likely to occur at sizes below a certain critical value. For example, the appearance of an emulsion can change from opaque to transparent when the droplet size is less than 80 nm (Wooster *et al.*, 2008). The stability of an emulsion to gravitational separation can increase when the droplet size falls below 100 nm (McClements and Rao, 2011). Consequently, a droplet diameter less than 100 nm is a suitable size range for defining nanoemulsions as having different properties from conventional emulsions.

In contrast, microemulsions are thermodynamically stable and contain even smaller particles with a size range of 2–50 nm in diameter (Flanagan and Singh, 2006; McClements, 2012). Microemulsions are usually formed by small molecule surfactant micelles in which oil molecules are incorporated into the hydrophobic core or between the surfactant tails. The surfactant micelles increase in size as oil droplets are added until they become saturated (McClements, 2012). A microemulsion is therefore a colloidal dispersion of small micelle spheroids composed of oil and surfactant molecules that are dispersed in an aqueous phase. However, for conventional emulsions and nanoemulsions, the surfactant is used to lower the interfacial tension at the droplet interface to stabilize the droplets formed via shear forces during homogenization (McClements, 1999). Clearly, the formation and properties of conventional emulsions, nanoemulsions and microemulsions are very different.

15.3 Designing nanoemulsions

15.3.1 Materials used for nanoemulsions

Like conventional emulsions, O/W nanoemulsions consist of an oil phase dispersed in a continuous aqueous phase containing some surfactants or emulsifiers that stabilize the dispersed oil phase (McClements, 1999). The aqueous phase is mostly water while the oil phase may contain non-polar components, such as triacylglycerol oils, free fatty acids, flavor oils, essential oils, mineral oils, fat substitutes, waxes, weighting agents, fat-soluble vitamins and bioactive lipophilic compounds (McClements and Rao, 2011).

Surfactants/emulsifiers Emulsifiers are used to improve the stability of emulsion. They include small molecule surfactants, phospholipids, proteins or polysaccharides. Most emulsifiers function by decreasing the interfacial tension of the oil and water phases and may confer electrostatic or steric stabilization (Henry *et al.*, 2009, 2010; Kralova and Sjöblom, 2009; McClements and Rao, 2011). Some of the emulsifiers used to produce nanoemulsions, in particular the small molecule surfactants, are more effective to form smaller droplets than protein or polysaccharide-based emulsifiers (Yin *et al.*, 2009; Qian and McClements, 2011). However, proteins and polysaccharides are able to impart better emulsion stability by electrostatic or steric repulsive forces (Chu *et al.*, 2007a; McClements and Rao, 2011).

Small molecule surfactants A variety of small molecule surfactants are available commercially to prepare food emulsions. These surfactants can be ionic, non-ionic or zwitterionic based on their electrical charges. The ionic surfactants can be negatively or positively charged but the non-ionic surfactants are not charged. The zwitterionic surfactants can have net negative, neutral or positive charges due to the ionizable groups on the molecules depending on pH changes (Hasenhuettl, 2008; Kralova and Sjöblom, 2009). Among these surfactants, non-ionic surfactants are most commonly used to prepare nanoemulsions. The non-ionic surfactants have lower toxicity and are more stable to pH changes and salt addition. Some of the non-ionic surfactants used to form nanoemulsions include sorbitan esters (e.g. Span and Tween series), polyoxyethylene ether (e.g. Brij^{TM}), monoglycerides (e.g. decaglycerol monolaurate), sugar esters (e.g. sucrose monolaurate, sucrose monomyristate, sucrose monopalmitate) and polyglycerol esters of monolaurate and monooleate series (Tan and Nakajima, 2005a, 2005b; Yuan *et al.*, 2008; Henry *et al.*, 2009; Yin *et al.*, 2009).

Of these surfactants, non-ionic polyoxyethylene sorbitan fatty acid esters (i.e. Tween surfactants) are more widely used. However, the series of Tween surfactants used depend on the emulsification method and their solubilization capacity in the oil or aqueous phase. Although Tween surfactants are structurally similar in their polyoxyethylene head group, they differ in the tail group of fatty acid esters. For instance, Tween 20 is a hydrophilic emulsifier with a medium-chain carbon tail of lauric acid whereas Tween 80 contains a long-chain carbon monooleate tail with higher oil solubilization capacity (Mahdi *et al.*, 2011). Consequently, Tween 20 is used more effectively to produce O/W nanoemulsion using high pressure homogenization whereas Tween 80 is also suitable for making O/W emulsion. In a previous study, Yuan *et al.* (2008) compared different types of Tween emulsifiers (Tween 20, 40, 60 and 80) to produce β-carotene nanoemulsions using high pressure homogenization. They showed that Tween 20 produced an emulsion with the smallest droplet size than those with higher molecular weight of Tween, due to higher hydrophilicity of Tween 20 to stabilize the droplets in the O/W emulsions.

Milk proteins Several milk proteins have been used to form emulsions, namely, caseins and whey proteins. Casein is a major protein found in milk, which consists of α_{S1}-, α_{S2}-, β- and κ-caseins. These caseins are linked by calcium ions and colloidal calcium phosphate (CCP) to form 'casein micelles' in milk (McClements, 1999; Garti, 2002; Livney, 2010). Structurally, caseins are highly disordered in their conformational structure with hydrophilic and hydrophobic groups unevenly distributed along their polypeptide chains (Livney, 2010; Singh, 2011). This explains why caseins possess excellent emulsifying properties. During emulsification, caseins readily adsorb at the surface of oil droplets in aqueous solution, decrease the interfacial tension at the droplet interface and stabilize the emulsion by electrostatic and steric repulsive forces (Chu *et al.*, 2007a). Caseins are available as sodium caseinate commercially. However, sodium caseinate does not contain CCP which makes the protein less aggregated (Garti, 2002).

Whey proteins are another group of milk proteins used to emulsify oil or fat in foods. They are globular proteins consisting mainly of β-lactoglobulin and α-lactalbumin with minor whey protein constituents of immunoglobulins, serum albumin and lactoferrin (Livney, 2010; Foegeding *et al.*, 2011). These protein fractions are able to form and stabilize emulsion by rapidly adsorbing onto the droplet interface, reducing the interfacial tension and forming a protective membrane to prevent droplet aggregation (Kulmyrzaev *et al.*, 2000). One of the important features of whey proteins is their solubility over a wide range of pH (Hosseinpour *et al.*, 2011; Singh, 2011). They can remain soluble even at pH near the isoelectric point (pI) if their native states have not been denatured. Whey proteins are commercially available as whey protein concentrate (WPC), whey protein isolate (WPI) and whey protein hydrolysate (WPH) with different protein concentrations and properties.

Both sodium caseinate and whey proteins were used to prepare β-carotene nanodispersions using emulsification and/or a solvent displacement method (Chu *et al.*, 2007a, 2007b). It was shown that sodium caseinate produced nanodispersions with smaller particle size and had better stability than those prepared with whey proteins due to the caseins' molecular structure and chemical properties. Caseins are structurally random, irregular and more flexible to adsorb onto β-carotene particles to form small droplets whereas whey proteins are highly ordered and have a rigid structure with less adsorption on the particles. Also, sodium caseinate-stabilized nanodispersions were shown to have higher zeta (ζ)-potential at pH 7 than whey protein-stabilized nanodispersions, resulting in an increase in the emulsion stability by preventing particle aggregation during storage.

Another milk protein that can be used to form and stabilize an O/W emulsion is lactoferrin. Lactoferrin has very different physicochemical properties from caseins and other major whey proteins. Lactoferrin is an iron-binding glycoprotein found as a minor whey protein in milk and mucosal secretions of mammals (Shimazaki, 2000). Bovine lactoferrin is a single chain polypeptide consisting of 689 amino acids with 17 disulfide bonds (Pierce *et al.*, 1991; Shimazaki, 2000). Due to a high level of basic amino acids, lactoferrin has a high isoelectric point (pI) of around pH 9 and contains high concentrations of positive charge on the molecule (Shimazaki, 2000).

Over the years, lactoferrin has been studied extensively for its molecular structure and biological functions (Shimazaki, 2000; Baker and Baker, 2009; González-Chavez *et al.*, 2009). However, the adsorption and emulsifying properties of lactoferrin have only been recently reported (Ye and Singh, 2007; Lesmes *et al.*, 2010; Tokle and McClements, 2011). It has been shown that lactoferrin is an excellent emulsifying agent which can produce a cationic emulsion. Previously, lactoferrin was studied in our laboratory to form O/W nanoemulsion using emulsification and a solvent evaporation method. The lactoferrin-stabilized nanoemulsions were compared to those prepared with WPI. The former exhibited better stability against pH changes. The nanoemulsions stabilized by WPI exhibited some aggregation at pH 4.5–5.5, which is near to the pI of whey proteins whereas the lactoferrin-stabilized nanoemulsions remained stable over the wide pH range studied (pH 2–12) (unpublished data).

Polysaccharides Polysaccharides are often used as thickeners, stabilizers and gelling agents in foods. Most polysaccharides are not surface active but they can stabilize emulsion by gelling or increasing the viscosity of the continuous phase (Dickinson, 2003, 2009; Sahin and Sumnu, 2006). However, some polysaccharides, such as gum Arabic and gum Ghatti, have some emulsifying properties due to the presence of protein moiety (Sahin and Sumnu, 2006; Kang *et al.*, 2011; Deshmukh *et al.*, 2012). These polysaccharides are able to adsorb onto the surface of oil droplets and stabilize them by electrostatic and steric repulsion to prevent droplet flocculation and coalescence (Dickinson, 2003).

A mixture of proteins and polysaccharides is often used to form and stabilize emulsion. The protein–polysaccharide emulsion can be formed using a protein emulsifier followed by the addition of polysaccharides to increase the viscosity of the continuous phase, thereby increasing the overall emulsion stability (Dickinson, 2003). Sun *et al.* (2007) studied the effect of xanthan gum on the stability of O/W emulsions formed by WPI. They found that the addition of xanthan gum increased the emulsion viscosity and inhibited creaming during storage. Some of these proteins and polysaccharides are also able to form complexes through electrostatic interactions and other interactions, such as hydrophobic interactions and hydrogen bonding (Weinbreck *et al.*, 2003; Ye *et al.*, 2006; Aryee and Nickerson, 2012). These protein–polysaccharide complexes can be used to form and stabilize emulsion. Recently, Stone and Nickerson (2012) studied the formation of protein–polysaccharide complexes using WPI and different types of carrageenan (κ, ι and λ). The complexes of WPI-carrageenan-stabilized emulsions showed an increase in the emulsion stability compared to those stabilized by either WPI or carrageenan alone.

Some nanoemulsions stabilized by polysaccharides, such as alginate and chitosan, have also been prepared (Choi *et al.*, 2011). The nanoemulsion was initially formed using a non-ionic surfactant (Tween 80) followed by coating with alginate and/or chitosan to form double or triple layer nanoemulsions. For triple layer nanoemulsions, alginate and chitosan were deposited successively onto the droplets to form the biopolymer coatings on the nanoemulsions through electrostatic interactions. The particle size of the double or triple layer nanoemulsions was similar around 20 nm, but their droplet electrical charges were different. The zeta (ζ)-potential of the single layer nanoemulsions stabilized by Tween 80 was −14.2 mV whereas the double layer nanoemulsions coated with alginate or chitosan had −31.7 mVand +26.3 mV, respectively. However, the ζ-potential of the triple layer nanoemulsions coated with alginate followed by chitosan in the outer layer was lower (−9.0 mV) than the other emulsions. This is because the positive and negative charges of the biopolymers cancelled each other due to charge neutralization. Consequently, the overall net charge of the triple layer nanoemulsions was much lower than the other emulsions. However, the triple layer nanoemulsions are coated by layers of biopolymers which can contribute to better steric stabilization.

Oil types Several types of oils have been used to prepare emulsions, including corn oil, soybean oil, coconut oil, palm oil and essential oil. Most of these oils are made up of triglycerides with long (LCT), medium (MCT) or short (SCT) chain fatty acids which can be saturated, monounsaturated or polyunsaturated (Chopra and Panesar, 2010). The type of oils used can affect the droplet size and stability of the resulting nanoemulsions due to the differences in the physicochemical characteristics, such as viscosity, interfacial tension, solubility, polarity, density and refractive index (McClements and Rao, 2011).

The formation of nanoemulsions using high-energy methods depends on the viscosity of the oil phase. In other words, the viscosity of oil can affect the mixing efficiency during homogenization to break up the oil phase into dispersed smaller oil droplets. Consequently, those triglyceride oils that consist of LCT or MCT are less efficient for producing nanoemulsions with smaller droplet size due to the high interfacial tension and viscosity (McClements and Rao, 2011). Previously, Chung *et al.* (2001) studied the influence of interfacial tension and viscosity of the oil phase on the formation of O/W emulsion using 18 different types of oils from vegetable and animal sources. In the study, the oil viscosity had little effect on the droplet size of emulsions as there was no correlation between them. However, the droplet size of emulsions decreased with increasing interfacial tension of the oils which was measured against water without any emulsifiers. However, the results of this study is not a definitive demonstration of oil types on the droplet size of emulsion as only vegetable and animal oils were used. More recently, there has been a growing interest in the use of essential oils to form nanoemulsions (Ghosh *et al.*, 2012; Salvia-Trujillo *et al.*, 2013). The essential oils, defined as 'volatile oils containing volatile aroma compounds', are obtained from plants. They have high polarity and low interfacial tension and viscosity which may form nanoemulsions with even smaller droplet size (McClements and Rao, 2011).

Previously, Wooster *et al.* (2008) compared the physical properties of LCT oil (peanut oil) and hexadecane on the formation and stability of nanoemulsions using SDS as a surfactant. The equilibrium interfacial tension of SDS at the peanut oil/water and hexadecane/water interface was 8 mN/m and 10 mN/m, respectively, but the viscosity of the peanut oil (50 MPa·s at 25 °C) was much higher than the hexadecane (3.1 MPa·s at 25 °C). As a consequence, the higher viscosity of the peanut oil formed larger droplets (~120 nm) than the hexadecane (~80 nm), due to a lower mixing efficiency of homogenization with less intense droplet disruption. However, the peanut oil emulsion was more stable against droplet aggregation and coalescence during storage due to their larger molar volume of 959 cm^3/mol, which makes them more insoluble in water to prevent Ostwald ripening. The findings from these studies suggest that the types of oil used can affect the formation and stability of emulsions. In other words, some oils are effective at producing small oil droplets while others may be more effective at stabilizing the droplets after formation. Therefore, one of the areas in the development of nanoemulsions is to investigate the types of edible oil on the formation and stability of emulsions. Some of these oils may also contain surface active fatty acids of different molar masses which can influence the interfacial tension of the dispersed oil phase.

Encapsulated components There are many potential applications of nanoemulsions in foods and beverages to encapsulate lipophilic components, including vitamins, flavours, colours, antioxidants and preservatives (McClements and Rao, 2011), that are difficult to incorporate in liquid food products. These lipophilic components can be mixed with the oil phase prior to emulsification. Alternatively, they can be dissolved in organic solvents, such as hexane and acetone when a solvent displacement technique is used.

Among these lipophilic components, bioactive compounds are of particular interest. Bioactive compounds are food components or food ingredients that confer health benefits to the human body, such as the prevention of cardiovascular diseases (CVD), hypertension, diabetes and some cancers (Onwulata, 2012). Some bioactive lipids with health benefits include omega (ω)-3 fatty acids, carotenoids, fat-soluble vitamins (e.g. vitamin E) and phytosterols. It has been shown that an increased intake of ω-3 fatty acids in the diet helps to reduce blood pressure, thrombosis, plasma triglyceride and inflammation and to prevent hypertension, CVD, hypertriglyceridaemia and other inflammatory diseases (e.g. arthritis, inflammatory bowel diseases, psoriasis) (Calder and Yaqoob, 2009). Carotenoids are antioxidants capable of scavenging singlet oxygen and free radicals to protect against diseases linked to oxidative stress, lipid peroxidation and free radicals (Wahlqvist and Wattanapenpaiboon, 2011). Phytosterols can help to lower blood cholesterol by inhibiting the intestinal absorption of cholesterol (Tiwari and Takhistov, 2012).

However, these bioactive lipids are unstable in food systems and are susceptible to light and oxidative deterioration. In addition, some bioactive lipids, such as carotenoids and phytosterols, have high melting points and are prone to crystallization (McClements *et al.*, 2007). This makes them even more difficult to incorporate into food products and requires the use of a delivery system. These bioactive compounds may be encapsulated in nanoemulsions for stabilization and better protection against degradation. Moreover, nanoemulsions are advantageous over other delivery systems as they are readily absorbed into the body due to their smaller size and larger surface area, which can enhance absorption and increase the bioavailability of the encapsulated bioactive lipids (McClements and Rao, 2011). One recent study that has shown the increased bioavailability of bioactive lipids by incorporating them in nanoemulsions is α-tocopherol administered in rats (Hatanaka *et al.*, 2010). The rats administered with α-tocopherol (10% w/w) loaded nanoemulsions (around 85 nm) had a higher blood plasma content of α-tocopherol than those fed with the control mixture of oil and α-tocopherol. This study showed that nanoemulsions can be used as an effective delivery system that improves the bioavailability of bioactive lipids.

15.3.2 Preparation methods of nanoemulsions

Nanoemulsions can be produced using high energy or low energy emulsification methods. The high energy method uses mechanical devices, such as the high pressure homogenizer, the microfluidizer and ultrasonic devices, to generate large disruptive forces to break up bulk oil or large oil droplets into smaller ones (Anton *et al.*, 2008). The low energy method can form small droplets or nanoemulsions under certain environmental conditions or emulsion composition by manipulating the physicochemical

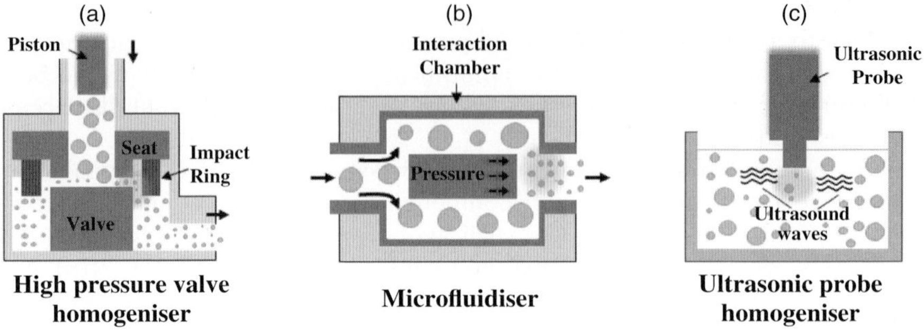

Figure 15.1 Schematic illustrations of mechanical devices used to produce nanoemulsion using high energy method (a) high pressure valve homogenizer (b) microfluidizer and (c) ultrasonic probe homogenizer. *Source:* Adapted from McClements, D.J. (2010). Reproduced with permission from Royal Society of Chemistry

properties of surfactant molecules (Anton *et al.*, 2008; Anton and Vandamme, 2009; McClements and Rao, 2011). This results in changes in the interfacial properties of an emulsion to form oil droplets spontaneously. The formation of nanoemulsions by low energy emulsification can be achieved by changing the temperature or system composition being described as phase inversion temperature (PIT) or phase inversion composition (PIC), which is described later.

High pressure homogenization In high pressure homogenization, a coarse emulsion containing large oil droplets is initially prepared by blending the oil and water phases using a high shear mixer before homogenizing them. During the subsequent homogenization process, the homogenizer forces the coarse emulsion to pass through narrow gaps (Figure 15.1a) under high pressures (3–20 MPa) to form a fine emulsion containing small droplets through a combination of shear, impact and cavitation forces (McClements, 1999; Anton *et al.*, 2008). The droplet size of the resulting fine emulsion depends on the homogenization pressures and the number of cycles used. The droplet size and size distribution of emulsions decrease with higher homogenization pressures and number of cycles used (McClements, 1999; Yuan *et al.*, 2008). However, the smallest droplet size that can be produced during homogenization is determined by the Laplace pressure (ΔP) in Equation 15.1 (McClements, 1999). The ΔP increases as the interfacial tension increases and the droplet size decreases. Consequently, it becomes more difficult to reduce the droplet size further once they reached a minimum droplet size.

$$\Delta P = \frac{4\gamma}{d} \tag{15.1}$$

where γ is the interfacial tension and d is the droplet diameter.

The effectiveness of the droplet disruption also depends on the design of the homogenizer valve. Several different types of homogenizer valves are used for different purposes. For instance, a spring loaded valve is used in commercial homogenizers to control the gap size (about 15–300 μm) for an emulsion to pass through. As the gap size decreases, the pressure drop across the valve increases, hence leading to the greater droplet disruption and formation of smaller droplets (McClements, 1999).

Some homogenizers are equipped with a two-stage homogenization valve to prevent re-coalescence of oil droplets for a narrower size distribution.

Microfluidizer Microfluidization uses very high pressures (up to 150 MPa) to form nanoemulsions (Jafari *et al.*, 2007). Like high pressure homogenization, a coarse emulsion is prepared first and then fed into the inlet of a microfluidizer. However, the emulsion is divided into two opposite streams in the interaction chamber of a microfluidizer (Figure 15.1b). The two streams of the emulsion can impinge each other (Figure 15.1b) at high velocity (300 m/s) and very high pressures to create large, intense disruptive forces to form small droplets (McClements, 1999; Jafari *et al.*, 2007; Anton *et al.*, 2008).

The formation of nanoemulsions using microfluidization was studied by several workers (Jafari *et al.*, 2007; Qian and McClements, 2011; Ahmed *et al.*, 2012; Li *et al.*, 2012; Salvia-Trujillo *et al.*, 2013). Some of the major factors affecting the droplet size of nanoemulsions produced by microfluidization were examined. Qian and McClements (2011) studied the emulsion composition and the microfluidization conditions on the formation of nanoemulsions. They found that the particle size of nanoemulsions decreased with increasing microfluidization pressures and cycles. However, the particle size did not decrease at higher pressures above 14 kBar (140 MPa) for six cycles. Further decrease in the particle size depends on the type and concentration of emulsifiers used. In another study, Jafari *et al.* (2007) showed that higher microfluidization pressures ($>$ 63 MPa) and number of cycles ($>$ 2 cycles) increased the droplet size of the emulsions containing 15% w/w *d*-limonene due to 'over processing'. During 'over processing', the newly formed droplets were small but the droplet size increased because the droplets re-coalesced faster than the rate of adsorption by the emulsifier at the droplet interface.

Ultrasonication The ultrasonication method uses ultrasound waves with a frequency higher than 20 kHz to generate imploding cavitation bubbles to cause intensive shock waves to break up large droplets into small ones (McClements, 1999; Anton *et al.*, 2008; Tang *et al.*, 2012). The ultrasonic device has a sonication probe to produce ultrasound waves (Figure 15.1c) to homogenize a pre-prepared coarse emulsion or a separate mixture of oil and water to reduce the oil droplet size (McClements, 1999; McClements and Rao, 2011). The size of the droplets depends on the sonication time and the energy used (Anton *et al.*, 2008; Ghosh *et al.*, 2012). In fact, it is possible to form a nanoemulsion using megasonic irradiation (Kamogawa *et al.*, 2004). The emulsion was sonicated at 40 kHz followed by a series of irradiation at 200 kHz and 1 MHz to form small droplets. Initially, the emulsion was sonicated at 40 kHz for 8 min and formed emulsion with droplet size of $\sim$232 nm. The droplet size decreased to $\sim$100 nm when subjected to another cycle of sonication at 200 kHz but did not decrease further at 1 MHz. This showed that higher frequency ($>$ 200 kHz) helps to break up the large droplets into smaller ones.

Several workers have reported on the formation of nanoemulsions using ultrasonication (Kentish *et al.*, 2008; Chalothorn and Warisnoicharoen, 2012; Ghosh *et al.*, 2012; Tang *et al.*, 2012). In these studies, some parameters such as emulsifier concentration, sonication time and energy (power) input were examined to optimize the processing conditions for the formation of nanoemulsions. They showed that an optimum condition used to produce flaxseed oil emulsions with small droplet size

(120 nm) using ultrasonic homogenization was either by batch or flow through sonication cell at 200 W nominal power (Kentish *et al.*, 2008). More recently, Ghosh *et al.* (2012) prepared nanoemulsions from food-grade ingredients using the ultrasonication method. They were able to form nanoemulsions with a very small droplet size (29.3 nm) using basil oil and Tween 80 at 20 kHz (750 W) for 15 min. The use of ultrasonication to produce nanoemulsions may seem to be superior, in terms of the droplet size and energy efficiency, when compared to high pressure homogenization or microfluidization. However, the variability of sonication conditions to produce nanoemulsions with small droplet size may be a problem for obtaining reproducible results.

In summary, nanoemulsions can be produced using various high energy methods such as high pressure homogenization, microfluidization and ultrasonication. Although these high energy methods are able to produce nanoemulsions, they are less energy efficient as a large amount of energy is required to produce small droplets and the energy is often dissipated as heat (Anton *et al.*, 2008). Moreover, the heat generated during processing may cause denaturation, chemical degradation and loss of bioactivity of heat labile components. Furthermore, the extent of particle size reduction using high energy is limited as it becomes increasingly difficult to reduce the particle size once they reached their minimum size due to Laplace pressure (McClements, 1999; Chu *et al.*, 2007b).

As well as the high energy methods described here, low energy methods have also been used to form emulsions. These are described in the next section.

Spontaneous emulsification Spontaneous emulsification is used to create emulsions or nanoemulsions by mixing two liquids together. The two liquids consist of an aqueous phase and a mixture of oil, surfactant and a water-miscible solvent. This method is used to form emulsions with small droplet size in a number of ways by changing the composition of the oil and water phases, environmental conditions (e.g. temperature, pH, ionic strength) or mixing conditions (e.g. stirring speed, rate and order of addition) (McClements and Rao, 2011; Yang *et al.*, 2012). The underlying mechanism for spontaneous emulsification to occur is the movement of some water miscible components from the oil to the water phase that generates turbulence to form small oil droplets (Anton and Vandamme, 2009). When the oil and water phases are mixed together, some water-miscible components move rapidly from the oil to the water phase. This creates interfacial turbulence and increases the interfacial area for the oil droplets to bud off from the oil–water interface and form nano-droplets (McClements and Rao, 2011) as illustrated in Figure 15.2.

In spontaneous emulsification, solvent displacement is commonly used to form nanoemulsions. This method consists of mixing an aqueous solution with a water-miscible organic solvent, such as ethanol and acetone, to form small droplets by rapid diffusion of the organic solvent in the aqueous phase (Chu *et al.*, 2007b, 2008). Previously, solvent displacement was used in high pressure homogenization to reduce the size of the emulsion droplets. This combined method of emulsification–solvent displacement has been used to prepare nanoemulsions.

Emulsification and solvent displacement/evaporation method Sometimes combining high and low energy methods may be more effective to form nanoemulsions. The droplet size of emulsions produced by high energy emulsification has been

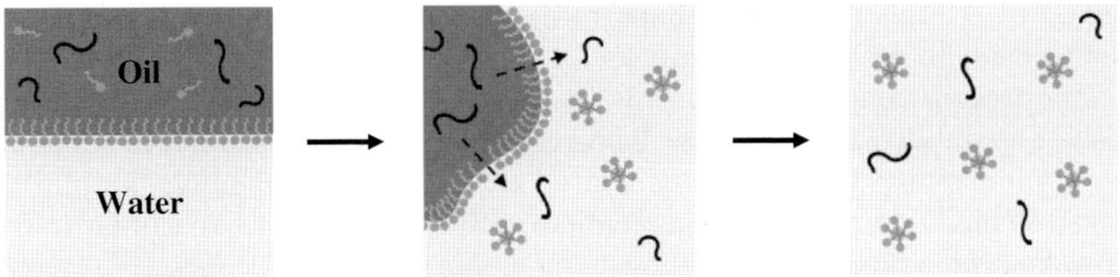

Figure 15.2 Schematic illustrations of mechanism for spontaneous emulsification when some water miscible components moved from the oil phase to water phase and oil droplet bud off from the oil-water interface to form nano-droplets. *Source:* Adapted from McClements, D.J. (2010). Reproduced with permission from Royal Society of Chemistry

shown to be further reduced using solvent displacement and evaporation (Lee and McClements, 2010). This method consists of an aqueous phase and an organic phase. The aqueous phase is a solution containing some emulsifiers and the organic phase is a mixture of organic solvent and some lipophilic component (e.g. oil). The aqueous and organic phases are mixed and homogenized to form an emulsion. During homogenization, the emulsifier in the aqueous phase adsorbs rapidly at the interface of the oil droplets to prevent droplet coalescence. If the solvent used is soluble or partially miscible in water, solvent displacement takes place *in situ* where the organic solvent moves from the oil droplets into the aqueous phase resulting in shrinkage of the droplet size. The size of the oil droplets can be further decreased when the organic solvent is removed from the emulsion droplets by evaporation under reduced pressure.

The emulsification–solvent displacement/evaporation method has been used to prepare nanodispersions containing β-carotene (Tan and Nakajima, 2005a, 2005b; Chu *et al.*, 2007a, 2008; Silva *et al.*, 2011). They showed that various food-grade emulsifiers, such as polyglycerol esters of fatty acids, Tween 20, whey proteins and caseinate can be used to prepare nanoemulsions. Hexane or acetone was used to prepare the O/W emulsions and microfluidized at very high pressure (140–160 MPa) to form very small β-carotene nanoparticles. In another study, the emulsification–solvent displacement/evaporation method was used to form whey protein-stabilized O/W nanoemulsions containing corn oil (Lee and McClements, 2010; Lee *et al.*, 2011). An amphiphilic volatile organic solvent (ethyl acetate) was used for the solvent displacement and evaporation. The authors observed nanoemulsions containing a droplet size of ~70 nm.

In our studies, an O/W emulsion stabilized by WPI was prepared with ethyl acetate (9.5% w/w) using high pressure homogenization followed by evaporation under reduced pressure to form small oil droplets (unpublished data). We observed that the droplet size (Z-Average) decreased from 93.7 ± 0.4 d·nm to 73.5 ± 0.0 d·nm with increasing WPI concentration from 0.3 to 1.0% w/w but the droplet size did not decrease any further at higher protein concentration (> 1% w/w). The effect of organic and aqueous phase ratios on the formation of nanoemulsions was also studied at two different organic phase ratios of 10 : 90 and 20 : 80. For nanoemulsions prepared at a higher organic phase ratio, the droplet size was larger (108.3 ± 0.9 d·nm) than those prepared at a lower organic phase ratio (73.5 ± 0.0 d·nm) at the same protein concentration used (1% w/w). This is probably due to insufficient emulsifier to stabilize the emulsion droplets and less mixing efficiency at a higher ratio of the organic phase. Consequently, a large amount of protein emulsifier (~5% w/w) was used at the higher organic phase ratio to achieve a droplet size similar to those at the lower organic phase ratio.

Phase inversion methods Nanoemulsions can be formed using phase inversion methods by inducing phase inversion from a W/O emulsion to an O/W emulsion system (or vice versa). Phase inversion can be achieved by manipulating the environmental conditions and the emulsion composition, such as temperature, ionic strength and pH (Solans and Solé, 2012). Some of the phase inversion methods include phase inversion temperature (PIT), phase inversion composition (PIC) and emulsion inversion point (EIP). These methods are discussed in the following sections.

Phase inversion temperature (PIT) The PIT method creates emulsions with small droplets by changing the surfactant curvature (molecular geometry) or relative solubility of non-ionic surfactants, usually polyoxyethylene (POE)-type, with temperature (Solans *et al.*, 2005; Solans and Solé 2012). The POE surfactant is a hydrophilic surfactant but becomes lipophilic as the temperature increases due to dehydration of the POE chains (Solans *et al.*, 2005). When the surfactants are added into a solution, they spontaneously associate with each other and form monolayers. The surfactants are assembled with an optimum curvature for the most efficient packing of the surfactant molecules to stabilize the emulsion (McClements, 1999). The optimum curvature of a monolayer depends on the critical packing parameter (CPP) of the surfactant in Equation 15.2.

$$CPP = \frac{v}{a_0 l_0} \tag{15.2}$$

where v is the molecular volume of the hydrophobic surfactant tail, a_0 is the surface area of the surfactant head group and l_0 is the chain length of the surfactant tail group.

The CPP can be used to relate to the physicochemical properties of the surfactants with changes in temperature. The temperature at which an emulsion is changed from an O/W to a W/O system (or vice versa) is known as the phase inversion temperature (PIT) (McClements, 1999). At temperatures below the PIT, the non-ionic surfactant has a relatively large head group (Figure 15.3a) with high water solubility. The CPP of the surfactant is less than 1 and the formation of an O/W emulsion is favored as the surfactant curvature is convex (Figure 15.3a) (Ee *et al.*, 2008; McClements and Rao, 2011). When the temperature increases, the surfactant becomes less soluble in water and the CPP increases (McClements and Rao, 2011). At the PIT, the CPP equals 1 and the emulsion breaks down to form a system consisting of a mixture of surfactant, oil and water organized into a liquid crystalline or lamellar phase with excess oil and excess water (Figure 15.3b). At this point, the interfacial tension is extremely low for emulsions to form small droplets by rapid cooling or heating to change the surfactant curvature to stabilize the droplets (Ee *et al.*, 2008; McClements and Rao, 2011; Solans and Solé, 2012). At temperatures above the PIT, the head group of the surfactant becomes smaller than the tail group, (Figure 15.3c) (CPP > 1), favoring the formation

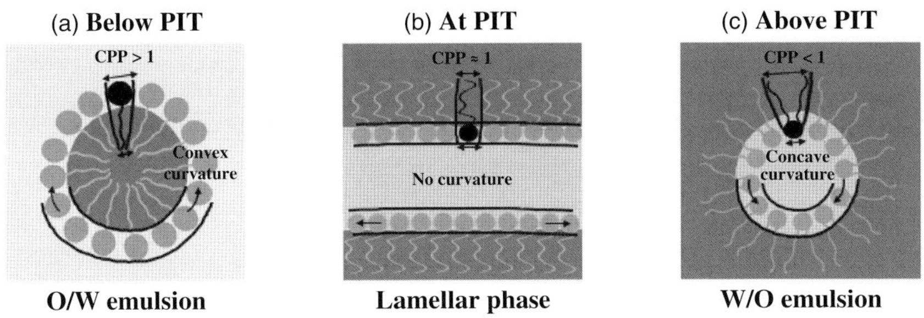

Figure 15.3 Schematic illustrations of temperature conditions on the spontaneous curvature of surfactant in emulsions. *Source:* Adapted from McClements, D.J. (2010). Reproduced with permission from Royal Society of Chemistry

of a W/O emulsion as the surfactant curvature is concave (Figure 15.3c) (McClements and Rao, 2011).

Previously, emulsification by the PIT method was used to form O/W nanoemulsions containing a mixture of oil (10% *n*-decane), water and non-ionic surfactant (4–8% Brij^{TM} 30) (Ee *et al.*, 2008). The oil phase containing the surfactant and the water phase were heated separately to a temperature above the PIT and mixed. The mixture of oil, surfactant and water was cooled slowly to the PIT around 33–38 °C. This was followed by rapid cooling to below the PIT (25 °C) to form nanoemulsions. The droplet size of the emulsions was measured at various temperatures near the PIT and during the cooling process at different surfactant concentrations. The droplet size of the emulsions did not decrease with different surfactant concentrations at temperatures near the PIT. However, the droplet size decreased with an increase in the surfactant concentration when the temperature was rapidly cooled to below the PIT (13–19 °C). The droplet size was approximately 35–54 nm. This study showed that small droplet size can be obtained by controlling the formation of the lamellar phase at the PIT with a rapid cooling (or heating) process to prevent droplet coalescence. The study also showed that the nanoemulsions formed by the PIT method was sensitive to temperature changes when the nanoemulsions were stored at different temperatures below or above the optimum temperature of 19 °C. The droplet size increased when they were stored at 11 °C (59–85 nm) or 25 °C (119–5440 nm). However, the destabilized emulsions were shown to be reverted to form small droplet size by adjusting the temperature back to the optimum temperature (19 °C).

Phase inversion composition (PIC) The PIC method is similar to the PIT method except the optimum curvature of the surfactant changes in the presence of electrolytes instead of temperature. Therefore, the PIC method can be used to produce nanoemulsions with ionic surfactants (McClements and Rao, 2011; Solans and Solé, 2012). In this method, the change in surfactant curvature is achieved by increasing or decreasing the ionic strength and/or pH of the system. The ionic strength of the system can be manipulated by adding salt or diluting in water. The addition of salt screens the electrical charges on the surfactant head group and increases the CPP of the ionic surfactant (CPP > 1) to favor the formation of W/O emulsions. The ionic strength can also be decreased by diluting in water to convert a W/O to an O/W emulsion (McClements and Rao, 2011). Similarly, the electrical charge of ionic surfactants can be changed by adjusting the pH of the system. The carboxyl group

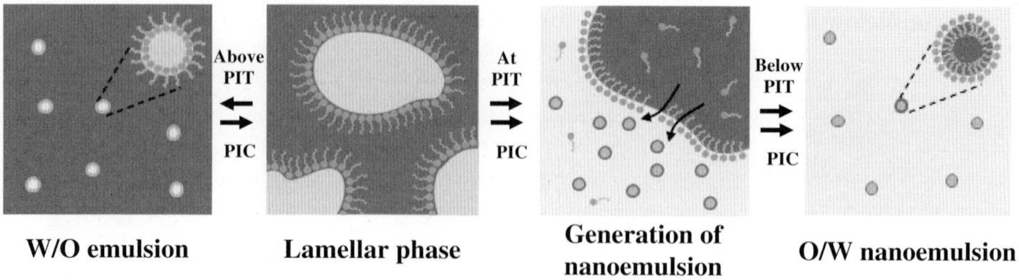

Figure 15.4 Schematic illustrations of the formation of nanoemulsions by the PIT or PIC method. For the PIT method, nanoemulsions are formed by rapid cooling or heating the lamellar phase to temperature below or above the PIT. For the PIC method, nanoemulsions are formed by the changes in the surfactant curvature in the lamellar phase. *Source:* Adapted from Anton & Vandamme, 2009

of ionic surfactants can be ionized (COO^-) by increasing the pH above the pK_a value. The ionized surfactant becomes soluble in water (CPP < 1) and forms O/W emulsions. However at pH below the pK_a value, the carboxyl groups are uncharged (COOH) and tend to form W/O emulsions (Solè *et al.*, 2006; Maestro *et al.*, 2008; McClements and Rao, 2011).

During addition of components, the ionic strength and/ or pH of the system are changed at a certain composition so that the electrical charge on the surfactant molecule and the surfactant curvature are changed. The surfactant curvature becomes zero and the emulsion breaks down to form a lamellar phase with a low interfacial tension and forms small droplets with a high surfactant curvature to stabilize them as the composition changes. As such, the PIC method is very similar to the PIT method as a surfactant curvature is produced during emulsification to form small droplets and stabilize the emulsion. A schematic illustration of the formation of nanoemulsions using the PIT or PIC method is shown in Figure 15.4.

The PIC method has many advantages over the PIT method. The nanoemulsions formed by the PIC method are less susceptible to temperature changes and more stable to droplet coalescence than those prepared by the PIT method. The PIC method can be used with other ionic surfactants whereas the PIT method is limited to only non-ionic POE type surfactants (Solans and Solè, 2012). The PIC method is more suitable for large scale production of nanoemulsions than the PIT method as the emulsion composition of the system can be changed more easily than manipulating the temperature.

Emulsion inversion point (EIP) The EIP method forms emulsions or nanoemulsions by changing the composition of the oil and water phase ratio (McClements and Rao, 2011). The EIP method is used to change an emulsion from W/O to O/W (and vice versa) by adding the dispersed phase progressively into the continuous phase until a critical level is reached. An O/W emulsion can be formed by increasingly adding water to the initial system of W/O emulsion. During each addition of water, some water droplets are formed and coalesced rapidly to exceed the oil droplets for phase inversion to occur. At the point of phase inversion, a lamellar phase with low interfacial tension is formed. The low interfacial tension helps to facilitate the formation of small droplets as the surfactant curvature changes from stabilizing a W/O emulsion to an O/W emulsion (Fernandez *et al.* 2004).

The formation of edible nanoemulsions using the EIP method was investigated for the emulsion composition, such as oil type, surfactant type and surfactant-to-oil ratio (SOR) and preparation conditions (Ostertag *et al.*, 2012). They found that MCT oils were more effective in producing smaller oil droplets than flavor oils (orange oil and limonene) and LCT oils (e.g. olive, grape seed, sesame, peanut and canola oils). For surfactant type, Tween 80 formed smaller droplet size than Tween 20 and Tween 85. However, a higher SOR of 2.5 formed emulsions with smaller droplet size using MCT and Tween 80. In the study, the formation of nanoemulsions using the EIP method was also compared to a high energy method using microfluidization at 12 000 psi (82 MPa) for three cycles. It was shown that microfluidization was more effective than the EIP method as microfluidization produced smaller droplet size ($d_{3,2} \sim 120$ nm) with much lower surfactant concentration than the EIP method ($d_{3,2} \sim 160$ nm).

Various emulsification methods can be used to form nanoemulsions by high energy or low energy approaches. The high energy emulsification methods are more commonly used to prepare nanoemulsions because they are adaptable to the different processing conditions. They can be used to form nanoemulsions using a variety of food grade ingredients but the low energy method is limited to the use of certain types of oils and surfactants. However, in some cases, the low energy method is more effective for producing smaller droplets. As such, there are considerable research efforts being focused on improving low energy methods to make them appealing to the food industry.

15.3.3 Techniques used to characterize nanoemulsions

This section describes some techniques that can be used to characterize the physicochemical properties of nanoemulsions.

Light scattering techniques The particle size and size distribution of emulsions can be measured using static or dynamic light scattering techniques. In static light scattering (SLS), the droplet size of an emulsion is measured by the scattering pattern of light produced by the droplets when a laser beam is passed through them. A suitable mathematical model based on Mie theory is used to predict the scattering pattern from the particle characteristics. The Mie theory is based on Maxwell's electromagnetic field equations and predicts the scattering intensities in particles by assuming that these particles are spherical and homogenous in dilute suspension (Horvath, 2009; Horne, 2011). This technique can be used to measure emulsions with particle sizes between 0.1 and 1000 μm in most food emulsions (Webb and Orr, 2006). However, SLS is less useful for measuring emulsions containing particles of less than 100 nm.

The dynamic light scattering (DLS) technique is capable of measuring particles with diameters between 3 and 5000 nm (McClements, 2007). This technique measures the particle size of the droplets when they move randomly in solution due to Brownian motion. During their movement, the intensity fluctuations of light scattered by the particles are measured to give the translational diffusion coefficient (D) and the Stokes–Einstein equation Equation 15.3 is used to calculate the droplet size of an emulsion (McClements, 1999, 2007; Horvath, 2009).

$$r = \frac{kT}{6\pi\eta_1 D} \qquad (15.3)$$

where r is the size of a particle in radius, K is the Boltzmann's constant, T is the absolute temperature and η_l is the viscosity of the continuous phase.

As a note of caution, importantly the light scattering techniques are unable to determine emulsion flocs unless the measurement is conducted in the presence of a dissociating agent, such as sodium dodecyl sulfate (SDS). The presence of emulsion flocs can give inaccurate information when reporting the particle size.

Microscopy A number of microscopy techniques have been used to study the microstructure of emulsions, including optical microscopy, laser scanning confocal microscopy (LSCM) and electron microscopy. Optical microscopy is commonly used to study the size, shape and microstructure of emulsion droplets (McClements, 1999). The LSCM technique is capable of providing better resolution as the laser beams are scanned across the sample to produce multiple optical sections that can be combined to generate a three-dimensional image. However, both optical microscopy and LSCM are not suitable for studying very small particles less than 200 nm. An electron microscope is used for nanoparticles and nanoemulsions, including transmission electron microscopy (TEM) and scanning electron microscopy (SEM). These electron microscopes use electron beams to generate the microscopic images of the samples. In TEM, the electron beams are transmitted through the sample and produce a two-dimensional image whereas in SEM, the electron beams are scanned across the surface of the sample in a raster scan pattern by scanning horizontally left to right to provide a three-dimensional structure (McClements, 1999; Klang *et al.*, 2012). Both TEM and SEM have been used by many researchers to study nanoparticles and nanodispersions (Tan and Nakajima, 2005a; Chu *et al.*, 2007a, 2007b). The previous work on β-carotene nanodispersions showed that these β-carotene particles had spherical morphology with diameters diameter between 20 and 200 nm (Chu *et al.*, 2007a, 2007b).

Although electron microscopy is a useful technique for studying the structure of emulsion droplets, the sample preparation methods can be complicated and tedious. Often, the emulsion droplets undergo structural changes during sample preparation, especially for TEM. This is because thin samples are necessary for the electron beams to pass through the sample for imaging. To overcome these problems, environmental SEM (ESEM) may be used for emulsions without any prior sample treatment to view the emulsions in their original state (McClements, 1999). Chu *et al.* (2007b) used resin embedding and freeze fracture replica methods to prepare β-carotene nanodispersions for TEM analysis. They found that the freeze fracture replica method provides higher resolution images than those from the resin embedding method. The negative staining method by TEM was also used to observe nanoemulsions formed with different layers of biopolymers (Choi *et al.*, 2011). The sample was placed on a copper grid and washed with water and drained off before staining with 2% uranyl acetate. The uranyl acetate was decanted and the sample was examined in a TEM microscope.

Electrical characteristics and zeta (ζ)-potential The electrical characteristics of emulsion droplets depend on the type of emulsifiers and the ionic strength of the emulsion continuous phase. The emulsion droplets are negatively charged when they are stabilized by anionic emulsifiers and positively charged when stabilized by cationic emulsifiers (Hasenhuettl, 2008). The electrical characteristics of emulsion droplets can be measured by the electrical charge (ζ-potential) of oil droplets in emulsions.

The ζ-potential measures the electrical potential at the 'shear plane' where counter ions are attached to the surface of the droplets (McClements and Rao, 2011). The droplet charge of emulsions can be measured by electrophoresis using an instrument where the electrical charges are measured from the particle velocity. Such an instrument uses light scattering technique to measure the particle velocity from the frequency fluctuations to calculate the ζ-potential (McClements, 1999).

The ζ-potential is a useful parameter to predict the stability of emulsion during storage. In general, a minimum ζ-potential value of ± 30 mV is required for an emulsion to be physically stable by electrostatic repulsion during storage. In a previous study, the ζ-potential of β-carotene nanodispersions stabilized by sodium caseinate was close to -30 mV but whey protein-stabilized nanodispersions had lower electrical charges of between -10 and -17 mV (Chu *et al.*, 2007a). Hence, it is expected that the nanodispersions stabilized by sodium caseinate would be more stable against droplet aggregation during storage. The observed difference in the electrical charge of these nanodispersions was due to the nature of the proteins used, as caseins have much higher negative charges than whey proteins at neutral pH (Chu *et al.*, 2007a).

However, the use of ζ-potential to evaluate the stability of emulsion is limited for those emulsions stabilized by hydrocolloids. This is because the ζ-potential measurement is taken at the 'shear plane' which is poorly defined in the droplets stabilized by hydrocolloids with low ζ-potential values measured (Dickinson, 2009). Moreover, hydrocolloids contribute to the emulsion stability by steric repulsion, which is not accounted for when ζ-potential is solely used to evaluate the emulsion stability (Dickinson, 2009).

In summary, although the techniques described earlier are useful to determine some characteristics in nanoemulsions, there are other powerful techniques that could be used to study more advanced properties of nanomaterials. For instance, X-ray photon correlation spectroscopy and rheo-small angle neutron scattering (SANS) are used to study the composition, structure and rheology of some nanoemulsions (Fryd and Mason, 2012).

Optical properties The appearance of nanoemulsions is distinctly different from that of conventional emulsions. Nanoemulsions can appear transparent or translucent to slightly opaque, depending on their particle size range and dispersed oil droplet concentration while conventional emulsions are turbid or opaque due to the larger size of oil droplets (Lee *et al.*, 2011; McClements and Rao, 2011). This is because the amount of scattered light from the droplets decreases when the size of droplet approaches or falls below the wavelength of light and the emulsions become transparent as more light can pass through them (McClements, 1999). The emulsions can change from opaque to transparent by reducing the droplet size from 120 to 80 nm (McClements, 2012). Thus, the small droplet size of nanoemulsions makes them appear transparent.

The optical properties of emulsions can be characterized by color (or opacity) and turbidity measurements (McClements, 1999). The color (or opacity) of an emulsion can be measured according to the Commission Internationale de L'Eclairage (CIE) L*a*b or the Munsell system (Sahin and Sumnu, 2006). In the color system, L* value is expressed in a range between 0 and 100 with 0 representing dark and 100 representing bright. The a* and b* values are color coordinates expressed numerically where +a* is red, –a* is green, +b* is yellow and –b* is blue. These values can be used to calculate the whiteness index (WI) of emulsions given in Equation 15.4. The WI is used to compare the transparency in different nanoemulsions. The WI decreases in nanoemulsions with small droplet size due to reduced light scattered effect (Salvia-Trujillo *et al.*, 2013).

$$WI = 100 - \left((100 - L)^2 + (a^2 + b^2)\right)^{0.5} \tag{15.4}$$

The turbidity of an emulsion can be measured using a UV-visible spectrophotometer over a range of wavelengths between 200 and 1000 nm (McClements, 1999). The emulsion turbidity is usually measured at a wavelength in the visible region (around 600 nm). During measurement, the intensity of light that passes through the emulsion sample is compared to the continuous phase. Emulsions with large particles of a certain size have higher turbidity because they can scatter more light to appear turbid or opaque (McClements, 1999). However, nanoemulsions containing very small particles less than 80 nm do not scatter light to the same extent (McClements and Rao, 2011). Thus, they appear transparent or translucent as more light can pass through them.

Interfacial properties The interface of an emulsion droplet is surrounded by an interfacial layer which is formed by some surface active components including small molecule surfactants and proteins. The type of surface active components adsorbed at the droplet interface determines the interfacial properties of an emulsion, such as the interfacial layer thickness, permeability, electrical charge, interactions, rheology, stability and environmental responsiveness (McClements and Rao, 2011). Some components may form a thick, fluid-like interfacial layer with low viscoelasticity while others may form a thin, elastic interfacial layer around the droplets. Other components such as surfactants may contribute to the electrical charge of emulsion droplets to become more or less positively or negatively charged (Hasenhuettl, 2008). Nevertheless, the interface of droplets in nanoemulsions and conventional emulsions may differ considerably. This is because the droplets in nanoemulsions are surrounded by an interfacial layer with about the same thickness as the droplet size ($\delta \approx r_n$) but the conventional emulsions have a comparatively thinner interfacial layer ($\delta << r_c$) due to their larger droplet size (McClements and Rao, 2011) as illustrated in Figure 15.5. Consequently,

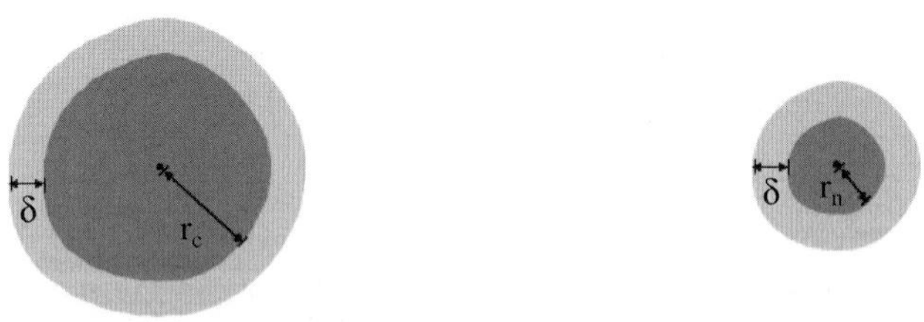

(a) **Conventional emulsion** ($\delta << r_c$)

(b) **Nanoemulsion** ($\delta \approx r_n$)

Figure 15.5 Schematic illustrations of the interfacial layer thickness (δ) on droplets radii (r) (a) from an oil droplet in a conventional emulsion and (b) from an oil droplet in a nanoemulsion. *Source:* Adapted from McClements, D.J. (2010). Reproduced with permission from Royal Society of Chemistry

nanoemulsions may have relatively higher proportion of the interfacial layer, which can exert a greater influence on the particle characteristics.

The interfacial characteristics of droplets can be manipulated when designing an emulsion as a delivery system. For instance, an emulsion can be designed to control the release of encapsulated components under changing environmental conditions, such as temperature, pH and ionic strength. This can be achieved by creating emulsions with multi-layer or mixed-layers at the interface. For example, the droplets in emulsions may be coated with a series of oppositely charged biopolymers through electrostatic interactions to create multi-layers around their droplets. Previously, Lesmes *et al.* (2010) studied the physical properties and *in vitro* lipase digestibility of protein-stabilized emulsions coated with lactoferrin and/or sodium caseinate. They found that the emulsions coated with a secondary layer of lactoferrin or sodium caseinate were more stable to pH changes (pH 3–7) and ionic strength (0–80 mM $CaCl_2$) but the lipid digestibility of oil droplets was similar to those in the primary emulsions. The study suggests that it is possible to increase the stability of emulsions to various environmental conditions without compromising the lipid digestibility by utilizing a series of different polyelectrolytes at the droplet interface.

Rheological properties Food emulsions have very different rheological behaviours. Some emulsions are dilute and fluid-like while others are viscous or highly viscoelastic (McClements, 1999; McClements and Rao, 2011). The rheological properties of an emulsion may depend on the composition, structure and droplet interactions (McClements and Rao, 2011). Consequently, nanoemulsions with small droplet size may have different rheological properties than most conventional emulsions. For instance, the small droplet size of nanoemulsions is thought to increase the emulsion viscosity due to higher particle interactions. Often, it is useful to have an understanding of the rheology of conventional emulsions as it is well established. Assuming food emulsions are being considered as a concentrated system, their viscosities can be described by the Krieger–Dougherty equation in Equation 15.5 (McClements, 1999).

$$\frac{\eta}{\eta_0} = \left(1 - \frac{\phi}{\phi_0}\right)^{-[\eta]\phi_0} \tag{15.5}$$

where η is the viscosity of the emulsion system, η_0 is the viscosity of the continuous phase, ϕ is the volume fraction of the dispersed phase, ϕ_0 is the maximum volume fraction of closely packed droplets and $[\eta]$ is the intrinsic viscosity which is 2.5 for spherical particles.

From the Krieger–Dougherty equation, the viscosity of an emulsion will increase when the volume fraction of its oil phase increases as the particles are more closely packed. When the volume fraction nears the droplet concentration where they are closely packed (around 0.4 to 0.6 for a non-flocculated emulsion), the emulsions are solid-like, viscoelastic or plastic (McClements and Rao, 2011). However, the rheological behaviour of nanoemulsions is different to that of conventional emulsions. Due to their smaller particle size, nanoemulsion droplets may have a thicker interfacial layer for repulsive interactions. The repulsive interactions prevent the droplets from coming in close proximity and consequently, the effective volume fraction (ϕ_{eff}) is substituted in the Krieger–Dougherty equation to replace ϕ in Equation 15.6

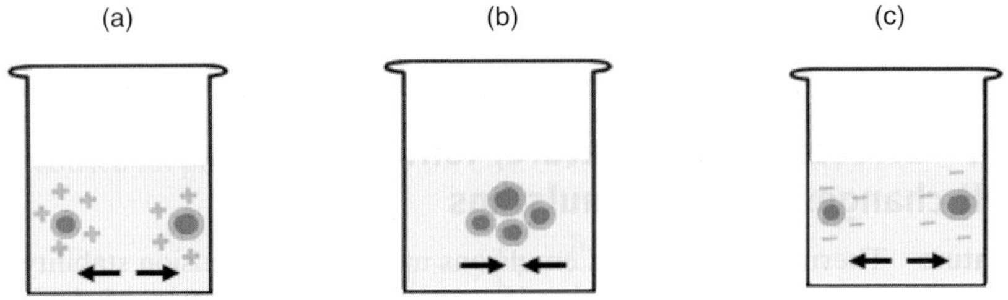

Figure 15.6 Schematic illustrations of emulsion droplet interactions at pH value (a) below the isoelectric point (pI), (b) near the isoelectric point and (c) above the isoelectric point of proteins

neutral with less electrostatic repulsive forces, leading to droplet aggregation (Figure 15.6b). When the pH is further increased above the pI, the carboxyl groups become negatively charged ($COOH \rightarrow COO^- + H^+$) and the amino groups remain neutral (NH_2). The overall net charge of the droplets is negative so they repel each other to form a stable emulsion (Figure 15.6c).

Some studies have shown that the stability and properties of protein-stabilized nanoemulsions can be affected by pH changes. The protein-stabilized emulsions are normally stable to pH changes above or below the pI of proteins but become unstable near to the pI due to less electrostatic repulsion. Qian *et al.* (2012) showed that the nanoemulsions stabilized by 2% β-lactoglobulin were stable at pH 3, 6, 7 and 8 but formed large aggregates at pH 4 and 5, which is near the pI of β-lactoglobulin. In another study, large aggregates were formed at pH 1, 9, 11 and 13 as the proteins were irreversibly denatured by extremely low or high pH values and lost their emulsifying properties (Chu *et al.*, 2008).

The stability of WPI-stabilized conventional emulsions and nanoemulsions during pH changes (pH 3–8) was also studied (Lee *et al.*, 2011). Both emulsions were unstable at pH values near to the pI of whey proteins (pH 4.5–5.5) but exhibited different phase separation behaviour. The conventional emulsions formed a cream layer on the top of their emulsions but the nanoemulsions settled down at the bottom. The observed difference in their phase separation behaviour can be explained by the overall particle density. Both emulsions contained a similar oil content of 0.5% w/w but the nanoemulsions (0.9% w/w) contained a higher amount of protein than the conventional emulsions (0.045% w/w). Consequently, the droplets in the nanoemulsions were coated by a thicker interfacial layer of protein which increases the particle density than the surrounding liquid for sedimentation to occur. However, the particle density of the conventional emulsions remained less than the surrounding liquid causing the formation of a cream layer.

15.3.5 Shelf life over long-term storage

The chemical stability of emulsions against lipid oxidation is an important factor when they are used to encapsulate and protect lipophilic components which are sensitive to oxygen, light and temperature. The lipid oxidation of protein-stabilized nanoemulsions and conventional emulsions containing menhaden oils during storage was carried out (Lee *et al.*, 2011). The thiobarbituric acid-reactive substance (TBARS) was determined to measure the lipid oxidation of emulsions. They found that the nanoemulsions have a higher oxidation rate than the conventional emulsions because of an increased surface area to volume ratio where more oil droplets are exposed to lipid oxidation. Furthermore, nanoemulsions are transparent systems and allow more light to penetrate, further increasing the rate of lipid oxidation (Tan and Nakajima, 2005a).

The long-term phase stability of emulsions is an important attribute. The phase stability of β-carotene nanodispersions at 4 °C for 12 weeks was investigated by Tan and Nakajima (2005a). The β-carotene nanodispersions were physically stable during storage for 12 weeks at 4 °C as their particle size did not increase but the β-carotene content was found to decrease due to oxidation during storage. The degradation of β-carotene was attributed to an increased surface area of nanoemulsions. Another study determined the storage stability of β-carotene-enriched nanoemulsions at different storage temperatures of 5, 20, 37 and 55 °C for 2 weeks (Qian *et al.*, 2012). The results also showed no significant change in their particle size but there was a greater loss of β-carotene at higher storage temperatures after 2 weeks. This suggests that further work to prolong storage of nanoemulsions and increase β-carotene stability is needed, for example using a controlled atmosphere.

15.4 Applications of nanoparticles and nanoemulsions

Nanotechnology can be used to improve or design foods with novel functionalities in tastes, flavors, textures and nutritional values. The current applications of nanotechnology are still mainly driven by the pharmaceutical and cosmetic industries. The applications of nanotechnology in food products are still in their infancy among food manufacturers. Nevertheless, the main applications are for delivery of bioactive food ingredients or nutraceuticals and for improving food functionalities, such as tastes, flavors, textures and nutritional values. These food products are likely to provide new ways to enhance health, beauty and wellness.

Some applications of nanotechnology for food products include:

- encapsulating bioactive ingredients in nano-delivery systems to increase delivery and bioavailability of the bioactive compounds;
- controlling the release of flavors in foods or masking off-flavors – this function allows the preferred flavor to be released when triggered by certain environmental conditions;
- creating a different visual appearance of food by changing optical clarity by reducing the particle size;
- modifying food texture to create highly viscous or gel-like texture in low or reduced fat products;
- improving the phase stability of food to increase the shelf life.

The application of nanotechnology for food and beverages is likely to result in innovative developments to enhance the functional and nutritional qualities of foods.

However, any new technological developments for use in food will inevitably raise some concerns over safety and the potential risks to health.

15.5 Potential health effects and risks

There are many viewpoints concerning the use of nanotechnology in foods and its potential risk to human health. The physicochemical properties of nanoparticles are fundamentally different compared to conventional ones, especially when the nanoparticles pass through the human gastrointestinal (GI) tract. The cellular uptake of particles in the GI tract has been shown to be higher for small particles as they have a greater ability to penetrate the mucus layer across the gut wall (Bouwmeester and Marvin, 2010). This may result in increased absorption and bioavailability of substances used in nanoparticles. As a result, the consumption of nano-foods may lead to certain health consequences that may be either beneficial or harmful. For example, bioactive components encapsulated in nanoemulsions can increase their bioavailability in foods, but some bioactive components may exhibit toxic effects when consumed at high levels due to greater absorption (Chaudhry *et al.*, 2010; McClements and Rao, 2011).

Moreover, nanoparticles may be absorbed directly into bloodstream in the human body as they may be able pass through the cell walls due to their relatively small size. This may pose certain risks to health as nanoparticles can reach unintended parts of the body where large particles are normally restricted. The nanoparticles are likely to enter these 'new' sites in the body and may act as a 'Trojan Horse' to translocate the encapsulated components, which may affect the physiology of human organs and human body. The nanoparticles may also adsorb or bind to various components in the body and act as a carrier to transport them across different parts of the body. This may pose potential harmful effects when undesirable contaminants or foreign substances are being transported (Bouwmeester and Marvin, 2010; Chaudhry *et al.*, 2010).

In addition, the use of some materials to prepare nanoparticles for food applications may not be suitable for human consumption due to their inherent toxicity. For examples, large amounts of surfactants or organic solvents are used to form nanoemulsions but these materials are potentially toxic and raise certain safety concerns. Therefore, all these concerns need to be considered when using nanotechnology in foods to deliver bioactive compounds and to improve their stability and bioavailability.

15.6 Conclusions

Nanotechnology can offer a variety of benefits to the food industry with many applications in the development of nano-structured materials such as nanoparticles or nanoemulsions. This review chapter attempts to provide an overview of the preparation of nanoemulsions and their physicochemical properties as well as some techniques used to characterize them. Nanoemulsions are shown to have many advantages over conventional emulsions, such as optical clarity, high kinetic stability and increased bioavailability. While nanoemulsions are considered to be one of the most promising delivery systems for food applications, its use is still limited while its effects on health and food safety are being investigated.

References

Ahmed, K., Li, Y., McClements, D.J. and Xiao, H. (2012). Nanoemulsion- and emulsion-based delivery systems for curcumin: Encapsulation and release properties. *Food Chemistry*, 132 (2), 799–807.

Anton, N. and Vandamme, T.F. (2009). The universality of low-energy nano-emulsification. *International Journal of Pharmaceutics*, 377 (1–2), 142–147.

Anton, N., Benoit, J. and Saulnier, P. (2008). Design and production of nanoparticles formulated from nano-emulsion templates – A review. *Journal of Controlled Release*, 128 (3), 185–199.

Aryee, F.N.A. and Nickerson, M.T. (2012). Formation of electrostatic complexes involving mixtures of lentil protein isolates and gum Arabic polysaccharides. *Food Research International*, 48 (2), 520–527.

Baker, E.N. and Baker, H.M. (2009). A structural framework for understanding the multifunctional character of lactoferrin. *Biochimie*, 91 (1), 3–10.

Bouwmeester, H. and Marvin, H.J.P. (2010). Potential risks of nanofood to consumers, in *Nanotechnologies in Food* (eds Q. Chaudhry, L. Castle and R. Watkins). The Royal Society of Chemistry, Cambridge, pp. 134–149.

Calder, P.C. and Yaqoob, P. (2009). Omega-3 polyunsaturated fatty acids and human health outcomes. *BioFactors*, 35 (3), 266–272.

Chalothorn, K. and Warisnoicharoen, W. (2012). Ultrasonic emulsification of whey protein isolate-stabilized nanoemulsions containing omega-3 oil from plant seed. *American Journal of Food Technology*, 7 (9), 532–541.

Chaudhry, Q., Watkins, R. and Castle, L. (2010). Nanotechnologies in the food arena: New opportunities, new questions, new concerns, in *Nanotechnologies in Food*. The Royal Society of Chemistry, Cambridge, pp. 1–17.

Choi, A.J., Kim, C.J., Cho, Y.J., Hwang, J.K. and Kim, C.T. (2011). Characterization of capsaicin-loaded nanoemulsions stabilized with alginate and chitosan by self-assembly. *Food Bioprocess Technology*, 4 (6), 1119–1126.

Chopra, H.K. and Panesar, P.S. (2010). *Food Chemistry*. Alpha Science International Ltd, Oxford.

Chu, B.S., Ichikawa, S., Kanafusa, S. and Nakajima, M. (2007a). Preparation of protein-stabilized β carotene nanodispersions by emulsification evaporation method. *Journal of American Oil Chemists' Society*, 84 (11), 1053–1062.

Chu, B.S., Ichikawa, S., Kanafusa, S. and Nakajima, M. (2007b). Preparation and characterization of β-carotene nanodispersions prepared by solvent displacement technique. *Journal of Agricultural and Food Chemistry*, 55 (16), 6754–6760.

Chu, B.S., Ichikawa, S., Kanafusa, S. and Nakajima, M. (2008). Stability of protein-stabilised β-carotene nanodispersions against heating, salts and pH. *Journal of the Science of Food and Agriculture*, 88 (10), 1769–1769.

Chung, H., Kim, T.W., Kwon, I.C. and Jeong, S.Y. (2001). Oil components modulate physical characteristics and function of the natural oil emulsions as drug or gene delivery system. *Journal of Controlled Release*, 71 (3), 339–350.

Deshmukh, A.S., Setty, C.M., Badiger, A.M. and Muralikrishna, K.S. (2012). Gum ghatti: A promising polysaccharide for pharmaceutical applications. *Carbohydrate Polymers*, 87 (2), 980–986.

Dickinson, E. (2003). Hydrocolloids at interfaces and the influence on the properties of dispersed systems. *Food Hydrocolloids*, 17 (1), 25–39.

Dickinson, E. (2009). Hydrocolloids as emulsifies and emulsion stabilizers. *Food Hydrocolloids*, 23 (6), 1473–1482.

Ee, S.L., Duan, X., Liew, J. and Nguyen, Q.D. (2008). Droplet size and stability of nano-emulsions produced by the temperature phase inversion method. *Chemical Engineering Journal*, 140 (1–3), 626–631.

Flanagan, J. and Singh, H. (2006). Microemulsions: A potential delivery system for bioactives in food. *Critical Reviews in Food Science and Nutrition*, 46 (3), 221–237.

Fernandez, P., André, V., Rieger, J. and Kühnie, A. (2004). Nano-emulsion formation by emulsion phase inversion. *Colloids and Surfaces A: Physicochemical Engineering Aspects*, 251 (1–3), 53–58.

Foegeding, E.A., Luck, P. and Vardhanabhuti, B. (2011). Milk protein products whey protein products, *Encyclopedia of Dairy Science*, 2nd edn. Academic Press, 873–878.

Fryd, M.M. and Mason, T.G. (2012). Advanced nanoemulsions. *Annual Review of Physical Chemistry*, 63, 493–518.

Garti, N. (2002). Food emulsifiers: Structure–reactivity relationships, design, and applications, in *Physical Properties of Lipids* (eds A.G. Marangoni and S.S. Narine). CRC Press, pp. 265–386.

Ghosh, V., Mukherjee, A. and Chandrasekaran, N. (2012). Ultrasonic emulsification of food-grade nanoemulsion formulation and evaluation of its bactericidal activity. *Ultrasonics Sonochemistry*, 20 (1), 338–344.

González-Chávez, S., Arévalo-Gallegos, S. and Rascón-Cruz, Q. (2009). Lactoferrin: Structure, function and applications. *International Journal of Antimicrobial Agents*, 33 (4), 301–308.

Gutiérrez, J.M., González, C., Maestro, A. *et al.* (2008). Nano-emulsions: New applications and optimization of their preparation. *Current Opinion in Colloid and Interface Science*, 13 (4), 245–251.

Hasenhuettl, G.L. (2008). Synthesis and commercial preparation of food emulsifiers, in *Food Emulsifiers and Their Applications*, 2nd edn (eds G.L. Hasenhuettl and R.W. Hartel). Springer Science + Business Media, New York, pp. 11–37.

Hatanaka, J., Chikamori, H., Sato, H. *et al.* (2010). Physiochemical and pharmacological characterization of α-tocopherol-loaded nano-emulsion system. *International Journal of Pharmaceutics*, 396 (1–2), 188–193.

Henry, J.V.L., Fryer, P.J., Frith, W.J. and Norton, I.T. (2009). Emulsification mechanism and storage instabilities of hydrocarbon-in-water sub-micron emulsions stabilised with Tweens (20 and 80), Brij 96v and sucrose monoesters. *Journal of Colloid and Interface Science*, 338 (1), 201–206.

Henry, J.V.L., Fryer, P.J., Frith, W.J. and Norton, I.T. (2010). The influence of phospholipids and food proteins on the size and stability of model sub-micron emulsions. *Food Hydrocolloids*, 24 (1), 66–71.

Horne, D.S. (2011). Analytical methods light scattering techniques, in *Encyclopaedia of Dairy Sciences*, 2nd edn. Academic Press, pp. 133–140.

Horvath, H. (2009). Gustav Mie and the scattering and absorption of light by particles: Historic developments and basics. *Journal of Quantitative Spectroscopy and Radiative Transfer*,10 (11), 787–799.

Hosseinpour, S., Izadi, M., Aminlari, M., Ramezani, R. and Tavana, M. (2011). Changes in the solubility and SDS-PAGE profile of whey proteins during storage at different temperatures: A kinetic study. *Journal of Food and Agriculture Science*, 1 (1), 15–21.

Hu, L., Mao, Z. and Gao, C. (2009). Colloidal particles for cellular uptake and delivery. *Journal of Materials Chemistry*, 19 (20), 3108–3115.

Jafari, S.M., He, Y. and Bhandari, B. (2007). Optimization of nano-emulsions production by microfluidisation. *European Food Research Technology*, 225 (5–6), 733–741.

Kamogawa, K., Okudaira, G., Matsumoto, M., Sakai, T., Sakai, M. and Abe, M. (2004). Preparation of oleic acid/water emulsions in surfactant-free condition by sequential processing using midsonic megasonic waves. *Langmuir*, 20 (6), 2043–2047.

Kang, J., Cui, S.W., Chen, J., Philips, G.O., Wu, Y. and Wang, Q. (2011). New studies on gum ghatti (*Anogeissus latifolia*) part I. Fractionation, chemical and physical characterization of the gum. *Food Hydrocolloids*, 25 (8), 1984–1990.

Kentish, S., Wooster, T.J., Ashokkumar, M. *et al.* (2008). The use of ultrasonics for nanoemulsion preparation. *Innovative Food Science and Emerging Technologies*, 9 (2), 170–175.

Klang, V., Matsko, N.B., Valenta, C. and Hofer, F. (2012). Electron microscopy of nanoemulsions: An essential tool for characterisation and stability assessment. *Micron*, 43 (2–3), 85–103.

Kulmyrzaev, A., Chanamai, R. and McClements, D.J. (2000). Influence of pH and $CaCl_2$ on the stability of dilute whey protein stabilized emulsions. *Food Research International*, 33 (1), 15–20.

Kralova, I and Sjöblom, J. (2009). Surfactants used in food industry: A review. *Journal of Dispersion Science and Technology*, 30 (9), 1363–1383.

Lee, S.J., Choi, S.J., Li, Y., Decker, E.A. and McClements, D.J. (2011). Protein-stabilized nanoemulsions and emulsions: comparison of physiochemical stability, lipid oxidation, and lipase digestibility. *Journal of Agricultural and Food Chemistry*, 59 (1), 415–427.

Lee, S.J. and McClements, D.J. (2010). Fabrication of protein-stabilized nanoemulsions using a combined homogenization and amphiphilic solvent dissolution/evaporation approach. *Food Hydrocolloids*, 24 (6–7), 560–569.

Lesmes, U., Baudot, P. and McClements, D.J. (2010). Impact of interfacial composition on physical stability and *in vitro* lipase digestibility of triacylglycerol oil droplets coated with lactoferrin and/or caseinate. *Journal of Agricultural and Food Chemistry*, 58 (13), 7962–7969.

Li, Y., Zheng, J., Xiao, H. and McClements, D.J. (2012). Nanoemulsion-based delivery systems for poorly water-soluble bioactive compounds: Influence of formation parameters on polymethoxyflavone crystallization. *Food Hydrocollods*, 27 (2), 517–528.

Livney, Y.D. (2010). Milk proteins as vehicles for bioactives. *Current Opinion in Colloid & Interface Science*, 15 (1–2), 73–83.

Maestro, A., Solè, I., González, C., Solans, C. and Gutiérrez, J.M. (2008). Influence of the phase behavior on the properties of ionic nanoemulsions prepared by the phase inversion composition method. *Journal of Colloid and Interface Science*, 327 (2), 433–439.

Mahdi, E.S., Sakeena, M.H.F., Abdulkarim, M.F. *et al.* (2011). Effect of surfactant and surfactant blends on pseudoternary phase diagram behaviour of newly synthesized palm kernel oil esters. *Drug Design, Development and Therapy*, 5, 311–323.

McClements, D.J. (1999). *Food Emulsions Principles, Practices, and Techniques*. CRC Press, Boca Raton, FL.

McClements, D.J. (2007). Critical review of techniques and methodologies for characterization of emulsion stability. *Critical Reviews in Food Science and Nutrition*, 47 (7), 611–649.

McClements, D.J. (2012). Nanoemulsions *versus* microemulsions: Terminology, differences, and similarities. *Soft Matter*, 8 (6), 1719–1729.

McClements, D.J. and Rao, J. (2011). Food-grade nanoemulsions: formulation, fabrication, properties, performance, biological fate, and potential toxicity. *Critical Reviews in Food Science and Nutrition*, 51 (4), 285–330.

National Science and Technology Council (2006). The National Nanotechnology Initiative Environmental, Health, and Safety Research Needs for Engineered Nanoscale Materials. http://www.nano.gov/sites/default/files/pub_resource/nni_ehs_research_needs.pdf?q=NNI_EHS_research_needs.pdf [accessed 28 July 2013].

Onwulata, C.I. (2012). Encapsulation of new active ingredients. *Annual Review of Food Science and Technology*, 3, 183–202.

Ostertag, F., Weiss, J. and McClements, D.J. (2012). Low-energy formation of edible nanoemulsions: Factors influencing droplet size produced by emulsion phase inversion. *Journal of Colloid and Interface Science*, 388 (1), 95–102.

Pierce, A., Colavizza, D., Benaissa, M. *et al.* (1991). Molecular cloning and sequence analysis of bovine lactotransferrin. *European Journal of Biochemistry*, 196 (1), 177–184.

Qian, C. and McClements, D.J. (2011). Formation of nanoemulsions stabilized by model food-grade emulsifiers using high-pressure homogenization: Factors affecting particle size. *Food Hydrocolloids*, 25 (5), 1000–1008.

Qian, C., Decker, E.A., Xiao, H. and McClements, D.J. (2012). Physical and chemical stability of β-carotene-enriched nanoemulsions: Influence of pH, ionic strength, temperature, and emulsifier type. *Food Chemistry*, 132 (3), 1221–1229.

Sahin, S. and Sumnu, S.G. (2006). *Physical Properties of Foods*. Springer Science + Business Media, New York.

Salvia-Trujillo, L., Rojas-Graü, M.A., Soliva-Fortuny, R. and Martín-Belloso, O. (2013). Effect of processing parameters on physiochemical and characteristics of microfluidised lemongrass essential oil–alginate nanoemulsions. *Food Hydrocolloids*, 30 (1), 401–407.

Shimazaki, K. (2000). Lactoferrin: A marvelous protein in milk? *Animal Science Journal*, 71 (4), 329–347.

Silva, H.D., Cerqueira, M.A., Souza, B.W.S. *et al.* (2011). Nanoemulsions of β-carotene using a high-enegy emulsification-evaporation technique. *Journal of Food Engineering*, 102 (2), 130–135.

Singh, H. (2011). Milk protein products functional properties of milk proteins, in *Encyclopadia of Dairy Sciences*, 2nd edn. Academic Press, pp. 887–893.

Solans, C., Izquierdo, P., Nolla, J. Azemar, N. and Garcia-Celma, M.J. (2005). Nano-emulsions. *Current Opinion in Colloid & Interface Science*, 10 (3–4), 102–110.

Solans, C. and Solè, I. (2012). Nano-emulsions: Formation by low-energy methods. *Current Opinion in Colloid & Interface Science*, 17 (5), 246–254.

Solè, I., Maestro, A, González, C., Solans, C and Gutiérrez, J.M. (2006). Optimization of nano-emulsion preparation by low-energy methods in an ionic surfactant system. *Langmuir*, 22 (20), 8326–8332.

Stone, A.K. and Nickerson, M.T. (2012). Formation and functionality of whey protein isolate-(kappa-, iota and lamda-type) carrageenan electrostatic complexes. *Food Hydrocolloids*, 27 (2), 271–277.

Sun, C., Gunasekaran, S. and Richards, M.P. (2007). Effect of xanthan gum on physiochemical properties of whey protein isolate stabilised oil-in-water emulsions. *Food Hydrocolloids*, 21 (4), 555–564.

Tadros, T., Izquierdo, P., Esquena, J. and Solans. (2004). Formation and stability of nano-emulsions. *Advances in Colloid and Interface Science*, 108–109, 303–318.

Tan, C.P. and Nakajima, M. (2005a). β-carotene nanodispersions: preparation, characterization and stability evaluation. *Food Chemistry*, 92 (4), 661–671.

Tan, C.P. and Nakajima, M. (2005b). Effect of polyglycerol esters of fatty acids on physiochemical properties and stability of β-carotene nanodispersions prepared by emulsification/evaporation method. *Journal of the Science of Food and Agriculture*, 85 (1), 121–126.

Tang, S.Y., Shridharan, P. and Sivakumar, M. (2012). Impact of process parameters in the generation of novel aspirin nanoemulsions – Comparative studies between ultrasound cavitation and microfluidiser. *Ultrasonics Sonochemistry*, 20 (1), 485–497.

Tiwari, R. and Takhistov, P. (2012). Nanotechnology-enabled delivery systems for food functionalization and fortification, in *Nanotechnology Research Methods for Foods and Bioproducts*) eds G.W. Padua and Q. Wang). John Wiley & Sons, Inc., pp. 55–101.

Tokle, T. and McClements, D.J. (2011). Physiochemical properties of lactoferrin stabilized oil-in-water emulsions: Effects of pH, salt and heating. *Food Hydrocolloids*, 25 (2), 976–982.

Wahlqvist, M.L. and Wattanapenpaiboon, N. (2011). Vitamins, vitamin-like compounds and phytonutrients, in *Food and Nutrition*, 3rd edn (ed. M.L. Wahlqvist). Allen & Unwin, New South Wales.

Webb, P.A. and Orr, C. (2006). Modern methods of particle characterization, part 1: Particle size. *American Ceramic Society Bulletin*, 85 (9), 24–27.

Weinbreck, F., Vries, R., Schrooyen, P. and Kruif, C.G. (2003). Complex coacervation of whey proteins and gum arabic. *Biomacromolecules*, 4 (2), 293–303.

Weiss, J. and McClements, D.J. (2000). Influence of Ostwald ripening on rheology of oil-in-water emulsions containing electrostatically stabilized droplets. *Langmuir*, 16 (5), 2145–2150.

Wooster, T.J., Golding, M. and Sanguansri, P. (2008). Impact of oil type on nanoemulsion formation and Ostwald ripening stability. *Langmuir*, 24 (22), 12758–12765.

Yang, Y., Marshall-Breton, C., Leser, M.E., Sher, A.A. and McClements, D.J. (2012). Fabrication of ultrafine edible emulsions: Comparison of high-energy and low-energy homogenization methods. *Food Hydrocolloids*, 29 (2), 398–406.

Ye, A., Flanagan, J. and Singh, H. (2006). Formation of stable nanoparticles via electrostatic complexation between sodium caseinate and gum arabic. *Biopolymers*, 8 (2), 121–133.

Ye, A. and Singh, H. (2007). Formation of multilayers at the interface of oil-in-water emulsion via interactions between lactoferrin and β-lactoglobulin. *Food Biophysics*, 2 (4), 125–132.

Yin, L.J., Chu, B.S., Kobayashi, I. and Nakajima, M. (2009). Performance of selected emulsifiers and their combinations in the preparation of β-carotene nanodispersions. *Food Hydrocolloids*, 23 (6), 1617–1622.

Yuan, Y., Gao, Y., Zhao, J. and Mao, L. (2008). Characterization and stability evaluation of β-carotene nanoemulsions prepared by high pressure homogenization under various emulsifying conditions. *Food Research International*, 41 (1), 61–68.

Zuidam, N.J. and Shimoni, E. (2010). Overview of microencapsulates for use in food products or processes and methods to make them, in *Encapsulation Technologies for Active Food Ingredients and Food Processing* (eds N.J. Zuidam and V. Nedović). Springer Science + Business Media, pp. 3–30.

IV
Health Benefits and Bioavailability of Functional Foods

16

Pharmacology and Health Benefits of Bioactive Food Sources

Maushmi S. Kumar[1] **and Shruti Mishra**[2]

[1]*Department of Pharmaceutical Biotechnology, Shobhaben Pratapbhai Patel School of Pharmacy and Technology Management, SVKM'S NMIMS (Deemed-to-be University), Mumbai, India*

[2]*Asian Institute of Technology, Pathum Thani, Thailand*

16.1 Introduction

From ancient times, food has been the most powerful tool available to heal chronic disease states and to cure and maintain health apart from surgery and medicines. The medicinal properties of foods have been recorded and extensively used in Asia and Europe. Ayurveda, a 5000 year old ancient Indian health science, mentions the benefits of food for therapeutic purposes. These foods not only provide calories but also communicate with our genes, which has given rise to an innovative field of study called nutrigenomics. Today, pharmaceutical and food researchers and industries share the desire to isolate and characterize new bioactive compounds from natural sources that can be used as new drugs, functional foods, nutraceuticals or dietary fibres. Due to recent research and an increased interest in the area, there are different terms which have been coined for food and food products. One of these terms is functional foods, which are defined as food products that have an added positive health benefit and provide the body with the required amount of vitamins, fats, proteins, carbohydrates, etc., needed for its healthy survival. The second class are known as a nutraceuticals, which are foods (or part of a food) that provide medical or health benefits, including the prevention and/or treatment of disease(s) and/or disorder(s). However, the term nutraceutical, as commonly used in marketing, has no regulatory definition. These bioactive components are derived from plant, food and microbial sources and provide medicinal benefits valuable to long-term health. Examples of these nutraceutical chemicals include probiotics, antioxidants and

Functional Foods and Dietary Supplements: Processing Effects and Health Benefits, First Edition.
Edited by Athapol Noomhorm, Imran Ahmad and Anil Kumar Anal.

sugar by 13.1, 16.3 and 21.4% and 3.2, 5.58 and 8.21%, respectively (Yadav *et al.*, 2002). The aqueous and methanol extracts of *M. koenigii* leaves exhibit a significant hypoglycaemic effect from the very first week in diabetic rat groups, which could be due to the presence of alanine, leucine, carbohydrate, niacin, iron and calcium in the aqueous extract and the various constituents in the volatile oil (indole alkaloids such as mahanine and mahanimbine, sesquiterpene such as cadinene and monoterpene such as dipentene) in the methanol extract of *M. koenigii.* The increase in plasma insulin concentration could also be due to the longer-lasting stimulant effect on β-cells of pancreatic islets or due to regeneration of pancreatic β-cells of *M. koenigii* (Vinuthan *et al.*, 2004). The *M. koenigii* leaves are also involved in decreasing oxidative stress and increasing paraoxonase1 activity both in liver and serum, associated with diabetes (Saha and Mazumder, 2013). However, as the antidiabetic property of the extract is not comparable to chlorpropamide, the plant extract cannot be used as a substitute for conventional antidiabetic drugs.

***Momordica charantia* (L.)** A very common remedy for DM in different cultures is *Momordica charantia* (karela or bitter gourd). A wide range of compounds have been isolated from *M. charantia,* of which, a polypeptide (*p*-insulin, was named as 'plant insulin'), the sterol glucoside mixture charantin and the pyrimidine nucleoside vicine have been identified as the orally antidiabetic principles for humans and animals. However, in a recent study, Ooi *et al.* (2012) concluded that the evidence on the effects of *M. charantia* for type 2 diabetes mellitus was statistically insignificant and insufficient and suggested further studies to address the issues of standardization and the quality control of preparations. Another study demonstrated that dry bitter gourd given at the 10% level in the diet improved diabetic status. Higher consumption in the diet was observed in control and diabetic rats fed bitter gourd and could be attributed to the high fibre content of bitter gourd (48% fibre) which makes it more palatable (Shetty *et al.*, 2005). Shibib *et al.* (1993) reported that the hypoglycaemic effect of bitter gourd is due to suppression of key gluconeogenic enzymes such as glucose-6-phosphatase and fructose-1,6-bisphosphatase on one hand and an accelerated glucose metabolism through glucose-6-phosphate dehydrogenase on the other. However, the mechanism of action of bitter gourd still remains unclear.

***Dioscorea opposita* (Thunb.)** The rhizomes of *Dioscorea opposita* Thunb. were traditionally used in diets to control blood sugar in China. Researchers confirmed that the water decoction of *D. opposita* has an anti-hyperglycaemic effect on experimental diabetic mice (Hao *et al.*, 1991). The chemical components dioscin and diosgenin of *D. opposite* may be the cause of medicinal effects. Polysaccharides were considered to be the active constituents. Rhizome extract significantly reduced insulin and glucose levels in the blood of dexamethasone-induced diabetic rats. The extract also increased mRNA expression of GLUT4 glucose transporter in 3T3-L1 adipocytes suggesting that *D. opposita* insulin sensitivity is associated with the regulation of GLUT4 expression (Gao *et al.*, 2007).

***Punica granatum* (L.)** *Punica granatum* is found to contain hydrolysable tannins as major active chemical constituents and phytoconstituents, namely, corilagin, ellagic acid, kaempferol, luteolin, myricetin, quercetin, quercimetrine and quercetin-3-*o*-rutinoside, which were previously isolated from the fruits of *P. granatum* (Jain *et al.*,

2011). The husk of *P. granatum* decreases concentration of glucose, triglyceride, cholesterol, low density lipoprotein (LDL) cholesterol, very low density lipoprotein (VLDL) cholesterol and increases high density lipoprotein (HDL) cholesterol and haemoglobin content in both normal and alloxan-diabetic rats treated with crude powder (Radhika *et al.*, 2011). The ethanolic extract of leaves of *P. granatum* at a dose of 500 mg/kg body weight produced significant antidiabetic activity in albino rats with alloxan-induced, non-insulin-dependent DM. It is highly effective in managing the complications associated with DM, such as hyperlipidaemia, and prevents the defects in lipid metabolism (Das and Barman, 2012).

***Ganoderma lucidum* (Leyss. ex. Fr.)** *Ganoderma lucidum* (GI) is commonly known as a medicinally potent mushroom. It has been widely used in China and other oriental countries for hundreds of years for the treatment of various diseases like hypertension, bronchial asthma, diabetes and cancer. Ganoderans A and B have been isolated and confirmed to have a hypoglycaemic activity. Studies have been carried out for understanding the GI polysaccharides (GI-PS) effect on STZ-induced mice. GI-PS produced a significant drop in fasting blood glucose levels in diabetic mice. One of the possible mechanisms of this anti-hyperglycaemic effect could be due to an insulin-release stimulatory effect. The treatments induced an increment in serum insulin levels, which might increase the renewal of β-cells in the pancreas or permit the recovery of partially destroyed β-cells and stimulate pancreatic insulin secretion (Li *et al.*, 2011). There are other studies that have shown that GI-PS can reduce and delay the absorption of glucose in rats (Cao and Guo, 2010).

***Prunella vulgaris* (L.)** Phytochemical studies indicate that *P. vulgaris* contains oleanolic, betulinic, ursolic, 2α, 3α-dihydroxyurs-12-en-28-oic, and 2α, 3α-ursolic acids, triterpenoids, flavonoids, tannins and anionic polysaccharide called prunellin (Fang *et al.*, 2005; Feng *et al.*, 2010). It *induces* anti-hyperglycaemic effects without stimulating insulin secretion. The anti-hyperglycaemic activity of the *P. vulgaris* may be due to any one or more of the constituents in the extract, for example, triterpenoids and flavonoids. The use of this plant for diabetes treatment is promising but the precise active substance(s), site(s) and mechanism(s) of its pharmacological effect are still to be determined (Zheng *et al.*, 2007). It was also reported that *Prunella vulgaris* significantly reduced the expressions of endothelin-1 and remarkably increased the expression of endothelial NO synthase in the aorta in *db/db* mice with type 2 diabetes (Hwang *et al.*, 2012). Water extract of *P. vulgaris* inhibits the activity of rat lens aldose reductase (rAR). Among the compounds isolated, caffeic acid ethylene ester and rosmarinic acid were demonstrated to possess strong AR inhibitory activity (Hong *et al.*, 2012).

***Stevia rebaudina* (Bert.) Hemsl.** Stevioside suppresses the postprandial blood glucose level in type 2 diabetic subjects by an average of 18%. The circulating insulin levels tend to be increased by stevioside but do not attain statistical significance. Stevioside reduces postprandial blood glucose and tends to potentiate the insulin secretion in patients with type 2 diabetes. Whether long-term administration of stevioside would improve the postprandial glycaemia and blood pressure enough to justify its use as a new treatment for type 2 diabetes remains to be proven (Gregerson *et al.*, 2004). *Stevia* extract also antagonizes the necrotic action of alloxan and has a revitalizing effect on pancreatic β-cells (Mishra *et al.*, 2011).

***Nelumbo nucifera* (Gaertn.)** *Nelumbo nucifera* rhizome extract showed antidiabetic and anti-inflammatory effects and contains the alkaloids liensinine, daurisoline and neferine and flavonoids as the main compounds that give medicinal effects (Mukherji *et al.*, 1997a, 1997b; Zhou *et al.*, 2009). Huang *et al.* (2011) have shown that the leaf methanolic extract regulated blood glucose levels in fasted normal mice and high-fat-diet-induced diabetic mice. The effects of active constituents quercetin and catechin on glucose-induced insulin secretion and blood glucose regulation have been evaluated resulting in quercetin having no effect on insulin secretion, but catechin causing significantly and dose-dependently enhanced insulin secretion. Orally administered catechin significantly reversed the glucose intolerance in high-fat-diet-induced diabetic mice. Thus catechin can be used in the control of hyperglycaemia in non-insulin-dependent DM through their action as insulin secretagogues in the future (Huang *et al.*, 2011). In another study, flower extract did not show any effect on haematological values and blood cell character in diabetic rats. However, it recovered the white blood cell (WBC) count in diabetic rats close to normal controls (Sakuljaitrong *et al.*, 2012).

***Psidium guajava* (L.)** *Psidium guajava* L. fruits are rich in dietary fibre associated with natural antioxidant compounds. The fruit contains a high percentage of vitamin C, carotene, vitamin B_1, B_2, B_6 and pectin. Antidiabetic activity based on higher concentrations of magnesium in the raw fruit peel of *P. guajava* has been found (Mishra and Sheshadri, 1967). The leaves of *P. guajava* inhibited the increase of plasma sugar level in alloxan-induced diabetic rats, during glucose tolerance testing (Rai *et al.*, 2007). Flavonoid glycosides such as strictinin, isostrictinin and pedunculagin are the effective constituents, which have been used in the clinical treatment of diabetes to improve the sensitivity of insulin (Maryuma *et al.*, 1985). The various fruit extracts inhibited glucose diffusion using an *in vitro* model of glucose absorption. In particular, methanol and aqueous extracts represent potential inhibitory glucose diffusion supplements that may be useful for allowing flexibility in meal planning in type 2 diabetes (Basha and Kumari, 2012). An α-glucosidase inhibiter was identified as dihydro-3,3′,4′,5,7-pentahydroxyflavone glycoside in *P. guajava* leaves, which might be responsible for the inhibitory activity towards α-glucosidase by guava plant extracts because of their hypoglycaemic activity (Alagesan *et al.*, 2012).

***Trigonella foenum-graecum* (L.)** *Trigonella foenum-graecum* leaves and seeds are widely used as a vegetable and spice respectively throughout India and have a long history of medicinal use in Ayurveda and Chinese medicine. Perera and Li (2012) have demonstrated that fenugreek seed extracts, powder and the gum of seeds and leaves can lower blood glucose and cholesterol levels in human and experimental diabetic animals. Its activity has been attributed to bioactive compounds like saponins, high fibre content, the amino acid 4-hydroxyisoleucine and the major alkaloid trigonelline. In recent studies, the ethanolic extracts of fenugreek herbs exhibited promising and safe antidiabetic activities in STZ induced type-1 DM in rats. The efficacy of these herbs was achieved by increasing insulin secretion and lowering blood glucose, lipid profiles, lipid peroxidation and nitric oxide levels. In addition, the plant extracts showed variable degrees of increases in HDL and GSH, resulting in capillary permeability normalization and accelerated wound healing (Wehash *et al.*, 2012). Another study by Puri *et al.* (2012) showed the antidiabetic effect of a compound GII – purified previously from the water extract of fenugreek seeds by Murthy and his colleagues (patented in India and USA) – in diabetic rabbits in 90 min for fasting blood sugar (FBG) and glucose tolerance (GTT) in the subdiabetic, moderately diabetic and severely diabetic groups. GII was found to improve blood glucose utilization in GTT and reduced FBG and HbA1C. The results indicated that a person with diabetes need not take GII daily once the FBG value becomes normal or near to normal. Patients might be able to take intermittent therapy with the potent product GII of the fenugreek seeds when the FBG value shows an increase.

Allii Cepa Bulbus Eating onions improved the metabolic status of diabetic patients – probably because of hypoglycaemic and hypocholesterolaemic effects – and mediated diabetic nephropathy by lowering blood cholesterol levels and decreasing lipid peroxidation. Its active principles showed that allyl propyl disulfide and *S*-methyl cysteine sulfoxide have an antidiabetic and anti-hyperlipidaemic effect, the latter being analogous to glibenclamide and insulin (Babu and Srinivasan, 1997, 1999; Andallu *et al.*, 2001). Onion extract reduced hyperglycaemia in a dose-dependent manner following a glucose tolerance test in a human study (Sharma *et al.*, 1997). *S*-Methyl cysteine sulfoxide isolated from onions produced a similar effect to insulin in a group of diabetic rats (Kumari *et al.*, 1995).

Allii Sativi Bulbus The bulbs of *Allium sativum* L. regulate blood sugar levels and are effective in lowering serum glucose levels in STZ-induced as well as alloxan-induced diabetic rats and mice. Most of the studies have shown that garlic can reduce blood glucose levels in diabetic mice, rats and rabbits. The hypoglycaemic action of garlic could possibly be due to an increase in pancreatic secretion of insulin from β-cells, release of bound insulin or enhancement of insulin sensitivity (Augusti and Sheela, 1996; Mathew and Augusti, 1973). Garlic has also been shown to reduce fasting blood glucose and HbA1C significantly compared to metformin and placebo and may be an effective addition to the family of antidiabetic agents (Ashraf *et al.*, 2011). Other metabolic complications like increased serum triglyceride, insulin and uric acid levels observed in diabetic rats were also normalized after garlic administration.

16.2.2 Cardiovascular diseases

Impressive developments are being made to verify the importance of bioactive compounds in reducing the risk of major chronic diseases and the underlying biological mechanisms that account for these disorders. Cardiovascular disease (CVD) is now the leading cause of death globally and is a growing health concern worldwide. Important risk factors for CVD include obesity, high blood cholesterol level, high blood pressure and type 2 diabetes. Eating a healthy diet, being physically active, not smoking and not drinking alcohol excessively can all help to reduce a person's risk of CVD (BNF, 2005). A number of studies have shown the relationship between the consumption of whole plant foods (e.g. fruit and vegetables, nuts, pulses, wholegrains) and CVD risk, and between plant-derived food components (e.g. dietary fibre) and CVD risk. Vegetable and fruit fibres (with pectin), garlic and oily seeds (walnut, almonds, etc.) and fish oils have lipid-lowering effects in humans, through both inhibition of fat absorption and suppression of hepatic cholesterol synthesis. A significant cardiovascular benefit of phytobioconstituents (polyphenols in wine, grapes and teas), vitamins (ascorbate, tocopherol) and minerals (selenium, magnesium) in foods is their capacity to scavenge free radicals produced during atherogenesis (Block *et al.,* 2001; Ferrari, 2004), which might be the mechanism underlying the effect.

Fish Potential mechanisms for the cardiovascular protective effects of *n*-3 fatty acids are suggested to be anti-inflammatory, antithrombotic (reduced platelet aggregability), antiarrhythmic (reducing the risk of potentially fatal cardiac arrhythmias), lowering of heart rate and blood pressure, hypotriglyceridaemic, and improved endothelial function (Mozaffarian, 2008). It has been established that fish oil, in clinically used doses (typically 4 g/day of eicosapentaenoic acid and docosahexaenoic acid) reduce high triglycerides. However, the role of omega-3 fatty acids in reducing mortality, sudden death, arrhythmias, myocardial infarction and heart failure has not yet been established (Weitz *et al.,* 2010). Omega-3 fatty acid reduces serum triglyceride levels by modulating VLDL and chylomicron metabolism. Literature reports that the end effect of fish oil is decreased hepatic secretion of VLDL – the major endogenous source of triglycerides (Harris, 1997).

Vegetables and fruits Fruit and vegetable intake has been associated with lower CVD risk. Soluble fibres including pectins from apples and citrus fruits, β-glucan from oats and barley, and fibres from flaxseed and psyllium are known to lower LDL cholesterol (Erkkila and Lichtenstein, 2006). Suggested mechanisms for lowering cholesterol are binding of bile acids and inhibition of cholesterol synthesis. Many nutrients and phytochemicals in fruits and vegetables, including fibre, potassium and folate, could be independently or jointly responsible for the apparent reduction in CVD risk. Functional aspects of fruits and vegetables, such as their low dietary glycaemic load and energy density, may also play a significant role (Bazzano, 2003).

Nuts and legumes Whole grains, like nuts, legumes and other edible seeds, contain many bioactive phytochemicals and various antioxidants. After cereals, nuts are the vegetable foods that are richest in fibre, which may partly explain their benefit on the lipid profile and cardiovascular health. Besides fat, the complex matrices of nuts contain many bioactive compounds: vegetable protein, fibre, minerals, tocopherols and phenolic compounds. By virtue of their unique composition, nuts are likely to benefit newer cardiovascular risk biomarkers, such as LDL oxidizability, soluble inflammatory molecules and endothelial dysfunction. Legumes offer a range of nutritional benefits: they provide plant protein, have the lowest glycaemic index, contain soluble fibre, contribute folate, are an antioxidants source, are rich in minerals like zinc, potassium, iron and magnesium, free of saturated fat and do not contain cholesterol. Beans also contain compounds called phytonutrients. Phytonutrients are non-essential compounds in foods that can provide health benefits and some phytonutrients found in beans have been reported to reduce risk factors associated with cardiovascular disease. Eating beans can help maintain desired weight, reduce blood glucose, insulin and cholesterol concentrations, and reduce the incidence and adverse consequences of diabetes. Thus, eating beans will help reducing the risk of premature atherosclerosis (heart attacks, strokes and peripheral vascular disease) (Rondini and Bennink, 2008).

Soy protein Soy protein is consumed as a component of traditional fermented and non-fermented soy foods, such as tofu, tempeh and miso, as well as whole soybeans, soynuts, soy milk, soy yogurt and soy cheese. The mechanisms by which soy modulates blood cholesterol and lipoprotein levels need further research. Several components associated with soy protein have been implicated in lowering cholesterol: trypsin inhibitors, phytic acid, saponins, isoflavones and fibre. Soy protein without the isoflavones seems to be less effective. Soy foods contain both copper and phytic acid and therefore may lower cholesterol levels by decreasing the ratio of zinc to copper. Saponin compounds may contribute to cholesterol lowering by increasing bile excretion (Sidhu and Oakenfull, 1986). Soy fibre has a hypocholesterolaemic effect when added to other foods but when added to soy protein it does not further enhance the hypocholesterolaemic effect of the protein (Potter *et al.*, 1993).

Cocoa and chocolates Dark chocolate (containing at least 60% cocoa solids) is rich in flavonoids which are known to have heart protecting effects, which has been only examined in short-term studies. In healthy adults, drinking flavonoid-rich cocoa improves NO-dependent vasorelaxation and flow-mediated dilation in the brachial arteries (Grassi *et al.*, 2005b). Administration of dark chocolate in essential hypertensives reduces ambulatory blood pressure and serum LDL cholesterol levels whereas white chocolate does not show any effects (Grassi *et al.*, 2005a). Furthermore, there is a clear reduction of the blood cholesterol levels as well as a significant rise of HDL cholesterol with reduction of circulating oxidized LDL (Baba *et al.*, 2007).

Whole grains Eating whole instead of refined grains substantially lowers total cholesterol, LDL (or bad) cholesterol, triglycerides and insulin levels. Any of these changes would be expected to reduce the risk for CVD. The mechanisms underlying the protective effect of whole grains on CVD risk include its effects on insulin sensitivity (McKeown *et al.*, 2002), blood pressure, lipids and inflammation (Lutsey *et al.*, 2007; Flint *et al.*, 2009). The bran and fibre present in whole grains make it more difficult for digestive enzymes to break down the complex starches into glucose. Soluble fibre helps in lowering cholesterol. Insoluble fibre helps in moving waste through the digestive tract. Fibre may also initiate the body's natural anticoagulants and so help in preventing the formation of small blood clots that can trigger heart attacks or strokes.

Coffee and tea Green tea has beneficial effects on CVD, but the results are inconsistent. The mechanism that might explain this beneficial effect of tea can be attributed to the improvement in the vascular endothelium. Endothelial function, including brachial artery flow-mediated dilation, is gaining increasing acceptance as a clinically relevant surrogate end-point for CVD risk. The results also vary in different regions. It has been reported in a meta-analysis that the incidence of myocardial infarction among individuals who consumed three cups of tea daily was not statistically significant and there has been large variability across studies (Peters *et al.*, 2001). The active constituents of coffee, like diterpenes such as kahweol and cafeastol, might be responsible for the cardioprotective effect. Coffee consumption may possibly reduce the risk of myocardial infarction, but data are as yet inconclusive (Panagiotakos *et al.*, 2003).

16.2.3 Cancer

Food can have both positive (carcinogenic) and negative (preventive) effects. Total calorie intake has a strong positive effect on cancer incidence. Vegetables rich in antioxidants and fibres tend to reduce cancer incidence. Carcinogenic plant alkaloids, mycotoxins and other food contaminants generated by heat-cooking like genotoxicants, including aromatic hydrocarbons (via combustion) and heterocyclic amines (HCAs) through reactions involving creatin(in)e, sugar and amino acids in meat, frequently enter our bodies (Sugimura, 2002). Pure curcumin and the crude ethanolic extract have also shown great potential in the prevention and cure of cancer. Curcumin has broad spectrum cancer chemopreventive activity in preclinical animal models (Naama *et al.,* 2010). There are many functional food items which might have a role in reducing the risk of cancer. The sulforaphane present in broccoli stimulates the body to produce its own protective enzymes and also neutralizes free radicals. Lycopene in tomatoes is potent antioxidant and might reduce the risk of prostate cancer. Limonene in oranges and lemons boosts levels of naturally occurring enzymes that may break down carcinogens. Allyl sulfides in garlic and onions boosts levels of naturally occurring enzymes that may help maintain a healthy immune system. Flavonoids inhibit enzymes that are the targets in anticancer treatment, like Cox I and II, eukaryotic DNA topoisomerase I and oestrogen 2- and 4-hydroxylases. Flavonoids reduce the activation of procarcinogen substrates to carcinogens by interacting with P450 enzymes, which makes them putative anticancer substances (Mukhtar *et al.,* 1988). Isoflavones (genistein and daidzein) from soybeans may act as anti-oestrogens, plugging up receptors for oestrogen, which may reduce the risk of oestrogen-dependent cancers and may inhibit the formation of blood vessels that assist tumour growth. Phytic acid in whole wheat may suppress the oxidative reactions in the colon that produce damaging free radicals. Lignans play a very important role in cancer. They are minor components in numerous edible plants and form the building blocks for the fibre lignin. In the gut, both lignin and lignans can be degraded by intestinal bacteria to enterolactone, the main lignan metabolite in the urine of mammals (Begum *et al.,* 2004). Lignans in flaxseed act as a phytoestrogen and may offer a reduced risk to certain kinds of cancer. Dairy products containing sphingomyelin and calcium may inhibit tumour cell growth and induce cell death. Conjugated linoleic acid (CLA) in beef and dairy may decrease the risk of certain cancer products, and at the same time may inhibit tumour cell growth and induce cell death. Polyphenols like catechin in tea may help block damage to DNA by neutralizing free radicals and reducing cancer risks. Bryostatin 1, a potent inhibitor of protein kinase C (PKC), acts in the phosphorylation of serine and threonine residues, and actually counteracts tumour promotion induced by phorbol esters. Emodin and aloe-emodin induce apoptosis, which involves disruption of the mitochondrial membrane potential, cytochrome C release and activation of Caspase 3. They also induce cell-cycle arrest, involving an increase in p53 expression level and accompanied by upregulation of p21 (Patel *et al.,* 2010).

16.3 Health benefits of specific bioactive compounds

The daily use of whole herbs in the diet, separate formulations of their bioactive compounds have been tested to ameliorate various disorders. Bioactive compounds are secondary plant/herb metabolites eliciting pharmacological or toxicological effects in humans and animals. These compounds may elicit different effects in humans and animals that eat the plants dependent on the plant species and the amount eaten. Plants with potent bioactive compounds are often characterized as both toxic and medicinal, and a beneficial or an adverse result may depend on the quantity eaten. For typical food plants with bioactive compounds with less pronounced effects, intake is usually regarded as beneficial and they are taken in ample amounts. The purified and concentrated formulations of these bioactives are aimed at treating disease conditions and balancing human health.

Sequoyitol is a patented antidiabetic natural compound extracted from *Taxus* sp. (US 20060135624). Both oral and subcutaneous administrations of sequoyitol improve hyperglycaemia and glucose intolerance in both *ob/ob* and STZ-treated mice. Sequoyitol directly improves glucose metabolism in hepatocytes and adipocytes by both insulin-dependent and insulin-independent mechanisms (Shen *et al.*, 2012). Curcumin, the main bioactive flavonoid derived from the rhizome of *Curcuma longa* has proven activity to treat CVD, inflammation and arthritis (Tan *et al.*, 2011). Gambogic acid is the principal active ingredient of gamboges, a resin from *Garcinia* species. It is effective against malignant tumours, breast cancer, lung cancer and liver cancer (Tan *et al.*, 2011). β-Elemene, a sesquiterpene mixture from Chinese herbs and plants is a potential candidate for anticancer therapeutic drugs (Tan *et al.*, 2011). Phlorotannins, sulfated chito-oligosaccharides, sulfated polysaccharides, lectins and bioactive peptides are some of the marine-derived anti-HIV agents (Vo and Kim, 2010). 1-Cinnamoyl-3,11-dihydroxymeliacarpin, a tetranortriterpenoid isolated from partially purified leaf extracts of *Melia azedarach* L., possesses antiviral and nuclear factor-kappaB modulating properties (Barquero *et al.*, 2006). Flavonoids and terpenoids from fruit sources have shown significant activities against atherosclerosis in both *in vitro* and *in vivo* studies (Surangi *et al.*, 2012). Dietary triterpenes are promising candidates for cardiac-related treatment owing to their antioxidant and antithrombotic activities (Allouche *et al.*, 2010). Flavonoids can be targeted against hypertension due to their potent angiotensin-converting enzyme (ACE) inhibitory activity (Balasuriya and Rupasinghe, 2011). Bioactive peptides isolated from marine sources such as fish protein hydrolysates, algal fucans, galactans and alginates possess anticoagulant, anticancer and hypocholesterolaemic activities (Lordan *et al.*, 2011). Bilberry anthocyanin-rich extract possesses potent activity against atherosclerosis development (Mauray *et al.*, 2012).

16.4 Polyherbal formulations

When two or more herbs are used in a formulation, it is known as polyherbal formulation. This is primarily done to achieve synergistic health effects. The combination of the selected herbs provide an effect greater than the sum of their individual effects.

In such cases, plant formulations and combined extracts of plants are used as a drug of choice rather than individual ones (Kumar, 2010), to find a suitable combination therapy for specific diseases. Here are some representative examples of polyherbal formulations for the above-mentioned diseases.

DIASOL is a polyherbal formulation which has been identified as an effective and safe antidiabetic formulation for type 2 diabetes. The formulation consists of extracts from the following plants: *Eugenia jambolana, Foenum graecum, Terminalia chebula,Quercus infectoria, Cuminum cyminum, Taraxacum officinale, Emblica officinalis, Gymnema sylvestre, Phyllanthrus nerui* and *Enicostemma littoral* (Babuji *et al.*, 2010). DB-12 is another polyherbal antidiabetic formulation which did not show any acute oral toxicity. It significantly reduced blood glucose levels and increased insulin and liver glycogen levels. *Momardica charantia, Ocimum sanctum, Azadirachta indica, Curcuma longa, Phyllantus amarus, Pterocarpus marsupium, Tinospora cordifolia, Eugenia jambolana* and *Emblica officinalis* are disclosed as the ingredients of the formulation (Babu *et al.*, 2012). DRF/AY/5001, a combination of *Gymnema sylvestre, Syzygium cuimini, Pterocarpus marsupium, Momordica charantia, Emblica officinalis, Terminalia belirica, Terminalia chebula* and *Asphaltum* helps to maintain good glycaemic and metabolic control (Mandlik *et al.*, 2008). BHUx, a patented polyherbal formulation, is a potent, multifactorial formulation against atherosclerosis, possibly through its anti-inflammatory, calcium channel-modulatory and antioxidant properties (Tripathi *et al.*, 2005). SJT ONC-1 is a combination of different proportions of extracts from stem bark of *Tecomella undulata, Bauhinia variegata, Oroxylum indicum* and leaves of *Indigofera tinctoria.* Its activity has been found to be comparable to the standard drug 5-fluorouracil and it has been identified as a prospective candidate for cancer therapy (Savjiyani *et al.*, 2012).

A polyherbal formulation made up from aqueous extracts of *Hippophae rhamnoides, Bacopa monerehii* and *Centella asiatica* proved to be effective against oxidative stress-induced liver problems and its efficacy should be further investigated in *in vivo* studies (Singh *et al.*, 2012). Another formulation consisting of *Tribulus terrestris, Piper nigrum* and *Ricinus communis* was effective against type 2 non-insulin-dependent DM in established animal models (Baldi and Goyal, 2011). *Kaishore guggulu* is one of the most famous ayurvedic formulations that is useful for balancing pitta in the musculoskeletal system. It has also been used for treatment of muscle pain (Lather *et al.*, 2011). A herbal mixture containing five ingredients – leaves of *Azadirachta indica* and *Gymnema sylvestre,* fruits of *Momordica charantia,* seeds of *Syzigium cumini* and *Trigonella foenum* – all in equal amounts, proved its efficacy as an antidiabetic and antioxidant agent and the combined activity seems to be more effective than the drug activities of the individual herbs (Katiyar *et al.*, 2012). Another formulation containing *Andrographis paniculata, Momardica charantia, Phyllanthus niruri, Terminallia chebula, Glycyrrhiza glabra* and *Punica granatum* is effective in the treatment and management of HIV-AIDS along with enhancement in body vitality and immunity (Choudhari *et al.*, 2011). Renalka syrup, another combination of potent herbs like *Tribulus terrestris, Crataeva magna, Hemidesmus indicus, Cyperus rotundus, Vetiveria zizanioides, Asparagus racemosus, Trikatu, Elettaria cardamomum* and *Kshara parpati* is found to be effective against a variety of urinary disorders (Desai and Palaniyamma, 2012). BHUx, a novel polyherbal formulation effective against hyperlipidaemia and atherosclerosis consisting of *Termenalia arjuna, Strychnox nux vomica, Boswellia serrata, Commiphora mukul* and *Semecarpus anacardium* is under clinical trials before it release into the commercial market as a functional food (Tripathi *et al.*, 2009). Qian-kun-nin, a Chinese herbal formulation is considered to have anti-infection, antitumour and immuno-enhancing properties and possess strong therapeutic potential for HIV treatment (Zhan *et al.*, 2000). Sudarshan churna, which contains *Swertia chirata* as the major (50%) ingredient along with other ingredients in equal proportion has antipyretic and antimicrobial activity (Singh *et al.*, 2011). In another study, a formulation containing chloroform and the petroleum ether and aqueous extracts of *Ferula asafetida, Momordica charantia* Linn and *Nardostachys jatamansi* demonstrated significant hepatoprotective activity (Dandagi *et al.*, 2008).

16.5 Standardization of the formulations

Standardization of such formulations is essential in order to assess the quality of the drugs. The stability parameters include physical, chemical, microbiological analysis such as UV-visible, thin-layer chromatography, high-performance liquid chromatography, high-performance thin-layer chromatography, gas chromatography–mass spectrometry, nuclear magnetic resonance and other methods. Environmental factors like climate and growth conditions, as well as the specific part of the plant used and its maturity stage will influence the composition of the formulation. An ayurvedic polyherbal formulation for DM, containing *Syzgium cumini, Mangifera indica, Ficus bengalensis, Ficus religiosa, Lawsonia inermis, Juglans nigra, Terminalia bellirica* and *Hibiscusrosa sinensis,* was studied and it was suggested that the following physicochemical factors should be used for standardization of the formulation: water-soluble, alcohol-soluble and ether-soluble extractive values, moisture content, bulk density, tapped density, Carr's index, Hausner's ratio, pH, water-soluble ash, acid-insoluble ash and organoleptic characteristics. The results obtained can be effectively used to set the limits for the reference standards and this can further lead to the quality control and quality assurance of these drugs (Maithani *et al.*, 2012).

16.6 How to get medicinal effects without actually eating medicines?

It is quite evident that these naturally occurring food derived compounds are a source of multiple health benefits. Unlike synthetic drugs, a single herb may possess multiple effects which can be exploited as a cure to target specific diseases. Due to the various drawbacks of synthetic drugs, Ayurveda has become a major focus for researchers. The disease curing techniques of Ayurveda are well proven. The established facts from Ayurveda justify further advanced research using modern techniques to develop significant health benefits using safe affordable treatments for everyone. These developments could replace the current reliance on tablets, which can become an inseparable part of people's lives and lead to dependence.

Natural and healthy substitutes are needed, which in conjunction with a healthy lifestyle, can help minimize the risk of contracting diseases. When, unfortunately, we are affected by diseases despite our efforts, nature has provided us with solutions to combat them.

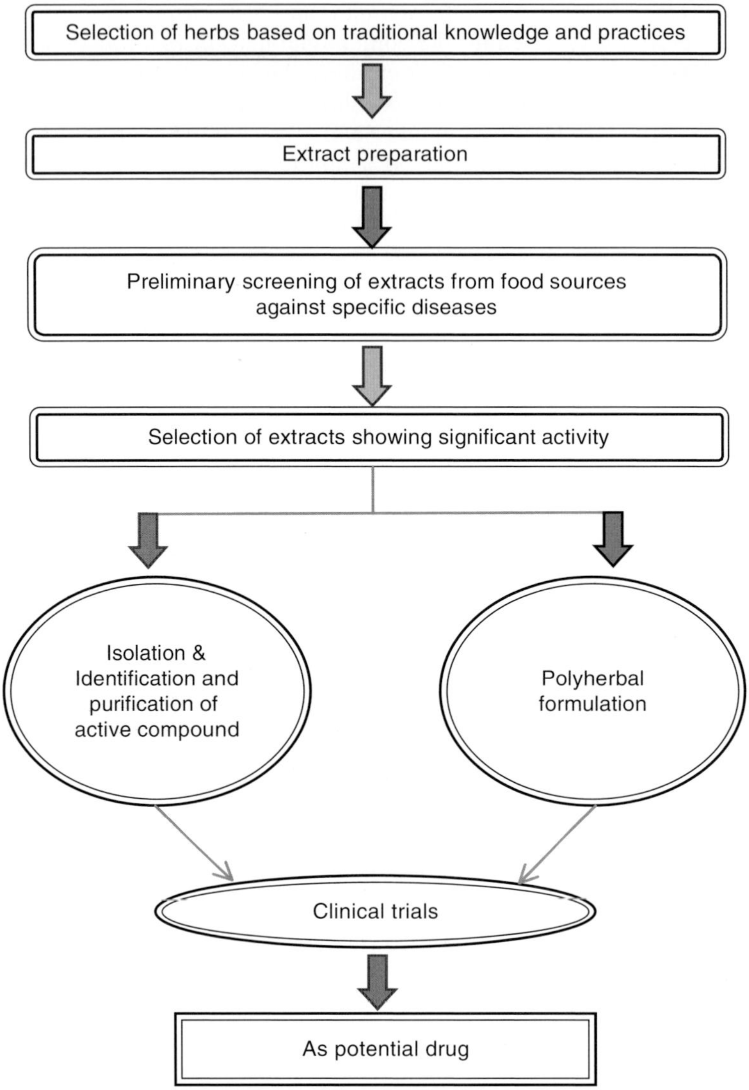

Figure 16.1 Approaches to obtain a potential drug from a food source

Figure 16.1 and Figure 16.2 explain the two approaches of acquiring health benefits from food/plant sources. Figure 16.1 explains how our traditional knowledge regarding herbs can be efficiently exploited to identify potential drugs. Since ancient times, the older generation has passed on information about the effectiveness of certain therapies. Based on these practices, various herbs/food compounds can be selected. There are well-established methods for the preliminary screening of herbs/food compounds against specific diseases using *in vitro* studies. Once an extract is selected based on its significant activity, it can be either taken for further purification purposes

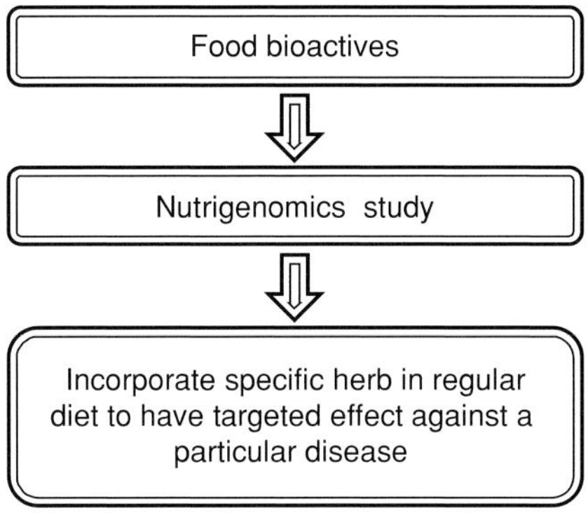

Figure 16.2 Futuristic approach to obtain benefits from bioactives in food sources

to identify the active compound or the herb can be part of a polyherbal formulation. Both the identified active compound and the polyherbal formulation can be taken up for further clinical studies in order to obtain potential drugs. Figure 16.2 explains about the nutrigenomic studies of bioactive compounds so that they can be directly incorporated into a regular diet against a specific disease. In this case there will be no need to take any drug, but a proven food bioactive will become the curing agent for a person as a part of his regular diet. There is a long way to go in such an approach but if successfully achieved, herbs will become an inherent part of one's diet.

Nutrigenomics, the use of a systems biology approach in nutrition and health science, has attracted both researchers and industrialists increasingly during this millennium. Genes are turned on and off according to metabolic signals that the nucleus receives from internal factors (e.g. hormones) and external factors (e.g. nutrients), which are among the most influential of environmental stimuli (Harland, 2005). Recently, nutrigenetics, as part of the acknowledged nutritional research, has shown that nutrients and other bioactive compounds in food interact with genetic factors. Nutrigenomics research is expected to identify biomarkers for health and their role for disease disposition. It will also play an important role in differentiating dietary responders and non-responders. Nutrition for the maintenance of individual health and the prevention of disease will be the major application outcome of nutrigenomics. The future of nutrigenomics suggests the interaction between the bioactive compounds and genes and accordingly each individual's diets would be tailored for disease prevention. If successfully achieved, a person may eat a defined dose of the bioactive compound from a food source for prevention of a particular disease. If we know how and why a drug affects genes, the doses of drugs can be decided accordingly. In such cases, a person can have the option of eating medicine separately or incorporating it into the diet as a natural process. Health conscious people can use the latter approach as part of a balanced lifestyle to combat the risk of contracting diseases. However, currently there is insufficient information and data on the affect of nutritional components on an individual's genes. We would also need to address ethical issues on the use of nutrigenomics study and data, with involvement of scientists, civic organizations and authorities before taking up these issues.

References

Alagesan, K., Thennarasu, P., Kumar, V., Sankarnarayanan, S. and Balsamy, T. (2012). Identification of α-glucosidase inhibitors from *Psidium guajava* leaves and *Syzygium cumini* Linn. seeds. *International Journal of Pharma Sciences and Research*, 3 (2), 316–322.

Allouche, Y., Beltrán, G., Gaforio, J.J., Uceda, M. and Mesa, M.D. (2010).Antioxidant and antiatherogenic activities of pentacyclic triterpenic diols and acids. *Food and Chemical Toxicology*, 48 (10), 2885–2890.

Andallu, B., Suryakantham, V. and Lakshmi, S.B. (2001).Effect of mulberry (*Morms indica* L) therapy on plasma and erythrocyte membrane lipids in patients with type 2 diabetes. *Clinical Chemical Acta*, 314, 47– 53.

Ashraf, R., Khan, R.A. and Ashraf, I. (2011). Effects of garlic on blood glucose levels and HbA1c in patients with type 2 diabetes mellitus. *Journal of Medicinal Plants Research*, 5 (13), 2922–2928.

Augusti, K.T. and Sheela, C.G. (1996). Antiperoxide effect of *S*-allyl cysteine sulfoxide, a insulin secretagogue, in diabetic rats. *Experientia*, 52, 115–20.

Baba, S., Natsume, M., Yasuda, A. *et al.* (2007). Plasma LDL and HDL cholesterol and oxidized LDL concentrations are altered in normo- and hypercholesterolemic humans after intake of different levels of cocoa powder. *The Journal of Nutrition*, 137 (6), 1436–1441.

Babu, P.S. and Srinivasan, K. (1997). Influence of dietary capsaicin and onion on the metabolic abnormalities associated with streptozotocin induced diabetes mellitus. *Molecular and Cellular Biochemistry*, 175, 49–57.

Babu, P.S. and Srinivasan, K. (1999). Renal lesions in streptozotocin-induced diabetic rats maintained on onion and capsaicin containing diets. *Journal of Nutritional Biochemistry*, 10, 477–483.

Babu, V., Kumbhar, P. and Varghese, A. (2012). Antidiabetic activity of a polyherbal formulation in animal models of diabetes. *International Journal of Pharmaceutical Research and Development*, 4 (6), 95–101.

Babuji, S.S.H., Sahu, D., Bahadur, V. and Kassim, T. (2010). Evaluation on safety and efficacy of a polyherbal antidiabetic formulation – DIASOL. *Asian Pacific Journal of Molecular Biology and Biotechnology*,18 (1), 59–61.

Baker, D. and Campbell, R.K. (1992).Vitamin and mineral supplementation in patients with diabetes mellitus. *Diabetes Education*, 18, 420–427.

Balasuriya, B.W.N. and Rupasinghe, V. (2011). Plant flavonoids as angiotensin converting enzyme inhibitors in regulation of hypertension *Functional Foods in Health and Disease*, 5, 172–188.

Baldi, A. and Goyal, S. (2011).Hypoglycemic effect of polyherbal formulation in alloxan induced diabetic rats. *Pharmacology online*, 3, 764–773.

Barquero, A.A., Michelini, F.M. and Alche, L.E. (2006). 1-Cinnamoyl-3,11-dihydroxymeliacarpin is a natural bioactive compound with antiviral and nuclear factor-kappaB modulating properties. *Biochemical and Biophysical Research Communications*, 344 (3), 955–962.

Basha, S.K. and Kumari, V.S. (2012). *In vitro* antidiabetic activity of *Psidium guajava* leaves extracts. *Asian Pacific Journal of Tropical Disease*, S98–S100.

Begum, A.N., Nicolle, C., Mila, I. *et al.* (2004). Dietary lignins are precursors of mammalian lignans in rats. *The Journal of Nutrition*, 134, 120–127.

Block, G., Mangels, A.R., Norkus, E.P. *et al.* (2001). Ascorbic acid status and subsequent diastolic and systolic blood pressure. *Hypertension*, 37 (2), 261–267.

Bazzano, L.A. (2003). Dietary intake of fruits and vegetables and risk of cardiovascular disease *Current Atherosclerosis Reports*, 5 (6), 492–499.

BNF (British Nutrition Foundation) (2005). Cardiovascular disease, diet, nutrition and emerging risk factors. Report of a British Nutrition FoundationTask Force (ed. S. Stanner). Blackwell Publishing, Oxford.

Cao, H. and Guo, X.Z. (2010).Therapeutic effects of *Ganoderma* polysaccharide on type 2 diabetes in rats. *Progress in Modern Biomedicine*, 12, 96–102.

Chandrika, U.G., Wedage, W.S., Wickramasinghe, S.M.D.N. and Fernando, W.S. (2006). Hypoglycaemic action of the flavonoid fraction of *Artocarpus heterophyllus* leaf. *African Journal of Traditional and Complementary Alternative Medicines*, 3 (2), 42–50.

Chen, J. and Seviour, R. (2007). Medicinal importance of fungal β-(1→3) (1→6)-glucans. *Mycological Research*, 111, 635–652.

Chen, J. and Raymond, K. (2008). β-glucans in the treatment of diabetes and associated cardiovascular risks.*Vascular Health Risk Management*, 4 (6), 1265–1272.

Choudhari, A.B., Rangari, V.D. and Darvekar, V.M. (2011). Formulation development for treatment and management of HIV AIDS. *International Journal of Pharmacy and Pharmaceutical Science*, 3 (1) 105–108.

Dandagi, P.M., Patil, M.B., Mastiholimath, V.S., Gadad, A.P. and Dhumansure, R.H. (2008). Development and evaluation of hepatoprotective polyherbal formulation containing some indigenous medicinal plants. *Indian Journal of Pharmaceutical Sciences*, 70 (2), 265–268.

Das, S. and Barman, S. (2012). Antidiabetic and antihyperlipidemic effects of ethanolic extract of leaves of *Punica granatum* in alloxan-induced non-insulin-dependent diabetes mellitus albino rats. *Indian Journal of Pharmacology*, 44 (2), 219–224.

Dinesh, K.B., Analava, M. and Manjunatha, M. (2010). Antidiabetic and hypolipidemic effect of mahanimbine (carbazole alkaloid) from *Murraya koenigii* (Rutaceae) leaves. *International Journal of Phytomedicine*, 2, 22–30.

Desai, M.G. and Palaniyamma, D. (2012). A Clinical review on a polyherbal formulation, renalka syrup in urinary tract infection. *Indian Journal of Clinical Practice*, 22, 12.

Erkkila, A.T. and Lichtenstein, A.H. (2006). Fibre and cardiovascular disease risk, how strong is the evidence? *Journal of Cardiovascular Nursing*, 21 (1), 3–8.

Fang, X., Yu, M.M., Yuen, W.H., Zee, S.Y. and Chang, R.C. (2005). 'Immune modulatory effects of *Prunella vulgaris* L. on monocytes/macrophages. *International Journal of Molecular Medicine*, 16 (6), 1109–1116.

Feng, L., Jia, X.B., Shi, F. and Chen, Y. (2010). Identification of two polysaccharides from *Prunella vulgaris* L. and evaluation on their anti-lung adenocarcinoma activity. *Molecules*, 15 (8), 5093–5103.

Ferrari, C.K. (2004). Functional foods, herbs and nutraceuticals, towards biochemical mechanisms of healthy aging. *Biogerontology*, 5 (5), 275–289.

Flint, A.J., Hu, F.B., Glynn, R.J. *et al.* (2009).Whole grains and incident hypertension in men. *American Journal of Clinical Nutrition*, 90 (3), 493–498.

Gao, X., Li, B., Jiang, H. *et al.* (2007). *Dioscorea opposita* reverses dexamethasone induced insulin resistance. *Fitoterapia*, 78 (1), 12–15.

Gandhi, G.R., Ignasumuthu, S. and Paulraj, M.G. (2012). Hypoglycemic and β-cells regenerative effects of *Aegle marmelos* (L.) Corr. bark extract in streptozotocin-induced diabetic rats. *Food and Chemical Toxicology,* 50 (5), 1667–1674.

Grassi, D., Lippi, C., Necozione, S. *et al.* (2005a). Short-term administration of dark chocolate is followed by a significant increase in insulin sensitivity and a decrease in blood pressure in healthy persons. *American Journal of Clinical Nutrition*, 81 (3), 611–614.

Grassi, D., Necozione, S. and Lippi, C. (2005b). Cocoa reduces blood pressure and insulin resistance and improves endothelium-dependent vasodilation in hypertensives. *Hypertension*, 46 (2), 398–405.

Gregersen, S., Jeppesen, P.B., Holst, J.J. and Hermansen, K. (2004). Anti-hyperglycemic effects of stevioside in type 2 diabetic subjects. *Metabolism*, 53 (1), 73–76.

Hao, Z.Q., Hang, B.Q. and Wang, Y. (1991). The anti-hyperglycemic effect of water decoction of *Dioscorea opposita* Thunb to experimental diabetic mice. *Journal of China Pharmaceutical University*, 22, 158–160.

Harland, J.I. (2005). *Nutrition and Genetics. Mapping Individual Health*. ILSI Europe Concise Monograph Series.

Harris, W.S. (1997). Review *n*-3 fatty acids and serum lipoproteins, human studies. *American Journal of Clinical Nutrition*, 65 (5 Suppl), 1645S–1654S.

Hong, M.L., Jin, K.K., Jai, M.J. *et al.* (2012). The inhibitory effect of *Prunella vulgaris* L. on aldose reductase and protein glycation. *Journal of Biomedicine and Biotechnology*, DOI: 10.1155/2012/928159.

Huang, C.F., Chen, Y.W., Yang, C.Y. *et al.* (2011). Extract of lotus leaf (*Nelumbo nucifera*) and its active constituent catechin with insulin secretagogue activity. *Journal of Agricultural and Food Chemistry*, 59 (4), 1087–1094.

Hwang, S.M., Kim, J.S., Lee, Y.J. *et al.* (2012). Antidiabetic atherosclerosis effect of *Prunella vulgaris* in db/db mice with type 2 diabetes. *American Journal of Chinese Medicine*, 40 (5), 937–951.

Jain, V., Viswanatha, G.L., Manohar, D. and Shivaprasad, H.N. (2012). Isolation of antidiabetic principle from fruit rinds of *Punica granatum*. *Evidence-Based Complementary and Alternative Medicine*, 2012, Article ID 147202, 11 pages. DOI: 10.1155/2012/147202.

Jamison, J.R. (2003). *Clinical Guide to Nutrition and Dietary Supplements in Disease Management*. Churchill-Livingston, Edinburgh, Scotland, 489 pp.

Jayawardena, R., Ranasinghe, P., Galappatthy, P. *et al.* (2012). Effects of zinc supplementation on diabetes mellitus, a systematic review and meta-analysis. *Diabetology and Metabolic Syndrome*, 4, 13.

Jenkins, A.L., Jenkins, D.J., Zdravkovic, U. *et al.* (2002). Depression of the glycemic index by high levels of β-glucan fibre in two functional foods tested in type 2 diabetes. *European Journal of Clinical Nutrition*, 56, 622–628.

Kamalakannan, N. and Prince, S.M. (2003). Hypoglycemic effect of water extracts of *Aegle marmelos* fruits in streptozotocin diabetic rats. *Journal of. Ethnopharmacology,* 87, 207–210.

Kamalakkanan, N. and Prince, P.S. (2005). Antihyperlipidaemic effect of *Aegle marmelos* fruit extract in streptozotocin-induced diabetes in rats. *Journal of the Science of Food and Agriculture*, 85, 569.

Karunanayake, E.H., Welihinda, J., Sirimanne, S.R. and Sinnadorai, G. (1984). Oral hypoglycemic activity of some medicinal plants of SriLanka. *Journal of Ethnopharmacology*, 11 (2), 223–231.

Katiyar, D.K., Mehrotra, A., Pant, K.K. and Ali, B. (2012). Study of hypoglycemic effects and antioxidant potential of polyherbal formulation in rats *Biomedical Research*, 23 (3), 444–449.

Kesari, A.N., Gupta, R.K., Singh, S.K., Diwakar, S. and Watal, S. (2006). Hypoglycemic and anti-hyperglycemic activity of *Aegles marmelos* seed extract in normal and diabetic rats. *Journal of Ethnopharmacology*, 107, 374–379.

Kiho, T., Morimoto, H., Sakushima, M. *et al.* (1995). Polysaccharides in fungi. XXXV. Anti diabetic activity of an acidic polysaccharide from the fruiting bodies of *Tremella aurantia*. *Biological and Pharmaceutical Bulletin*, 18, 1627–1629.

Kim, Y.W., Kim, K.H., Choi, H.J. *et al.* (2005). Antidiabetic activity of β-glucans and their enzymatically hydrolyzed oligosaccharides from *Agaricus blazei*. *Biotechnology Letters*, 27, 483–487.

Kowluru, R.A. and Kanwar, M. (2007). Effects of curcumin on retinal oxidative stress and inflammation in diabetes. *Nutrition and Metabolism*, 4, 8–12.

Kumar, J. (2010). Herbal medicine for type 2 diabetes. *International Journal of Diabetes Developing Countries*, 30, 111–112.

Kumari, M., Survase, S. and Singhal, R. (2008). Production of schizophyllan using *Schizophyllan commune* NRCM. *Bioresource Technology*, 99 (5), 1036–1043.

Kumari, K., Mathew, B.C. and Augusti, K.T. (1995). Antidiabetic and hypolipidaemic effects of S-methyl cysteine sulfoxide isolated from *Allium cepa* Linn. *Indian Journal of Biochemistry and Biophysics*, 32, 49–54.

Lather, A., Gupta, V., Bansal, P. *et al.* (2011). An Ayurvedic polyherbal formulation kaishore guggulu. *A Review. International Journal of Pharmaceutical and Biological Archives*, 2 (1), 497–503.

Li, F., Zhang, Y. and Zhong, Z. (2011). Anti-hyperglycemic effect of *Ganoderma lucidum* polysaccharides on streptozotocin-induced diabetic mice. *International journal of Molecular Science*, 12, 6135–6145.

Lordan, S., Ross, R.P. and Stanton, C. (2011). marine bioactives as functional food ingredients, potential to reduce the incidence of chronic diseases. *Drugs*, 9 (6), 1056–1100.

Ludwig, D.S. (2003). Dietary glycaemic index and the regulation of body weight. *Lipids*, 38, 117–121.

Lutsey, P.L., Jacobs, D.R., Kori, S. *et al.* (2007). Whole grain intake and its cross-sectional association with obesity, insulin resistance, inflammation, diabetes and subclinical CVD, the MESA Study. *British Journal of Nutrition*, 98 (2), 397–405.

Maithani, J., Agarwal, K., Sharma, V. and Saini, P. (2012). Preparation and standardization of a polyherbal formulation. *Journal of Advanced Scientific Research*, 3 (2), 84–85.

Mandlik, R.V., Desai, S.K. and Naik, S.R. (2008). Antidiabetic activity of a polyherbal formulation (DRF/AY/5001). *Indian Journal of Experimental Biology*, 46, 599–606.

Maryuma, Y., Matsuda, H., Matsuda, R. *et al.* (1985). Study on *Psidium guajava* L. (I) Antidiabetic effect and effective components of the leaf of *Psidium guajava* L. (Part I). *Shoyakugaku Zasshi*, 39, 261–269.

Maity, P., Hansda, D., Bandyopadhyay, U. and Mishra, D.K. (2009). Biological activities of crude extracts and chemical constituents of Bael, *Aegle marmelos* (L.) Corr. *Indian Journal of Experimental Biology*, 47, 849–861.

Mathew, P.T. and Augusti, K.T. (1973). Studies on the effect of allicin (diallyl disulphide-oxide) on alloxan diabetes I. Hypoglycaemic action and enhancement of serum insulin effect and glycogen synthesis. *Indian Journal of Biochemistry and Biophysics*, 10, 209–212.

Mauray, A., Felgines, C., Morand, C. *et al.* (2012). Bilberry anthocyanin-rich extract alters expression of genes related to atherosclerosis development in aorta of apo E-deficient mice. *Nutrition, Metabolism and Cardiovascular Diseases*, 22 (1), 72–80.

McKeown, N.M., Meigs, J.B., Liu, S., Wilson, P.W.F. and Jacques, P.F. (2002). Whole-grain intake is favorably associated with metabolic risk factors for type 2 diabetes and cardiovascular disease in the Framingham Offspring Study. *American Journal of Clinical Nutrition*, 76 (2), 390–398.

Mishra, K. and Seshadri, T.R. (1967). Chemical components of the fruits of *Psidium guajava*. *Phytochemistry*, 7, 641–645.

Mishra, H., Soni, M., Silawat, N. *et al.* (2011). Antidiabetic activity of medium-polar extract from the leaves of *Stevia rebaudiana* Bert. (Bertoni) on alloxan-induced diabetic rats. *Journal of Pharmacy and Bioallied Sciences*, 3 (2), 242–248.

Mooradian, A., Failla, M., Hoogwerf, B. *et al.* (1994). Selected vitamin and minerals in diabetes. *Diabetes Care*, 17 (5), 464–479.

Mukherjee, P.K., Saha, K., Das, J., Pal, M. and Saha, B.P. (1997). Studies on the anti-inflammatory activity of rhizomes of *Nelumbo nucifera*. *Planta Medica*, 63, 367–369.

Mukherjee, P.K., Saha, K. and Saha, B.P. (1997). Effect of *Nelumbo nucifera* rhizome extract on blood sugar level in rats. *Journal of Ethnopharmacolog*, 58, 207–213.

Mukhtar, H., Das, M., Khan, W.A. and Bik, D.P. (1988). Exceptional activity of tannic acid among naturally occurring plant phenols in protecting against 7,12-dimethybenz(*a*)anthraxcene-, benzo(*a*)pyrene-, 3-methylcholanthrene-, and *N*-methyl-*N*-nitrosourea-induced skin tumourigenesis in mice. *Cancer Research*, 48, 2361–2365.

Mozaffarian, D. (2008). Fish and *n*-3 fatty acids for the prevention of fatal coronary heart disease and sudden cardiac death. *American Journal of Clinical Nutrition*, 87 (6), 1991S–1996S.

Naama, J.H., Al-Temimi, A.A. and Al-Amiery, A.A.H. (2010). Study the anticancer activities of ethanolic curcumin extract. *African Journal of Pure and Applied Chemistry*, 4 (5), 68–73.

Nishiyama, T., Mae, T., Kishida, H. *et al.* (2005). Curcuminoids and sesquiterpenoids in turmeric (*Curcuma longa* L.) suppress an increase in blood glucose level in type 2 diabetic KK-AMice. *Journal of Agricultural and Food Chemistry*, 53 (4), 959–963.

Ooi, C.P., Yassin, Z. and Hamid, T.A. (2012). *Momordica charantia* for type 2 diabetes mellitus. *Cochrane Database of Systematic Reviews*, 8 (Art. No.: CD007845), DOI: 10.1002/14651858.CD007845.pub3.

Pan, M.H., Lin-Shiiau, S.Y. and Lin, J.K. (2000). Comparative studies on the suppression of nitric oxide synthase by curcumin and its hydrogenated metabolites through down-regulation of Ikappa Bkinase and NFkappaB activation in macrophages. *Biochemical Pharmacology*, 60, 1665–1676.

Panagiotakos, D.B., Pitsavos, C., Chrysohoou, C. *et al.* (2003). The J-shaped effect of coffee consumption on the risk of developing acute coronary syndromes, the CARDIO2000 case-control study. *The Journal of Nutrition*, 133 (10), 3228–3232.

Panchatcharam, M., Miriyala, S., Gayathri, VS. and Suguna, L. (2006). Curcumin improves wound healing by modulating collagen and decreasing reactive oxygen species. *Molecular and Cell. Biochemistry*, 290, 87–96.

Patel, B., Das, S., Prakash, R. and Yasir, M. (2010). Natural bioactive compound with anticancer potential. *International Journal of Advances in Pharmaceutical Sciences*, 1, 32–41.

Perera, P.K. and Li, Y. (2012). Functional herbal food ingredients used in type 2 diabetes mellitus. *Pharmagnosy Reviews*, 6 (11), 37–45.

Peters, U., Poole, C. and Arab, L. (2001). Does tea affect cardiovascular disease? A meta-analysis. *American Journal of Epidemiology*, 154 (6), 495–503.

Ponnachan, P.T.C., Paulose, C.S. and Panikkar, K.R. (1993). Effect of leaf extract of *Aegle marmelos*in diabetic rats. *Indian Jouranl of Experimental Biology*, 31, 345–347.

Potter, S.M., Bakhit, R.M. and Essex-Sorlie, D. (1993). Depression of plasma cholesterol in men by consumption of baked products containing soy protein. *American Journal of Clinical Nutrition*, 58, 501–506.

Puri, D., Prabhu, K.M. and Murthy, P.S. (2012). Antidiabetic effect of GII compound purified from fenugreek (*Trigonella foenum graecum* Linn) seeds in diabetic rabbits. *Indian Journal of Clinical Biochemistry*, 27 (1), 21–27.

Radhika, S., Smila, K.H. and Muthezhilan, R. (2011). Antidiabetic and hypolipidemic activity of *Punica granatum* Linn on alloxan induced rats. *World Journal of Medical Sciences*, 6 (4), 178–182.

Rai, P.K., Rai, N.K., Rai, A.K. and Watal, G. (2007). Role of LIBS in elemental analysis of *P. guajava* responsible for glycemic potential. *Instrument Science and Technology*, 35, 507–522.

Rondini, E.A. and Bennink, M.R. (2008). Beans and Cardiovascular Disease. http//www.ontariobeans.on.ca/documents/BeansandCardiovascularDisease.pdf [accessed 17 July 2013].

Sachdewa, A., Raina, D., Srivatsava, A. and Khemani, L.D. (2001). Effect of *Aegle marmelos* and *Hibis cusrosasinensis* leaf extract on glucose tolerance in glucose induced hyperglycemic rats (Charlesfoster). *Journal of Environmental Biology*, 22, 53–57.

Saha, A. and Mazumder, S. (2013). An aqueous extract of *Murraya koenigii* leaves induces paraoxonase 1 activity in streptozotocin induced diabetic mice. *Food & Function*, 4, 420–425.

Sajithlal, G., Chithra, P. and Chandrakasan, G. (1998). Effect of curcumin on the advanced glycation and cross-linking of collagen in diabetic rats. *Biochemistry and Pharmacology*, 56, 1607–1614.

Sakuljaitrong, S., Chomko, S., Talubmook, C., Buddhakala, N. (2012). Effect of flower extract from lotus (*Nelumbo nucifera*) on haematological values and blood cell characteristics in streptozotocin-induced diabetic rats. *ARPN Journal of Science and Technology*, 2 (11), 1049–1054.

Saris, W.H. (2003). Glycemic carbohydrate and body weight regulation. *Nutrition Reviews*,61, S10–S16.

Savjiyani, J.V., Dave, H., Trivedi, S., Rachchh, M.A. and Gokani, R.H. (2012). Evaluation of anti cancer activity of polyherbal formulation. *International Journal of Cancer Research*, 8 (1), 27.

Sharma, S.S., Kochupilla, I.V. and Gupta, S.K. (1997). Antiemetic efficacy of ginger (*Zingiber officinale*) against cisplatin-induced emesis in dogs. *Journal of Ethnopharmacology*, 57, 93–96.

Sharma, S., Kulkarni, S.K. and Chopra, K. (2006). Curcumin, the active principle of turmeric (*Curcuman longa*), ameliorates diabetic nephropathy in rats. *Clinical and Experimental Pharmacology and Physiology*, 33, 940–945.

Shetty, A.K., Suresh Kumar, G., Sambaiah, K. and Salimath, P.V. (2005). Effect of bitter gourd (*Momordica charantia*) on glycaemic status in streptozotocin induced diabetic rats. *Plant Foods for Human Nutrition*, 60, 109–112.

Shanmugasundaram, E.R.B., Gopinath, K.L. Shanmugasundaram, K.R. and Rajendran, V.M. (1990). Possible regeneration of the islets of Langerhans in streptozotocin-diabetes rats given *Gymnema sylvestre* leaf extracts. *Jouran of Ethnopharmacology*, 30, 265–279.

Shen, H., Shao, M., Cho, K.W. *et al.* (2012). Herbal constituent sequoyitol improves hyperglycemia and glucose intolerance by targeting hepatocytes, adipocytes, and βcells *American Journal of Physiology: Endocrinology and Metabolism*, 302 (8), E932–E940.

Shibib, B.A., Khan, L.A. and Rahman, R. (1993). Activity of *Coccinia indica* and *Momordica charantia* in diabetic rats: Depression of the hepatic gluconeogenic enzymes glucose-6-phosphatase and fructose-1,6-bisphosphatase and elevation of both liver and red-cell shunt enzyme glucose-6-phosphate. *Biochemical Journal*, 292, 267–270.

Sidhu, G.S. and Oakenfull, D.G. (1986). A mechanism for the hypocholesterolemic activity of saponins. *British Journal of Nutrition*, 55, 643–649.

Singh, A.K., Nagpal, D. and Attrey, D.P. (2012). Characterization of a prepared poly-herbal formulation and comparison of its DPPH scavenging activity with other marketed formulations. *European Journal of Biological Sciences*, 4 (3), 68–72.

Singh, B., Gupta, V., Bansal, P., Kumar, D. and Krishna, C.M. (2011). Pharmacological potential of polyherbal formulation, sudarshan churna – A review. *International Journal of Ayurvedic Medicine*, 2, 2.

Sugimura, T. (2002). Food and cancer. *Toxicology*, 181–182, 17–21.

Sukandar, E.Y., Permana, H., Adnyana, I.K. *et al.* (2010). Clinical study of turmeric (*Curcuma longa* L.) and garlic (*Allium sativum* L.) extracts as anti-hyperglycemic and antihyperlipidemic agent in type-2 diabetes-dyslipidemia patients. *International Journal of Pharmacology*, 6 (4), 456–463.

Surangi,H., Thilakarathna, H.P. and Rupasinghe, V. (2012). Anti-atherosclerotic effects of fruit bioactive compounds: A review of current scientific evidence. *Canadian Journal of Plant Science*, 92 (3), 407–419.

Tan, W., Li, J., Mingqing, H. *et* al. (2011). Anti-cancer natural products isolated from Chinese medicinal herbs. *Chinese Medicine*, (6) 27.

Tapola, N., Karvonen, H., Niskanen, L. *et al.* (2005). Glycemic responses of oat bran products in type 2 diabetic patients. *Nutrition, Metabolism and Cardiovascular Disease*, 15, 255–261.

Tembhurne, S.V. and Sakarkar, D.M. (2009). Hypoglycemic effects of fruit juice of *Murraya koenigii* (l) in alloxan induced diabetic mice. *International Journal of Pharm Tech Research*, 1 (4), 1589–1593.

Tripathi, Y.B. (2009). BHUx, a patented polyherbal formulation to prevent hyperlipidemia and atherosclerosis. *Recent Patents on Inflammation & Allergy Drug Discovery*, 3 (1), 49–57.

Vinuthan, M.K., Kumar, G.V., Ravindra, J.P., Jayaprakash and Narayana, K. (2004). Effect of extracts of *Murraya koenigii* leaves on the levels of blood glucose and plasma insulin in alloxan-induced diabetic rats. *Indian Journal of Physiology & Pharmacology*, 48 (3), 348–352.

Vo, T.S. and Kim, S.K. (2010). Potential anti-HIV agents from marine resources, an overview. *Marine Drugs*, 8 (12), 2871–2892.

Weber, W.M., Hunsaker, L.A., Roybal, C.N. *et al.* (2006). Activation of NF kappa B is inhibited by curcumin and related enones. *Bioorganics & Medicinal Chemistry*, 14, 2450–2461.

Wehash, F.E., Ismail, I., Abo-Ghanema and Rasha, M.S. (2012). Some physiological effects of *Momordica charantia* and *Trigonella foenum-graecum* extracts in diabetic rats as compared with Cidophage®. *World Academy of Science, Engineering and Technology*, 64, 1206–1214.

Weitz, D., Weintraub, H., Fisher, E. and Schwartzbard, A.Z. (2010). Fish oil for the treatment of cardiovascular disease. *Cardiology Review*, 18 (5), 258–263.

Yadav, S., Vats, V., Dhunnoo, Y. and Grover, J.K. (2002). Hypoglycemic and anti-hyperglycemic activity of *Murraya koenigii* leaves in diabetic rats. *Journal of Ethnopharmacology*, 82 (2), 111–116.

Zhan, L., Yue, S.T., Xue, Y.X., Attele, A.S. and Yuan, C.S. (2008). Effects of qian-kun-nin, a Chinese herbal medicine formulation, on HIV positive subjects, a pilot study. *American Journal of Chinese Medicine*, 28 (3–4), 305–312.

Zheng, J., Jiguo, H., Baoping, J., Ye, L. and Zhang, X. (2007). Anti-hyperglycemic activity of *Prunella vulgaris* L. in streptozotocin-induced diabetic mice. *Asia Pacific Journal of Clinical Nutrition*, 16 (Suppl 1), 427–431.

Zhou, T., Luo, D., Li, X. and Luo, Y. (2009). Hypoglycemic and hypolipidemic effects of flavonoids from lotus (*Nelumbo nucifera* Gaertn) leaf in diabetic mice. *Journal of Medicinal Plants Research*, 3, 290–293.

17 Potential Cardio-protective Effects of Functional Foods

Eman M. Alissa[1] and Gordon A. Ferns[2]

[1]*Faculty of Medicine, King AbdulAziz University, Jeddah, Kingdom of Saudi Arabia*
[2]*Division of Medical Education, Brighton and Sussex Medical School, Sussex, UK*

17.1 Introduction

Cardiovascular disease (CVD) is now the leading cause of death globally and is a growing health concern (De Backer *et al.*, 2003). Lifestyle-related conditions, such as obesity, hyperlipidaemia, type 2 diabetes and hypertension, are also widespread and becoming more prevalent globally (Alberti *et al.*, 2009). Lifestyle choices, including diet, are important in the pathogenesis of CVD as they are major determinants of CVD risk factors such as blood pressure and blood lipid levels, although they have been less extensively investigated.

The role of dietary factors has been largely investigated by altering the content of a specific food component known to increase the risk (i.e. sodium or saturated fats) (McGill, 1979) or by large longitudinal cohort studies in which baseline dietary intake was related to cardiovascular outcomes (He *et al.*, 2003; Bernstein *et al.*, 2010).

Functional foods are defined as foods that in addition to supplying nutrients offer potential health benefits that can enhance the well-being of individuals. They affect one or more target functions in the body, beyond their nutritional effects, to either improve health and/or reduce the risk of disease (Ferrari, 2004).

Nutraceuticals are another term that has been used to designate foods that may be used for disease prevention and health promotion. The interest in nutraceuticals for cardiovascular prevention was stimulated by the observation of an association between the consumption of vitamin E and a reduced cardiovascular event rate (Rimm *et al.*, 1993; Stampfer *et al.*, 1993).

Functional Foods and Dietary Supplements: Processing Effects and Health Benefits, First Edition.
Edited by Athapol Noomhorm, Imran Ahmad and Anil Kumar Anal.

Epidemiologic studies have previously demonstrated an association between certain dietary patterns and cardiovascular health. Nutritional research into the cardioprotective potential of their dietary components may support the development of functional foods and nutraceuticals.

17.2 The protective effect of diet in CVD

It has been proposed that CVD can be prevented by lifestyle changes, including diet (Stampfer *et al.*, 2000). Early evidence for the role of diet in CVD came from data on trends in food consumption and ecological studies that has shown associations between CVD prevalence and fat intake (McGill, 1979). Moreover, excessive consumption of foods that are calorie-dense, nutritionally poor, highly processed and rapidly absorbable can lead to systemic inflammation, reduced insulin sensitivity and a cluster of metabolic abnormalities, including obesity, hypertension, dyslipidaemia and glucose intolerance (Srinath Reddy and Katan, 2004). More recently, research has focused on the effects of wholefoods (Folsom *et al.*, 2007). An integrated approach combining lifestyle modification with the correct pharmacologic treatment is sought to reduce cardiovascular risk factors, to improve vascular health and to reduce healthcare expenditure (Aldana *et al.*, 2007).

While epidemiological studies have identified a relationship between diet and CVD, there is still considerable uncertainty about the relationship between specific dietary components and cardiovascular risk. Observational, prospective cohort studies suggest that a higher dietary intake, or supplementation of antioxidants is associated with a lower risk of CVD and mortality but the evidence from clinical trials is still largely negative (Kris-Etherton *et al.*, 2004). The inconsistent results that indicate the apparent protective effects of nutrients as part of dietary intake and the lack of effectiveness of a single nutrient supplementation in trials has led to a focus on whole foods, or modified diets as being protective against CVD (Huang and Sumpio, 2008).

Oxidative stress may be defined as a disturbance in the pro-oxidant/antioxidant balance that favours oxidation. Oxidative stress is involved in the aetiology of several chronic diseases including CVD, some cancers and neurodegenerative disorders (Ferrari and Torres, 2003). Dietary antioxidants (both water- and lipid-soluble), comprise an important component of the antioxidant defence system.

Beyond their normal occurrence in cells and tissues of living organisms, free radicals and reactive oxygen species are also produced in the foods people consume every day, inducing undesirable reactions such as oxidation of lipids, proteins, nucleic acids and carbohydrates.

An impaired capacity to scavenge free radicals and reactive species may be a consequence of decreased levels of antioxidant cellular defence systems or excessive free radicals production, which is common in the brain, liver, heart and other important target organs in humans and animals (Tian *et al.*, 1998; Forster *et al.*, 2000).

Nonetheless, high doses of some antioxidant vitamins have been reported to have potentially adverse vascular effects. In primary and secondary prevention trials, treatment with supplements of β-carotene, vitamin A and vitamin E has been reported to increase mortality and the potential role of vitamin C and selenium on mortality needs further study (Miller *et al.*, 2005; Bjelakovic *et al.*, 2007).

17.3 Functional foods with health-related properties

The conflicting results between the apparent protective effects of nutrients as part of entire food intake and the lack of effectiveness of single nutrient supplementation in trials has led to a focus on whole foods as being protective against CVD. Populations consuming a large proportion of plant-based foods, including fruits and vegetables, or those with a high intake of seafood are known to have a lower incidence of CVD and certain types of cancer (Block *et al.*, 1992).

Functional foods contain physiologically active components either from plant or animal sources and are often marketed with the claim of their ability to reduce heart disease risk focusing primarily on established risk factors, that is blood cholesterol, diabetes and hypertension. Functional foods are suspected of exerting their cardio-protective effects through lipid lowering effects, antioxidant actions and/or decreased homocysteine levels (Table 17.1).

Vegetable and fruit fibres (with pectin), garlic and oily seeds (walnut, almonds, etc.) and fish oils have lipid-lowering effects in humans, by either inhibiting fat absorption or suppressing hepatic cholesterol synthesis. Homocysteine increases the risk of both cardiovascular and cerebrovascular disorders (Mattson, 2003), perhaps by enhancing arteriolar constriction and decreasing endothelial vasodilation (Smolders *et al.*, 2004). A higher intake of folate, antioxidant vitamins, whole grains and phytochemicals has been reported to abrogate the deleterious vascular effects of homocysteine (Broekmans *et al.*, 2000; McKeown *et al.*, 2002). However, a recent clinical trial did not find any beneficial effect of homocysteine reduction on major vascular events (Esfahani *et al.*, 2011). A significant cardiovascular benefit of phytochemicals (polyphenols in wine, grapes and teas), vitamins (ascorbate, tocopherol) and minerals (selenium, magnesium) in foods (Block *et al.*, 2001; Ferrari, 2004) is thought to be related to their ability to scavenge free radicals. The most frequently investigated functional foods that have been studied in cardiovascular patients include: long-chain *n*-3 fatty acids, dietary fibre, phytochemicals as well as nutrients based on or enriched with vegetable proteins, mainly soy.

17.3.1 Fish and fish oils

Individuals with a high intake of dietary fish, or fish oil supplements have a low rate of CVD (Kromhout *et al.*, 1995; He *et al.*, 2004). Although fish contains various nutrients with potentially favourable effects on health, attention has been particularly focused on the omega-3 (*n*-3) fatty acids. However, *n*-3 fatty acids may also be derived from plants as alpha-linolenic acid (ALA, 18:3 *n*-3), eicosapentaenoic acid (EPA, 20:5 *n*-3) and docosahexaenoic acid (DHA, 22:6 *n*-3). Both EPA and DHA are found in oily fish, such as salmon, lake trout, tuna and herring and fish-derived products (fish oils). *n*-3 Fatty acids precursor, α-linolenic acid, is typically found in various plants (e.g. spinach), seeds (nuts and flaxseeds) and oils derived from them (canola, walnut oils). Generally, very little ALA is converted to EPA and even less to DHA and therefore direct intake of the latter two is optimal.

Diets in which cold water fish such as mackerel, salmon, halibut and trout are the main staple are associated with reduced incidence of CVD. Studies of susceptible men

Table 17.1 Potential cardiovascular protective effects of functional foods

Potential mechanism(s)	Functional food(s)	Bioactive compound(s)	Reference(s)
Lowering blood cholesterol	Nuts	Tocopherols, omega-3 fatty acids Fibre and polyphenols	Sabate and Ang, 2009 Albert, *et al.*, 2002
	Legumes	Fibre and phytochemicals	Erkkilä and Lichtenstein, 2006 Darmadi-Blackberry, *et al.*, 2004
	Fruits and vegetables	Fibre (pectin, cellulose) Tocopherols Resveratrol and quercetin	Chopra, *et al.*, 2000 Liu, *et al.*, 2002 Genkinger, *et al.*, 2004
	Whole grains	β-glucan	Lutsey, *et al.*, 2007
	Margarine	Phytosterols	Hicks and Moreau, 2001
	Fish oil	Omega-3 fatty acids	Dyerberg *et al.*, 2004
	Vegetable oils	Tocopherols	Kushi, *et al.*, 1996
	Soy proteins	Genistein and daidzein	Anderson, *et al.*, 1995 Harland and Haffner, 2008
	Dark chocolate	Flavonoid	Grassi, *et al.*, 2005b Baba, *et al.*, 2007
	Tea	Quercetin	Sumpio, *et al.*, 2006
Inhibition of LDL oxidation	Fish	Omega-3 fatty acids	Lee and Wander, 2005
	Green leafy vegetables, fruits	Carotenoids Vitamin C	Chopra, *et al.*, 2000 Sesso, *et al.*, 2008 Aguirre and May, 2008
	Pomegranate	Polyphenols	Davidson, *et al.*, 2009
	Grapes and red wines	Resveratrol	Perez-Jimenez and Saura-Calixto, 2008
	Tomato	Lycopene	Engelhard, *et al.*, 2006
	Extra-virgin olive oil	Polyphenolics and oleic acid	Psaltopoulou, *et al.*, 2004
	Green tea	Polyphenolics	Hooper, *et al.*, 2008
	Soy proteins	Genistein, daidzein and glycitin	Wiseman, *et al.*, 2000
	Dark chocolate	Flavonoid and anthocyanins	Grassi, *et al.*, 2005b
Lowering blood triglycerides	Fish	Omega-3 fatty acids	Durrington *et al.*, 2001 Dyerberg *et al.*, 2004 Harris, *et al.*, 2008
	Whole grains	Flaxseed	Mellen, *et al.*, 2008
	Fruits and vegetables	Ascorbic acid	Osganian, *et al.*, 2003b
Decreasing blood pressure	Fish	Omega-3 fatty acids	Mozaffarian, 2008
	Legumes	Fibre	He *et al.*, 1995
	Whole grains	Fibre and phytochemicals	Flint, *et al.*, 2009
	Ginseng	Ginsenosides	Savica, *et al.*, 2010
	Onion and garlic	Quercetin	Lee, *et al.*, 2009
	Green and black teas	Polyphenols	Hooper, *et al.*, 2008
	Grapes and red wines	Grape polyphenols	Perez-Jimenez and Saura-Calixto, 2008
	Dark chocolate	Flavonoid	Grassi, *et al.*, 2005b

Table 17.1 (*Continued*)

Potential mechanism(s)	Functional food(s)	Bioactive compound(s)	Reference(s)
Lowering blood homocysteine	Fruits and vegetables	Folate Vitamin C Phytochemicals	Samman, *et al.*, 2003 Jenkins, *et al.*, 2002 Broekmans, *et al.*, 2000
	Whole grains	Fibre and phytochemicals	Jacobs, *et al.*, 2000
	Nuts, seeds and oils	Vitamin E	Ros, *et al.*, 2004
Antioxidant action	Green leafy vegetables and fruits	Carotenoids Tocopherol, tocotrienols Vitamin C Flavonoids Indoles Lutein	Krinsky and Johnson, 2005 Aguirre and May, 2008 Sesso, *et al.*, 2008 Bazzano, *et al.*, 2003 Prior and Cao, 2000 Genkinger, *et al.*, 2004
	Tomatoes	Lycopene	Engelhard, *et al.*, 2006
	Vegetable oils	Tocopherols	Kushi, *et al.*, 1996
	Grapes and red wines	Anthocyanins, catechins, cyanidins, flavonols, myricetin, resveratrol and quercetin	Perez-Jimenez and Saura-Calixto, 2008
	Strawberries and raspberries	Cyaniding	
	Soy proteins	Genistein and daidzein	Sacks, *et al.*, 2006
	Brazil nuts, grains and seeds	Vitamin E Selenium	Ros, *et al.*, 2004
	Green and black teas	Polyphenols	Mink, *et al.*, 2007
Anti-inflammatory action	Fish	Omega-3 fatty acids	Ueeda, *et al.*, 2008
	Nuts, seeds and oils	Vitamin E	Singh, *et al.*, 2005 Kushi, *et al.*, 1996
	Legumes	Polyphenols	Lutsey, *et al.*, 2007
	Tea	Catechins	Sumpio, *et al.*, 2006
	Peppers	Capsaicin	
	Fruits and vegetables	Quercetin	Lupton and Turner, 2003
	Grapes and red wines	Anthocyanins, catechins, cyanidins, flavonols, myricetin and quercetin	Perez-Jimenez and Saura-Calixto, 2008
Endothelial function	Fish	Omega-3 fatty acids	Ueeda, *et al.*, 2008
	Nuts	Polyphenols	Ros, *et al.*, 2004
	Citrus fruits and vegetables	Vitamin C Polyphenols	Aguirre and May, 2008
	Grapes and red wines	Anthocyanins, catechins, cyanidins, flavonols, myricetin and quercetin	Perez-Jimenez and Saura-Calixto, 2008
	Dark chocolate	Flavonoid	Grassi, *et al.*, 2005a
Platelets aggregation	Grapes and red wines	Anthocyanins, catechins, cyanidins, flavonols, myricetin and quercetin	Perez-Jimenez and Saura-Calixto, 2008 Mink, *et al.*, 2007

from Holland, Japan and the United States showed that sudden death from coronary artery disease is substantially lower when 1–2 fish meals are consumed weekly (Albert *et al.*, 1998). Despite the established beneficial effect of fatty fish consumption on CHD, the species and amount of fish consumed, as well as the preparation method, have an impact on their potential benefit (Bjerregaard *et al.*, 2010). The concomitance of low amounts of *n*-3 fatty acids in our average diet and the need for prolonged administration for prevention and treatment has led to the development of selected preparations (enriched foods or special formulations, e.g. *n*-3 fatty acids incorporated into cows' milk). These should allow the combination of acceptability and adequate bioavailability despite their relatively low contents of *n*-3 fatty acids. *n*-3 fatty acids are therefore being incorporated into a number of commercially available, natural foods that, due to their structural features, appear to be particularly suited as efficient fatty acid vehicles (Carrero *et al.*, 2004). However, it has been argued that the environmental contaminants found in certain fish, for example methylmercury, polychlorinated biphenyls and dioxins, may diminish the health benefits of fish-derived *n*-3 fatty acids (Mozaffarian and Rimm, 2006).

The cardiovascular protective effects of *n*-3 fatty acids may be related to several properties: they are anti-inflammatory, anti-thrombotic (reduced platelet aggregability) and anti-arrhythmic (reducing the risk of potentially fatal cardiac arrhythmias); furthermore, they lower heart rate and blood pressure, plasma triglycerides levels (Harris *et al.*, 2008) and improve endothelial function (Mozaffarian, 2008).

Fish oil supplements have favourable effects on lipid profile and blood pressure (Durrington *et al.*, 2001; Dyerberg *et al.*, 2004). The former appears to be due to decreased hepatic triglyceride secretion combined with enhanced clearance of triglycerides from plasma. Moreover, fish ingestion has been related to a reduced risk of death from myocardial infarction, which may relate to beneficial effects of EPA and DHA on plaque stability (probably related to the content of inflammatory cells) and modulation of endothelial function (Ueeda *et al.*, 2008). EPA and DHA have also been shown to lower oxidative susceptibility of low-density lipoprotein cholesterol (LDL-C), which could help to reduce the risk of CVD (Lee and Wander, 2005). While research has mainly concentrated on the effects of the long-chain compounds (EPA and DHA), the role of *n*-3 ALA should also be considered. Data on the effects of ALA on CVD outcomes are somewhat limited (Hu *et al.*, 1999; Campos *et al.*, 2008), as some researchers suggest potential cardiovascular protection by this unsaturated fatty acid (Djoussé *et al.*, 2005).

A meta-analysis of 65 studies demonstrated that *n*-3 fatty acids lowered triglyceride levels in a dose-dependent manner; with the triglyceride lowering being proportional to baseline levels (Kris-Etherton *et al.*, 2002). However, there was a large inter-study variability in response to the treatment that is possibly due to the dose or relative amounts of *n*-3 fatty acids, the duration of study, the prior health status of participants, diet and other confounding factors. The FDA evaluated the data and determined that, although there is scientific evidence supporting the claim, further studies will be helpful in substantiating it. The large heterogeneity within studies with *n*-3 fatty acids supplementation for the response to triglycerides is likely to be attributable to genetic variability within the study population. Nevertheless, these particular intervention studies are largely short-term and have generally used a higher dose of *n*-3 fatty acids compared to the clinical outcome studies. Furthermore, studies are also required to determine whether individuals of a specific genotype may benefit more from n-3 fatty acids. Clinical studies also need to determine whether the reduction in CVD risk factors is due to EPA, DHA or the combination of both and the dosage of the effective components (He *et al.*, 2004).

17.3.2 Fruit and vegetables

The literature is consistent in reporting the beneficial effects of diets rich in vegetables and fruits on CVD risk (Liu *et al.*, 2000; Joshipura *et al.*, 2001; Dauchet *et al.*, 2006; He *et al.*, 2007). An inadequate intake of fruit and vegetables has been linked to a higher incidence of CVD (Lock *et al.*, 2005). The benefits of fruit and vegetables seem to be dose related and the frequency of fruit and vegetable intake has been associated with lower CVD risk (Pietinen *et al.*, 1996; Rosengren *et al.*, 2009).

The mechanisms by which fruit and vegetables exert their protective effects are not entirely clear but are likely to include their content of antioxidants and anti-inflammatory constituents. Their folate content may also reduce plasma homocysteine (Broekmans *et al.*, 2000). The antioxidants in fruit and vegetables decrease the susceptibility of LDL particles to oxidation (Chopra *et al.*, 2000). Potassium may also have a protective role on the incidence of CVD as mounting evidence indicates an inverse association between dietary intake of fruit and vegetables and blood pressure (He and Whelton, 1997; Savica *et al.*, 2010). Bioactive components in fruit and vegetables include: carotenoids, vitamin C, citrus flavonoids and limonoids, essential oils containing monoterpenes, fibre, magnesium and potassium. The totality of the evidence supports the current Dietary Guidelines for Americans to increase fruit and vegetable consumption to at least five and possibly up to nine portions per day (Report of the DGA, 2010).

Soluble fibres including pectins from apples and citrus fruits, β-glucan from oats and barley, fibres from flaxseed and psyllium are known to lower LDL-C (Erkkilä and Lichtenstein, 2006). It has been shown that 3 g of β-glucan reduces serum cholesterol, by 5% (Ripsin *et al.*, 1992). On the basis of these findings, the FDA awarded the first food-specific health claim in 1997 for oats and oat products. Psyllium husk is used as an additive in several other products such as cereals and supplements. The FDA extended the soluble fibre health claim to psyllium fibre in 1998. The cholesterol-lowering effects of soluble fibre are proposed to be due to their binding of bile acids and inhibition of cholesterol synthesis. However, in the Health Professionals Follow-Up Study, only cereal fibre and not fruit or vegetable fibre, was found to be inversely associated with the risk of stroke (Liu *et al.*, 2002).

Although fruits and vegetables should provide the main staple of a healthy diet, the specific polyphenol content of fruit and vegetables is very variable and is affected by how they are prepared and their variable absorption efficiency confound the ability to provide clear-cut dietary and clinical recommendations of polyphenol-rich fruits and vegetables in the nutritional prevention of heart disease. Furthermore, several studies have not demonstrated significant protective effects of fruit and vegetables on mortality, although most show protective trends. These include a study of adults in Maryland (Genkinger *et al.*, 2004), the Kuopio Ischaemic Heart Disease Risk Factor (KIHD) study among middle-aged Finnish men (Rissanen *et al.*, 2003) and the Adventist Health Study (Fraser *et al.*, 1992). These studies may have had insufficient power, or inadequate ranges of intake to observe significant effects.

17.3.3 Garlic

Garlic is known for its antibacterial activity, but has also been reported to reduce the incidence of CVD, hypercholesterolaemia and hypertension (Alder and Holub, 1997). The characteristic aroma and taste of garlic is due to an abundance of organosulfur compounds (e.g. allicin), which are probably responsible for the various beneficial health effects of garlic. Garlic bulbs contains the amino acid alliin, which is converted to allicin, that spontaneously decomposes to numerous sulfur-containing compounds, some of which have been shown to inhibit tumorigenesis and to reduce cancer risk in humans (Dorant *et al.*, 1993).

17.3.4 Nuts and legumes

Nuts are complex foods containing cholesterol-lowering mono- and polyunsaturated fatty acids, arginine (a precursor of the vasodilator nitric oxide), soluble fibre and several antioxidant polyphenols (Sabate and Ang, 2009). Almonds, hazelnuts, Brazil nuts, peanuts, walnuts, pistachios, pine nuts and pecans have all been shown to have a beneficial effect. Large prospective studies have demonstrated that the consumption of 1–4 servings of nuts per week was associated with about a 40% reduction in risk of coronary heart disease, after adjusting for conventional risk factors such as hypertension, smoking, diabetes and hyperlipidaemia (Hu and Stampfer, 1999). Postprandial vascular reactivity is characterized by decreased bioavailability of nitric oxide and increased expression of pro-inflammatory cytokines and cellular adhesion molecules (Ros *et al.*, 2004). Prospective data from the Physicians' Health Study (Albert *et al.*, 2002) have indicated a reduced risk of sudden cardiac death associated with nut consumption.

Legumes are also complex foods, rich in soluble fibres and polyphenols, as well as folic acid. Legumes were the only food group predictive of survival among five long-lived elderly cohorts in Japan, Sweden, Greece and Australia (Darmadi-Blackberry *et al.*, 2004). Furthermore, cumulative evidence from experimental research indicates that the cholesterol-lowering effect of legumes is probably due to the combined effects of several bioactive components, such as protein, soluble and insoluble fibres, and phytosterols (Martins *et al.*, 2005). A recent interventional trial in humans has shown that lupin kernel flour added to bread has a positive effect on blood pressure: both the fibre and the protein were suggested to be responsible (Lee *et al.*, 2009).

17.3.5 Whole grains

Whole grain products contain intact grain kernels rich in fibre and trace nutrients. They are nutritionally important because they contain phyto-protective substances that might work synergistically to reduce cardiovascular risk.

The potential protective role of whole grains was first evaluated in the early 1970s (Morris *et al.*, 1977). Based on the results of the prospective Iowa Women's Health Study, that demonstrated cereal fibre had different associations with total mortality, depending on whether the fibre came from foods that contained primarily whole grain or refined grain (Jacobs *et al.*, 2000). A more recent meta-analysis based on seven qualifying prospective cohort studies focused on whole grain consumption and cardiovascular outcomes reported that the inverse association between dietary whole grains and incident CVD was strong and consistent across trials (Bazzano *et al.* 2003; Lupton and Turner, 2003; Streppel *et al.*, 2005; Mellen *et al.*, 2008).

The mechanisms underlying the protective effect of whole grains on CVD risk include its effects on insulin sensitivity (McKeown *et al.*, 2002), blood pressure (Flint *et al.*, 2009), lipids and inflammation (Lutsey *et al.*, 2007). Although the anti-inflammatory mechanism is not clear, it may be related to higher intakes of antioxidant nutrients present in the germ of whole grains. As compared to refined grains, whole grains have a reduced glycaemic response following ingestion (i.e. the post-prandial rise in blood glucose is lessened) and reductions in postprandial glucose surges have been associated with reduced reactive oxygen generation after a meal and reduced postprandial inflammation and CVD risk (McKeown *et al.*, 2002).

17.3.6 Soy proteins

Soy is the main source of protein in the Japanese diet, in which it is consumed in the form of miso soup and tofu. Soy products are rich in polyunsaturated fatty acids, fibre, vitamins and minerals and have a low saturated fat content (Sacks *et al.*, 2006). Soybeans and soy foods contain many phytochemicals that are considered to be effective in preventing and ameliorating chronic diseases such as cancer, CVD and osteoporosis and it appears to alleviate menopausal symptoms. The phytochemicals in soybeans include phytoestrogens (e.g. genistein, daidzein and glycitein and their glucosides), phytosterols, tocophenols, saponins, phenolic acids, lecithins, protease inhibitors and phytic acid.

Prospective observational studies in vegetarians (Burslem *et al.*, 1978), in Chinese women (Zhang *et al.*, 2003) and in a Japanese population (Nagata *et al.*, 1998), have all shown a reduction of total cholesterol and LDL-C as well as of ischaemic and cerebrovascular events with a daily soy protein intake of more than 6 g, compared with less than 0.5 g. In 1999, the FDA approved a health claim for soy protein on the grounds that daily consumption of at least 25 g of soy protein tends to reduce the risk of CVD. A large number of clinical studies were summarized in a meta-analysis (Anderson *et al.*, 1995) and confirmed that serum LDL-C concentrations are modified, the effects being related to baseline blood cholesterol levels. The results of this meta-analysis were criticized recently, since more recent studies appeared not to confirm the very powerful cholesterol-reducing effect of soy proteins (Sacks *et al.*, 2006). A recent systematic review of the available randomized controlled studies, most conducted in subjects with moderate hypercholesterolaemia, confirmed that a modest intake of soy protein (25 g) produces a highly significant reduction of total cholesterol and LDL-C levels equivalent to ca. 6% LDL reduction (Harland and Haffner, 2008). Old studies were based on the effects in severely hypercholesterolaemic individuals, whereas patients with hypercholesterolaemia in the very highest range (>335 mg/l (>8.68 mmol/L) have not been selected for treatment in more recent studies. The exact mechanism by which soy protein exerts its hypocholesterolaemic effect has not yet been fully elucidated, but may involve enhanced synthesis of the LDL receptor and inhibition of cholesterol biosynthesis (Cho *et al.*, 2007).

Soy products contain several isoflavonoids (genistein, daidzein, glycitin) that are natural phytoestrogens able to inhibit LDL oxidation, thus decreasing the risk of atherosclerosis (Wiseman, 1999). Some studies have reported a decrease in susceptibility of LDL particles to oxidation with increased soy protein consumption (Wiseman *et al.*, 2000; Jenkins *et al.*, 2002). A meta-analysis of randomized controlled trials has shown that soy isoflavones can lower serum total and LDL cholesterol in humans (Taku, *et al.*, 2007). However, no dose–response effect between soy isoflavones and changes in LDL or HDL cholesterol levels was identified. The efficacy of soy foods and isoflavone supplements on blood lipids in clinical trials is less clear. These contradictory data may be due to poorer responses in hypercholesterolaemic subjects compared to their normocholesterolaemic control counterparts (Sacks *et al.*, 2006). Recent clinical trials with soy protein in postmenopausal women have also shown similar inconsistencies (Ho *et al.*, 2007). Clearly additional studies are needed to determine whether there are differences among whole food, soy protein and isoflavone extracts.

Comparisons between different animal or clinical studies are hampered by the lack of standardization of soy nomenclature, the different formulations, doses, routes of administration, time and duration of exposure (Cederroth and Nef, 2009).

17.3.7 Dark chocolate

Cocoa is a flavonoid-rich food, containing compounds such as (–)epicatechin that has been recently investigated for its possible role in the prevention of CVD (Ding *et al.*, 2006; Galleano *et al.*, 2009). In healthy adults, drinking flavonoid-rich cocoa may improve nitric oxide-dependent vaso-relaxation and flow-mediated dilation in the brachial arteries (Grassi *et al.*, 2005a). Administration of dark chocolate in essential hypertensives reduced ambulatory blood pressure and serum LDL-C levels whereas white chocolate had no significant effects (Grassi *et al.*, 2005b). Furthermore there was a clear reduction of the blood cholesterol levels as well as a significant rise of HDL cholesterol in addition to a marked reduction of circulating oxidized LDL (Baba *et al.*, 2007).

17.3.8 Coffee and tea

The active constituents of coffee likely to be responsible for a cardio-protective effect are diterpenes, such as kahweol and cafestol. Coffee consumption may reduce the risk of myocardial infarction, but data are as yet inconclusive (Christensen *et al.*, 2001; Panagiotakos *et al.*, 2003). A dose–response decrease in cardiovascular risk and heart disease mortality was reported for daily caffeine intake in patients with type 2 diabetes (Bidel *et al.*, 2006; Greenberg *et al.*, 2007).

The harvested fresh tea leaf is unusually rich in polyphenols (ca. 30% dry weight), however, this changes with processing. The phenolic constituents in green tea differ from that of black tea. In green teas, especially those of Japanese production, most of the polyphenols survive whereas in black tea production the transformations are much more extensive, with some 90% destruction of the flavan-3-ols in processing (Riemersma *et al.*, 2001). Green tea consumption appears to be protective against CVD and cancer (Sumpio *et al.*, 2006), but results are again inconsistent. Catechins are the principal polyphenols in tea and they are present as four major types; epicatechin, epicatechin-3-gallate, epigallocatechin and epigallocatechin-3-gallate, which are flavonoid derivatives. It has been reported in a meta-analysis that the incidence of myocardial infarction among individuals who consumed three cups of tea daily was not statistically significant and there has been large variability across studies (Peters *et al.*, 2001). There were regional differences in this meta-analysis, with increasing tea consumption associated with an increased risk for coronary heart disease in the United Kingdom and for stroke in Australia, whereas the risk decreased in other regions, particularly in continental Europe. The hypothesis that addition of milk to tea (as typically done in United Kingdom and Australia) abolishes its plasma antioxidant potential may only partially explain these geographic differences.

17.3.9 Dairy products

Dairy products, such as milk, cheese and yogurt, are among the best sources of several important vitamins and minerals. Based on the current scientific evidence, the 2010 DGA stated, 'Moderate evidence shows that intake of milk and milk products is associated with a reduced risk of CVD and type 2 diabetes and with lower blood pressure in adults' (USDA, 2010). These effects may be attributable to milk fat, vitamin D, calcium, magnesium, potassium, whey proteins, or the combination of these as part of the unique nutrient package that dairy food provides. However, well-controlled trials evaluating the effects of dairy foods as a whole (including the effects of saturated fatty acids from milk fat and salt from cheese) on the development of CVD are necessary to verify the results from observational and prospective research and to better understand the effects on chronic disease risk.

The fermented dairy products, such as yogurt and sour milk are categorized as 'probiotics' which are defined as live microbial food supplements, which beneficially affect the host animal by improving its intestinal microbial balance (Farnworth, 2000). Probiotics have attracted considerable attention, primarily because they display anticarcinogenic, hypocholesterolaemic and antagonistic action against intestinal pathogens (Mital and Garg, 1995). Fermentable carbohydrates that serve as nutrient substrates for the beneficial microflora of the gut make up a class of 'prebiotics' which have been defined as nondigestible food ingredients that beneficially affect the host by selectively stimulating the growth and/or activity of one or a limited number of bacteria in the colon and thus improve host health (Farnworth, 2000).

17.4 Bioactive dietary compounds with cardio-protective potentials

Early research evaluated the benefits of plant-derived foods based on their vitamin C, vitamin E and carotenoid content (Block *et al.*, 1992). More recent work has noted the possible correlation of benefits with individual compounds (Prior and Cao, 2000). However, the effects of testing them alone may be related to the synergistic action of the various other bioactive compounds present in the source materials (Omenn *et al.*, 1996). The main doubt about their efficacy, whether they should be consumed in a whole food diet or provided in a supplemental form remains to be answered and will be discussed later. In each family of bioactive compounds there are usually many members that are present as discussed later. Furthermore it is well known that in biological systems these compounds operate synergistically and that large intakes of a single antioxidant may have a deleterious effect overall (Abudu *et al.*, 2004).

17.4.1 Phytochemicals

Plant foods contain many bioactive compounds known as 'phytochemicals'. Some groups of phytochemicals that have, or appear to have, significant health benefits are: carotenoids, phenolic compounds (flavonoids, phytoestrogens, phenolic acids), phytosterols and phytostanols, tocotrienols, organosulfur compounds and non-digestible carbohydrates (dietary fibre and prebiotics). Isoflavones are found in high concentration in soybean, soybean products (e.g. tofu) and red clover. Lignans are mainly found in flaxseed.

17.4.2 Polyphenol compounds

Polyphenol compounds include simple phenols and flavonoids, which are found in fruits, vegetables and nuts and their products. They possess important antioxidant properties. Polyphenols have been shown in *in vivo* studies to exert anti-atherosclerotic effects in the early stages of atherosclerosis development (e.g. decreased LDL oxidation); improve endothelial function and increase nitric oxide release (potent vasodilator); modulate inflammation and lipid metabolism (i.e. hypolipidaemic effect); improve antioxidant status; and, protect against atherothrombotic episodes including myocardial ischaemia and platelet aggregation (Perez-Jimenez and Saura-Calixto, 2008; Davidson *et al.*, 2009).

Flavonoids Plant-derived flavonoids are the most common group of polyphenols in the human diet (e.g. proanthocyanidins, quercetin and epicatechin) and are contained in vegetables and fruits as well as in beverages such as cocoa, tea and wine. Some isoflavones like lignans are phytoestrogens, a group of non-steroidal plant constituents that elicit oestrogen-like biological response. They are associated as minor components with dietary fibre in food items that include oilseeds, cereal grains, vegetables, fruits and legumes. Like other phenolic compounds, phytoestrogens have antioxidant activity and like oestrogens, they can influence lipoprotein metabolism and enhance vascular reactivity.

Intake of flavonoids has been associated with decreased cardiovascular mortality and general mortality among elderly Dutch individuals (Geleijnse *et al.*, 2002). Several prospective studies have reported inverse associations between flavonoid intake and CVD incidence or mortality (Hertog *et al.* 1993; Knekt *et al.*, 1996; Mukamal *et al.*, 2002). Of the cardiovascular protective mechanisms of flavonoids, several have been proposed to explain their anti-inflammatory properties. These include: their antioxidant activity and their properties as chelators for transitional metal ions (copper and iron that catalyze lipid oxidation); their inhibition of platelet aggregation; and modulation of eicosanoid generation and nitric oxide synthesis; their inhibitory effects on superoxide production; and beneficial effects on lipid profile (Lichtenstein, 1998, Mink *et al.*, 2007) and modulation of pro-inflammatory gene expression (Prior and Cao, 2000; Jiang and Dusting, 2003; Garcia-Lafuente *et al.*, 2009).

A systematic review of the effectiveness of different flavonoid subclasses and flavonoid-rich foods on CVD concluded that some flavonoid-rich foods, including chocolate or cocoa, red wine or grape and green or black tea may have some measurable effects on CVD risk factors, including a reduction in blood pressure and a favourable influence on endothelial function (Hooper *et al.*, 2008).

The beneficial effects of red wine are thought to result from high concentrations of polyphenols, which are extracted from grape skins during fermentation and have antioxidant properties. The principal compounds in red wine include flavonols such as quercetin, catechin, anthocyanins, phenolic acids including caffeic acid and the stilbene resveratrol. Red wine appears to be the richest source of resveratrol, which is believed to have antioxidant, anti-inflammatory, anti-proliferative and anti-angiogenic properties, hence the benefit in many disorders where oxidative stress plays an important role (Catalgol *et al.*, 2012). Despite the evidence for the effectiveness of wine against CVD, a US study demonstrated that consumption of red wine did not significantly reduce coronary risk (Klatsky *et al.*, 1997). It should also be pointed out that excessive consumption of alcoholic beverages has been linked to the development of several types of cancer, such as breast cancer (Bowlin *et al.*, 1997), as well as cirrhosis of the liver.

Nevertheless, there still exists uncertainty as to whether or not flavonoids are the only bioactive compounds mediating the enhanced vascular reactivity. This is in part due to the fact that flavonoid-rich food and plant extracts contain many potentially bioactive compounds and information ensuing from investigations in humans using specific, chemically pure flavonoids is rare. Therefore the observed effects on vascular function may potentially, at least in part, be related to compounds other than flavonoids contained in these foods/extracts. On the other hand, because phytoestrogens compete with oestrogen for binding to oestrogen receptors, their use could have beneficial effects in preventing osteoporosis and sex hormone-mediated malignancy, such as breast and prostate cancer. This might be the reason why the populations that consume large quantities of soy products daily (e.g. inhabitants of Far Eastern countries) generally have a reduced risk of oestrogen-dependent cancers and lower incidence of postmenopausal hot flushes and night sweating compared to Western women. However, it should be noted that no conclusive evidence has so far emerged about the therapeutic efficacy of isoflavones in reducing the incidence of CVD and breast cancer and in preventing the loss of bone mineral density in menopausal women.

Plant sterols and stanols Plant sterols or phytosterols are structurally similar and functionally analogous to the animal sterol, cholesterol. A less abundant class of related compounds is the plant stanols or phytostanols, which are completely saturated forms of phytosterols. Dietary sources include vegetable oils, nuts, seeds and grains but the amounts are often insufficient to have significant cholesterol-lowering effects (Berger *et al.*, 2004). Furthermore they have been incorporated into foods with a high fat content, such as spreads (margarines) and salad dressings. Phytosterols and phytostanols inhibit intestinal absorption of cholesterol (Hicks and Moreau, 2001). HDL cholesterol and/or VLDL cholesterol have generally not been significantly affected by the intake of stanols/ sterols. The effects of sterols/ stanols on LDL cholesterol have been found to be additive to diets and/or cholesterol-lowering drugs (Normen *et al.*, 2005). This has been the basis for the development of phytosterol-enriched functional foods. Similar efficacy has been observed between plant sterols and stanols when they are esterified, which is the form added to foods (Demonty *et al.*, 2009). The FDA expanded the scope of a phytosterol heart health claim in 2003. The agency allowed a broader range of food products and dietary supplements to bear the heart health claim in labelling when they are formulated with 0.65 g of phytosterol ester or 0.4 g of free phytosterol per serving. Because plant sterols and stanols can reduce fat-soluble vitamins, it is necessary to consume plant sterols and stanols with an appropriate intake of fruit and vegetables, including carotenoids (Quílez *et al.*, 2003). There are also concerns about margarines containing plant sterols and stanols, related to the energy intake associated with consuming >2 g daily (Wolfs *et al.*, 2006).

Vitamin C The powerful antioxidant functions of vitamin C serve to reduce tissue reactive oxygen species concentrations, which in the atherosclerotic condition help prevent endothelial dysfunction, inhibit vascular smooth muscle proliferation and reduce oxidized LDL cholesterol (Aguirre and May, 2008). Several prospective studies have assessed the role of vitamin C, both dietary and supplemental, in CVD, with conflicting results (Knekt *et al.*, 2004). Despite its role as an antioxidant, vitamin C has been identified as a pro-oxidant under conditions of high oxidative stress (Ye and Song, 2008). Most clinical trials have incorporated vitamin C into a mixture including vitamin E and β-carotene, with largely null results in relation to CVD (Cook *et al.*, 2007; Sesso *et al.*, 2008). Nutrients and bioactive compounds in foods act synergistically or antagonistically in the complex food matrix to deliver the established health effects of foods.

Carotenoids There are several plant-derived carotenoids in the human diet, for example β-carotene, α-carotene, lutein, zeaxanthin and lycopene. Carotenoids have been proposed to have health-promoting effects: immune-enhancement and reduction of the risk of developing degenerative diseases such as cancer, CVD and cataracts (Gaziano and Hennekens, 1993, Krinsky and Johnson, 2005). These physiological activities have been attributed to their ability to quench singlet oxygen and interact with free radicals (Palace *et al.*, 1999). The carotenoids, particularly lycopene and β-carotene, are dietary antioxidants that function to reduce oxidative stress *in vivo* and blood markers of inflammation (Engelhard *et al.*, 2006). Evidence for a role of carotenoids in CVD first stemmed from studies that showed that higher intakes of fruit and vegetables were associated with a lower risk of CVD (Liu *et al.*, 2001). However, studies on the association between dietary carotenoids and CVD risk have been inconsistent. Women who regularly eat large amounts of lycopene, are reported to be less prone to developing CVD, since this phytochemical has the strongest antioxidant activities in the cardiovascular system (Agarwall and Rao, 2000). Results from the KIHD study confirmed that lower serum lycopene levels were associated with enhanced risk of atherosclerosis in the common carotid artery (Rissanen *et al.*, 2003). An inverse relationship between lycopene in tomato products and the risk of cancers was also documented in a review of more than 30 studies (Giovannucci, 1999). These protective associations were not evident for other carotenoids like lutein, zeaxanthin, or β-cryptoxanthin that were suggested to have a potential preventive effect against macular degeneration (Osganian *et al.*, 2003a).

Conversely, large placebo-controlled studies using single antioxidants or combinations to prevent CVD have not shown antioxidant supplementation to be beneficial, but sometimes rather harmful, as exemplified by the incidence of increased lung cancer in those receiving β-carotene supplements in a study of more than 25 000 middle-aged male Finnish smokers (Albanes *et al.*, 1996). Despite overwhelming evidence from epidemiological studies on the role of carotenoids in CVD, however, clinical trials have failed to demonstrate a beneficial effect (Vivekananthan *et al.*, 2003; Bjelakovic *et al.*, 2007).

Vitamin E In addition to its role as a free radical scavenger, vitamin E is a potent anti-inflammatory agent, especially at high doses (Singh *et al.*, 2005). Mounting evidence supports the strong inverse association between plasma vitamin E and CVD (Gey *et al.*, 1991) and between vitamin E intake and risk of coronary heart disease (Kushi *et al.*, 1996). Nevertheless, clinical trials failed to support the role of vitamin E supplementation in preventing CVD (Bolton-Smith *et al.*, 1992). Subsequent meta-analyses and systematic reviews of more than 90 trials showed similar null results (Eidelman *et al.*, 2004; Shekelle *et al.*, 2004). A dose–response meta-analysis showed increased risk of high-dose vitamin E ($\geq$400 IU/day) on total mortality (Miller *et al.*, 2005). There are many potential explanations for these largely negative effects that include the use of the most appropriate form and/or dose of vitamin E. This may be essential to obtain effective reduction of oxidative stress. As with carotenoids, the contrast between the results of observational and interventional studies suggests that the protective effects of α-tocopherol occur in the presence of other nutrients and therefore, it is most effective and safe when obtained from foods.

Antioxidant vitamin supplementation The term 'dietary supplement' can be defined as a product that is intended to supplement the diet with one or more of the following ingredients: a vitamin, a mineral, an herb or other botanical, an amino acid, intended for ingestion in pill, capsule, tablet, or liquid form (Kalra, 2003). It should be noted that nutraceuticals differ from dietary supplements in the following aspects (i) nutraceuticals must not only supplement the diet but should also aid in the prevention and/or treatment of disease; and (ii) nutraceuticals are used as conventional foods or as sole items of a meal or diet (Kalra, 2003).

In view of the potentially damaging role of free radicals and reactive oxygen species in the pathophysiology of atherosclerosis, supplementation with antioxidants (vitamins A, C, E, folic acid, β-carotene, selenium, zinc) was expected to be protective. Some supplements (for example marine *n*-3 fatty acids and niacin) are effective in improving CVD risk factors. Others (like B-vitamins; folate, vitamin B_{12}, vitamin B_6, antioxidants; vitamin E and selenium) have shown little effect on CVD mortality and morbidity despite promising *in-vitro* studies and antioxidant supplements may even have adverse effects. Trace elements with antioxidant properties such as copper and selenium may become strongly pro-oxidant both *in vivo* and *in vitro* as a consequence of their physical properties. Vitamins A, C and E can also become pro-oxidant when present in low concentrations and near transition metal ions.

It was initially thought that antioxidant vitamins would provide a simple approach to counteract increased oxidative stress by cardiovascular risk factors. Epidemiologic studies have reported that a high dietary intake of foods rich in vitamin E (Rimm *et al.*, 1993), vitamin C (Osganian *et al.*, 2003b) and β-carotene (Osganian *et al.*, 2003a), have been inversely associated with the incidence of coronary artery disease. Nevertheless, firm recommendations to take antioxidant supplements to treat or prevent CVD or metabolic diseases require evidence derived from randomized controlled trials with vitamin supplements, which were found to be disappointing (Brigelius-Flohe *et al.*, 2005). Indeed, only one trial has shown a reduction in myocardial infarction and cardiac events (Stephens *et al.*, 1996), whereas all the others have shown no effect or detrimental effects. Within five trials, such antioxidant supplementation was associated with increased all-cause mortality and two have shown higher risk of fatal CHD (ATBC and CARET). Indeed, those controversial results by no means invalidate the role of oxidative stress in CVD; rather, they suggest that very high supplementation with antioxidant vitamins may not represent an optimal strategy to prevent vascular damage induced by oxidative stress and lipid oxidation. Several factors ought to be considered, which may have contributed to cloud the results of clinical trials, like choosing the optimal dose and form of vitamins, the use of single vitamin(s) or in combination, the timing of antioxidant administration, etc. (Blumberg and Frei, 2007).

17.5 Dietary patterns and reduced risk of chronic diseases

Eating habits and dietary trends have health, environmental and social impacts. Some diet plans demonstrated the ability to reduce cardiovascular risk (Ornish *et al.*, 1998). Despite the high levels of interest in the relationship between diet and health, the traditional approach in nutritional epidemiology has mainly focused on the effects of individual nutrients or foods. However, individuals do not consume nutrients in isolation but, rather, meals consisting of a variety of foods with combinations of nutrients that are likely to be interactive or synergistic. Indeed, much less concern has been focused on dietary patterns because of their complex nature. The mechanisms by which these diets reduce inflammatory risk are not well understood but may relate to high intakes of food items containing antioxidant nutrients and polyphenols that reduce free radical concentrations throughout tissues.

Patterns of consuming food vary significantly across nations and this might contribute differently to the apparent differences in the health of populations on the continent.

17.6 Conclusion

The relationship between dietary factors and CVD has been a major focus of health research for almost half a century. Epidemiological and clinical studies indicate that the risk of CVD is reduced by a diet rich in fruits, vegetables, unrefined grains, fish and low-fat dairy products and low in saturated fats and sodium (Aldana *et al.*, 2007). Other foods such as mono- and polyunsaturated fats, brans, nuts, plant sterols and soy proteins have all been shown to have a favourable effect on lipid profile and blood pressure (Jensen *et al.*, 2004; Srinath Reddy and Katan, 2004).

Novel dietary approaches to cardiovascular prevention are of major significance in clinical research and practice. However, nutrition is a very complex research topic and it is not clear whether an individual component of the diet or a combination of nutrients and dietary habits may be responsible for any cardio-protective effects. The advances in the knowledge of both the disease processes and healthy dietary components have provided new avenues to develop dietary strategies to prevent and/or to treat CVD. It is now evident, based on the extensive scientific evidence, that functional foods have broad ranging physiologic effects *in vivo* that lessen inflammatory cascades and vascular reactivity. These effects are as powerful as pharmaceutical interventions, yet much safer. Albeit that many of these functional foods have been found to have high therapeutic potential, future studies should include well-designed clinical trials assessing different combinations of these nutrients to realize the possible additive and/or synergistic effects on health outcomes. Many functional foods have antioxidant and anti-inflammatory activities, by mechanisms that may require further investigation. Therefore, these functional foods should be incorporated into a healthy diet to provide cardiovascular benefits; and hence lower cardiovascular risk.

Emerging evidence for a potential role of antioxidant vitamins in atherosclerotic progression implies that the effect of micronutrients is complex and not likely due to a single nutrient in isolation. Therefore, the use of vitamin supplements is not recommended. Rather, efforts should be targeted to increasing the consumption of vitamin-rich fruit and vegetables.

References

Abudu, N., Miller, J.J., Attaelmannan, M. and Levinson, S.S. (2004). Vitamins in human arteriosclerosis with emphasis on vitamin C and vitamin E. *Clinica Chimica Acta*, 339 (1–2), 11–25.

Agarwall, S. and Rao, A.V. (2000). Tomato lycopene and its role in human health and chronic diseases. *Canadian Medical Association Journal*, 163, 739–744.

Aguirre, R. and May, J.M. (2008). Inflammation in the vascular bed, importance of vitamin C. *Pharmacology Therapy*, 119, 96–103.

Albanes, D., Heinonen, O.P., Taylor, P.R. *et al.* (1996). Alpha-tocopherol and beta-carotene supplements and lung cancer incidence in the alpha tocopherol, beta-carotene cancer prevention study: effects of base-line characteristics and study compliance. *Journal of the National Cancer Institute*, 88, 1560–1570.

Albert, C.M., Gaziano, J.M., Willett, W.C. *et al.* (2002). Nut consumption and decreased risk of sudden cardiac death in the Physicians' Health Study. *Archives of Internal Medicine*, 162, 1382–1387.

Albert, C.M., Hennekens, C.H., O'Donnell, C.J. *et al.* (1998). Fish consumption and risk of sudden cardiac death. *JAMA*, 279, 23–28.

Alberti, K.G., Eckel, R.H., Grundy, S.M. *et al.* (2009). Harmonizing the metabolic syndrome. A joint interim statement of the International Diabetes Federation Task Force on Epidemiology and Prevention; National Heart, Lung and Blood Institute; American Heart Association; World Heart Federation; International Atherosclerosis Society; and International Association for the Study of Obesity. *Circulation*, 120, 1640–1645.

Aldana, S.G., Greenlaw, R., Salberg, A. *et al.* (2007). The effects of an intensive lifestyle modification program on carotid artery intima-media thickness: A randomized trial. *American Journal of Health Promotion*, 21, 510–516.

Alder, A. and Holub, B. (1997). Effect of garlic and fish oil supplementation on serum lipid and lipoprotein concentrations in hypercholesteromic men. *The American Journal of Clinical Nutrition*, 65, 445–450.

Anderson, J.W., Johnstone, B.M. and Cook-Newell, M.E. (1995). Meta-analysis of the effects of soy protein intake on serum lipids. *New England Journal of Medicine*, 333, 276–282.

Baba, S., Natsume, M., Yasuda, A. *et al.* (2007). Plasma LDL and HDL cholesterol and oxidized LDL concentrations are altered in normo- and hypercholesterolemic humans after intake of different levels of cocoa powder. *The Journal of Nutrition*, 137, 1436–1441.

Bazzano, L.A., Serdula, M.K. and Liu, S. (2003). Dietary intake of fruits and vegetables and risk of cardiovascular disease. *Current Atherosclerosis Reports*, 5 (6), 492–499.

Berger, A., Jones, P.J. and Abumweis, S.S. (2004). Plant sterols, factors affecting their efficacy and safety as functional food ingredients. *Lipids in Health and Disease*, 7, 3–5.

Bernstein, A.M., Sun, Q., Hu, F.B. *et al.* (2010). Major dietary protein sources and risk of coronary heart disease in women. *Circulation*, 122 (9), 876–883.

Bidel, S., Hu, G., Qiao, Q. *et al.* (2006). Coffee consumption and risk of total and cardiovascular mortality among patients with type 2 diabetes. *Diabetologia*, 49, 2618–2626.

Bjelakovic, G., Nikolova, D., Gluud, L.L. *et al.* (2007). Mortality in randomized trials of antioxidant supplements for primary and secondary prevention: Systematic review and meta-analysis. *JAMA*, 297, 842–857.

Bjerregaard, L.J., Joensen, A.M., Dethlefsen, C. *et al.* (2010). Fish intake and acute coronary syndrome. *European Heart Journal*, 31, 29–34.

Block, G., Mangels, A.R., Norkus, E.P. *et al.* (2001). Ascorbic acid status and subsequent diastolic and systolic blood pressure. *Hypertension*, 37, 261–267.

Block, G., Patterson, B. and Suber, A. (1992). Fruits, vegetables and cancer prevention, a review of the epidemiological evidence. *Nutrition and Cancer*, 18, 1–29.

Blumberg, J.B. and Frei, B. (2007). Why clinical trials of vitamin E and cardiovascular diseases may be fatally flawed. Commentary on 'The relationship between dose of vitamin E and suppression of oxidative stress in humans'. *Free Radical Biology & Medicine*, 43, 1374–1376.

Bolton-Smith, C., Woodward, M. and Tunstall-Pedoe, H. (1992). The Scottish Heart Health Study. Dietary intake by food frequency questionnaire and odds ratios for coronary heart disease risk. II. The antioxidant vitamins and fibre. *European Journal of Clinical Nutrition*, 46, 85–93.

Bowlin, S., Leske, M., Varma, A. *et al.* (1997). Breast cancer risk and alcohol consumption: results from a large case-control study. *International Journal of Epidemiology*, 26, 915–923.

Brigelius-Flohe, R., Kluth, D. and Banning, A. (2005). Is there a future for antioxidants in atherogenesis? *Molecular Nutrition and Food Research*, 49, 1083–1089.

Broekmans, W.M.R., Klöpping-Ketelaars, I.A.A., Schuurman, C.R.W.C. *et al.* (2000). Fruits and vegetables increase plasma carotenoids and vitamins and decrease homocysteine in humans. *The Journal of Nutrition*, 130, 1578–1583.

Burslem, J., Schonfeld, G., Howald, M.A. *et al.* (1978). Plasma apoprotein and lipoprotein lipid levels in vegetarians. *Metabolism*, 27, 711–719.

Campos, H., Baylin, A. and Willett, W.C. (2008). Alpha-linolenic acid and risk of nonfatal acute myocardial infarction. *Circulation*, 118, 339–345.

Carrero, J.J., Baró, L., Fonollá, J. *et al.* (2004). Cardiovascular effects of milk enriched with omega-3 polyunsaturated fatty acids, oleic acid, folic acid and vitamins E and B6 in volunteers with mild hyperlipidemia. *Nutrition*, 20, 521–527.

Catalgol, B., Batirel, S., Taga, Y. and Ozer, N.K. (2012). Resveratrol: French paradox revisited. *Frontiers in Pharmacology*, 3, 141.

Cederroth, C.R. and Nef, S. (2009). Soy, phytoestrogens and metabolism: A review. *Molecular and Cellular Endocrinology*, 304, 30–42.

Cho, S., Juillerat, M. and Lee, C. (2007). Cholesterol lowering mechanisms of soy protein hydrolysate. *Journal of Agriculture and Food Chemistry*, 55, 10599–10604.

Chopra, M., O'Neill, M.E., Keogh, N. *et al.* (2000). Influence of increased fruit and vegetable intake on plasma and lipoprotein carotenoids and LDL oxidation in smokers and nonsmokers. *Clinical Chemistry*, 46, 1818–1829.

Christensen, B., Mosdol, A., Retterstol, L. *et al.* (2001). Abstention from filtered coffee reduces the concentrations of plasma homocysteine and serum cholesterol – a randomized controlled trial. *American Journal of Clinical Nutrition*, 74, 302–307.

Cook, N.R., Albert, C.M., Gaziano, J.M. *et al.* (2007). A randomized factorial trial of vitamins C and E and beta carotene in the secondary prevention of cardiovascular events in women:

results from the Women's Antioxidant Cardiovascular Study. *Archives of Internal Medicine*, 167, 1610–1618.

Darmadi-Blackberry, I., Wahlqvist, M.L., Kouris-Blazos, A. *et al.* (2004). Legumes: The most important dietary predictor of survival in older people of different ethnicities. *Asia Pacific Journal of Clinical Nutrition*, 13, 217–220.

Dauchet, L., Amouyel, P., Hercberg, S. and Dallongeville, J. (2006). Fruit and vegetable consumption and risk of coronary heart disease: A meta-analysis of cohort studies. *The Journal of Nutrition*, 136, 2588–2593.

Davidson, M.H., Maki, K.C., Dicklin, M.R. *et al.* (2009). Effects of consumption of pomegranate juice on carotid intima-media thickness in men and women at moderate risk for coronary heart disease. *American Journal of Cardiology*, 104, 936–942.

De Backer, G., Ambrosioni, E., Borch-Johnsen, K. *et al.* (2003). European guidelines on cardiovascular disease and prevention in clinical practice. *Atherosclerosis*, 171, 145–155.

DeFelice, S.L. (1995). The nutraceutical revolution, its impact on food and industry R & D. *Trends in Food Science and Technology*, 6, 59–61.

Demonty, I., Ras, R., van der Knaap, H. *et al.* (2009). Continuous dose–response relationship of the LDL-cholesterol-lowering effect of phytosterol intake. *The Journal of Nutrition*, 139, 271–284.

Ding, E.L., Hutfless, S.M., Ding, X. *et al.* (2006). Chocolate and prevention of cardiovascular disease, a systematic review. *Nutrition and Metabolism (London)*, 3, 2.

Djoussé, L., Arnett, D.K., Carr, J.J. *et al.* (2005). Dietary linolenic acid is inversely associated with calcified atherosclerotic plaque in the coronary arteries, the National Heart, Lung and Blood Institute Family Heart Study. *Circulation*, 111, 2921–2926.

Dorant, E., van den Brandt, P., Goldbohm, R. *et al.* (1993). Garlic and its significance for the prevention of cancer in humans: A critical review. *The British Journal of Cancer*, 67, 424–429.

Durrington, P.N., Bhatnagar, D., Mackness, M.I. *et al.* (2001). An omega-3 polyunsaturated fatty acid concentrate administered for one year decreased triglycerides in simvastin treated patients with coronary heart disease and persisting hypertriglyveridaemia. *Heart*, 85, 544–548.

Dyerberg, J., Eskersen, D.C, Anderson, P.W. *et al.* (2004). Effect of trans- and *n*-3 unsaturated fatty acids on cardiovascular risk markers in healthy males. An 8 weeks dietary intervention study. *European Journal of Clinical Nutrition*, 58, 1062–1070.

Eidelman, R.S., Hollar, D., Hebert, P.R. *et al.* (2004). Randomized trials of vitamin E in the treatment and prevention of cardiovascular disease. *Archives of Internal Medicine*, 164, 1552–1556.

Engelhard, Y.N., Gazer, B. and Paran, E. (2006). Natural antioxidants from tomato extract reduce blood pressure in patients with grade-1 hypertension: a double-blind, placebo-controlled pilot study. *American Heart Journal*, 151, 100.e6–100.e1.

Erkkilä, A. and Lichtenstein, A. (2006). Fiber and cardiovascular disease risk: How strong is the evidence? *Journal of Cardiovascular Nursing*, 21, 3–8.

Esfahani, A., Wong, J.M., Truan, J. *et al.* (2011). Health effects of mixed fruit and vegetable concentrates: A systematic review of the clinical interventions. *Journal of the American College of Nutrition*, 30 (5), 285–94.

Farnworth, E.R. (2000). Probiotics and probiotics, in *Handbook of Nutraceuticals and Functional Foods* (ed. R.E.C. Wildman). CRC Press, Boca Raton, FL, pp. 407–422.

Ferrari, C.K.B. (2004). Functional foods, herbs and nutraceuticals, towards biochemical mechanisms of healthy aging. *Biogerontology* 5, 275–89.

Ferrari, C.K.B. and Torres, E.A.F.S. (2003). Biochemical pharmacology of functional foods and prevention of chronic diseases of aging. *Biomedical Pharmacotherapy*, 57, 251–60.

Flint, A.J., Hu, F.B., Glynn, R.J. *et al.* (2009). Whole grains and incident hypertension in men. *American Journal of Clinical Nutrition*, 90, 493–498.

Folsom, A.R., Parker, E.D. and Harnack, L.J. (2007). Degree of concordance with DASH diet guidelines and incidence of hypertension and fatal cardiovascular disease. *American Journal of Hypertension*, 20, 225–232.

Forster, M.J., Sohal, B.H. and Sohal, R.S. (2000). Reversible effects of long-term caloric restriction on protein oxidative damage. *Journal of Gerontol Series A: Biological Sciences and Medical Sciences*, 55, B522–B529.

Fraser, G.E., Sabate, J., Beeson, W.L. and Strahan, T.M. (1992). A possible protective effect of nut consumption on risk of coronary heart disease. *The Adventist Health Study. Archives of Internal Medicine*, 152, 1416–1424.

Galleano, M., Oteiza, P.I. and Fraga, C.G. (2009). Cocoa, chocolate and cardiovascular disease. *Journal of Cardiovascular Pharmacology*, 54 (6), 483–490.

Garcia-Lafuente, A., Guillamón, E. and Villares, A. *et al.* (2009). Flavonoids as anti-inflammatory agents: Implications in cancer and cardiovascular disease. *Inflammation Research*, 58, 537–552.

Gaziano, J.M. and Hennekens, C.H. (1993). The role of beta-carotene in the prevention of cardiovascular disease. *Annals of the New York Academy of Science*, 691, 148–155.

Geleijnse, J.M., Launer, L.J., Van der Kuip, D.A. *et al.* (2002). Inverse association of tea and flavonoid intakes with incident myocardial infarction: The Rotterdam Study. *American Journal of Clinical Nutrition*,. 75 (5), 880–886.

Genkinger, J.M., Platz, E.A., Hoffman, S.C. *et al.* (2004). Fruit, vegetable, and antioxidant intake and all-cause, cancer, and cardiovascular disease mortality in a community-dwelling population in Washington County, Maryland. *American Journal of Epidemiology*, 160, 1223–1233.

Gey, K.F., Puska, P., Jordan, P. and Moser, U.K. (1991). Inverse correlation between plasma vitamin E and mortality from ischemic heart disease in cross-cultural epidemiology. *American Journal of Clinical Nutrition*, 53, 326S–334S.

Giovannucci, E. (1999). Tomatoes, tomato-based products, lycopene, and cancer: Review of the epidemiologic literature. *Journal of the National Cancer Institute*, 91, 317–31.

Grassi, D., Lippi, C., Necozione, S. *et al.* (2005b). Short-term administration of dark chocolate is followed by a significant increase in insulin sensitivity and a decrease in blood pressure in healthy persons. *American Journal of Clinical Nutrition*, 81, 611–614.

Grassi, D., Necozione, S., Lippi, C. *et al.* (2005a). Cocoa reduces blood pressure and insulin resistance and improves endothelium-dependent vasodilation in hypertensives. *Hypertension*, 398–405.

Greenberg, J.A., Dunbar, C.C., Schnoll, R. *et al.* (2007). Caffeinated beverage intake and the risk of heart disease mortality in the elderly: A prospective analysis. *American Journal of Clinical Nutrition*, 85, 392–398.

Harland, J. and Haffner, T. (2008). Systematic review, metaanalysis and regression of randomised controlled trials reporting an association between an intake of circa 25 g soya protein per day and blood cholesterol. *Atherosclerosis*, 200, 13–27.

Harris, W.S., Miller, M., Tighe, A.P. *et al.* (2008). Omega-3 fatty acids and coronary heart disease risk: Clinical and mechanistic perspectives. *Atherosclerosis*, 197, 12–24.

He, F.J., Nowson, C.A., Lucas, M. and MacGregor, G.A. (2007). Increased consumption of fruit and vegetables is related to a reduced risk of coronary heart disease: Meta-analysis of cohort studies. *Journal of Human Hypertension*, 21, 717–728.

He, J., Klag, M., Whelton, P. *et al.* (1995). Dietary macronutrients and blood pressure in southwestern China. *Journal of Hypertension*, 13 (11), 1267–1274.

He, K., Merchant, A., Rimm, E.B. *et al.* (2003). Dietary fat intake and risk of stroke in male US healthcare professionals: 14 year prospective cohort study. *BMJ*, 327 (7418), 777–782.

He, K., Song, Y., Daviglus, M.L. *et al.* (2004). Accumulated evidence on fish consumption and coronary heart disease mortality: A meta-analysis of cohort studies. *Circulation*, 109, 2705–2711.

Hertog, M.G., Hollman, P.C., Katan, M.B. *et al.* (1993). Intake of potentially anticarcinogenic flavonoids and their determinants in adults in The Netherlands. *Nutrition and Cancer*, 20, 21–29.

Hicks, K.B. and Moreau, R.A. (2001). Phytosterols and phytostanols: Functional food cholesterol busters. *Food Technology*, 55, 63–67.

Ho, S.C., Chen, Y.M., Ho, S.S. and Woo, J.L. (2007). Soy isoflavone supplementation and fasting serum glucose and lipid profile among postmenopausal Chinese women: A double-blind, randomized, placebo controlled trial. *Menopause*, 14, 905–12.

Hooper, L., Kroon, P.A., Rimm, E.B. *et al.* (2008). Flavonoids, flavonoid-rich foods and cardiovascular risk: A meta-analysis of randomized controlled trials. *American Journal of Clinical Nutrition*, 88, 38–50.

Hu, F.B. and Stampfer, M.J. (1999). Nut consumption and risk of coronary heart disease: A review of epidemiologic evidence. *Current Atherosclerosis Reports*, 1, 204–209.

Hu, F.B., Stampfer, M.J., Manson, J.E. *et al.* (1999). Dietary intake of alpha-linolenic acid and risk of fatal ischemic heart disease among women. *American Journal of Clinical Nutrition*, 69, 890–897.

Huang, C.L. and Sumpio, B.E. (2008). Olive oil, the mediterranean diet and cardiovascular health. *Journal of the American College of Surgeons*, 207, 407–416.

Jacobs, D.R., Pereira, M.A., Meyer, K.A. and Kushi, L.H. (2000). Fiber from whole grains, but not refined grains, is inversely associated with all-cause mortality in older women: The Iowa women's health study. *Journal of the American College of Nutrition*, 19, 326S–330S.

Jenkins, D.J., Kendall, C.W., Jackson, C.J. *et al.* (2002). Effects of high- and low-isoflavone soyfoods on blood lipids, oxidized LDL, homocysteine, and blood pressure in hyperlipidemic men and women. *American Journal of Clinical Nutrition*, 76, 365–372.

Jensen, M.K., Koh-Banerjee, P., Hu, F.B. *et al.* (2004). Intake of whole grains, bran, and germ and the risk of coronary heart disease in men. *American Journal of Clinical Nutrition*, 80, 1492–1499.

Jiang, F. and Dusting, G.J. (2003). Natural phenolic compounds as cardiovascular therapeutics: Potential role of their anti-inflammatory effects. *Current Vascular Pharmacology*, 1, 135–156.

Joshipura, K.J., Hu, F.B., Manson, J.E. *et al.* (2001). The effect of fruit and vegetable intake on risk for coronary heart disease. *Annals of Internal Medicine*, 134, 1106–1114.

Kalra, E.K. (2003). Nutraceutical–Definition and Introduction. *AAPS PharmSci*, 5, 25.

Klatsky, A., Armstrong, M. and Friedman, G. (1997). Red wine, white wine, liquor, beer, and risk for coronary artery disease hospitalization. *The American Journal of Cardiology*, 80, 416–420.

Knekt, P., Jarvinen, R., Reunanen, A. *et al.* (1996). Flavonoid intake and coronary mortality in Finland: A cohort study. *BMJ*, 312, 478–481.

Knekt, P., Ritz, J., Pereira, M.A. *et al.* (2004). Antioxidant vitamins and coronary heart disease risk: A pooled analysis of 9 cohorts. *American Journal of Clinical Nutrition*, 80, 1508–1520.

Krinsky, N.I. and Johnson, E.J. (2005). Carotenoid actions and their relation to health and disease. *Molecular Aspects of Medicine*, 26, 459–516.

Kris-Etherton, P.M., Harris, W.S. and Appel, L.J. (2002). American Heart Association. Nutrition Committee. Fish consumption, fish oil, omega-3 fatty acids, and cardiovascular disease. *Circulation*, 106, 2747–2757.

Kris-Etherton, P.M., Lichtenstein, A.H., Howard, B.V. *et al.* (2004). Nutrition Committee of the American Heart Association Council on Nutrition, Physical Activity, and Metabolism. Antioxidant vitamin supplements and cardiovascular disease. *Circulation*, 110, 637–641.

Kromhout, D., Feskens, E.J. and Bowles, C.H. (1995). The protective effect of a small amount of fish on coronary heart disease mortality in an elderly population. *International Journal of Epidemiology*, 24, 340–345.

Kushi, L.H., Folsom, A.R., Prineas, R.J. *et al.* (1996). Dietary antioxidant vitamins and death from coronary heart disease in postmenopausal women. *New England Journal of Medicine*, 334, 1156–1162.

Lee, Y., Mori, T., Puddey, I. *et al.* (2009). Effects of lupin kernel flour-enriched bread on blood pressure: A controlled intervention study. *American Journal of Clinical Nutrition*, 89, 766–772.

Lee, Y.-S. and Wander, R.C. (2005). Reduced effect on apoptosis of 4-hydroxyhexenal and oxidized LDL enriched with *n*-3 fatty acids from postmenopausal women. *Journal of Nutrition and Biochemistry*, 16, 213–221.

Lichtenstein, A.H. (1998). Soy protein, isoflavones and cardiovascular disease risk. *The Journal of Nutrition*,128 (10), 1589–1592.

Liu, S., Buring, J.E., Sesso, H.D. *et al.* (2002). A prospective study of dietary fibre intake and risk of cardiovascular disease among women. *Journal of the American College of Cardiology*, 39, 49–56.

Liu, S., Lee, I.M., Ajani, U. *et al.* (2001). Intake of vegetables rich in carotenoids and risk of coronary heart disease in men: The Physicians' Health Study. *International Journal of Epidemiology*, 30, 130–135.

Liu, S., Manson, J.E., Lee, I.M. *et al.* (2000). Fruit and vegetable intake and risk of cardiovascular disease: The Women's Health Study. *American Journal of Clinical Nutrition*, 72, 922–928.

Lock, K., Pomerleau, J., Causer, L. *et al.* (2005). The global burden of disease attributable to low consumption of fruit and vegetables: Implications for the global strategy on diet. *Bulletin of the World Health Organization*, 83, 100–108.

Lupton, J.R. and Turner, N.D. (2003). Dietary fibre and coronary disease: Does the evidence support an association? *Current Atherosclerosis Reports*, 5 (6), 500–505.

Lutsey, P.L., Jacobs, Jr, D.R., Kori, S. *et al.* (2007). Whole grain intake and its cross-sectional association with obesity, insulin resistance, inflammation, diabetes and subclinical CVD, the MESA Study. *British Journal of Nutrition*, 98, 397–405.

Martins, J.M., Riottot, M., de Abreu, M.C. *et al.* (2005). Cholesterol-lowering effects of dietary blue lupin (*Lupinus angustifolius* L.). in intact and ileorectal anastomosed pigs. *Journal of Lipid Research*, 46, 1539–1547.

Mattson, M.P. (2003). Will caloric restriction and folate protect against AD and PD? *Neurology*, 60, 690–695.

McGill, H.C. (1979). The relationship of dietary cholesterol to serum cholesterol concentration and to atherosclerosis in man. *American Journal of Clinical Nutrition*, 32, 2664–2702.

McKeown, N.M., Meigs, J.B., Liu, S. *et al.* (2002). Whole-grain intake is favorably associated with metabolic risk factors for type 2 diabetes and cardiovascular disease in the Framingham Offspring Study. *American Journal of Clinical Nutrition*, 76, 390–8.

Mellen, P.B., Walsh, T.F. and Herrington, D.M. (2008). Whole grain intake and cardiovascular disease: A meta-analysis. *Nutrition, Metabolism and Cardiovascular Disease*, 18, 283–290.

Miller, E.R., 3rd, Pastor-Barriuso, R., Dalal, D. *et al.* (2005). Meta-analysis: High-dosage vitamin E supplementation may increase all-cause mortality. *Annals of Internal Medicine*, 142, 37–46.

Mink, P.J., Scrafford, C.G., Barraj, L.M. *et al.* Flavonoid intake and cardiovascular disease mortality: A prospective study in postmenopausal women. *American Journal of Clinical Nutrition*, 85, 895–909.

Mital, B. and Garg, S. (1995). Anticarcinogenic, hypocholesterolemic and antagonistic activities of *Lactobacillus acidophilus*. *Critical Reviews in Microbiology*, 21, 175–214.

Morris, J.N., Marr, J.W. and Clayton, D.G. (1997). Diet and heart: A postscript. *BMJ*, 2, 1307–14.

Mozaffarian, D. (2008). Fish and *n*–3 fatty acids for the prevention of fatal coronary heart disease and sudden cardiac death. *American Journal of Clinical Nutrition*, 87, 1991S–1996S.

Mozaffarian, D. and Rimm, E.B. (2006). Fish intake, contaminants and human health: Evaluating the risks and the benefits. *JAMA*, 296, 1885–1899.

Mukamal, K.J., Maclure, M., Muller, J.E. *et al.* Tea consumption and mortality after acute myocardial infarction. *Circulation*, 105, 2476–2481.

Nagata, C., Takatsuka, N., Kurisu, Y. *et al.* (1998). Decreased serum total cholesterol concentration is associated with high intake of soy products in Japanese men and women. *The Journal of Nutrition*, 128, 209–213.

Normen, L., Holmes, D. and Frohlich, J. (2005). Plant sterols and their role in combined use with statins for lipid lowering. *Current Opinions on Investigational Drugs*,6, 307–316.

Omenn, G.S., Goodman, G.E., Thionquist, M.D. *et al.* (1996). Effects of a combination of beta-carotene and vitamin A on lung cancer and cardiovascular disease. *New England Journal of Medicine*, 334, 1150–1155.

Osganian, S.K., Stampfer, M.J., Rimm, E. *et al.* (2003a). Vitamin C and risk of coronary heart disease in women. *Journal of the American College of Cardiology*, 42, 246–252.

Osganian, S.K., Stampfer, M.J., Rimm, E. *et al.* (2003b). Dietary carotenoids and risk of coronary artery disease in women. *American Journal of Clinical Nutrition*, 77, 1390–1399.

Palace, V.P., Khaper, N., Qin, Q. and Singal, P.K. (1999). Antioxidant potentials of vitamin A and carotenoids and their relevance to heart disease. *Free Radical Biology and Medicine*, 26, 746–761.

Panagiotakos, D.B., Pitsavos, C., Chrysohoou, C. *et al.* (2003). The J-shaped effect of coffee consumption on the risk of developing acute coronary syndromes: The CARDIO2000 case-control study. *The Journal of Nutrition*, 133, 3228–3232.

Perez-Jimenez, J. and Saura-Calixto, F. (2008). Grape products and cardiovascular disease risk factors. *Nutrition Research Reviews*, 21 (2), 158–173.

Peters, U., Poole, C. and Arab, I. (2001). Does tea affect cardiovascular disease? A meta-analysis. *American Journal of Epidemiology*, 154, 495–503.

Pietinen, P., Rimm, E.B., Korhonen, P. *et al.* (1996). Intake of dietary fiber and risk of coronary heart disease in a cohort of Finnish men. The Alpha-Tocopherol, Beta-Carotene Cancer Prevention Study. *Circulation*, 94, 2720–2727.

Prior, R.L. and Cao, G. (2000). Antioxidant phytochemicals in fruits and vegetables: Diet and health implications. *Horticultural Science*, 35, 588–592.

Psaltopoulou, T., Naska, A., Orfanos, P. *et al.* (2004). Olive oil, the Mediterranean diet, and arterial blood pressure: The Greek European prospective investigation into cancer and nutrition (EPIC). study. *American Journal of Clinical Nutrition*, 80, 1012–1018.

Quílez, J., Rafecas, M., Brufau, G. *et al.* (2003). Bakery products enriched with phytosterol esters, alpha-tocopherol and beta-carotene decrease plasma LDL-cholesterol and maintain plasma beta-carotene concentrations in normocholesterolemic men and women. *The Journal of Nutrition*, 133 (10), 3103–9.

Riemersma, R.A., Rice-Evans, C.A., Tyrrell, R.M. *et al.* (2001). Tea flavonoids and cardiovascular health. *QJM*, 94 (5), 277–282.

Rimm, E.B., Stampfer, M.J., Ascherio, A. *et al.* (1993). Vitamin E consumption and the risk of coronary heart disease in men. *New England Journal of Medicine*, 328, 1450–1456.

Ripsin, C.M., Keenan, J.M., Jacobs, D.R., Jr *et al.* (1992). Oat products and lipid lowering. A meta-analysis. *JAMA*, 267, 3317–3325.

Rissanen, T.H., Voutilainen, S., Nyyssönen, K. *et al.* (2003). Serum lycopene concentrations and carotid atherosclerosis, the Kuopio Ischemic Heart Disease Factor Study. *American Journal of Clinical Nutrition*, 77, 133–138.

Ros, E., Núñez, I., Pérez-Heras, A. *et al.* (2004). A walnut diet improves endothelial function in hypercholesterolemic subjects: A randomized crossover trial. *Circulation*, 109, 1609–1614.

Rosengren, A., Subramanian, S.V., Islam, S. *et al.* (2009). Education and risk for acute myocardial infarction in 52 high, middle and low-income countries, INTERHEART case-control study. *Heart*, 95 (24), 2014–2022.

Sabate, J. and Ang, Y. (2009). Nuts and health outcomes, new epidemiologic evidence. *American Journal of Clinical Nutrition*, 89 (suppl), 1S–6S.

Sacks, F.M., Lichtenstein, A., Van Horn, L. *et al.* (2006). Soy protein, isoflavones and cardiovascular health: An American heart association science advisory for professionals from the nutrition committee. *Circulation*, 113, 1034–1044.

Samman, S., Sivarajah, G., Man, J.C. *et al.* (2003). A mixed fruit and vegetable concentrate increases plasma antioxidant vitamins and folate and lowers plasma homocysteine in men. *The Journal of Nutrition*, 133, 2188–2193.

Savica, V., Bellinghieri, G., Kopple, J.D. (2010). The effect of nutrition on blood pressure. *Annual Review of Nutrition*, 30, 365–401.

Sesso, H.D., Buring, J.E., Christen, W.G. *et al.* (2008). Vitamins E and C in the prevention of cardiovascular disease in men: The Physicians' Health Study II randomized controlled trial. *JAMA*, 300, 2123–2133.

Singh, U., Devaraj, S. and Jialal, I. (2005). Vitamin E, oxidative stress and inflammation. *Annual Review of Nutrition*, 25, 151–174.

Shekelle, P.G., Morton, S.C., Jungvig, L.K. *et al.* (2004). Effect of supplemental vitamin E for the prevention and treatment of cardiovascular disease. *Journal of General and Internal Medicine*, 19, 380–9.

Smolders, R.G., Sipkema, P., Kenemans, P. *et al.* (2004). Homocysteine impairs oestrogen induced vasodilation in isolated rat arterioles. *Menopause*, 11, 98–103.

Srinath Reddy, K. and Katan, M.B. (2004). Diet, nutrition and the prevention of hypertension and cardiovascular diseases. *Public Health and Nutrition*, 7, 167–86.

Stampfer, M.J., Hennekens, C.H., Manson, J.E. *et al.* (1993). Vitamin E consumption and the risk of coronary disease in women. *New England Journal of Medicine*, 328, 1444–1449.

Stampfer, M.J., Hu, F.B., Manson, J.E. *et al.* (2000). Primary prevention of coronary heart disease in women through diet and lifestyle. *New England Journal of Medicine*, 343, 16–22.

Stephens, N.G., Parsons, A., Schofield, P.M. *et al.* (1996). Randomised controlled trial of vitamin E in patients with coronary disease: Cambridge heart antioxidant study (CHAOS). *Lancet*, 347, 781–786.

Streppel, M.T., Arends, L.R., van 't Veer, P. *et al.* (2005). Dietary fibre and blood pressure: A meta-analysis of randomized placebo-controlled trials. *Archives of Internal Medicine*, 165 (2), 150–156.

Sumpio, B.E., Cordova, A.C., Berke-Schlessel, D.W. *et al.* (2006). Green tea, the 'Asian paradox,' and cardiovascular disease. *Journal of the American College of Surgeons*, 202, 813–825.

Taku, K., Umegaki, K., Sato, Y. *et al.* (2007). Soy isoflavones lower serum total and LDL cholesterol in humans: A meta-analysis of 11 randomized controlled trials. *American Journal of Clinical Nutrition*, 85, 1148–56.

Tian, L., Cai, Q. and Wei, H. (1998). Alterations of antioxidant enzymes and oxidative damage to macromolecules in different organs of rats during aging. *Free Radical Biology and Medicine*, 24, 1477–84.

Ueeda, M., Doumei, T., Takaya, Y. *et al.* (2008). Serum N-3 polyunsaturated fatty acid levels correlate with the extent of coronary plaques and calcifications in patients with acute myocardial infarction. *Circulation Journal*, 72, 1836–1843.

USDA (2010). United States Department of Health and Human Services. *Dietary guidelines for Americans 2010*, 7th edn. Government Printing Office, Washington, DC.

Vivekananthan, D.P., Penn, M.S., Sapp, S.K. *et al.* (2003). Use of antioxidant vitamins for the prevention of cardiovascular disease: Meta-analysis of randomised trials. *Lancet*, 361, 2017–2023.

Ye, Z. and Song, H. (2008). Antioxidant vitamins intake and the risk of coronary heart disease, meta-analysis of cohort studies. *European Journal of Cardiovascular Prevention and Rehabilitation*, 15, 26–34.

Wiseman, H. (1999). The bioavailability of non-nutrient plant factors: Dietary flavonoids and phyto-oestrogens. *Proceedings of the Nutrition Society*, 58, 139–146.

Wiseman, H., O'Reilly, J.D., Adlercreutz, H. *et al.* (2000). Isoflavone phytoestrogens consumed in soy decrease F(2)-isoprostane concentrations and increase resistance of low-density lipoprotein to oxidation in humans. *American Journal of Clinical Nutrition*, 72, 395–400.

Wolfs, M., de Jong, N., Ocké, M.C. *et al.* (2006). Effectiveness of customary use of phytosterol/stanol-enriched margarines on blood cholesterol lowering. *Food Chemistry and Toxicology*, 44, 1682–1688.

Zhang, X., Shu, X.O., Gao, Y.T. *et al.* (2003). Soy food consumption is associated with lower risk of coronary heart disease in Chinese women. *The Journal of Nutrition*, 133, 2874–2878.

Index

Functional Foods and Dietary Supplements: Processing Effects and Health Benefits, First Edition.
Edited by Athapol Noomhorm, Imran Ahmad and Anil Kumar Anal.